Clinical Gynecologic Endocrinology and Infertility

Fourth Edition

Clinical Gynecologic Endocrinology and Infertility

Fourth Edition

Leon Speroff
Robert H. Glass
Nathan G. Kase

WILLIAMS & WILKINS
BALTIMORE · HONG KONG · LONDON · MUNICH
PHILADELPHIA · SYDNEY · TOKYO

Editor: Carol-Lynn Brown
Associate Editor: Victoria M. Vaughn
Copy Editor: Harry Finkelstein
Design: Norman W. Och
Illustration Planning: Lorraine Wrzosek
Production: Charles E. Zeller

Graphics by Nancy A. Burgard, Kayo Parsons-Korn, and Don Moyer

Copyright © 1989
Williams & Wilkins
428 East Preston Street
Baltimore, Maryland, 21202, USA

Accurate indications, adverse reactions, and dosage schedules for drugs are provided in this book, but it is possible that they may change. The reader is urged to review the package information data of the manufacturers of the medications mentioned.

Printed in the United States of America

First Edition 1973

Library of Congress Cataloging in Publication Data

Speroff, Leon, 1935–
    Clinical gynecologic endocrinology & infertility / Leon Speroff, Robert H. Glass, Nathan G. Kase.—4th ed.
    p. cm.

    Includes bibliographical references and index.
    ISBN 0-683-07897-6
    1. Endocrine gynecology.   2. Infertility—Endocrine aspects.   I. Glass, Robert H., 1932–   II. Kase, Nathan G., 1930–   .   III. Title.   IV. Title: Clinical gynecologic endocrinology and infertility.
RG159.S62   1988   618.1—dc19   88-12072
                                    CIP

91 92 93
6 7 8 9 10

Preface

The Fourth Edition! How could it be? It seems like just yesterday that we were meeting on Thursday evenings in a typically small Yale office to plan the first edition. (Dedicated to that nostalgic memory, the blue on the cover of this edition is Yale blue). Perhaps most symbolic of the many changes and advances since then is the fact that much of the manuscript for the first edition was typed on a Royal portable typewriter. This edition was composed on an IBM PC, using Wordstar 2000 (a total of over 1.74 million bytes and 226 thousand words), and has been printed directly from floppy disks. There is no paper manuscript in existence!

While the technique is now electronic, the basic approach and philosophy are the same. This book continues to be a formulation derived from our teaching and clinical activities. We review physiologic principles and then present our methods of clinical management, which are based on a foundation of those principles. We continue to believe that an encyclopedic style burdens rather than informs.

The progress in basic science at the molecular level over the last few years has been nothing short of awesome. We are just entering an era in which these basic science accomplishments will be translated into patient management. Clinical endocrinology will undergo considerable change similar to that now taking place in basic endocrinology. Therefore, while this book provides a compilation of up-to-date information, the clinician, now more than ever, must be alert to changes and developments reported in the current literature.

The book continues to be dedicated to the improvement of patient care, and we hope that it will aid you to accomplish that goal.

Leon Speroff, M.D.
Portland, Oregon

Robert H. Glass, M.D.
San Francisco, California

Nathan G. Kase, M.D.
New York, New York

Contents

Preface   v

Physiology of Female
Reproduction

Chapter 1:   1
**Hormone Biosynthesis, Metabolism, and
Mechanism of Action**
How hormones are formed and metabolized, and how
hormones work.

Chapter 2:   51
Neuroendocrinology
How reproductive events are perceived, integrated, and
acted upon by the central nervous system.

Chapter 3:   91
Regulation of the Menstrual Cycle
The cyclic changes in ovarian and pituitary hormones, and
what governs the patterns of these hormonal changes.

Clinical Endocrinology

Chapter 4:   121
The Ovary from Conception to Senescence
Correlation of morphology with reproductive and
steroidogenic functions. A consideration of the physiology
of the menopause and hormone replacement therapy.

Chapter 5:   165
Amenorrhea
Differential diagnosis of amenorrhea of all types utilizing
procedures available to all physicians. The problems of
galactorrhea and pituitary adenomas.

Chapter 6:   213
Anovulation
How loss of ovulation can occur and the clinical
expressions of anovulation. The polycystic ovary.

Chapter 7:   233
Hirsutism
The biology of hair growth; the diagnosis and management
of hirsutism.

Chapter 8:   265
Dysfunctional Uterine Bleeding
A physiologic basis for medical management without
primary surgical intervention.

Chapter 9:   283
The Breast
The factors involved in physiologic lactation and the
differential diagnosis of galactorrhea. The endocrinology of
breast cancer.

Chapter 10:
The Endocrinology of Pregnancy   317
The steroid and protein hormones of pregnancy, perinatal
thyroid physiology, and fetal pulmonic maturation.

Chapter 11:
Prostaglandins   351
The biochemistry of prostaglandins, and significant roles in
reproduction.

Chapter 12:
Normal and Abnormal Sexual Development   379
Normal and abnormal sexual differentiation, and the
differential diagnosis of ambiguous genitalia.

Chapter 13:
Abnormal Puberty and Growth Problems   409
Abnormalities that produce accelerated or retarded sexual
maturation, and growth problems in adolescents.

Chapter 14:
Obesity   445
The physiology of adipose tissue, and the problem of
obesity.

Chapter 15:
Steroid Contraception   461
A survey of the risks and benefits of steroid contraception.
Methods for patient management.

Infertility   **Chapter 16:**
Sperm and Egg Transport, Fertilization, and   499
Implantation
Mechanisms of the first days of conception.

Chapter 17:
Investigation of the Infertile Couple   513
An approach to the problem of infertility. The proper
diagnostic tests and their correct interpretation.

Chapter 18:
Endometriosis and Infertility   547
Diagnosis and suitable treatment for the individual patient.

Chapter 19:
Male Infertility   565
Principles of male infertility, including analysis of semen,
treatment, and therapeutic insemination.

Chapter 20:
Induction of Ovulation   583
Programs for clomiphene, bromocriptine, GnRH, and
Pergonal administration.

Chapter 21:
In Vitro Fertilization   611
An overview of the latest technological achievements.

Appendix   **Chapter 22:**   621
                  Clinical Assays
Methods and interpretations of laboratory assays that are
useful in gynecologic endocrine diagnosis.

Index   651

1

Hormone Biosynthesis, Metabolism, and Mechanism of Action

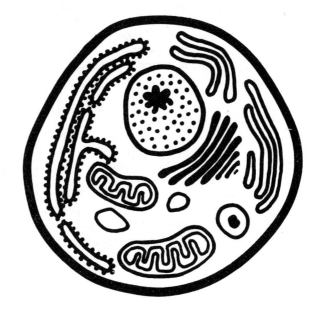

To begin a clinical book with a chapter on biochemistry only serves to emphasize that competent clinical judgment is founded upon a groundwork of basic knowledge. On the other hand, clinical practice does not require a technical and sophisticated proficiency in a basic science. *The purpose of this chapter, therefore, is not to present an intensive course in biochemistry, but rather to present a selective review of the most important principles of how hormones are formed and metabolized, and how hormones work.* This information is essential for the development of the physiological concepts to follow, and it is intended that certain details, which we all have difficulty remembering, will be available in this chapter for reference.

The classical definition of a hormone is a substance which travels from a special tissue, where it is released into the bloodstream, to distant responsive cells where the hormone exerts its characteristic effects. What was once thought of as a simple voyage is now appreciated as an odyssey which becomes more complex as new facets of the journey are unraveled in research laboratories throughout the world.

Indeed, the notion that hormones are products only of special tissues is being challenged. Complex hormones and hormone receptors have been discovered in primitive, unicellular organisms, suggesting that endocrine glands are a late development of evolution. The widespread capability of cells to make hormones explains the puzzling discoveries of hormones in strange places, such as gastrointestinal hormones in the brain, reproductive hormones in intestinal secretions, and the ability of cancers to unexpectedly make hormones. Hormones and neurotransmitters were and are a means of communication. Only when animals evolved into complex organisms did special glands develop to produce hormones which could be used in a more sophisticated fashion. Furthermore, hormones must have appeared even before plants and animals diverged because there are many plant substances similar to hormones and hormone receptors. Therefore it is not surprising that every cell should contain genes necessary for hormonal expression, and cancer cells, because of their dedifferentiation, can uncover gene expression and in inappropriate locations and at inappropriate times, make hormones.

Hormones, therefore, are substances which provide a means of communication. The classic endocrine hormones travel through the bloodstream to distant sites, but cellular communication is also necessary at local sites. Two words which are now encountered relatively more frequently are paracrine and autocrine, depicting a more immediate form of communiction:

Paracrine Communication. Intercellular communication involving the local diffusion of regulating substances from a cell to nearby (contiguous) cells.

Autocrine Communication. Intracellular communication whereby a single cell produces regulating substances which in turn act upon receptors on or within the same cell.

Let us follow an estradiol molecule throughout its career, and in so doing gain an overview of how hormones are formed, how hormones work, and how hormones are metabolized. Estradiol begins its life-span with its synthesis in a cell specially suited for this task. For this biosynthesis to take place, the proper enzyme capability must be present along with the proper precursors. In the human female the principal sources of estradiol are the granulosa cells of the developing follicle and the corpus luteum. These cells possess the ability to turn on steroidogenesis in response to specific stimuli. The stimulating agents are the gonadotropins, follicle-stimulating hormone (FSH) and luteinizing hormone (LH). The initial step in the process which will give rise to estradiol is the transmission of the message from the stimulating agents to the steroid-producing mechanisms within the cells.

Messages which stimulate steroidogenesis must be transmitted through the cell membrane. This is necessary because gonadotropins, being large glycopeptides, do not ordinarily enter cells, but must communicate with the cell by joining with specific receptors on the cell membrane. In so doing they activate a sequence of communication. A considerable amount of investigation has been devoted to determining the methods by which this communication takes place. E. M. Sutherland received the Nobel Prize in 1971 for proposing the concept of a second messenger.

Gonadotropin, the first messenger, activates an enzyme in the cell membrane called adenylate cyclase. This enzyme transmits the message by catalyzing the production of a second messenger within the cell, cyclic adenosine 3'5'-monophosphate (cyclic AMP). The message passes from LH to cyclic AMP, much like a baton in a relay race.

Cyclic AMP, the second messenger, initiates the process of steroidogenesis, leading to the synthesis and secretion of the hormone, estradiol. This notion of message transmission has grown more and more complex with the appreciation of new physiological concepts such as the heterogeneity of peptide hormones, the up and down regulation of cell membrane receptors, and the regulation of adenylate cyclase activity.

Secretion of estradiol into the bloodstream directly follows its synthesis. Once in the bloodstream, estradiol exists in two forms, bound and free. A majority of the hormone is bound to protein carriers, albumin and sex steroid hormone binding globulin. The purpose of this binding is not totally clear. The biologic activity of a hormone may be limited by binding in the blood, thereby avoiding extreme or sudden reactions. In addition, binding may prevent unduly rapid metabolism, allowing the hormone to exist for the length of time necessary to ensure a biologic effect. This reservoir-like mechanism avoids peaks and valleys in hormone levels and allows a more steady state of hormone action.

The biologic and metabolic effects of a hormone are determined by a cell's ability to receive and retain the hormone. The estradiol which is not bound to a protein, but floating freely in the bloodstream, readily enters cells by rapid diffusion. For estradiol to produce its effect, however, it must be grasped by a receptor within the cell. Only those cells which contain estradiol-specific receptors will respond to estradiol. The job of the receptor is to aid in the transmission of the hormone's message to the nuclear chromatin. The result is production of messenger RNA leading to protein synthesis and a cellular response characteristic of the hormone.

Once estradiol has accomplished its mission, it is probably released back into the bloodstream. It is possible that estradiol can perform its duty several times before being cleared from the circulation by metabolism. On the other hand, many molecules will be metabolized without ever having the chance to produce an effect. Unlike estradiol, other hormones, such as testosterone, are metabolized and altered within the cell in which an effect is produced. In the latter case, a steroid is released into the bloodstream as an inactive compound. Clearance of steroids from the blood varies according to the structure of the molecules.

Cells which are capable of clearing estradiol from the circulation accomplish this by biochemical means (conversion to estrone and estriol, moderately effective and very weak estrogens, respectively) and conjugation to products which are water-soluble and excreted in the urine and bile (sulfo- and glucuro-conjugates).

Thus, a steroid hormone has a varied career packed into a short lifetime, and it is now appropriate to review the important segments of this life-span in greater detail.

Nomenclature

All steroid hormones are of basically similar structure with relatively minor chemical differences leading to striking alterations in biochemical activity. The basic structure is the perhydrocyclopentanephenanthrene molecule. It is composed of three 6-carbon rings and one 5-carbon ring. One ring is benzene, two rings naphthalene, and three rings phenanthrene; add a cyclopentane (5-carbon ring) and you have the perhydrocyclopentanephenanthrene structure of the steroid nucleus.

The sex steroids are divided into 3 main groups according to the number of carbon atoms they possess. The 21-carbon series includes the corticoids and the progestins and the basic structure is the *pregnane* nucleus. The 19-carbon series includes all the androgens and is based on the *androstane* nucleus, whereas the estrogens are 18-carbon steroids based on the *estrane* nucleus.

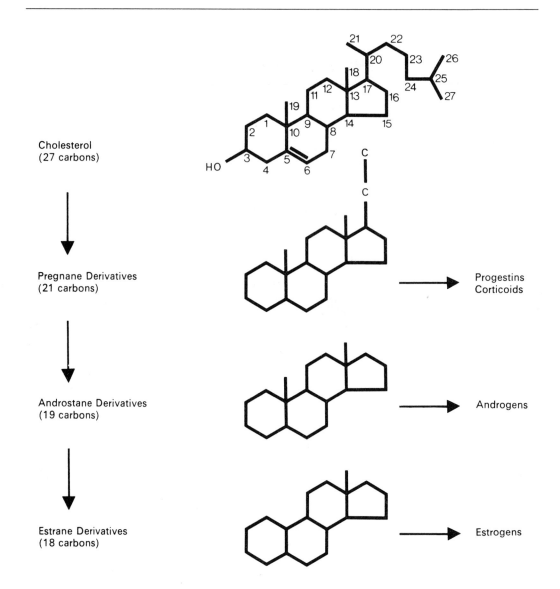

Cholesterol
(27 carbons)

Pregnane Derivatives
(21 carbons)

Progestins
Corticoids

Androstane Derivatives
(19 carbons)

Androgens

Estrane Derivatives
(18 carbons)

Estrogens

4

There are 6 centers of asymmetry on the basic ring structure, and there are 64 possible isomers. Almost all naturally occurring and active steroids are nearly flat, and substituents below and above the plane of the ring are designated alpha (α) (dotted line) and beta (β) (solid line), respectively. Changes in the position of only one substituent can lead to inactive isomers. For example, 17-epitestosterone is considerably weaker than testosterone, the only difference being a hydroxyl group in the α position at C-17 rather than in the β position.

Progesterone

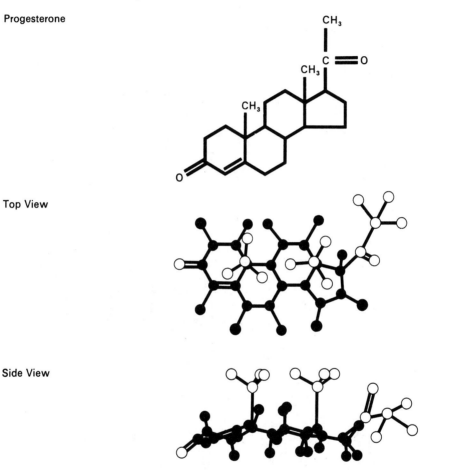

Top View

Side View

The convention of naming steroids uses the number of carbon atoms to designate the basic name (e.g. pregnane, androstane, or estrane). The basic name is preceded by numbers which indicate the position of double bonds and the name is altered as follows to indicate 1, 2, or 3 double bonds: -ene, -diene, and -triene. Following the basic name, hydroxyl groups are indicated by the number of the carbon attachment, and 1, 2, or 3 hydroxyl groups are designated -ol, -diol, or -triol. Ketone groups are listed last with numbers of carbon attachments, and 1, 2, or 3 groups designated -one, -dione, or -trione. Special designations include: dehydro, elimination of 2 hydrogens; deoxy, elimination of oxygen; nor, elimination of carbon; delta or Δ , location of double bond.

Estrone
1,3,5(10)-Estratriene-3β-ol-17-one

Testosterone
4-Androstene-17β-ol-3-one

Progesterone
4-Pregnene-3,20-dione

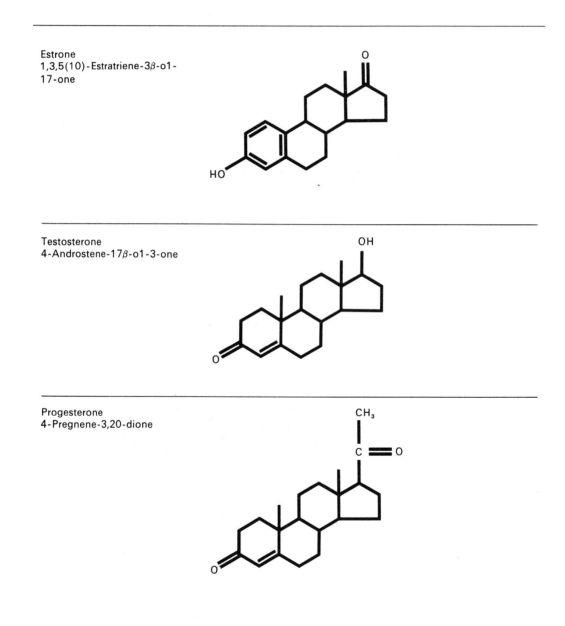

Lipoproteins and Cholesterol

Cholesterol is the basic building block in steroidogenesis. All steroid-producing organs except the placenta can synthesize cholesterol from acetate. Progestins, androgens, and estrogens, therefore, can be synthesized in situ in the various ovarian tissue compartments from the 2-carbon acetate molecule via cholesterol as the common steroid precursor. However, the major resource is blood cholesterol which enters the ovarian cells and can be inserted into the biosynthetic pathway, or stored in esterified form for later use. The cellular entry of cholesterol is mediated via a cell membrane receptor for low-density lipoprotein (LDL), the bloodstream carrier for cholesterol.

Lipoproteins are large molecules that facilitate the transport of nonpolar fats in a polar solvent, the blood plasma. There are 5 major categories of lipoproteins according to their charge and density (flotation during ultracentrifugation). They are derived from each other in the following cascade of decreasing size and increasing density:

Chylomicrons. Large, cholesterol (10%) and triglyceride (90%) carrying particles formed in the intestine after a fatty meal.

Very Low-Density Lipoproteins (VLDL). Also carry cholesterol, but mostly triglyceride; more dense than chylomicrons.

Intermediate-Density Lipoproteins (IDL). Formed (for a transient existence) with the removal of some of the triglyceride from the interior of VLDL particles.

Low-Density Lipoproteins (LDL). The end products of VLDL catabolism, formed after further removal of triglyceride leaving approximately 50% cholesterol; the major carriers (2/3) of cholesterol in the plasma and thus a strong relationship exists between elevated LDL levels and cardiovascular disease.

High-Density Lipoproteins (HDL). The smallest and most dense of the lipoproteins with the highest protein and phospholipid content; HDL levels are inversely associated with atherosclerosis (high levels are protective).

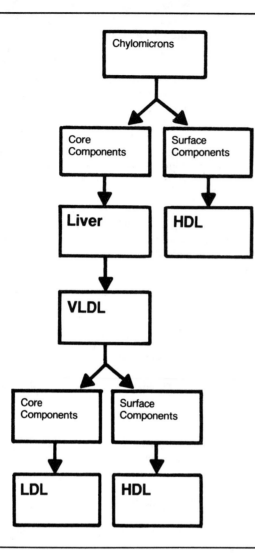

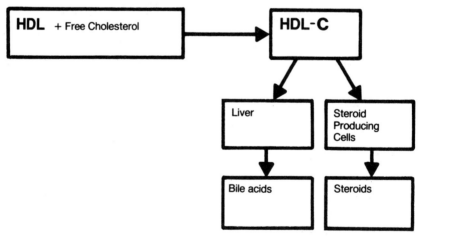

The lipoproteins contain 4 ingredients: 1) cholesterol in two forms: free cholesterol on the surface of the spherical lipoprotein molecule, and esterified cholesterol in the molecule's interior; 2) triglyceride in the interior of the sphere; 3) phospholipid and 4) protein: electrically charged substances on the surface of the sphere and responsible for miscibility with plasma and water. The surface proteins, called *apoproteins,* constitute the sites which bind to the lipoprotein receptor molecules on the cell surfaces. The principal protein of LDL is apoprotein B, and apoprotein A-I is the principal apoprotein of HDL. These protein moieties of the lipoprotein particles are strongly related to the risk of cardiovascular disease, and genetic abnormalities in their synthesis or structure can result in atherogenic conditions.(1)

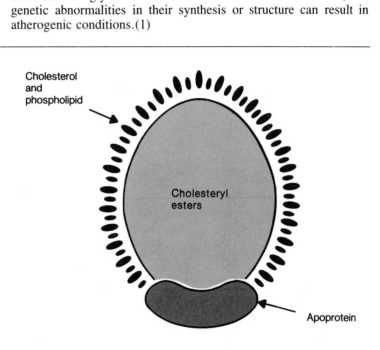

The distribution of the lipoproteins within the LDL and HDL categories indicates subpeaks or subfractions. HDL_2 is a fraction with more lipid than protein, and with less density. HDL_2 is strongly associated with cardiovascular disease.

The lipoproteins are a major reason for the disparity in arteriosclerosis risk between men and women. Throughout adulthood, the blood HDL-cholesterol level is about 10 mg/dl higher in women, and this difference continues through the postmenopausal years. Total and LDL-cholesterol levels are lower in premenopausal women than in men, but after menopause they rise rapidly.

LDL is removed from the blood by organ (mainly liver) receptors which recognize one of the surface apoproteins. The liver is the favored site for this process because it contains the largest number of LDL receptors as well as a unique high affinity receptor for one of the apoproteins, apoprotein E. The lipoprotein bound to the cell membrane receptor is internalized and degradated. When these LDL receptors are saturated or deficient, LDL is taken up by "scavenger" cells (most likely derived from macrophages) in other tissues, most notably the arterial intima. Thus these cells can become the nidus for atherosclerotic plaques.

The protective nature of HDL is due to its ability to pick up free cholesterol from cells or other circulating lipoproteins. In so doing, HDL acquires apoprotein E and this apoprotein E-rich, lipid-rich HDL is known as HDL_c. Thus HDL converts lipid-rich scavenger cells back to their low-lipid state, and carries the excess cholesterol to sites (mainly liver) where it can be metabolized.

Another method by which HDL removes cholesterol from the body focuses on the uptake of free cholesterol from cell membranes. The free cholesterol is esterified and moves to the core of the HDL particle. This lipid-rich particle is the HDL_2 subfraction. Thus both HDL_2 and HDL_c can remove cholesterol by delivering cholesterol to sites for utilization (steroid-producing cells) or metabolism and excretion (liver).

Understanding the role of the cell surface receptors for the homeostasis of cholesterol (discussed later in this chapter), the work of the 1985 Nobel Laureates, M.S. Brown and J.L. Goldstein, revolutionized our concepts of cholesterol, lipoprotein metabolism, and hormonal action at the cell membrane.(2) In their Nobel lecture, Brown and Goldstein paid tribute to cholesterol as the most highly decorated small molecule in biology.

The relationship between cholesterol levels and death from cardiovascular disease is strong and continuous, i.e., increasing risk with increasing levels.(3) Levels of cholesterol less than 200 mg/dl are associated with a lower risk of atherosclerosis. When LDL-cholesterol levels are below 100 mg/dl (equivalent to an approximate total cholesterol level of 170 mg/dl), heart attacks are rare. LDL-cholesterol levels rise above 100 mg/dl only in people who eat a diet rich in saturated animal fats and cholesterol. Cholesterol, smoking, and hypertension are additive or even multiplicative risk factors for coronary heart disease. Adding one of these risk factors to the other decreases the age at which a critical degree of coronary atherosclerosis is achieved by about 10 years.(4)

An important NIH angiographic study demonstrated that lowering of total cholesterol levels and improving the ratio of total cholesterol to HDL correlated with lack of progression of coronary atherosclerosis.(5) In a clinical trial using cholestyramine (a bile-acid binding resin that facilitates cholesterol excretion from the intestine, causing an increase in the liver's demand for cholesterol which in turn leads to increased production of liver LDL receptors) to lower LDL levels in men, there was a 2% decrease in risk of first heart attacks for every 1% fall in total cholesterol levels.(6,7) The benefit could be attributed both to a lowering of LDL-cholesterol and an increase in HDL levels.

The latest (12 year) Framingham Study report confirmed that total cholesterol and HDL-cholesterol levels are strongly related to the development of cardiovascular disease in both men and women.(8) An important observation in this report was the recognition that at all levels of total cholesterol (including those below 200 mg/dl) HDL-cholesterol showed a strong inverse association with the incidence of cardiovascular disease.

For good cardiovascular health, the blood concentration of cholesterol must be kept low and its escape from the bloodstream must be prevented. The problem of cholesterol transport is solved by esterifying the cholesterol and packaging the ester within the cores of plasma lipoproteins. The delivery of cholesterol to cells is in turn solved by lipoprotein receptors. After binding the lipoprotein with its package of esterified cholesterol, the complex is delivered into the cell by receptor-mediated endocytosis, where the lysosomes liberate cholesterol for use by the cell.

Major protection against atherosclerosis depends upon the high affinity of the receptor for LDL and the ability of the receptor to recycle multiple times, thus allowing large amounts of cholesterol to be delivered while maintaining a healthy low blood level of LDL. Cells can control their uptake of cholesterol by increasing or decreasing the number of LDL receptors according to the intracellular cholesterol levels.

There are 3 important clinical points:

1. Atherosclerotic disease is related to increased LDL and decreased HDL-cholesterol concentrations.

2. Lowering LDL levels and raising HDL levels can reduce the incidence of atherosclerotic disease.

3. Atherosclerosis is not a disease limited to aging people. It begins in early childhood, and its manifestation later in life can be influenced by health care behavior during younger years.

All adults should have a screening measurement of total cholesterol and the lipoproteins. Familial hypercholesterolemia is not always associated with a family history of premature cardiovascular disease. Dietary efforts to lower cholesterol and change the LDL:HDL ratio should be directed to any individual with a cholesterol level over 200 mg/dl. Brown and Goldstein postulate that the LDL receptor evolved under dietary conditions of a lower fat intake, and that the high fat, high cholesterol modern diet may suppress the production of LDL receptors, thereby allowing cholesterol to rise to levels associated with cardiovascular disease.

Steroidogenesis

The overall steroid biosynthesis pathway shown in the figure is based primarily on the pioneering work of K.J. Ryan and his co-workers. These pathways follow the fundamental pattern displayed by all steroid-producing endocrine organs. As a result, it should be no surprise that the normal human ovary produces all 3 classes of sex steroids: estrogens, progestins, and androgens. The importance of ovarian androgens is appreciated, not only as obligate precursors to estrogens, but also as clinically important secretory products. The ovary differs from the testis in its fundamental complement of critical enzymes and, hence, its distribution of secretory products. The ovary is distinguished from the adrenal gland in that it is deficient in 21-hydroxylase and 11β-hydroxylase enzymes. Glucocorticoids and mineralocorticoids, therefore, are not produced in normal ovarian tissue.

11

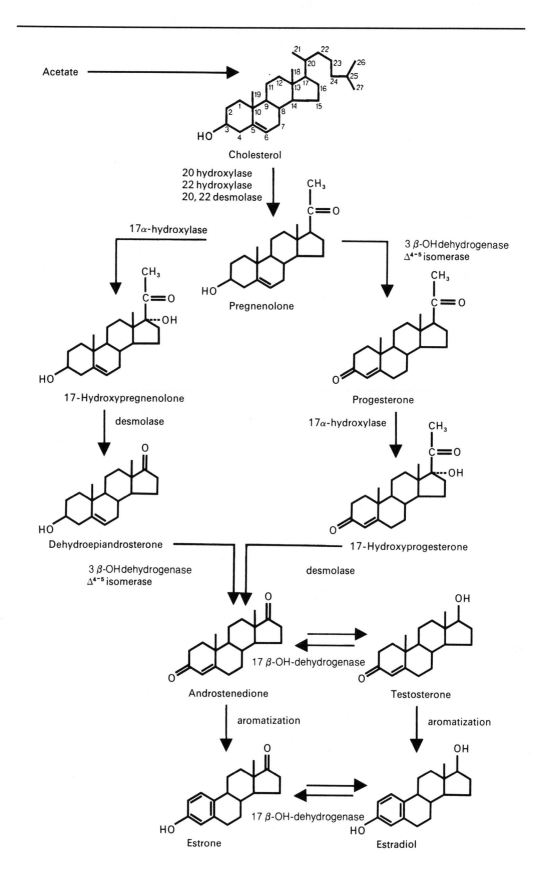

Cholesterol

20 hydroxylase
22 hydroxylase
20, 22 desmolase

17α-hydroxylase

3 β-OHdehydrogenase
Δ⁴⁻⁵ isomerase

Pregnenolone

17-Hydroxypregnenolone

desmolase

Progesterone

17α-hydroxylase

Dehydroepiandrosterone

3 β-OHdehydrogenase
Δ⁴⁻⁵ isomerase

desmolase

17-Hydroxyprogesterone

Androstenedione

17 β-OH-dehydrogenase

Testosterone

aromatization

aromatization

Estrone

17 β-OH-dehydrogenase

Estradiol

During steroidogenesis, the number of carbon atoms in cholesterol or any other steroid molecule can be reduced but never increased. The following reactions may take place:

1. Cleavage of a side chain (desmolase reaction).

2. Conversion of hydroxyl groups into ketones or ketones into hydroxyl groups (dehydrogenase reactions).

3. Addition of OH group (hydroxylation reaction).

4. Creation of double bonds (removal of hydrogen).

5. Addition of hydrogen to reduce double bonds (saturation).

Conversion of cholesterol to pregnenolone involves hydroxylation at the carbon 20 and 22 positions (20-hydroxylase and 22-hydroxylase enzymes), with subsequent cleavage of the side chain (20,22-desmolase). Conversion of cholesterol to pregnenolone takes place within the mitochondria. It is a rate-limiting step in the steroid pathway and is one of the principal effects of LH stimulation.

It is important to note that once pregnenolone is formed further steroid synthesis in the ovary can proceed by one of 2 pathways, either via Δ^5-3β-hydroxysteroids or via the Δ^4-3-ketone pathway. The first (the Δ^5 pathway) proceeds by way of pregnenolone and dehydroepiandrosterone (DHA) and the second (the Δ^4 pathway) via progesterone and 17α-hydroxyprogesterone.

The conversion of pregnenolone to progesterone involves two enzyme steps: the 3β-hydroxysteroid dehydrogenase and Δ^{4-5} isomerase reactions which convert the 3-hydroxyl group to a ketone and transfer the double bond from the 5-6 position to the 4-5 position. Once the Δ^{4-5} ketone is formed, progesterone is hydroxylated at the 17 position to form 17α-hydroxyprogesterone. 17α-Hydroxyprogesterone is the immediate precursor of the C-19 (19 carbons) series of androgens in this pathway. By peroxide formation at C-20, followed by epoxidation of the C-17, C-20 carbons, the side chain is split off forming androstenedione. The 17-ketone may be reduced to a 17β-hydroxyl to form testosterone by 17β-hydroxysteroid dehydrogenase. Both C-19 steroids (androstenedione and testosterone) are rapidly converted to corresponding C-18 phenolic steroid estrogens (estrone and estradiol) by microsomal enzymes in a process referred to as aromatization. This process includes hydroxylation of the angular 19-methyl group, followed by oxidation, loss of the 19-carbon as formaldehyde, and ring A aromatization (dehydrogenation).

As an alternative, pregnenolone can be directly converted to the Δ^5-3β-hydroxy C-19 steroid, DHA, by 17α-hydroxylation followed by desmolase cleavage of the side chain. With formation of the Δ^4-3-ketone, DHA is converted into androstenedione. It is thought that conversion of each of the Δ^5 compounds to their corresponding Δ^4 compounds can occur at any step; however, the principal pathways are via progesterone and DHA. Regardless of the precursor source, C-19 Δ^4-3-ketone substrates proceed to estrogens as noted above.

13

There is a menstrual midcycle increase in circulating levels of androstenedione and testosterone, probably arising from LH stimulation of ovarian stromal tissue. The stromal compartment of the ovary is derived from cells which originally comprised the thecal layer of developing follicles. This tissue responds to gonadotropins (LH and human chorionic gonadotropin [HCG]) with increased steroidogenesis. Postmenopausally, when only stromal tissue remains active, androstenedione and testosterone secretion is increased for a few years, until even this compartment of the ovary becomes atrophic.

The Two-Cell System

The two-cell system is a logical explanation of the events involved in ovarian follicular steroidogenesis and development.(9) This explanation brings together recent information on the site of specific steroid production, along with the appearance and importance of hormone receptors. The following facts are important:

1. FSH receptors are present on the granulosa cells.

2. FSH receptors are induced by FSH itself.

3. LH receptors are present on the theca cells and initially absent on the granulosa cells, but, as the follicle grows, FSH induces the appearance of LH receptors on the granulosa cells.

4. FSH induces aromatase enzyme activity in granulosa cells.

5. Granulosa cells contain estrogen and androgen specific receptors.

6. Estrogen enhances FSH activity.

The above facts combine into the two-cell system to explain the sequence of events in ovarian follicular growth and development. The initial change from a primordial follicle is independent of hormones, and the stimulus governing this initial step in growth is unknown. Continued growth, however, depends upon FSH stimulation. As the granulosa responds to FSH, growth is associated with an increase in FSH receptors, a specific effect of FSH itself, but an action which is enhanced very significantly by estradiol. The theca cells are characterized by steroidogenic activity in response to LH, specifically resulting in androgen production. Aromatization of androgens to estrogens is a distinct activity within the granulosa layer induced by FSH. Androgens produced in the theca layer, therefore, must diffuse into the granulosa layer. In the granulosa layer they are converted to estrogens, and the increasing level of estradiol in the peripheral circulation reflects release of the estrogen back toward the theca layer and into blood vessels.

The estradiol produced by the cooperative effort of the 2 cells, theca and granulosa, plays an important role in enhancing the activity of FSH, thus promoting the growth and function of its own follicle. As the follicle approaches ovulation, LH receptors begin to appear on the granulosa layer, induced by FSH in another action enhanced by estradiol. After ovulation the dominance of the luteinized granulosa layer is dependent upon preovulatory induction of an adequate number of LH receptors, and therefore, dependent upon adequate FSH action. Prior to ovulation the granulosa layer is

14

characterized by aromatization activity and conversion of the theca androgens to estrogens, an FSH-mediated activity. After ovulation the granulosa layer secretes progesterone and estrogens directly into the bloodstream, an LH-mediated activity.

Granulosa and theca cells each have an androgen aromatase system which can be demonstrated in vitro. However, in vivo, the activity of the granulosa layer in the follicular phase is several hundred times greater than the in vitro activity of the theca layer, and therefore, the granulosa is the main biosynthetic source of estrogen in the growing follicle.(10) The rate of aromatization in the granulosa layer is directly related to the androgen substrate made available by the theca cells. Hence, estrogen secretion by the follicle prior to ovulation is the result of combined LH and FSH stimulation of the 2 cell types, the theca and the granulosa.

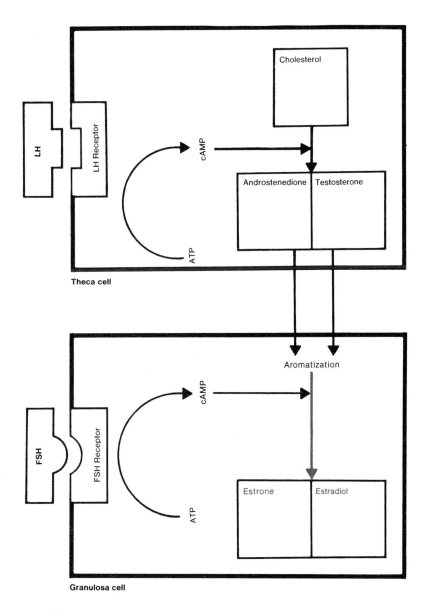

15

Blood Transport of Steroids

While circulating in the blood a majority of the principal sex steroids, estradiol and testosterone, is bound to a β-globulin, a protein carrier, known as sex hormone binding globulin (SHBG). Another 10-40% is loosely bound to albumin, leaving only about 1% unbound and free. Hyperthyroidism, pregnancy, and estrogen administration all increase SHBG levels, whereas corticoids, androgens, progestins, and growth hormone decrease SHBG. Transcortin, also called corticosteroid binding globulin, is a plasma glycoprotein which binds cortisol, progesterone, deoxycorticosterone, corticosterone, and some of the other minor corticoid compounds. Normally about 75% of circulating cortisol is bound to transcortin, 15% is loosely bound to albumin, and 10% is unbound or free.

The biologic effects of the major sex steroids are determined by the unbound portion, known as the free hormone. In other words, the active hormone is unbound and free while the bound hormone is inactive. This concept is not without controversy. The hormone-binding protein complex may be involved in an active uptake process at the target cell plasma membrane. The albumin-bound fraction of steroids may also be available for cellular action. Routine assays determine the total hormone concentration, bound plus free, and special steps are required to measure the active free level of testosterone, estradiol, and cortisol.

Estrogen Metabolism

Androgens are the common precursors of estrogens. 17β-Hydroxysteroid dehydrogenase activity converts androstenedione to testosterone which is not a major secretory product of the normal ovary. It is rapidly demethylated at the C-19 position and aromatized to estradiol, the major estrogen secreted by the human ovary. Estradiol also arises to a major degree from androstenedione via estrone, and estrone itself is secreted in significant daily amounts. Estriol is the peripheral metabolite of estrone and estradiol, and not a secretory product of the ovary. The formation of estriol is typical of general metabolic "detoxification," conversion of biologically active material to less active forms.

The conversion of steroids in peripheral tissues is not always a form of inactivation. Free androgens are peripherally converted to free estrogens, for example, in skin and adipose cells. The work of Siiteri and MacDonald (11) showed that enough estrogen can be derived from circulating androgens to produce bleeding in the postmenopausal woman. In the female the adrenal gland remains the major source of circulating androgens, in particular androstenedione. In the male, almost all of the circulating estrogens are derived from peripheral conversion of androgens.

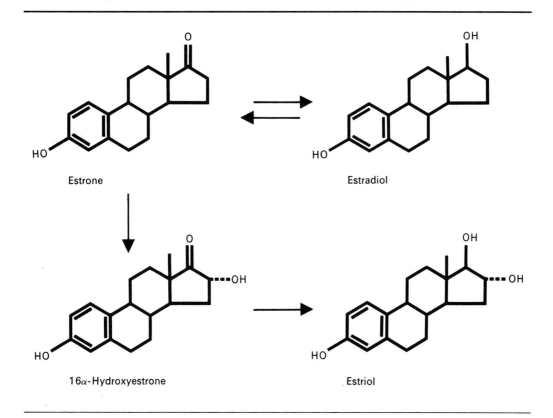

Estrone

Estradiol

16α-Hydroxyestrone

Estriol

It can be seen, therefore, that the pattern of circulating steroids in the female is influenced by the activity of various processes outside the ovary. Because of the peripheral contribution to steroid levels, the term *secretion rate* is reserved for direct organ secretion, whereas *production rate* includes organ secretion plus peripheral contribution via conversion of precursors. The *metabolic clearance rate (MCR)* equals the volume of blood which is cleared of the hormone per unit of time. The *blood production rate (PR)* then equals the metabolic clearance rate multiplied by the concentration of the hormone in the blood.

MCR = Liters/Day

PR = MCR × Concentration

PR = Liters/Day × Amount/Liter = Amount/Day

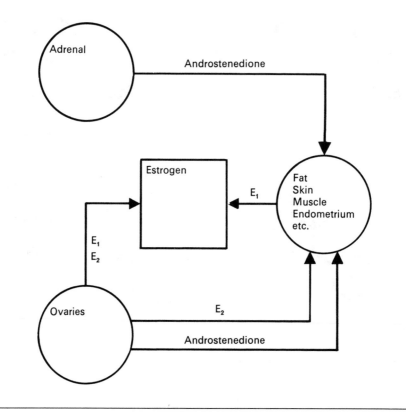

In the normal nonpregnant female, estradiol is produced at the rate of 100-300 μg/day. The production of androstenedione is about 3 mg/day and the peripheral conversion (about 1%) of androstenedione to estrone accounts for about 20-30% of the estrone produced per day. Since androstenedione is secreted in milligram amounts, even a small percent conversion to estrogen results in a significant contribution to estrogens which exist and function in microgram amounts. Thus, the circulating estrogens in the female are the sum of direct ovarian secretion of estradiol and estrone, plus peripheral conversion of C-19 precursors.

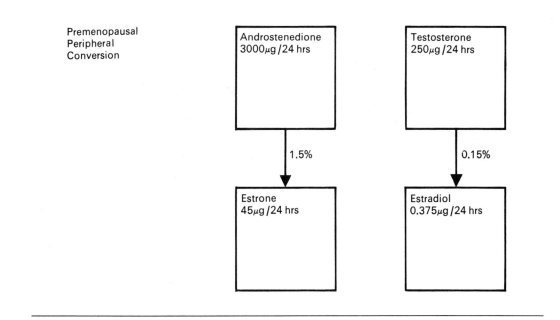

Premenopausal Peripheral Conversion

| Androstenedione 3000μg /24 hrs | → 1.5% → | Estrone 45μg /24 hrs |

| Testosterone 250μg /24 hrs | → 0.15% → | Estradiol 0.375μg /24 hrs |

Progesterone Metabolism

Peripheral conversion of steroids to progesterone is not seen in the nonpregnant female, rather the production rate is a combination of secretion from the adrenal and the ovaries. Including the small contribution from the adrenal, the blood production rate of progesterone in the preovulatory phase is about 2-3 mg/day. During the luteal phase, production increases to 20-30 mg/day. The metabolic fate of progesterone, as expressed by its many excretion products, is more complex than estrogen. About 10-20% of progesterone is excreted as pregnanediol.

Pregnanediol glucuronide is present in the urine in concentrations less than 1 mg/day until ovulation. Postovulation pregnanediol excretion reaches a peak of 3-6 mg/day, which is maintained until 2 days prior to menses. The assay of pregnanediol in the urine now has little use.

Newer methods of assay utilizing binding proteins or antibodies to measure plasma levels of progesterone are more sensitive and more precise. In the preovulatory phase in adult females, in all prepubertal females, and in the normal male, the blood levels of progesterone are at the lower limits of assay sensitivity: less than 100 ng/dl. After ovulation, i.e. during the luteal phase, progesterone ranges from 500 to 2000 ng/dl. In congenital adrenal hyperplasia, progesterone blood levels can be as high as 50 times above normal.

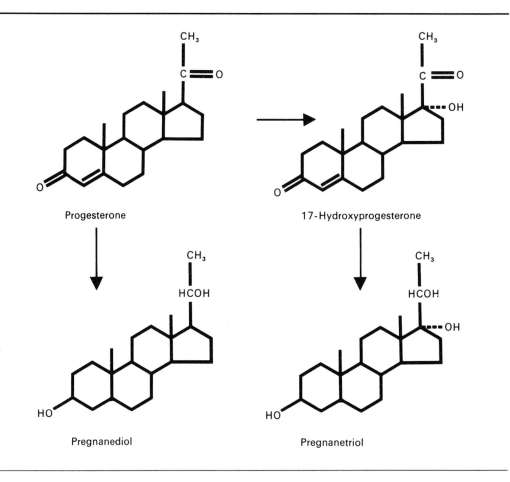

Progesterone

17-Hydroxyprogesterone

Pregnanediol

Pregnanetriol

Pregnanetriol is the chief urinary metabolite of 17α-hydroxyprogesterone, and has clinical significance in the adrenogenital syndrome, where an enzyme defect results in accumulation of 17α-hydroxyprogesterone and increased excretion of pregnanetriol. The plasma or serum assay of 17α-hydroxyprogesterone is a more sensitive and accurate index of this enzyme deficiency than pregnanetriol. Normally the blood level of 17α-hydroxyprogesterone is less than 100 ng/dl, although after ovulation and during the luteal phase of a normal menstrual cycle, a peak of 200 ng/dl can be reached. In syndromes of adrenal hyperplasia, values can be 50-400 times normal.

Androgen Metabolism

The major androgen products of the ovary are dehydroepiandrosterone (DHA) and androstenedione which are secreted mainly by stromal tissue. With excessive accumulation of stromal tissue or in the presence of an androgen-producing tumor, testosterone becomes a significant secretory product. Occasionally, a nonfunctioning tumor can induce stromal proliferation and increased androgen production. The normal accumulation of stromal tissue at midcycle results in a rise in circulating levels of androstenedione and testosterone at the time of ovulation.

The adrenal cortex produces 3 groups of steroid hormones, the glucocorticoids, the mineralocorticoids, and the sex steroids. The sex steroids represent intermediate by-products in the synthesis of glucocorticoids and mineralocorticoids, and excessive secretion of the

Hormones circulate in extremely low concentrations and, in order to respond with specific and effective actions, target cells require the presence of special mechanisms. There are 2 types of hormone action at the cellular level. One mediates the action of tropic hormones (peptide and glycoprotein hormones) at the cell membrane level and involves adenylate cyclase activity. In contrast, the smaller steroid hormones enter cells readily, and the basic mechanism of action involves specific receptor molecules. It is the affinity and specificity of the receptors together with the large concentration of receptors in cells which allow a small amount of hormone to produce a biologic response.

The specificity of the reaction of tissues to steroid hormones is due to the presence of intracellular receptor proteins.(13,14) Different types of tissues, such as liver, kidney, and uterus, respond in a similar manner. The mechanism includes: 1) diffusion across the cell membrane, 2) transfer across the nuclear membrane to the nucleus and binding to receptor protein, 3) interaction of a hormone-receptor complex with nuclear DNA, 4) synthesis of messenger RNA (mRNA), 5) transport of the mRNA to the ribosomes, and finally, 6) protein synthesis in the cytoplasm which results in specific cellular activity. Each of the major classes of steroid hormones, including estrogens, progestins, androgens, glucocorticoids, and mineralocorticoids, has been shown to act according to this general mechanism.

The classic receptor model was developed in the second half of the 1960s by E.V. Jensen and J. Gorski. This concept assigned a primary role to receptors located in the cytoplasm.

Steroid hormones are rapidly transported across the cell membrane by simple diffusion. The factors responsible for this transfer are unknown, but the concentration of free (unbound) hormone in the bloodstream seems to be an important and influential determinant of cellular function. Once within the cell, assuming the cell is responsive to steroid hormone, the hormone is quickly bound by a protein *cytoplasmic* receptor.

In the classic concept, the physiological response to steroid hormones required movement of the hormone and receptor into the nucleus to interact with DNA, leading to the production of messenger RNA (gene transcription). This movement was known as *translocation*. The classic view further held that during this process, *transformation* occurred. Transformation refers to a conformational change of the hormone-receptor complex revealing or producing a binding site which was necessary in order for the complex to bind to the chromatin. It's important to note that the process of translocation was always hypothetical, supported only by circumstantial evidence.

Transformation, the change from an inactive to an active complex, was distinguished by physical parameters such as sedimentation rates, migration during ultracentrifugation through solutions of varying sucrose density. With estrogen receptors, transformation was associated with a change in sedimentation rate from 4S to 5S, smaller and larger molecules, respectively. The progesterone cytoplasmic receptor is 7S in size and is transformed to a smaller 5.5S form. It

sex steroids occurs only with neoplastic cells or in association with enzyme deficiencies. Under normal circumstances, adrenal gland production of the sex steroids is less significant than gonadal production of androgens and estrogens.

There is no circadian cycle of the major sex steroids in the female. However, short-term variations in the blood levels due to episodic secretion require multiple sampling for absolutely accurate assessment. *Although frequent sampling is necessary for a high degree of accuracy, a random sample is sufficient to determine whether a level is within a normal range.*

The testosterone binding capacity is decreased by androgens. Hence, the binding capacity in men is lower than that in normal women; the binding globulin level in women with increased androgen production is also depressed. Androgenic effects are dependent upon the unbound fraction which can move freely from the vascular compartment into the target cells. Routine assays determine the total hormone concentration, bound plus free. Thus, a total testosterone concentration may be in the normal range in a woman who is hirsute or even virilized, but, since the binding globulin level is depressed by the androgen effects, the percent free and active testosterone is elevated. The need for a specific assay for the free portion of testosterone can be questioned since the very presence of hirsutism or virilism indicates increased androgen effects. In the face of hirsutism, one can reliably interpret a normal testosterone level as compatible with decreased binding capacity and increased active free testosterone.

Both total and unbound testosterone are normal in only a few women with hirsutism. In these cases, the hirsutism, heretofore regarded as idiopathic, most likely results from excessive intracellular androgen effects (specifically increased intracellular conversion of testosterone to dihydrotestosterone).

The production rate of testosterone in the normal female is 0.2-0.3 mg/day, and approximately 50% arises from peripheral conversion of androstenedione to testosterone, whereas 25% is secreted by the ovary and 25% by the adrenal.

Reduction of the Δ^4 unsaturation in testosterone is very significant, producing derivatives very different in their spatial configuration and activity. The 5β derivatives are not androgenic: however, the 5α derivative is extremely potent. Indeed, dihydrotestosterone (DHT), the 5α derivative, is the principal androgenic hormone in a variety of target tissues and is formed within the target tissue itself.

In men, the majority of circulating DHT is derived from testosterone which enters a target cell and is converted by means of 5α-reductase to DHT. In women, because the production rate of androstenedione is greater than testosterone, blood DHT is primarily derived from androstenedione.(12) Thus in women, the skin production of DHT may be predominantly influenced by androstenedione.

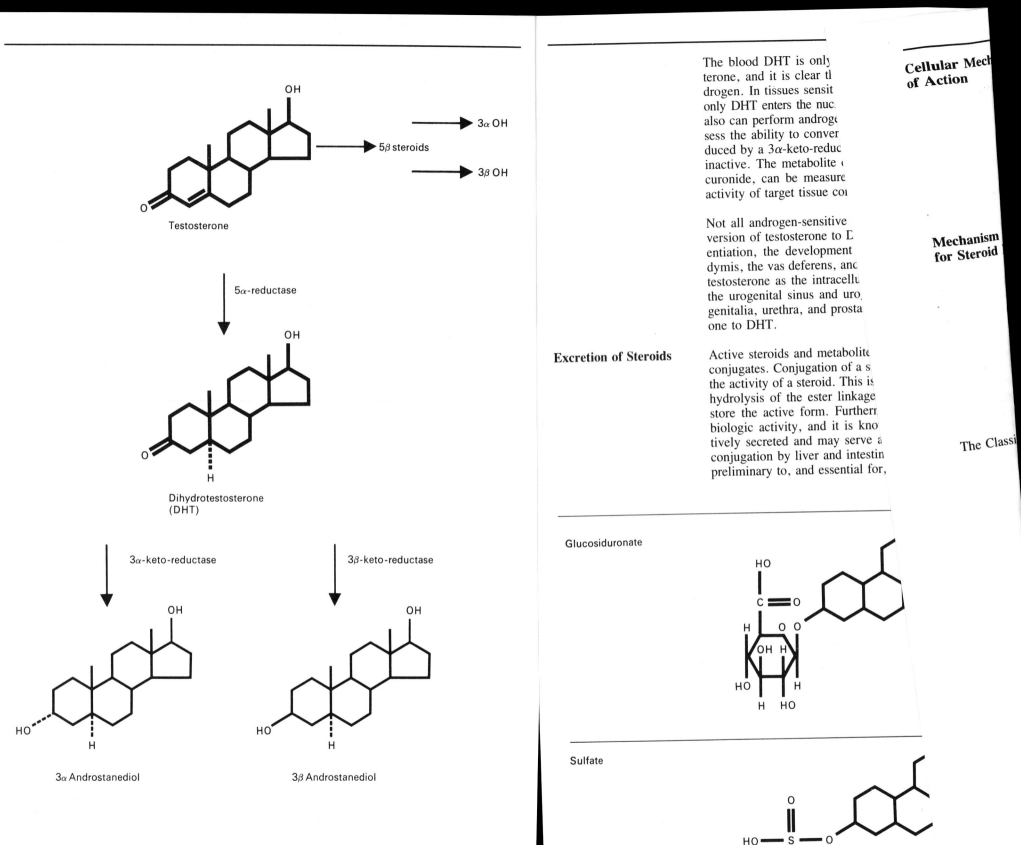

Testosterone

5α-reductase

Dihydrotestosterone
(DHT)

3α-keto-reductase 3β-keto-reductase

3α Androstanediol 3β Androstanediol

3α OH

5β steroids

3β OH

The blood DHT is only
terone, and it is clear th
drogen. In tissues sensit
only DHT enters the nuc
also can perform androge
sess the ability to conver
duced by a 3α-keto-reduc
inactive. The metabolite
curonide, can be measure
activity of target tissue co

Not all androgen-sensitive
version of testosterone to L
entiation, the development
dymis, the vas deferens, and
testosterone as the intracellu
the urogenital sinus and uro
genitalia, urethra, and prosta
one to DHT.

Excretion of Steroids

Active steroids and metabolite
conjugates. Conjugation of a s
the activity of a steroid. This is
hydrolysis of the ester linkage
store the active form. Furtherm
biologic activity, and it is kno
tively secreted and may serve a
conjugation by liver and intestin
preliminary to, and essential for,

**Mechanism
for Steroid**

The Classi

Glucosiduronate

Sulfate

22

23

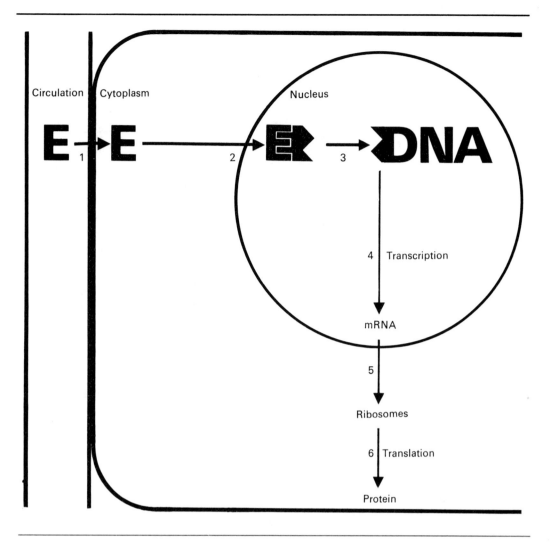

Circulation | Cytoplasm | Nucleus

E →[1] E ——→ [2] ER →[3] DNA

4 | Transcription

mRNA

5

Ribosomes

6 | Translation

Protein

is a complex (a dimer) of two nonidentical subunits, one of which is keyed to specific nonhistone proteins in the chromatin and thus is responsible for finding the appropriate nuclear binding site, allowing the other subunit to bind directly to DNA and initiate transcription. Androgens and progestins crossreact for their receptors, but do so only when present in pharmacological concentrations.

Once in the nucleus, the hormone-receptor complex moves along the chromosome until the site for gene activation (DNA acceptor site) is encountered. The number of high affinity DNA acceptor sites is in the order of several thousand per nucleus, and there is a much larger number of low affinity sites. The specific binding of the hormone-receptor complex with DNA results in RNA polymerase initiation of transcription. Transcription leads to translation, mRNA-mediated protein synthesis on the ribosomes. The principal action of steroid hormones is the regulation of intracellular protein synthesis by means of the receptor mechanism. In target tissues which respond to steroid hormones by growth (e.g. endometrium) nuclear binding and prolonged nuclear retention directly lead to increased DNA synthesis.

An important action of estrogen is its modification of its own and other steroid hormone activity by affecting receptor concentration. Estrogen increases target tissue responsiveness to itself and to progestins and androgens by increasing the concentration of its own receptor and that of the intracellular progestin and androgen receptors. This process is called *replenishment*. Progesterone and clomiphene, on the other hand, limit tissue response to estrogen by blocking the replenishment mechanism, thus decreasing over time the concentration of estrogen receptors. Replenishment is very responsive to the available amount of steroid and receptors. Small amounts of receptor depletion and small amounts of steroid in the blood activate the mechanism.

Biologic activity is maintained only while the nuclear site is occupied with the hormone-receptor complex. The dissociation rate of the hormone and its receptor as well as the half-life of the nuclear chromatin-bound complex are factors in the biologic response. One reason only small amounts of estrogen need be present in the circulation is the long half-life of the estrogen hormone-receptor complex. Indeed, a major factor in the potency differences among the various estrogens (estradiol, estrone, estriol) is the length of time the estrogen-receptor complex occupies the nucleus. The higher rate of dissociation with the weak estrogen (estriol) can be compensated for by continuous application to allow prolonged nuclear binding and activity. Cortisol and progesterone must circulate in large concentrations because their receptor complexes have short half-lives in the nucleus. The classic concept suggested that after receptors had done their job they were recycled for use again. But receptor *recycling* was never proven.

The New Concept

The classic receptor model was based on the fact that unoccupied receptor was found in the cytosol, and after a steroid hormone was administered, the receptor was found in the nucleus (concomitant with a loss of receptor from the cytosol). The new concept (15,16) has 2 principal ideas:

1. The receptor is a nuclear protein at all times, occupied or unoccupied.

2. The receptor, occupied or unoccupied, is immobilized by association with some structural element in the nucleus.

Monoclonal antibodies to receptors have been found only in the nuclei.(17-19) Furthermore, there was no evidence of translocation (specifically there was no significant change in nuclear staining intensity following treatment of cells or animals with hormone). *Previous conclusions, i.e. the classic two step model, were, therefore, due to the fact that unoccupied receptors are so loosely bound to nuclear material that disruption of the cell causes the receptor to move into the cytosol. The classic model was based upon an artifactual finding.*

The new concept does not change the idea of transformation, which is now called *activation*. It simply says that the changes in transformation (activation) take place in the nucleus. The result is a change from a loosely bound (low affinity) receptor to a tightly bound (high affinity) receptor. New studies argue that the change is complex, involving more than one specific modification.

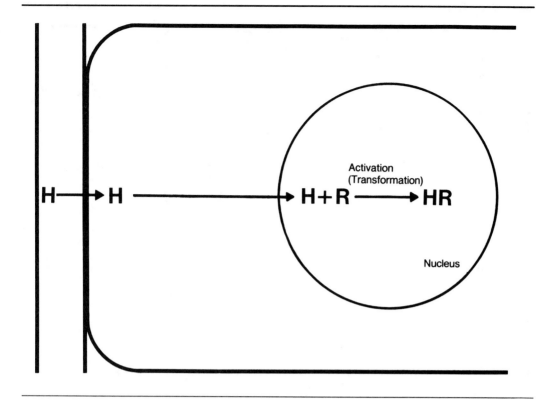

Studies with steroid hormone receptors indicate that the receptor has 3 domains. At the carboxy terminus of the molecule is the hormone-binding domain and at the nitrogen terminus is a modulating domain of uncertain function.(20) In the middle is the DNA binding site. Activation involves a change in size which is partly due to the loss of receptor binding factors (nuclear proteins which inhibit activation), dephosphorylation, and a conformational change leading to the unmasking of high affinity DNA binding sites. The progesterone receptor is very similar to the glucocorticoid receptor, but it is composed of 2 dissimilar subunits, while the glucocorticoid receptor has similar subunits. The androgen receptor molecule appears to be a monomer, but it has the same 3 domains: steroid binding site, DNA binding site, and a third fragment of uncertain nature.

The estrogen receptor, when unoccupied by estrogen, exists in the nucleus loosely bound in the monomer state. Each monomer has only one binding site for a molecule of estrogen. The complete complementary DNA of the estrogen receptor has been cloned and sequenced.(21) The human estrogen receptor, with its 3 domains, has a spatial separation between the steroid-binding site and the DNA-binding site. It is the DNA-binding domain which determines specific function of the hormone-receptor complex (the specific message transmitted). With estrogen binding, activation involves the formation of a dimer.(22) Previous studies assigning size according to ultracentrifugation reflected conformational changes which were both artifactual and due to activation.

One of the aspects of activation is an increase in affinity for estrogen. This is an action of estrogen, and it is greatest with estradiol

27

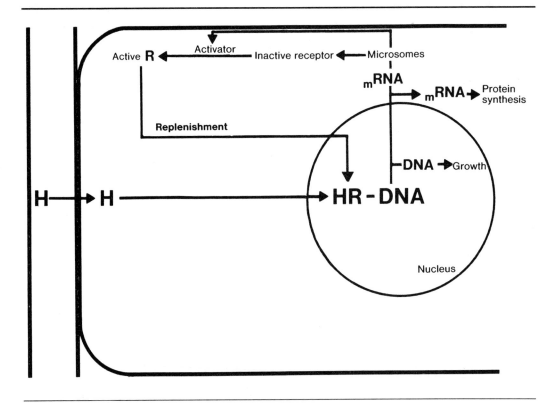

and least with estriol. This action of estradiol, the ability of binding at one site to affect another site, is called *cooperativity*. An increase in affinity is called positive cooperativity. The biologic advantage of positive cooperativity is that this increases the receptor's ability to respond to small changes in the concentration of the hormone. One of the anti-estrogen actions of clomiphene is its property of negative cooperativity, the inhibition of the transition from a low affinity to a high affinity state. The relatively long duration of action exhibited by estradiol is due to the high affinity state achieved by the receptor.

Replenishment, the synthesis of steroid receptors, obviously still takes place in the cytoplasm, but it must be quickly followed by transportation into the nucleus. There is an incredible nuclear traffic.(23) The nuclear membrane contains 3,000 to 4,000 pores. A cell synthesizing DNA imports about one million histone molecules from the cytoplasm every 3 minutes. If the cell is growing rapidly, about 3 newly assembled ribosomes will be transported every minute in the other direction. The typical cell can synthesize 10,000 to 20,000 different proteins. How do they know where to go? The answer is that these proteins have signals attached.

Proteins are synthesized as precursor proteins carrying with them specific amino acid sequences that are recognized by the organelles in the cytoplasm. These sequences are called leader sequences, and they are cleaved after the protein enters the organelle. This raises the possibility that some diseases are due to poor traffic control. This can be true of some acquired diseases as well, e.g. Reye's syndrome, an acquired disorder of mitochondrial enzyme function.

The fate of the hormone-receptor complex after gene activation is now referred to as hormone-receptor *processing*. In the case of estrogen receptors, processing involves the conversion of high affinity estrogen receptor sites to a rapidly dissociating form followed by loss of binding capacity which is completed in about 6 hours.(24) The rapid turnover of estrogen receptors has clinical significance. The continuous presence of estrogen is an important factor for continuing response.

The best example of the importance of these factors is the difference between estradiol and estriol. Estriol has only 20-30% affinity for the estrogen receptor compared to estradiol; therefore, it is rapidly cleared from a cell. But if the effective concentration is kept equivalent to that of estradiol, it can produce a similar biologic response.(25) In pregnancy, where the concentration of estriol is very great, it can be an important hormone, not just a metabolite.

One of the puzzles in clinical medicine has been why large doses of estrogen can produce a regression of an estrogen-sensitive breast cancer. This is a direct pharmacological effect on receptor replenishment. The nuclear estrogen receptor concentration drops rapidly in the presence of pharmacological levels of estrogen.(26)

The depletion of estrogen receptors in target tissues by progestational agents is the fundamental reason for adding progestins to estrogen replacement programs. The progestins accelerate the turnover of pre-existing receptors, and this is followed by inhibition of estrogen-induced receptor synthesis. Using monoclonal antibody immunocytochemistry, this action has been pinpointed to the interruption of transcription in estrogen-regulated genes.(27) The mechanism is different for androgen anti-estrogen effects. Androgens do not involve depletion of estrogen receptors, but in some way decrease estrogen-induced RNA activity in the cytoplasm. (28)

The cellular mechanism is more complex for androgens. Androgens can work in any one of three ways:

1. By intracellular conversion of testosterone to dihydrotestosterone (DHT).

2. By testosterone itself.

3. By intracellular conversion of testosterone to estradiol (aromatization).

In those cells which respond only to DHT, only DHT will be found within the nucleus activating messenger RNA production. Because testosterone and DHT bind to the same high affinity androgen receptor, why is it necessary to have the DHT mechanism? One explanation is that this is a mechanism for amplifying androgen action, because the androgen receptor preferentially will bind DHT (greater affinity). The anti-androgens, including cyproterone acetate, spironolactone, and even cimetidine, bind to the androgen receptor with about 20% of the affinity of testosterone.(29) This weak affinity is characteristic of binding without activation of the biologic response.

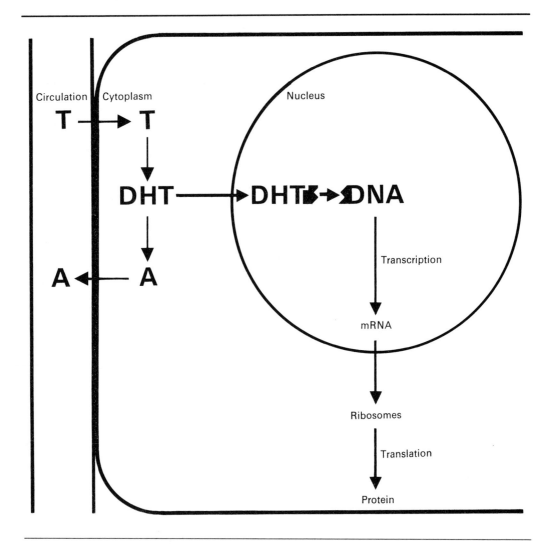

Progestins not only compete for androgen receptors, but also compete for the metabolic utilization of the 5α-reductase enzyme. The dihydroprogesterone which is produced, in turn also competes with testosterone and DHT for the androgen receptor. A progestin, therefore, can act both as an anti-androgen and as an anti-estrogen.

Tissues which exclusively operate via the testosterone pathway are the derivatives of the wolffian duct, whereas hair follicles and derivatives of the urogenital sinus require the conversion of testosterone to DHT. The hypothalamus actively converts androgens to estrogens; hence, aromatization may be necessary for certain androgen feedback messages in the brain.

The syndrome of testicular feminization (androgen insensitivity) represents a congenital abnormality in the androgen intracellular mechanism. There is either a defect in receptor production or an abnormality in receptor function. In either event, there is a failure in nuclear binding of androgens. What was once a confusing picture is now easily understood as a progressive increase in androgen receptor action. At one end, there is a complete absence of androgen binding—complete testicular feminization. In the middle is a spectrum of clinical presentations representing varying degrees of abnormal receptors and binding, while at the other end, it has been suggested that about 25% of men with normal genitalia, normal family histories, and infertility due to azoospermia have a receptor disorder. (30)

Mechanism of Action for Tropic Hormones

Tropic hormones include the releasing hormones originating in the hypothalamus, and a variety of peptides and glycoproteins released by the anterior pituitary gland. The specificity of the tropic hormone depends upon the presence of a receptor in the cell membrane of the target tissue. Tropic hormones do not enter the cell to stimulate physiologic events but simply unite with a receptor on the surface of the cell. Union with the receptor activates the adenylate cyclase enzyme within the membrane wall leading to the conversion of adenosine 5'-triphosphate (ATP) within the cell to cyclic AMP. Specificity of action and/or intensity of stimulation can be altered by changes in the structure or concentration of the receptor at the cell wall binding site. In addition to changes in biological activity due to target cell alterations, changes in the molecular structure of the tropic hormone can interfere with cellular binding and physiological activity.

The cell's mechanism for sensing the low concentrations of circulating tropic hormone is to have an extremely large number of receptors but to require only a very small percentage (as little as 1%) to be occupied by the tropic hormone. The cyclic AMP released is specifically bound to a cytoplasm receptor protein, and this cyclic AMP-receptor protein complex activates a protein kinase. The protein kinase is thought to be present in an inactive form as a tetramer, containing 2 regulatory subunits and 2 catalytic subunits. Binding of cyclic AMP to the regulatory units releases the catalytic units, the regulatory units remaining as a dimer. The catalytic units catalyze the phosphorylation of cellular proteins such as enzymes and mitochondrial, microsomal, and chromatin proteins. The physiologic event follows this cyclic AMP-mediated energy-producing event. Cyclic AMP is then degraded by the enzyme phosphodiesterase into the inactive compound, 5'-AMP.

Acute responses such as increased steroidogenesis do not operate through gene transcription but rather through phosphorylation. Long-term effects of peptide hormones, such as differentiation and growth, do operate through nuclear activity, and cyclic AMP may exert an effect on RNA polymerase activity (transcription) as well as on translation. Because LH can stimulate steroidogenesis without apparent changes in cyclic AMP (at low hormone concentrations), it is possible that an independent pathway exists; i.e. a mechanism independent of cyclic AMP. Mechanisms independent of cyclic AMP could include ion flow, calcium distribution, and changes in phospholipid metabolism.

The cyclic AMP system can be regarded as an example of evolutionary conservation. Rather than developing new regulatory systems, certain critical regulators have been preserved from bacteria to mammals. How is it that a single intracellular mediator can regulate different events? This is accomplished by turning on different biochemical events. There are numerous possibilities governed by

31

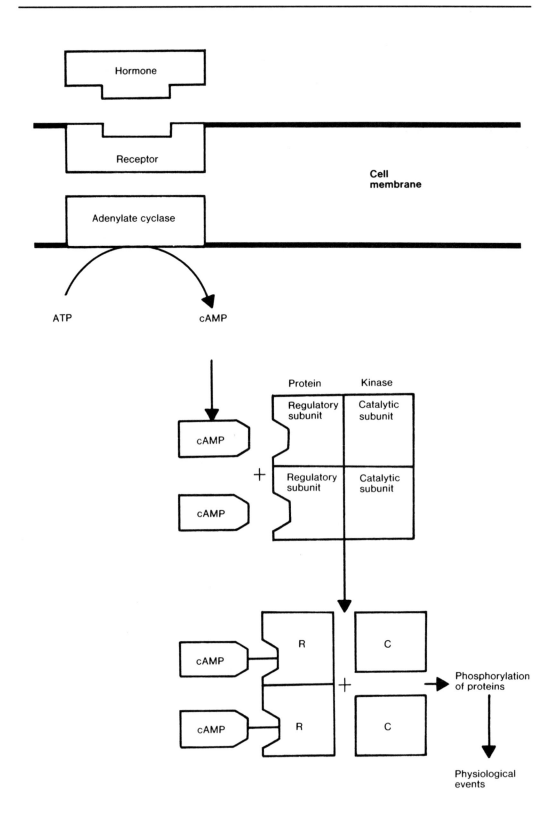

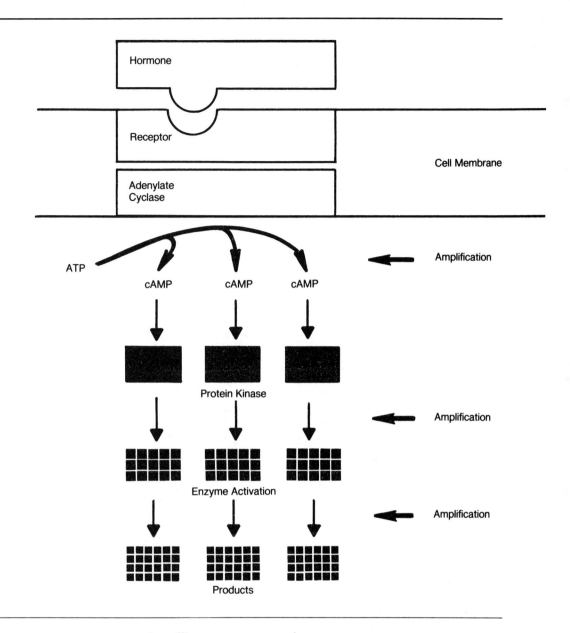

the cell's own gene expression.

The cyclic AMP system provides a method for amplification of the faint hormonal signal swimming in the sea of the bloodstream. Each cyclase molecule produces a lot of cyclic AMP; the protein kinases activate a large number of molecules which in turn lead to an even greater number of products. This is an important part of the sensitivity of the endocrine system. This is a major reason why only a small percentage of the cell membrane receptors need be occupied in order to generate a response.

Prostaglandins have been implicated in the cyclic AMP mechanism. Because prostaglandins stimulate adenylate cyclase activity and cyclic AMP accumulation, a role is implied for prostaglandins in transmitting the message from the exterior cell wall to the interior cell wall and the adenylate cyclase enzyme. Despite the effect on adenylate cyclase, prostaglandins appear to be synthesized after the action of cyclic AMP. This implies that tropic hormone stimulation of cyclic AMP occurs first; cyclic AMP then activates prostaglandin synthesis, and finally, intracellular prostaglandin moves to the cell wall to facilitate the response to the tropic hormone.

In addition, prostaglandins and cyclic GMP (cyclic guanosine 3'5'-monophosphate) may participate in an intracellular negative feedback mechanism governing the degree of, or direction of, cellular activity (e.g. the extent of steroidogenesis or shutting off of steroidogenesis after a peak of activity is reached). In other words, the level of cellular function may be determined by the interaction among prostaglandins, cyclic AMP, and cyclic GMP.

The intracellular calcium concentration is also a regulator of both cyclic AMP and cyclic GMP levels.(31) Activation of the surface receptor either opens a channel in the cell membrane which lets calcium ions into the cell, or calcium is released from internal stores (the latter is especially the case in muscle). This calcium flux is an important intracellular mediator of response to hormones, functioning itself as a second messenger in the nervous system and in muscle.

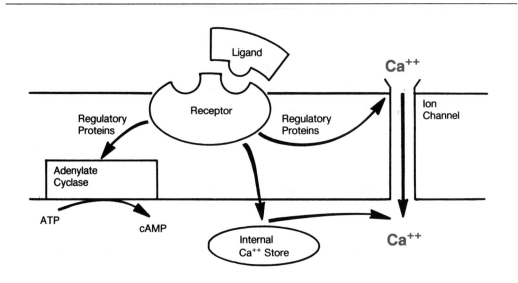

The calcium messenger system is linked to hormone-receptor function by means of a specific enzyme, phospholipase C, which catalyzes the hydrolysis of polyphosphatidylinositols, specific phospholipids in the cell membrane. Activation of this enzyme by hormone binding to its receptor leads to the generation of 2 intracellular messengers, inositol trisphosphate and diacylglycerol, which initiate the function of the 2 parts of the calcium system. The first is a calcium activated protein kinase responsible for sustained cellular responses, and the second part involves a regulator called calmodulin responsible for acute responses.

Calmodulin has been identified in all animal and plant cells that have been examined, therefore, it is a very ancient protein. It is a single polypeptide chain of 148 amino acid residues whose se-

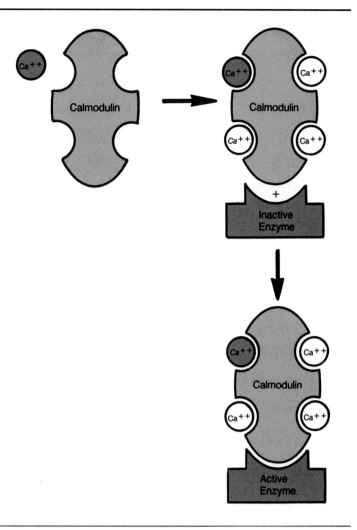

quence and structural and functional properties are similar to those of troponin C, the substance which binds calcium during muscle contractions, facilitating the interaction between actin and myosin. The calmodulin molecule has 4 calcium binding sites, and binding with calcium gives a helical conformation which is necessary for biologic activity. A typical animal cell contains more than 10 million molecules of calmodulin, constituting about 1% of the total cell protein. The calcium regulatory protein, calmodulin, serves as an intracellular calcium receptor and modifies calcium transport, the calcium regulation of cyclic nucleotide and glycogen metabolism, and such processes as secretion and cell motility. Thus, calmodulin serves a role analogous to that of troponin C, mediating calcium's actions in noncontractile tissues, and cyclic AMP works together with calcium and calmodulin in the regulation of intracellular metabolic activity.

There are differences among the tropic hormones. Oxytocin, insulin, growth hormone, prolactin, and human placental lactogen (HPL) do not utilize the adenylate cyclase mechanism. The message of these hormones is somehow passed directly to nuclear and cytoplasmic metabolic sites. Gonadotropin releasing hormone (GnRH) is calcium dependent in its mechanism of action.

Regulation of Tropic Hormones

Modulation of the peptide hormone mechanism is an important biologic system for enhancing or reducing target tissue response. This regulation of tropic hormone action currently has 3 major components:

1. Heterogeneity of the hormone.

2. Up and down regulation of receptors.

3. Regulation of adenylate cyclase.

Heterogeneity

The preciseness of the chemical make-up of the tropic hormones is an essential element in determining the ability of the hormone to mate with its receptor. The glycopeptides (FSH, LH, TSH, and HCG) all share a common α chain, an identical structure containing 92 amino acids. The β chains (or the β subunits) differ in both amino acid and carbohydrate content, conferring the specificity inherent in the relationship between hormones and their receptors. Therefore, the specific biologic activity of a glycopeptide hormone is determined by the β subunit.

β-HCG is the largest β subunit, containing a larger carbohydrate moiety and 145 to 150 amino acid residues including a unique carboxyl terminal tail piece of 28 to 30 amino acid groups. It is this unique part of the HCG structure which allows the production of highly specific antibodies and the utilization of highly specific radioimmunological assays.

The rate-limiting step in the synthesis of gonadotropins and TSH may be the availability of β units, since excess α units can be found in blood and in tissue. The half-life of α-HCG is 6-8 minutes, that of whole HCG about 12 hours. All human tissues appear to make HCG as a whole molecule, but the placenta is different in having the ability to glycosylate the protein, thus reducing its rate of metabolism and giving it biological activity through a long half-life. The carbohydrate components are comprised of fructose, galactose, mannose, galactosamine, glucosamine, and sialic acid. Whereas the other sugars are necessary for hormonal function, sialic acid is the critical determinant of biological half-life. Removal of terminal sialic acid residues in HCG, FSH, and LH leads to very rapid elimination from the circulation.

The glycopeptide hormones can be found in the pituitary existing in a variety of forms, differing in their carbohydrate makeup. Removal of carbohydrate residues from the FSH molecule produces forms of FSH with antagonistic properties. Treatment of women with a GnRH antagonist yields circulating levels of deglycosylated FSH that binds to gonadal receptors but exerts no biological activity.(32) Thus, the pituitary can secrete forms of the glycopeptide hormones which can function as naturally occurring antihormones.

Certain clinical conditions may be associated with alterations in the usual chemical structure of the glycopeptides, resulting in an interference with the ability to bind to receptors and stimulate biological activity. In addition to deglycosylation and the formation of anti-

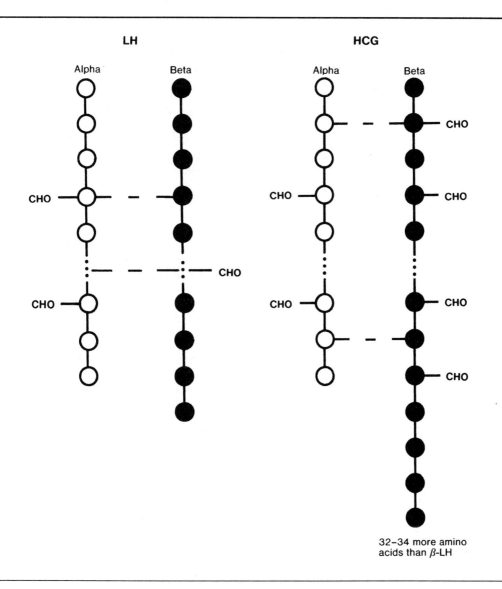

LH

Alpha　　Beta

HCG

Alpha　　Beta

CHO

CHO　—○— – – —●— CHO

CHO　—○　　　　●— CHO

– – —:—:— CHO

CHO　—○　　　　●— CHO

CHO　—○— – – —●

●— CHO

32–34 more amino
acids than β-LH

hormones, gonadotropins can be produced with an increased carbohydrate content. A low estrogen environment in the pituitary gland, for example, favors the production of so-called big gonadotropins, gonadotropins with an increased carbohydrate component and, as a result, decreased biological activity.

At midcycle (periovulatory), there is an increased secretion of free α-subunits in response to GnRH, and in anovulatory women, estrogen administration amplifies the α-subunit response to GnRH.(33) This again indicates that the pituitary response to GnRH is intensely modulated by the hormonal milieu, especially the estrogen environment.

The carbohydrate component, therefore, affects biological activity in two ways: 1) metabolic clearance and half-life, and 2) biological activity. The latter action focuses on two functions for the hormone-receptor complex: binding and activation. One structural domain of HCG is important for binding and another for triggering the biological response. Carbohydrate residues, especially the sialic acid residues, are important in both domains. Removal of the carbohydrate moiety of either subunit diminishes the gonadotropic activity of HCG. Specific studies indicate that the carbohydrate component plays a critical role in activation, specifically for coupling of the adenylate cyclase system.(34,35) Furthermore, new findings reveal that the α subunit also plays an important role in accomplishing normal receptor binding and activation. (36,37) Neither subunit alone can effectively bind to the receptor with high affinity or exert biological effect. In other words, binding and activation occur only when the hormone is in the combined α-β form.

Using recombinant DNA technology, it has been demonstrated that there is a single human gene for the expression of the α subunit. There are at least 7 genes for the β subunit of HCG, but only one for β-LH. It is thought that β-HCG evolved from β-LH, and the unique amino acid terminal extension of β-HCG arose by reading a gene similar to β-LH.(38) Interestingly, rodents do not have chorionic gonadotropin expression, and it has been suggested that development of HCG from LH took place sometime before the evolution of the horse.

Up and Down
Regulation

Positive or negative modulation of receptors by homologous hormones is known as up and down regulation. Little is known regarding the mechanism of up regulation, however hormones such as prolactin and GnRH can increase the cell membrane concentration of their own receptors.

Theoretically, deactivation of the hormone-receptor complex could be accomplished by dissociation of the complex, or loss of receptors from the cell, either by shedding (externally) or by internalization of the receptors into the cell. It is the process of *internalization* which is the major biological mechanism by which polypeptide hormones down regulate their own receptors and thus limit hormonal activity. As a general rule, an excess concentration of a tropic hormone such as LH or GnRH will stimulate the process of internalization, leading to a loss of receptors in the cell membrane and a decrease in biological response. We now understand that the principal reason for the episodic (pulsatile) secretion of hormones is to avoid down regulation and to maintain, if not up regulate, its receptors. The pulse frequency is a key factor, therefore, in regulating receptor number; however, further effects on target tissue response also occur at sites distal to receptors.(39)

It is believed that receptors are randomly inserted into the cell membrane after intracellular synthesis. The polypeptide receptor may be viewed as having 2 important sites, an external binding site which is specific for a polypeptide hormone, and an internal site which plays a role in the process of internalization. When the receptor is bound to a polypeptide hormone and when high concentrations of the hormone are present in the circulation, the hormone-receptor

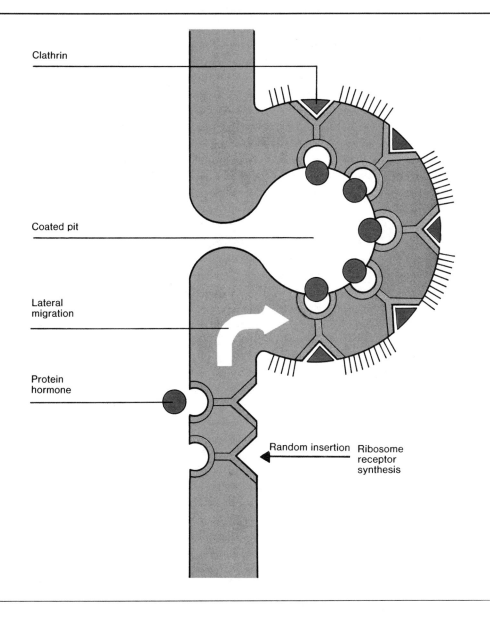

Clathrin

Coated pit

Lateral
migration

Protein
hormone

Random insertion   Ribosome
receptor
synthesis

complex moves through the cell membrane in a process called lateral migration. Lateral migration carries the complex to a specialized region of the cell membrane, *the coated pit*. Each cell in target tissues contains from 500 to 1500 coated pits. Lateral migration thus concentrates hormone-receptor complexes in the coated pit (*clustering*), allowing increased internalization of the complex via the special mechanism of receptor-mediated endocytosis. (40) The time course for this process (minutes rather than seconds) is too slow to explain the immediate hormone-induced responses, but other cellular events may be mediated by this mechanism which circumvents the intracellular messenger, cyclic AMP.

The coated pit is a lipid vesicle hanging on a basket of specific proteins, called *clathrins,* (from the Latin "clathra" meaning "lattice"). The unit is a network of hexagons and pentagons, thus looking like a soccer ball. The internal margin of the pit has a brush border, hence the name coated pit. The clathrin protein network may serve to localize the hormone-receptor complexes by binding to the internal binding site on the receptor.

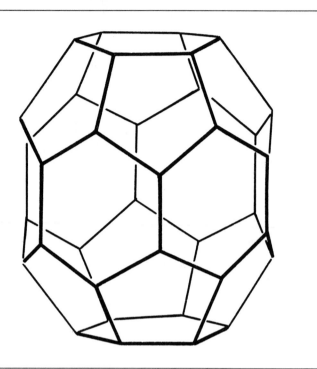

When fully occupied, the coated pit invaginates, pinches off, and enters the cell as a coated vesicle also called a receptosome. The coated vesicle is delivered to the lysosomes where the structure then undergoes degradation, releasing the substance (e.g. a polypeptide hormone) and the receptor. The receptor may be recycled, i.e. it may be reinserted into the cell membrane and used again. On the other hand, the receptor and the hormone may be metabolized, thus decreasing that hormone's biologic activity. The internalized hormones may also mediate biologic response by influencing cellular organelles such as the Golgi apparatus, the endoplasmic reticulum, and even the nucleus. Nuclear membranes from human ovaries bind HCG and LH and there follows an enzyme response which is involved in the transfer of mRNA from nucleus to the cytoplasm.(41)

Besides down regulation of polypeptide hormone receptors, the process of internalization can be utilized for other cellular metabolic events, including the transfer into the cell of vital substances such as iron or vitamins. Hence, cell membrane receptors can be separated into 2 classes. (42)

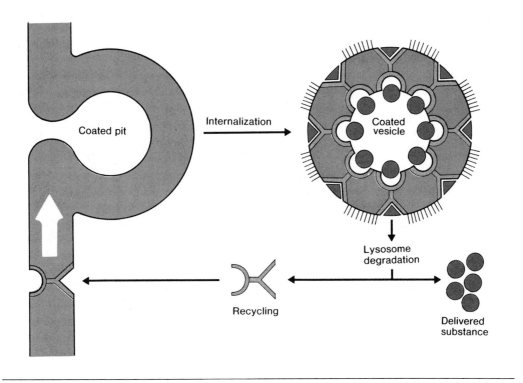

The Class I receptors are randomly distributed in the cell membrane and transmit information to modify cell behavior. For these receptors, internalization is a method for down regulation by degradation in lysosomes. Because of this degradation, recycling is usually not a feature of this class of receptors. Hormones which utilize this category of receptors include: FSH, LH, HCG, GnRH, TSH, TRH, and insulin. For these hormones, the coated pit can be viewed as a trap to immobilize hormone-receptor complexes. The fate of the hormone, however, can vary from tissue to tissue. In some target tissues, HCG is internalized and the HCG-receptor complex is transferred intact from the coated vesicle into the lysosomes for dissociation and degradation. In other tissues, especially the placenta, it is thought that the HCG-receptor complex is recycled back to the cell surface as a means of transporting HCG across the placenta into both maternal and fetal circulations.(43)

The Class II receptors are located in the coated pits and binding leads to internalization, thus providing the cell with required factors, or the removal of noxious agents from the biologic fluid bathing the cell, or the transfer of substances through the cell (transendocytosis). These receptors are spared from degradation and can be recycled. Examples of this category include: low-density lipoproteins (LDL) which supply cholesterol to steroid-producing cells, cobalamin and transferrin which supply vitamin B_{12} and iron, respectively, and the transfer of immunoglobulins across the placenta to provide fetal immunity.

41

A closer look at LDL and its receptor is informative. The low-density lipoprotein particle is a sphere. It contains in its center about 1500 molecules of cholesterol which are attached as esters to fatty acids. This core is contained by a bilayer lipid membrane. Protein binding proteins (the apoproteins) project on the surface of this membrane, and it is these proteins which the receptor must recognize.

Remember, this is an important story, because all cells which produce steroids must use cholesterol as the basic building block. Such cells do not contain and cannot synthesize enough cholesterol, and therefore must bring cholesterol into the cell from the bloodstream. LDL is the principal messenger delivering the cholesterol. Experimental evidence, however, indicates that HDL-cholesterol as well as LDL can provide cholesterol to steroid producing cells.(44)

Recent studies have revealed that different cell surface receptors and proteins contain surprisingly similar structural parts.(45) For example, the receptor for LDL contains a region that is homologous to the precursor of epidermal growth factor, and another region that is homologous to a component of complement. The LDL receptor is a "mosaic protein." There are regions of proteins derived from the exons of different gene families. This is an example of a protein that evolved as a new combination of pre-existing functional units of other proteins.

The LDL Receptor

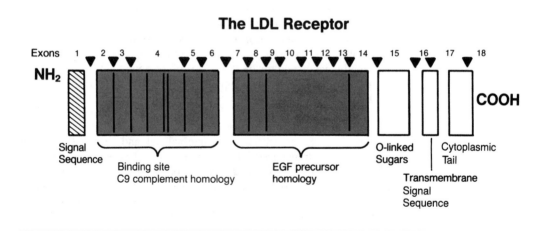

The LDL receptor is synthesized as a precursor of 860 amino acids. The precursor includes 22 amino acids which constitute a hydrophobic signal sequence that is cleaved prior to its insertion into the cell surface. This signal sequence presumably directs the protein where to go in the cell. This leaves an 839 amino acid protein which has 5 recognizable areas called domains.

1. NH$_2$-terminal of 292 amino acids, composed of a sequence of 40 amino acids repeated with some variation some 7 times. This domain is the binding site for LDL and is located on the external surface of the cell membrane.

42

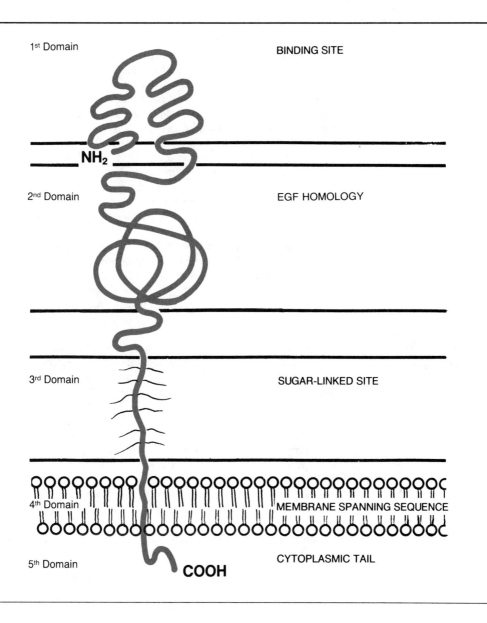

1st Domain   BINDING SITE

NH₂

2nd Domain   EGF HOMOLOGY

3rd Domain   SUGAR-LINKED SITE

4th Domain   MEMBRANE SPANNING SEQUENCE

5th Domain   CYTOPLASMIC TAIL

COOH

2. Approximately 400 amino acids homologous to epidermal growth factor precursor.

3. The sugar-linked site.

4. 22 Hydrophobic amino acids that cross the cell membrane. Deletion of the transmembrane signal sequence (found in a naturally occurring mutation) results in an LDL receptor which is secreted from the cell instead of being inserted into the membrane.

5. Cytoplasmic tail of 50 amino acids which is located internally and serves to cluster LDL receptors in coated pits.

When the coated pit is fully occupied with LDL, in the process called endocytosis, a coated vesicle is delivered into the cell. The vesicle moves to the Golgi system and then is routed by an unknown mechanism (although a similar coated pit system in the Golgi appears to be involved) to the lysosomes where the structure undergoes degradation, releasing cholesterol esters and the receptor. The receptor may be recycled or degraded. Synthesis and insertion of new LDL receptors are a function of LH in the gonads, and ACTH in the adrenal. This process is relatively fast. It has been calculated that the coated pit system turns over an amount of cell surface equivalent to the total amount of plasma membrane every 30-90 minutes.(23) The LDL receptor makes one round trip every 10 minutes during its 20-hour life-span for a total of several hundred trips.(2)

A genetic defect in receptors for LDL can lead to a failure in internalization and hyperlipidemia. Autoantibodies to membrane receptors can compete with a hormone for binding to the receptor and result in specific diseases, e.g. myasthenia gravis with antibodies to acetylcholine receptors, Graves' disease with antibodies to TSH receptors, and asthma with antibodies to adrenergic receptors.

Regulation of
Adenylate Cyclase

The biologic activity of a polypeptide hormone (such as FSH or LH) can be altered by the heterogeneity of the molecules, up and down regulation of the receptors, and finally, by modulation of the activity of the enzyme, adenylate cyclase.

In a useful concept of how this enzyme works, adenylate cyclase is considered to be composed of 2 protein units, a guanyl nucleotide regulatory unit and a catalytic unit. (46,47) The regulatory unit is a coupling protein, regulated by guanine nucleotides (specifically GTP), and therefore it is called GTP binding protein or G protein for short. The catalytic unit converts ATP to cyclic AMP. The receptor and the nucleotide regulatory unit are structurally linked, but inactive until the hormone binds to the receptor. Upon binding, the complex of hormone, receptor, and nucleotide regulatory unit is activated leading to an uptake of guanosine 5'-triphosphate (GTP) by the regulatory unit. The activation and uptake of GTP result in an active enzyme which can convert ATP to cAMP. This result can be viewed as the outcome of the regulatory unit *coupling* with the catalytic unit, forming an intact complete enzyme. Enzyme activity is then terminated by hydrolysis of the GTP to guanosine 5'-diphosphate (GDP) returning the enzyme to its inactive state. Quick action and acute control of adenylate cyclase are assured because the G protein is a GTPase which self activates upon binding of GTP.

This receptor complex can be the site of abnormal function. Cholera toxin is an enzyme that alters the G protein so that it no longer hydrolyzes its bound GTP. Once activated by a hormone-receptor complex, it remains irreversibly turned on, and in the GI tract this turn on of cyclic AMP results in massive efflux of sodium and water into the gut. A genetic deficiency of the coupling protein has been reported, responsible for the manifestations of at least certain types of pseudohypoparathyroidism. Finally, some manifestations of abnormal thyroid function are due to the ability of thyroid hormone to alter receptor coupling.

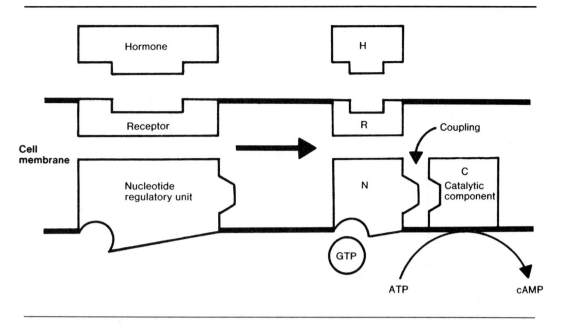

The ability of the hormone-receptor complex to work through a common messenger (cyclic AMP) and produce contrasting actions (stimulation and inhibition) is thought to be due to the presence of both stimulatory nucleotide regulatory units and inhibitory nucleotide regulatory units. Thus, stimulating agents may work through specific stimulatory units.

Another way to explain stimulating and inhibiting actions at the adenylate cyclase level focuses on the mechanism of coupling. LH stimulates steroidogenesis in the corpus luteum and works through the coupling of stimulatory regulatory units to the catalytic units of adenylate cyclase.

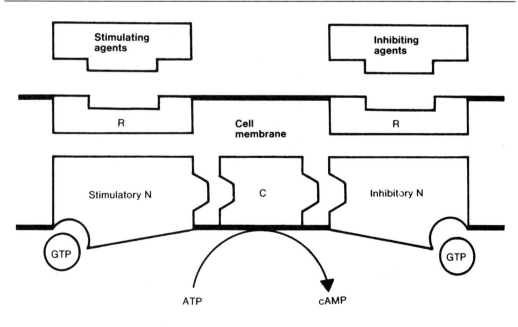

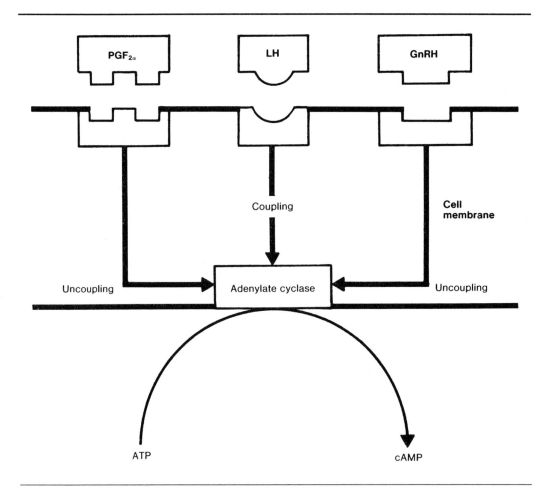

Both prostaglandin $F_{2\alpha}$ and GnRH are directly luteolytic, inhibiting luteal steroidogenesis through a mechanism which follows binding to specific receptors. This luteolytic action (in the rodent) may be exerted via inhibitory regulatory units which lead to uncoupling with the catalytic units, thus interfering with gonadotropin action. It should be noted, however, that in human tissue GnRH is not luteolytic and has no effect on adenylate cyclase activity in luteal membranes.(48)

Increasing concentrations of tropic hormones, such as gonadotropins, are directly associated with desensitization of adenylate cyclase independently of the internalization of receptors. Desensitization is a rapid, acute change without loss of receptors in contrast to the slower process of internalization and true receptor loss. The desensitization process probably involves uncoupling, perhaps through hydrolysis of GTP, thus returning the active enzyme to its inactive state.

References

1. **Freedman DS, Srinivasan SR, Shear CL, Franklin FA, Webber LS, Berenson GS,** The relation of apolipoproteins A-I and B in children to parental myocardial infarction, New Eng J Med 315:721, 1986.

2. **Brown MS, Goldstein JL,** A receptor-mediated pathway for cholesterol homeostasis, Science 232:34, 1986.

3. **Stamler J, Wentworth D, Neaton JD,** Is relationship between serum cholesterol and risk of premature death from coronary heart disease continuous and graded? JAMA 256:2823, 1986.

4. **Grundy SM,** Cholesterol and coronary heart disease, JAMA 256:2849, 1986.

5. **Levy RI, Brensike JF, Epstein SE, et al,** The influence of changes in lipid values induced by cholestyramine and diet on progression of coronary artery disease: results of the NHLBI Type II coronary intervention study, Circulation 69:325, 1984.

6. **The Lipid Research Clinics Program,** The Lipid Research Clinics Coronary Primary Prevention Trial Results: I. Reduction in the incidence of coronary heart disease, JAMA 251:351, 1984.

7. **The Lipid Research Clinics Program,** The Lipid Research Clinics Coronary primary prevention trial results: II. The relationship of reduction in incidence of coronary heart disease to cholesterol lowering, JAMA 251:365, 1984.

8. **Castelli WP, Garrison RJ, Wilson PWF, Abbott RD, Kalousdian S, Kannel WB,** Incidence of coronary heart disease and lipoprotein cholesterol levels, JAMA 256:2835, 1986.

9. **Erickson GF,** An analysis of follicle development and ovum maturation, Seminars Reprod Endocrinol 4:233, 1986.

10. **Hillier SG, Reichert LE Jr, Van Hall EV,** Control of preovulatory follicular estrogen biosynthesis in the human ovary, J Clin Endocrinol Metab 52:847, 1981.

11. **Siiteri PK, MacDonald PC,** Role of extraglandular estrogen in human endocrinology, in *Handbook of Physiology, Section 7, Endocrinology*, Geiger SR, Astwood EB, Greep RO, editors, American Physiology Society, Washington, DC, 1973, pp 615-629.

12. **Silva PD, Gentzschein EEK, Lobo RA,** Androstenedione may be a more important precursor of tissue dihydrotestosterone than testosterone in women, Fertil Steril 48:419, 1987.

13. **Muldoon TG,** Steroid hormone receptor dynamics: the key to tissue responsiveness, in *Molecular Mechanism of Steroid Hormone Action*, Modugdil VK, editor, Walter de Gruyter & Co., Berlin, 1985, pp 173-197.

14. **King RJB,** Structure and function of steroid receptors, J Endocrinol 114:341, 1987.

15. **Walters MR,** Steroid hormone receptors and the nucleus, Endocrin Rev 6:512l, 1985.

16. **Gorski J, Welshons WV, Sakai D, Hansen J, Walent J, Kassis J, Shull J, Stack G, Campen C,** Evolution of a model of estrogen action, Rec Prog Hor Res 42:297, 1986.

17. **King WJ, Greene GL,** Monoclonal antibodies localize oestrogen receptor in the nuclei of target cells, Nature 307:745, 1984.

18. **Welshons WV, Lieberman ME, Gorski J,** Nuclear localization of unoccupied oestrogen receptors, Nature 307:747, 1984.

19. **Press MF, Greene GL,** Localization of progesterone receptor with monoclonal antibodies to the human progestin receptor, Endocrinology 122:1165, 1988.

20. **Waterman ML, Adler S, Nelson C, Greene GL, Evans RM, Rosenfeld MG,** A single domain of the estrogen receptor confers deoxyribonucleic acid binding and transcriptional activation of the rat prolactin gene, Mol Endocrinol 2:14, 1988.

21. **Green S, Walter P, Kumar V, Krust A, Bornert J-M, Argos P, Chambon P,** Human oestrogen receptor cDNA: sequence, expression and homology to v-*erb*-A, Nature 320:134, 1986.

22. **Scholl S, Lippman ME,** The estrogen receptor in MCF-7 cells: evidence from dense amino acid labeling for rapid turnover and a dimeric model of activated nucleic receptor, Endocrinology 115:1295, 1984.

23. **Willingham MC, Pastan I,** Endocytosis and membrane traffic in cultured cells, Rec Prog Hor Res 40:569, 1984.

24. **Strobl JS, Kasid A, Huff KK, Lippman ME,** Kinetic alterations in estrogen receptors assocated with estrogen receptor processing in human breast cancer cells, Endocrinology 115:1116, 1984.

25. **Katzenellenbogen BS,** Biology and receptor interactions of estriol and estriol derivatives in vitro and in vivo, J Steroid Biochem 20:1033, 1984.

26. **Umans RS, Weichselbaum RR, Johnson CM, Little JB,** Effects of estradiol concentration on levels of nuclear estrogen receptors in MCF-7 breast tumor cells, J Steroid Biochem 20:605, 1984.

27. **DeSombre ER, Kuivanen PC,** Progestin modulation of estrogen-dependent marker protein synthesis in the endometrium, Sem Oncol 12:Suppl 1:6, 1985.

28. **Hung TT, Gibbons WE,** Evaluation of androgen antagonism of estrogen effect by dihydrotestosterone, J Steroid Biochem 19:1513, 1983.

29. **Tindall DJ, Chang CH, Lobl TJ, Cunningham, GR,** Androgen antagonists in androgen target tissues, Pharmacol Ther 24:367, 1984.

30. **Griffin JE, Wilson JD,** Disorders of androgen receptor function, Ann NY Acad Sci 438:61, 1984.

31. **Rasmussen H,** The calcium messenger system, New Eng J Med 314:1094,1164, 1986.

32. **Dahl KD, Bicsak TA, Hsueh AJW,** Naturally occurring antihormones: Secretion of FSH antagonists by women treated with a GnRH analog, Science 239:72, 1988.

33. **Rezai P, Scommegna A, Zbella EA, Lessing J, Barenner S, Weiss G, Benveniste R,** Free α-subunit response to gonadotropin-releasing hormone in women with polycystic ovaries, Fertil Steril 47:249, 1987.

34. **Richardson MC, Masson GM, Sairam MR,** Inhibitory action of chemically deglycosylated human chorionic gonadotrophin on hormone-induced steroid production by dispersed cells from human corpus luteum, J Endocrinol 101:327, 1984.

35. **Sairam MR, Bhargavi GN,** A role for glycosylation of the alpha subunit in transduction of biological signal in glycoprotein hormones, Science 229:65, 1985.

36. **Hwang J, Menon KMJ,** Spatial relationships of the human chorionic gonadotropin (hCG) subunits in the assembly of the hCG-receptor complex in the luteinized rat ovary, Proc Natl Acad Sci 81:4667, 1984.

37. **Merz WE, Dorner M,** Studies on structure-function relationships of human choriogonadotropins with C-terminally shortened alpha subunits. I. receptor binding and immunologic properties, Biochemica et Biophysica Acta 844:62, 1985.

38. **Fiddes JC, Talmadge K,** Structure, expression, and evolution of the genes for the human glycoprotein hormones, Rec Prog Hor Res 40:43, 1984.

39. **Katt JA, Duncan JA, Herbon L, Barkan A, Marshall JC,** The frequency of gonadotropin-releasing hormone stimulation determines the number of pituitary gonadotropin-releasing hormone receptors, Endocrinology 116:2113, 1985.

40. **Goldstein JL, Anderson RGW, Brown MS,** Coated pits, coated vesicles, and receptor-mediated endocytosis, Nature 279:679, 1979.

41. **Toledo A, Ramani N, Rao ChV,** Direct stimulation of nucleoside triphosphatase activity in human ovarian nuclear membranes by human chorionic gonadotropin, J Clin Endocrinol Metab 65:305, 1987.

42. **Kaplan J,** Polypeptide-binding membrane receptors: analysis and classification, Science 212:14, 1981.

43. **Ascoli M,** Lysosomal accumulation of the hormone-receptor complex during receptor-mediated endocytosis of human chorionic gonadotropin, J Cell Biol 99:1242, 1984.

44. **Parinaud J, Perret B, Ribbes H, Chap H, Pontonnier G, Douste-Blazy L,** High density lipoprotein and low density lipoprotein utilization by human granulosa cells for progesterone synthesis in serum-free culture: Respective contributions of free and esterified cholesterol, J Clin Endocrinol Metab 64:409, 1987.

45. **Sudhof TC, Goldstein JL, Brown MS, Russell DW,** The LDL receptor gene: a mosaic of exons shared with different proteins, Science 228:815, 1985.

46. **Rodbell M,** The role of hormone receptors and GTP-regulatory proteins in membrane transduction, Nature 284:17, 1980.

47. **Gilman AG,** Guanine nucleotide-binding regulatory proteins and dual control of adenylate cyclase, J Clin Invest 73:1, 1984.

48. **Rojas FJ, Asch RH,** Effects of luteinizing hormone-releasing hormone agonist and calcium upon adenyl cyclase activity of human corpus luteum membranes, Life Sci 36:841, 1985.

2 Neuroendocrinology

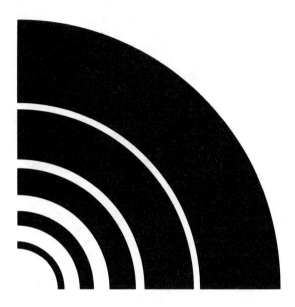

There are two major sites of action within the brain which are important in the regulation of reproductive function, the hypothalamus and the pituitary gland. In the past, the pituitary gland was viewed as the master gland. Then a new concept emerged in which the pituitary was relegated to a subordinate role as part of an orchestra, with the hypothalamus as the conductor, responding to both peripheral and central nervous system messages and exerting its influence by means of neurotransmitters transported to the pituitary by a portal vessel network. However, recent developments now indicate that the complex sequence of events known as the menstrual cycle is controlled by the sex steroids produced within the very follicle destined to ovulate. The hypothalamus and its direction are essential for the operation of the entire mechanism, but the endocrine function which leads to ovulation is brought about by steroid feedback on the anterior pituitary.

A full understanding of this feature of reproductive biology will benefit the clinician who faces problems in gynecologic endocrinology. With this understanding, the clinician can comprehend the hitherto mysterious, but significant, effects of stress, diet, exercise, and other diverse influences on the pituitary-gonadal axis. Furthermore, we will be prepared to make advantageous use of the numerous neuropharmacologic agents that are the dividends of neuroendocrine research. *To these ends, this chapter offers a clinically oriented review of the current status of reproductive neuroendocrinology.*

**Hypothalamic-
Hypophyseal Portal
Circulation**

In order to influence the anterior pituitary gland, the brain requires a means of transmission or connection. A direct nervous connection does not exist. The blood supply of the anterior pituitary, however, originates in the capillaries which richly lace the median eminence area of the hypothalamus. The direction of the blood flow in this hypophyseal portal circulation is from the brain to the pituitary. Section of the neural stalk which interrupts this portal circulation leads to inactivity and atrophy of the gonads, along with a decrease in adrenal and thyroid activity to basal levels. With regeneration of the portal vessels, anterior pituitary function is restored. Thus, the anterior pituitary gland is under the influence of the hypothalamus by means of neurohormones released into this portal circulation. There also exists retrograde flow so that pituitary hormones can be delivered directly to the hypothalamus, creating the opportunity for pituitary feedback upon the hypothalamus.

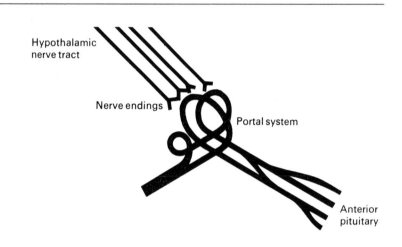

**The Neurohormone
Concept**

A considerable body of evidence has accumulated indicating that influence of the pituitary by the hypothalamus is achieved by materials secreted in the cells of the hypothalamus and transported to the pituitary by the portal vessel system. In addition to the stalk section experiments cited above, transplantation of the pituitary to ectopic sites (e.g. under the kidney capsule) results in failure of gonadal function. With retransplantation to an anatomic site under the median eminence, followed by regeneration of the portal system, normal pituitary function is regained. This retrieval of gonadotropic function is not accomplished if the pituitary is transplanted to other sites in the brain. Hence, there is something very special about the blood draining the basal hypothalamus. An exception to this overall pattern of positive influence is the control of prolactin secretion. Stalk secretion and transplantation cause release of prolactin from the anterior pituitary, implying a negative hypothalamic control. Furthermore, cultures of anterior pituitary tissue release prolactin in the absence of hypothalamic tissue or extracts.

Neuroendocrine agents originating in the hypothalamus have positive stimulatory impact on growth hormone, thyroid stimulating hormone (TSH), ACTH, as well as gonadotropins, and represent the individual neurohormones of the hypothalamus. The neurohor-

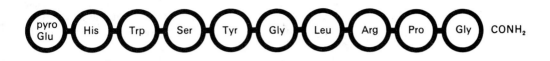

mone which controls gonadotropins is called gonadotropin releasing hormone, GnRH. The neurohormone which controls prolactin is called prolactin inhibiting hormone, and is probably dopamine. In addition to their effects on the pituitary, behavioral effects within the brain have been demonstrated for several of the releasing hormones. Thyrotropin releasing hormone (TRH) antagonizes the sedative action of a number of drugs and also has a direct antidepressant effect in humans. GnRH evokes mating behavior in male and female animals.(1)

Initially, it was believed that there were two separate releasing hormones for follicle-stimulating hormone (FSH) and luteinizing hormone (LH). It is now apparent that there is a single neurohormone (GnRH) for both gonadotropins. Purified or synthesized GnRH stimulates both FSH and LH secretion. The divergent patterns of FSH and LH in response to a single GnRH are due to the modulating influences of the endocrine environment, specifically the feedback effects of steroids on the anterior pituitary gland.

GnRH is a decapeptide with a similar structure in all mammals. Substitution of amino acids at the 2 or 3 positions yields antagonists, while substitution at the 6 or 10 positions produces agonists. Clinical applications include both stimulation and suppression. Induction of ovulation is the best example of stimulation. Suppression of pituitary secretion of gonadotropins by a GnRH agonist (down regulation) or antagonist can be utilized for the treatment of endometriosis, uterine leiomyomata, or precocious puberty.

Small neuroendocrine peptides share common large precursor polypeptides, called polyproteins or polyfunctional peptides. These proteins can serve as precursors for more than one biologically active peptide. The precursor protein for GnRH has been found to also contain a 56 amino acid sequence called GAP (GnRH-associated peptide).(2) GAP occupies the carboxy-terminal region of the precursor and is a potent inhibitor of prolactin secretion as well as a stimulator of gonadotropins.

There is a syndrome of hereditary hypogonadism in the mouse which is due to a deletion of the distal half of the gene responsible for the common precursor of GnRH and GAP. Interestingly the normal architecture of neurons and circuits necessary for GnRH function is not affected by this gene deletion. This syndrome has been completely cured by the introduction of an intact GnRH gene into the genome of the hypogonadal mouse.(3) The degree of human hypogonadism is due to varying levels of impaired hypothalamic secretion of GnRH.(4) The implications for the treatment of this problem with genetic engineering in men and women are obvious and enormous.

The Hypothalamus and GnRH Secretion

The hypothalamus is the part of the diencephalon, at the base of the brain, which forms the floor of the third ventricle and part of its lateral walls. Within the hypothalamus are peptidergic neural cells which secrete the releasing and inhibiting hormones. These cells share the characteristics of both neurons and endocrine gland cells. They respond to signals in the bloodstream, as well as to neurotransmitters within the brain, in a process known as neurosecretion. In neurosecretion, a neurohormone or neurotransmitter is synthesized on the ribosomes in the cytoplasm of the neuron, packaged into a granule in the Golgi apparatus, and then transported by active axonal flow to the neuronal terminal for secretion into a blood vessel or across a synapse.

In primates, the primary network of GnRH cell bodies is located within the medial basal hypothalamus. Most of these can be seen within the arcuate nucleus where GnRH is synthesized in GnRH neurons. The delivery of GnRH to the portal circulation is via an axonal pathway, the GnRH tuberoinfundibular tract.

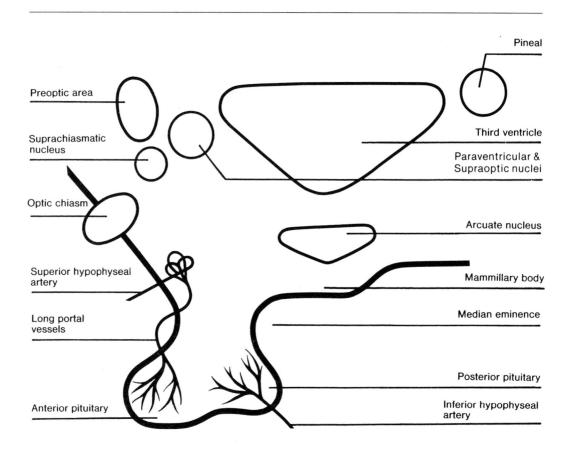

Fibers, identified with immunocytochemical techniques using antibodies to GnRH, also can be visualized in the posterior hypothalamus, descending into the posterior pituitary, and in the anterior hypothalamic area, projecting to sites within the limbic system.(5) However, lesions which interrupt GnRH neurons projecting to regions other than the median eminence do not affect gonadotropin release. Only lesions of the arcuate nucleus in the monkey lead to gonadal atrophy and amenorrhea.(6) Therefore, the arcuate nucleus can be viewed with the median eminence as a unit, the key locus within the hypothalamus for GnRH secretion into the portal circulation. The other GnRH neurons may be important for a variety of behavioral responses.

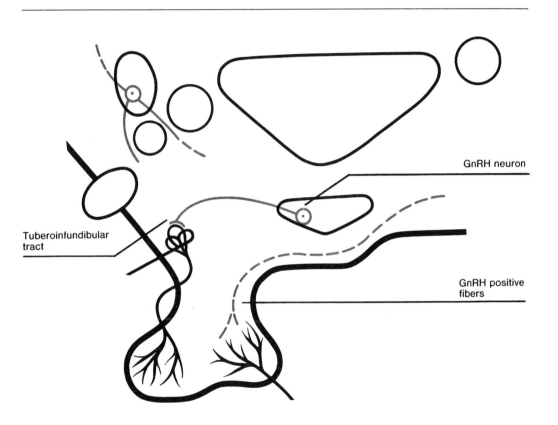

GnRH neuron

Tuberoinfundibular tract

GnRH positive fibers

GnRH Secretion

The half-life of GnRH is only 2-4 minutes. Therefore, control of the reproductive cycle depends upon constant release of GnRH. This function, in turn, depends upon the complex and coordinated inter-relationships among this releasing hormone, other neurohormones, the pituitary gonadotropins, and the gonadal steroids. The interplay among these substances is governed by feedback effects, both positive stimulatory and negative inhibitory. *The long feedback loop* refers to the feedback effects of circulating levels of target gland hormones, and this occurs both in the hypothalamus and the pituitary. *The short feedback loop* indicates a negative feedback of gonadotropins on pituitary secretion, presumably via inhibitory effects on GnRH in the hypothalamus. *Ultrashort feedback* refers to inhibition by the releasing hormone on its own synthesis. These signals as well as signals from higher centers in the central nervous system may modify GnRH secretion through an array of neurotransmitters, primarily dopamine, norepinephrine, and endorphin, but also serotonin and melatonin.

Dopamine and norepinephrine are synthesized in the nerve terminals by decarboxylation of dihydroxyphenylalanine (DOPA), which in turn is synthesized by hydroxylation of tyrosine. Dopamine is the immediate precursor of norepinephrine, but dopamine itself may function as a key neurotransmitter in the hypothalamus and the pituitary.

A most useful concept is to view the arcuate nucleus as the central site of action, releasing GnRH into the portal circulation in pulsatile fashion. In a classic series of experiments, it was demonstrated that normal gonadotropin secretion requires pulsatile GnRH discharge in frequency and amplitude within a critical range.(7)

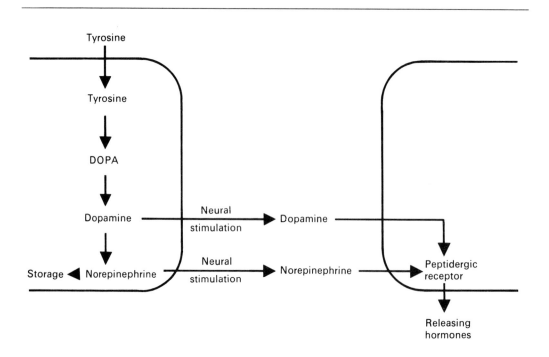

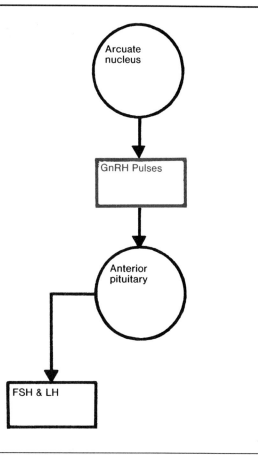

Experimental manipulations have indicated that the critical range of GnRH pulsatile secretion is rather narrow. The administration (to monkeys) of 1 μg GnRH per minute for 6 minutes every hour (1 pulse per hour) produces a portal blood concentration about equal to the peak concentration of GnRH in human portal blood, about 2 ng/ml. Increasing the frequency to 2 and 5 pulses per hour extinguishes gonadotropic secretion. A similar decline in gonadotropin secretion is obtained by increasing the dose of GnRH. Decreasing the pulse frequency decreases LH secretion, but increases FSH secretion.

Like GnRH, gonadotropins are also secreted in pulsatile fashion. Initiation of the pulsatile pattern of gonadotropin secretion occurs just before puberty with night time increases in LH. After puberty, pulsatile secretion is maintained throughout the 24-hour period, but it varies in both amplitude and frequency. The pulsatile secretion of gonadotropins is due to the pulsatile release of GnRH into the portal system.(8) In puberty, arcuate activity begins with a low frequency of GnRH release and proceeds through a cycle of acceleration of frequency, characterized by passage from total inactivity, to nocturnal activation, to the full adult pattern. The progressive changes in FSH and LH reflect this activation of GnRH pulsatile secretion.

| Timing of GnRH Pulses | The measurement of LH pulses is utilized as an indicator of GnRH pulsatile secretion (the long half-life of FSH precludes its use for this purpose).(9) The characteristics of LH pulses (and presumably of GnRH pulses) during the menstrual cycle are as follows: (10) |

LH pulse mean amplitude:

Early follicular phase: 6.5 mIU/ml.

Midfollicular phase: 5.1 mIU/ml.

Late follicular phase: 7.2 mIU/ml.

Early luteal phase: 14.9 mIU/ml.

Mid luteal phase: 12.2 mIU/ml.

Late luteal phase: 7.6 mIU/ml.

LH pulse mean frequency:

Early follicular phase: 94 minutes.

Late follicular phase: 71 minutes.

Early luteal phase: 103 minutes.

Late luteal phase: 216 minutes.

Despite the handicap of the long half-life, it has been ascertained that FSH secretion is correlated with LH secretion. Thus pulsatile secretion is more frequent but smaller in amplitude during the follicular phase compared to the luteal phase. It should be emphasized that these numbers are not inviolate. There is considerable variability between and within individuals and a large normal range exists. (11)

The anterior pituitary gland also appears to have a pulsatile pattern of its own. While pulses of significant amplitude are linked to GnRH, small amplitude pulses of high frequency represent spontaneous secretion (at least as demonstrated in isolated pituitary glands in vitro).(12) It is not known whether this has any importance in vivo, and at the present time, the major secretory pattern is thought to reflect GnRH.

Control of GnRH Pulses

Normal menstrual cycles require the maintenance of the pulsatile release of GnRH within a critical range of frequency and amplitude. This pulsatile release is mediated by a catecholaminergic mechanism and can be modified by gonadal steroids and endorphins. In addition, a leukotriene, LTC_4, is found in GnRH neurons, playing a still to be determined role.(13)

The Dopamine Tract. Cell bodies for dopamine synthesis can be found in the arcuate and periventricular nuclei. The dopamine tuberoinfundibular tract arises within the medial basal hypothalamus and projects to the median eminence.

The administration of dopamine by intravenous infusion to men and women is associated with a suppression of circulating prolactin and gonadotropin levels.(14) Dopamine does not exert a direct effect on gonadotropin secretion by the anterior pituitary, thus this effect is mediated through GnRH release in the hypothalamus. While the exact chemical nature of the prolactin inhibiting hormone is still not known, evidence is rather overwhelming that dopamine is the hypothalamic inhibitor of prolactin secretion and is directly secreted into the portal blood, thus behaving like a neurohormone.(15) Therefore, dopamine may directly suppress arcuate GnRH activity, and also be transported via the portal system to directly and specifically suppress pituitary prolactin secretion. The hypothalamic tuberoinfundibular dopamine pathway is not the only dopamine pathway in the CNS, and it is only one of two major dopamine pathways in the hypothalamus. But it is this pathway which directly participates in the regulation of prolactin secretion. Ergot derivatives, such as bromocriptine, used clinically to treat high prolactin levels, activate dopaminergic receptors and directly inhibit the secretion of prolactin in a fashion identical to dopamine. Whether the peptide associated with GnRH (GAP) plays a role in physiologic prolactin regulation is not known.

Many studies, including specific *in vitro* systems, have indicated that dopamine stimulates the release of GnRH from the hypothalamus.(16) This appears to be a paradox, but it simply indicates that the ultimate GnRH response reflects the complex interactions of steroids and neurotransmitters. For an understanding of clinical problems, it is best to view dopamine as an inhibitor of both GnRH and prolactin.

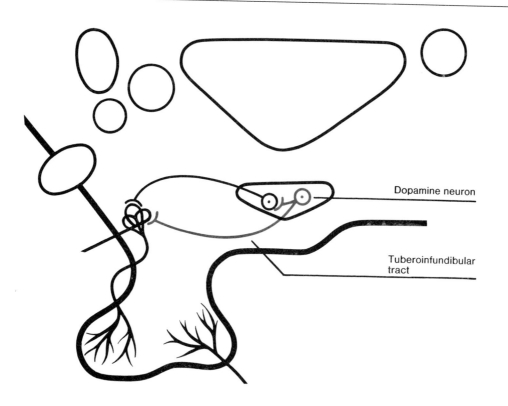

Dopamine neuron

Tuberoinfundibular tract

The story is further complicated by an apparent direct stimulation of prolactin secretion by GnRH.(17) This action is thought to represent a paracrine interaction between the pituitary gonadotropes and lactotropes, occurring independently of FSH and LH.

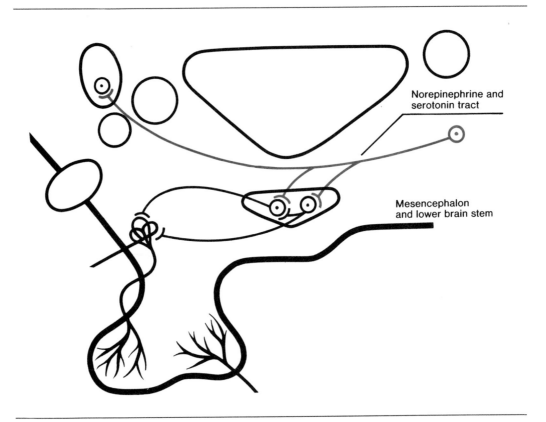

Norepinephrine and serotonin tract

Mesencephalon and lower brain stem

The Norepinephrine Tract. Most of the cell bodies which synthesize norepinephrine are located in the mesencephalon and lower brainstem. These cells also synthesize serotonin. Axons for amine transport ascend into the medial forebrain bundle to terminate in various brain structures including the hypothalamus.

The current concept is that the biogenic catecholamines regulate GnRH pulsatile release. Norepinephrine is thought to exert stimulatory effects on GnRH, while dopamine and serotonin exert inhibitory effects. Little is known, however, about the role of serotonin. The probable mode of action of catecholamines is to change the frequency (and perhaps the amplitude) of GnRH discharge. Thus, pharmacologic or psychologic factors that affect pituitary function probably do so by altering catecholamine synthesis or metabolism, and thus the pulsatile release of GnRH.

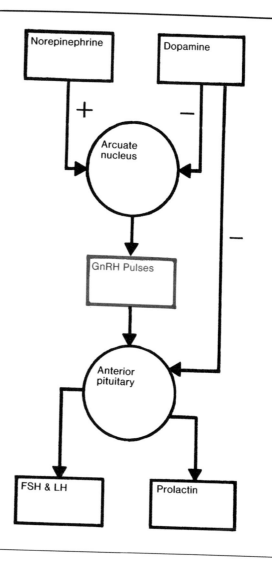

The following clinical observations illustrate the preceding physiologic mechanisms: Pseudocyesis, with high LH and prolactin secretion, can be explained by a lack of dopamine activity in the hypothalamus, thus luteal function and galactorrhea are maintained. Amenorrhea on a central basis can be due to a decrease in GnRH pulses below the critical frequency, caused, perhaps, by excessive dopamine in the hypothalamus. Marijuana use is associated with decreased gonadotropins and reproductive function due to a decrease in GnRH pulsatile release in the hypothalamus.

Brain Peptides

There are a large variety of peptides which may function as neurotransmitters.(18) Examples include the following:

Neurotensin. A brain peptide which is vasodilatory, alters pituitary hormone release, and lowers body temperature.

Cholecystokinin. An intestinal hormone which is found in the brain and may be involved in the regulation of behavior, satiety, and fluid intake.

Vasoactive Intestinal Peptide (VIP). High levels of this peptide are found in the cerebral cortex, and it is also found in the hypothalamus. VIP causes vasodilation, stimulates conversion of glycogen to glucose, enhances lipolysis and insulin secretion, stimulates pancreatic and intestinal secretion, and inhibits the production of gastric acid.

Thyroid Releasing Hormone (TRH). TRH is found in many areas of the brain. It elicits behavioral excitation and anorexia in animals, and may cause mood enhancement in humans.

Somatostatin. This hypothalamic peptide inhibits the release of growth hormone, prolactin, and TSH from the pituitary. It is also a typical gut-brain peptide, being found in neurons throughout the brain, stomach, intestine, and pancreas. It inhibits secretion of glucagon, insulin, and gastrin. It is also located in sensory neurons and may be a transmitter of pain sensation.

The Endogenous Opiates. The most fascinating peptide group is the endogenous opioid peptide family.(19) β-Lipotropin is a 91 amino acid molecule which was first isolated from the pituitary in 1964. Its function remained a mystery for over 10 years until receptors for opioid compounds were identified, and by virtue of their existence, it was postulated that endogenous opioid compounds must exist and serve important physiological roles. Endorphin was a word coined to denote morphine-like action and endogenous origin in the brain.

The Endogenous Opioid Peptides

Opiate production is regulated by gene transcription and the synthesis of precursor peptides, and at a post-translational level where the precursors are processed into the various bioactive smaller peptides. (20) All opiates derive from one of 3 precursor peptides:

Proopiomelanocortin (POMC)–the source of endorphins.

Proenkephalin A–the source of several enkephalins.

Proenkephalin B (Prodynorphin)–yields dynorphins.

POMC was the first precursor peptide to be identified. It is made in the anterior and intermediate lobes of the pituitary, in the hypothalamus and other areas of the brain, in the sympathetic nervous system, and in other tissues including the gonads, the placenta, the gastrointestinal tract, and the lungs. The highest concentration is in the pituitary gland.

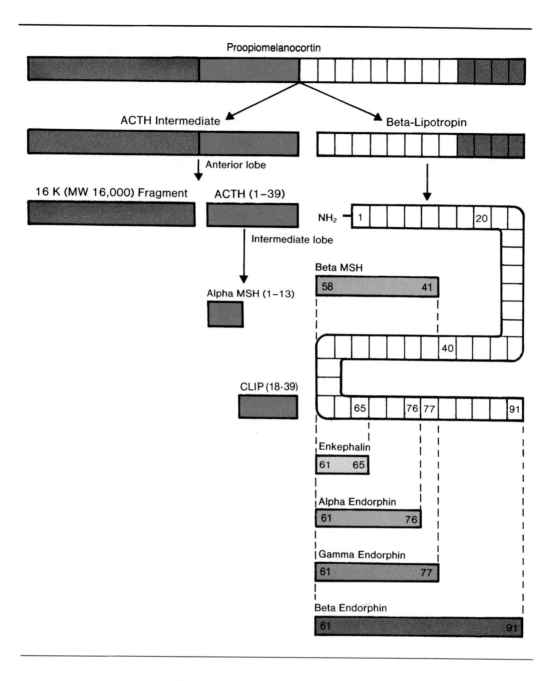

Proopiomelanocortin is split into 2 fragments, an ACTH intermediate fragment and β-lipotropin. β-Lipotropin has no opioid activity, but is broken down in a series of steps to β-melanocyte stimulating hormone (β-MSH), enkephalin, and α-, γ-, and β-endorphins.

Enkephalin and the α- and γ-endorphins are as active as morphine on a molar basis, while β-endorphin is 5-10 times more potent. In the adult pituitary gland, the major products are ACTH and β-lipotropin, with only small amounts of endorphin. Thus ACTH and β-lipotropin blood levels show similar courses, and they are major secretion products of the anterior pituitary in response to stress. In the intermediate lobe of the pituitary (which is prominent only during fetal life), ACTH is cleaved to CLIP (corticotropin-like intermediate lobe peptide) and β-MSH. In the placenta and adrenal medulla, POMC processing yields α-MSH-like and β-endorphin peptides. β-endorphin has also been detected in the ovaries and in the testes.

In the brain, the major products are the opiates, with little ACTH. In the hypothalamus the major product is β-endorphin in the region of the arcuate nucleus and the ventromedial nucleus. Therefore, the pituitary system is a system for secretion into the circulation while the hypothalamic system allows for distribution via axons to regulate other brain regions and the pituitary gland. β-endorphin is actively secreted into the hypophyseal portal circulation.

β-Endorphin is appropriately considered a neurotransmitter, a neurohormone, and a neuromodulator. β-Endorphin influences a variety of hypothalamic functions, including regulation of reproduction, temperature, cardiovascular and respiratory function, as well as extrahypothalamic functions such as pain perception and mood. POMC gene expression in the anterior pituitary is controlled mainly by adrenal hormones, stimulated by CRH (corticotropin releasing hormone) and influenced by the feedback effects of glucocorticoids. In the hypothalamus, regulation of POMC gene expression is via the sex steroids. In the absence of sex steroids, little, if any, secretion occurs.

Proenkephalin A is produced in the adrenal medulla, the brain, the posterior pituitary, the spinal cord, and the gastrointestinal tract. It yields several enkephalins: methionine-enkephalin, leucine-enkephalin, and other variants. The enkephalins are the most widely distributed endogenous opioid peptides in the brain, and are probably mainly involved as inhibitory neurotransmitters in the modulation of the autonomic nervous system. Proenkephalin B, found in the brain (concentrated in the hypothalamus) and the gastrointestinal tract, yields dynorphin, an opioid peptide with high analgesic potency and behavioral effects, as well as α-neoendorphin, β-neoendorphin, and leumorphin. The last 13 amino acids of leumorphin constitute another opioid peptide, rimorphin. The proenkephalin B products probably function in a similar fashion as endorphin.

It is easier to simply say that there are 3 classes of opiates: enkephalins, endorphin, and dynorphin.

Opioid peptides are able to act through different receptors, although specific opiates bind predominantly to one of the various receptor types. Naloxone, used in most human studies, does not bind exclusively to any one receptor type, and thus results with this antagonist are not totally specific. Localization of opioid receptors explains many of the pharmacological actions of the opiates. Opioid receptors are found in the nerve endings of sensory neurons, in the limbic system (site of euphoric emotions), in brainstem centers for reflexes such as respiration, and widely distributed in the brain and the spinal cord.

Opioid Receptors:

Name	Principal Opiate	Naloxone Antagonism
mu	endorphin	sensitive
kappa	endorphin dynorphin	sensitive
delta	enkephalin	resistant
epsilon	endorphin	sensitive
sigma	?	very resistant

Summary of Body Functions Affected by Opioid Peptides:

-Pain
-Respiratory Function
-Feeding and Drinking Behavior
-Sexual Behavior and Function
-Learning
-Memory
-Temperature
-Blood Pressure
-Hormone Regulation

Opioid Peptides and the Menstrual Cycle. The opioid tone is an important part of menstrual function and cyclicity. (21) While estradiol alone increases endorphin secretion, the highest levels of endorphin occur with sequential replacement therapy of both estradiol and progesterone (in ovariectomized monkeys). Endogenous endorphin levels, therefore, increase throughout the cycle, from nadir levels during menses, to highest levels during the luteal phase. Normal cyclicity thus requires sequential periods of high (luteal phase) and low (during menses) hypothalamic opioid activity.

A reduction in LH pulse frequency is linked to increased endorphin release. Naloxone increases both the frequency and the amplitude of LH pulses. *Thus, the endogenous opiates inhibit gonadotropin secretion by suppressing the hypothalamic release of GnRH.* Opiates have no effect on the pituitary response to GnRH. The gonadal steroids modify endogenous opioid activity, and the negative feedback of steroids on gonadotropins appears to be mediated by endogenous opiates. Because the fluctuating levels of endogenous opiates in the menstrual cycle are related to the changing levels of estradiol and progesterone, it is attractive to speculate that the sex steroids directly stimulate endogenous opioid receptor activity. There is an absence of opioid effect on postmenopausal and oophorectomized levels of gonadotropins, and the response to opiates is restored with the administration of estrogen, progesterone, or both.(22) Both estrogen and progesterone alone increase endogenous opiates, but estrogen enhances the action of progesterone, explaining the maximal suppression of GnRH and gonadotropin pulse frequency during the luteal phase due to peak stimulation of hypothalamic endogenous opioid activity.(23,24) Experiments with naloxone administra-

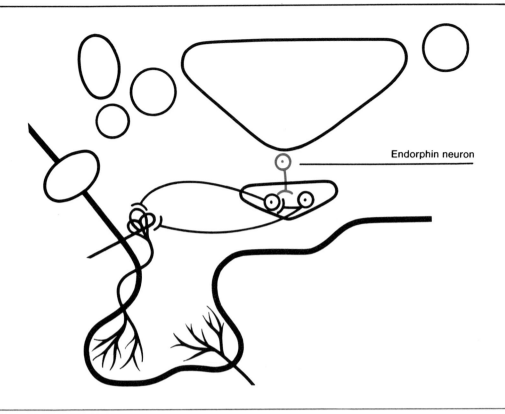

Endorphin neuron

tion suggest that the suppression of gonadotropins during pregnancy and the recovery during the postpartum period reflect steroid-induced opioid inhibition, followed by a release from central opioid suppression.

The principal endogenous opiates affecting GnRH release are β-endorphin and dynorphin, and it is probable that the major effect is modulation of the catecholamine pathway, but principally norepinephrine. The action does not involve dopamine receptors, acetylcholine receptors, or alpha-adrenergic receptors. On the other hand, endorphin may affect GnRH release directly, without the involvement of any intermediary neuroamine.

A change in opioid inhibitory tone is not thought to be important in the changes of puberty because the responsiveness to naloxone does not develop until after puberty. A change in opioid tone does seem to mediate the hypogonadotropic state seen with elevated prolactin levels, exercise, and other conditions of hypothalamic amenorrhea, while endogenous opioid inhibition does not seem to play a causal role in delayed puberty or hereditary problems such as Kallman's Syndrome.(25,26) Experimental evidence indicates that corticotropin-releasing hormone (CRH) directly inhibits hypothalamic GnRH secretion, perhaps by augmenting endogenous opioid secretion. Women with hypothalamic amenorrhea demonstrate hypercortisolism, suggesting that this could be the pathway by which stress interrupts reproductive function.(27) Cumming concludes that most studies indicate an exercise-induced increase in endogenous opiates, but a significant impact on mood remains to be substantiated.(28) He notes that *runners' high* is more common in California than in Canada (euphoria is hard to come by running at below freezing temperatures).

Administration of morphine, enkephalin analogs, and β-endorphin causes release of prolactin. The effect is mediated by inhibition of dopamine secretion in the tuberinfundibular neurons in the median eminence. Most studies have reported no effect of naloxone on basal, stress-induced, or pregnant levels of prolactin, nor on secretion by prolactinomas. Thus a physiological role for endogenous opioid regulation of prolactin does not appear to exist in men and women. However, suppression of GnRH secretion associated with hyperprolactinemia does appear to be mediated by endogenous opiates.(29)

Opiates stimulate TSH and growth hormone release, but naloxone has no major effects, and a physiological role is unlikely. Opiates can be localized in the hypothalamus together with oxytocin and vasopressin.

Every pituitary hormone appears to be modulated by opiates. Physiological effects are important with ACTH, gonadotropins, and possibly vasopressin. Opioid compounds have no direct action on the pituitary, nor do they alter the action of releasing hormones on the pituitary.

POMC-like mRNA is present in the ovary and the placenta. (30) Expression is regulated by gonadotropins in the ovary, but not in the placenta. Reasons for endorphin presence in these tissues are not yet apparent. High concentrations of all of the members of the POMC family are found in human ovarian follicular fluid, but only β-endorphin shows significant changes during the menstrual cycle, reaching highest levels just before ovulation.(31)

Catecholestrogens

Catecholestrogens have two faces, a catechol side and an estrogen side. The enzyme which converts estrogens to catecholestrogens is richly concentrated in the hypothalamus, hence there are higher concentrations of catecholestrogens than estrone and estradiol in the hypothalamus and pituitary gland.

Because catecholestrogens have two faces, they have the potential for interacting with both catecholamine and estrogen-mediated systems.(32) To be specific, catecholestrogens can inhibit tyrosine hydroxylase (which would decrease catecholamines) and compete for catechol-o-methyltransferase (which would increase catecholamines). Since GnRH, estrogens, and catecholestrogens are located in similar sites, it is possible that catecholestrogens may serve to interact between catecholamines and GnRH secretion.

67

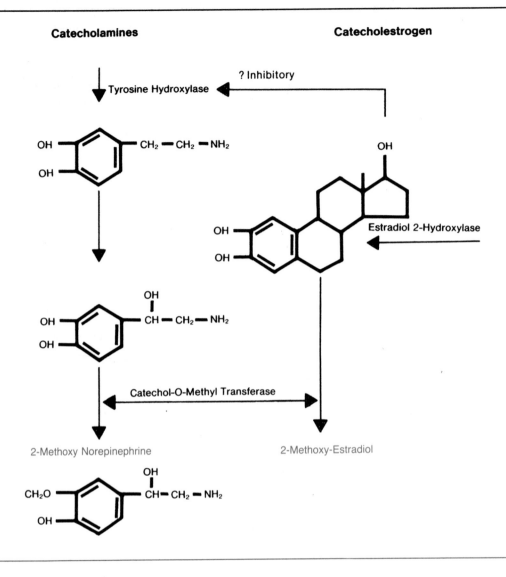

Catecholamines

Catecholestrogen

? Inhibitory

Tyrosine Hydroxylase

OH — CH$_2$ — CH$_2$ — NH$_2$

OH

OH

OH

Estradiol 2-Hydroxylase

OH

OH

OH

OH — CH — CH$_2$ — NH$_2$

Catechol-O-Methyl Transferase

2-Methoxy Norepinephrine

2-Methoxy-Estradiol

OH

CH$_2$O — CH — CH$_2$ — NH$_2$

OH

Summary: Control of GnRH Pulses

The key concept is that normal menstrual function requires GnRH pulsatile secretion in a critical range of frequency and amplitude.(8,9,33) The normal physiology and pathophysiology of the menstrual cycle, at least in terms of central control, can be explained by mechanisms which affect the pulsatile secretion of GnRH. The pulses of GnRH appear to be directly under the influence of a dual catecholaminergic system: norepinephrine facilatory and dopamine inhibitory. In turn, the catecholamine system can be influenced by endogenous opioid activity. The feedback effects of steroids may be mediated through this system via catecholsteroid messengers.

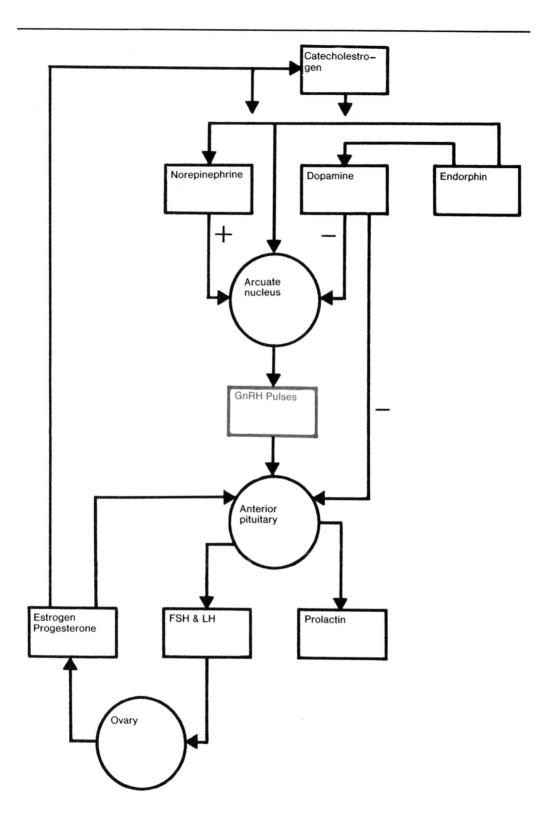

Tanycytes

A significant pathway for hypothalamic influence may be via the cerebrospinal fluid (CSF). Tanycytes are specialized ependymal cells whose ciliated cell bodies line the third ventricle over the median eminence. The cells terminate on portal vessels, and they can transport materials from ventricular CSF to the portal system, e.g. substances from the pineal gland, or vasopressin, or oxytocin. Tanycytes change morphologically in response to steroids, and exhibit morphological changes during the ovarian cycle.

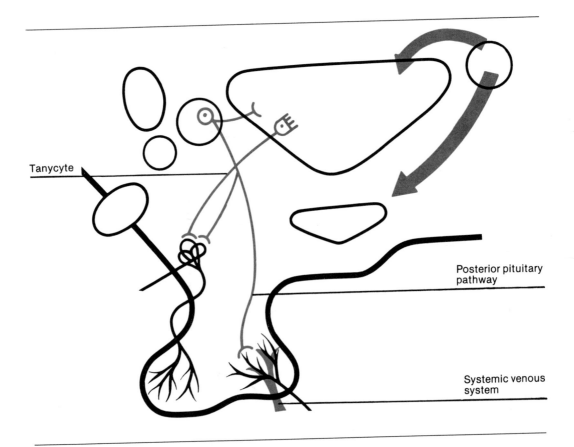

Tanycyte

Posterior pituitary pathway

Systemic venous system

The Posterior Pituitary Pathway

The posterior pituitary is a direct prolongation of the hypothalamus via the pituitary stalk, whereas the anterior pituitary arises from pharyngeal epithelium which migrates into position with the posterior pituitary. Separate neurosecretory cells in both the supraoptic and paraventricular nuclei make vasopressin, oxytocin, and their transport peptide, neurophysin.(34) Both oxytocin and vasopressin consist of 9 amino acid residues. In the human, vasopressin contains arginine, unlike animals which have lysine vasopressin. The neurophysins are polypeptides with a molecular weight of about 10,000. There are two distinct neurophysins, estrogen-stimulated neurophysin known as neurophysin I, and nicotine-stimulated neurophysin, known as neurophysin II.

The neurons secrete two large protein molecules, a precursor called pro-pressophysin which contains vasopressin and its neurophysin, and a precursor called pro-oxyphysin, which contains oxytocin and its neurophysin.(35) It is thought that neurophysin I is specifically

70

related to oxytocin, and neurophysin II accompanies vasopressin. Because of this unique packaging, the hormones and their neurophysins are stored together and released at the same time into the circulation. The only known function for the neurophysins is axonal transport for oxytocin and vasopressin.

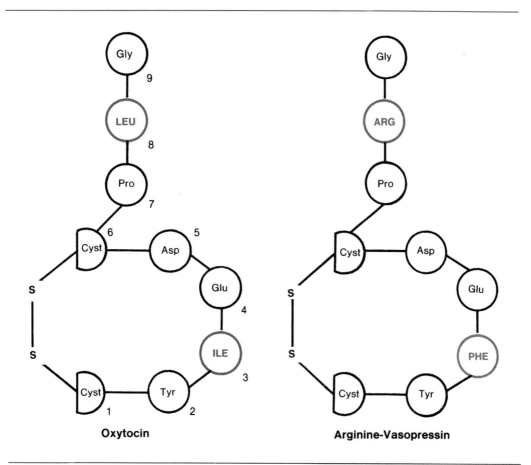

Oxytocin   Arginine-Vasopressin

The posterior pathway is complex and not limited to the transmission of vasopressin and oxytocin to the posterior pituitary. The transportation of vasopressin and oxytocin to the posterior pituitary occurs via nerve tracts which emanate from the supraoptic and paraventricular nuclei and descend through the median eminence to terminate in the posterior pituitary. However, these hormones are also secreted into the cerebrospinal fluid and directly into the portal system. Therefore, vasopressin and oxytocin can reach the anterior pituitary and influence, in the case of vasopressin, ACTH secretion, and in the case of oxytocin, gonadotropin secretion. Vasopressin acts synergistically with corticotropin releasing hormone to cause an increased yield of ACTH. Vasopressin and oxytocin-like materials are also found in the ovary, the oviduct, the testis, and the adrenal gland, suggesting that these neurohypophyseal peptides have roles as paracrine or autocrine hormones.(36) The concentrations of these substances in the cerebrospinal fluid exhibit a circadian rhythm (with peak levels occurring during the day), suggesting a different mechanism for CSF secretion compared to posterior pituitary release.(37)

Neurophysin II is called nicotine neurophysin because the administration of nicotine or hemorrhage increases the circulating levels. Neurophysin I is called estrogen neurophysin because estrogen administration increases the levels in the peripheral blood, and peak levels of both neurophysin I and oxytocin are found at the time of the LH surge.(38) The rise in estrogen neurophysin begins 10 hours after the rise in estrogen, precedes that of the LH surge, and the elevation of neurophysin lasts longer than the LH surge. Because GnRH and oxytocin are competing substrates for hypothalamic degradation enzymes, it has been hypothesized that oxytocin in the portal blood at the midcycle may inhibit the metabolism of GnRH, thus increasing the amount of GnRH available. Furthermore, oxytocin may have direct actions on the pituitary, ovary, uterus, and fallopian tube during ovulation.

Neurophysin-containing pathways have been traced from the hypothalamic nuclei to various centers in the brainstem and the spinal cord. In addition, behavioral studies suggest a role for vasopressin in learning and memory. Administration of vasopressin has been associated with improvement in memory in brain-damaged human subjects, and enhanced cognitive responses (learning and memory) in both young, normal individuals and depressed patients.

Both oxytocin and vasopressin circulate as the free peptides. The half-life of vasopressin is 3-6 minutes and that of oxytocin 5-17 minutes (a mean of 10 minutes). Three major stimuli for vasopressin secretion are changes in osmolality of the blood, alterations in blood volume, and psychogenic stimuli such as pain and fear. The osmoreceptors are located in the hypothalamus; the volume receptors are in the left atrium, aortic arch, and carotid sinus. Angiotensin II also produces a release of vasopressin, suggesting another mechanism for the link between fluid balance and vasopressin. Cortisol may modify the osmotic threshold for the release of vasopressin.

The major functions of vasopressin involve the regulation of osmolality and blood volume. Vasopressin is a powerful vasoconstrictor and antidiuretic hormone. Vasopressin release increases when plasma osmolality rises and is inhibited by water loading (resulting in diuresis). Diabetes insipidus is a condition due to the loss of water because of a lack of vasopressin action in the tubules of the kidney, all secondary to a defect in synthesis or secretion of vasopressin. The opposite condition is the continuous and autonomous secretion of vasopressin, the syndrome of inappropriate ADH (antidiuretic hormone) secretion. This syndrome, with its resultant retention of water, is associated with a variety of brain disorders as well as the production of vasopressin and its precursor by malignant tumors.

Oxytocin stimulates muscular contractions in the uterus and myoepithelial contractions in the breast. Thus it is involved in parturition and the letdown of milk. The release of oxytocin is so episodic that it is described as spurts. Ordinarily, there are about 3 spurts every 10 minutes. Oxytocin is released during coitus, probably by the Ferguson reflex (vaginal and cervical stimulation), but also by olfactory, visual, and auditory pathways. Perhaps oxytocin has some role in muscle contractions during orgasm.(39) In the male, release of oxytocin during coitus may contribute to sperm transport during ejaculation.

During pregnancy, maternal plasma oxytocin increases with gestational age, as do amniotic fluid levels. Fetal urine and meconium contain large amounts of oxytocin. During labor, maternal levels increase from the first stage to the second stage, but decline during the third stage. The major mechanism is thought to be the Ferguson reflex.

Umbilical artery levels of oxytocin are always higher than umbilical vein levels, except when oxytocin is administered. Since oxytocin readily crosses the placenta, it is likely that during normal labor, fetal oxytocin crosses into the maternal compartment, and during oxytocin administration there is a reverse movement into the fetal compartment. It appears that fetal oxytocin plays a major role during the first stage of labor, while maternal oxytocin is significant during the second stage.(40)

Oxytocin is released in response to suckling, mediated through impulses generated at the nipple and transmitted via the 3rd, 4th, and 5th thoracic nerves to the spinal cord up to the hypothalamus. In addition to causing milk ejection, the reflex is responsible for the uterine contractions associated with breast feeding. Opioid peptides inhibit oxytocin release and this may be the means by which stress, fear, and anger inhibit milk output in lactating women.

The Brain and Ovulation

The Classic Concept. Classic studies in a variety of rodents indicated the presence of feedback centers in the hypothalamus that responded to steroids with the release of GnRH. The release of GnRH was the result of the complex, but coordinated, relationships among the neurohormones, the pituitary gonadotropins, and the gonadal steroids designated by the time-honored terms positive and negative feedback.

FSH levels were thought to be largely regulated by a negative inhibitory feedback relationship with estradiol. In the case of LH, there existed both a negative inhibitory feedback relationship with estradiol, and a positive stimulatory feedback with high levels of estradiol. The feedback centers were located in the hypothalamus, and they were called the tonic and cyclic centers. The tonic center controlled the day to day basal level of gonadotropins, and was responsive to the negative feedback effects of steroids. The cyclic center in the female brain was responsible for the midcycle surge of gonadotropins, a response mediated by the positive feedback of estrogen. Specifically, the midcycle surge of gonadotropins was thought to be due to an outpouring of GnRH in response to the positive feedback action of estradiol on the cyclic center of the hypothalamus.

This classic concept was not inaccurate. The problem was that the concept accurately described events in the rodent, but the mechanism is different in the primate.

73

The Present Concept. In the primate, the "center" for the mid-cycle surge of gonadotropins has moved from the hypothalamus to the pituitary. Experiments in the monkey have clearly demonstrated that GnRH, originating in the hypothalamus, plays a permissive role. Its pulsatile secretion is an important prerequisite for normal pituitary function (33), but the feedback responses regulating gonadotropin levels are controlled by ovarian steroid feedback on the anterior pituitary cells.

The present concept is derived from experiments in which the medial basal hypothalamus (MBH) is either destroyed (7) or the hypothalamus is surgically separated from the pituitary.(41) In a typical (and now classic) experiment, lesion of the MBH by radiofrequency waves was followed by loss of LH levels as the source of GnRH was eliminated.(6) Administration of GnRH by an intravenous pump restored LH secretion. The administration of estradiol was then able to produce both negative and positive feedback responses, clearly actions that must be directly on the anterior pituitary because the hypothalamus was absent and GnRH was being administered in a steady and unchanging frequency and dose.

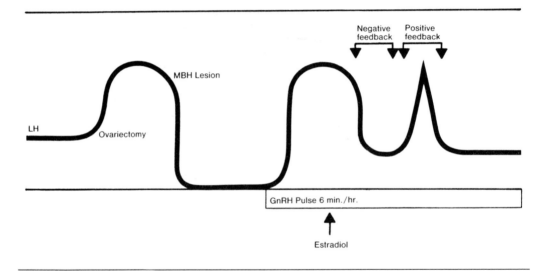

Administration of GnRH intravenously, as a bolus, produces an increase in blood levels of LH and FSH within 5 minutes, reaching a peak in about 20-25 minutes for LH and 45 minutes for FSH. Levels return to pretreatment values after several hours. When administered by constant infusion at submaximal doses, there is first a rapid rise with a peak at 30 minutes, followed by a plateau or fall between 45 and 90 minutes, then a second and sustained increase at 225-240 minutes. This biphasic response suggests the presence of two functional pools of pituitary gonadotropins.(42) The readily releasable pool (secretion) produces the initial response, and the later response is dependent upon a second, reserve pool of stored gonadotropins.

Synthesis of gonadotropins takes place on the rough endoplasmic reticulum. The hormones are packaged into secretory granules by the Golgi cisternae of the Golgi apparatus, and then stored as secretory granules. Secretion requires migration (activation) of the

74

mature secretory granules to the cell membrane where an alteration in membrane permeability results in extrusion of the secretory granules in a process which involves calcium and cyclic AMP changes in response to GnRH.

There are three principal positive actions of GnRH on gonadotropin elaboration:

1. Synthesis and storage (the reserve pool) of gonadotropins.

2. Activation, movement of gonadotropins from the reserve pool to a pool ready for direct secretion.

3. Immediate release (direct secretion) of gonadotropins.

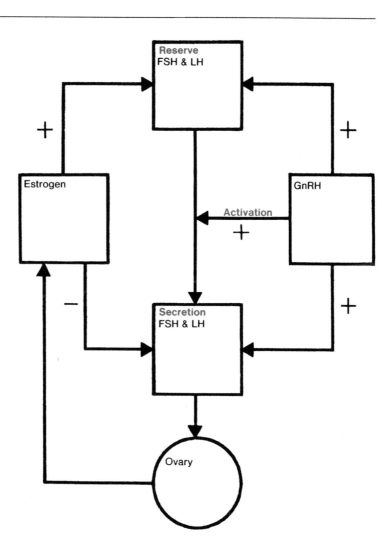

Secretion, synthesis, and storage change during the cycle. At the beginning of the cycle, when estrogen levels are low, both secretion and storage levels are low. With increasing levels of estradiol, a greater increase occurs in storage, with little change in secretion. Thus, in the early follicular phase, estrogen has a positive effect on the synthesis and storage response, building up a supply of gonadotropins in order to meet the requirements of the midcycle surge. Premature release of gonadotropins is prevented by a negative (inhibitory) action of estradiol on the pituitary secretory response to GnRH.

As the midcycle approaches, subsequent responses to GnRH are greater than initial responses, indicating that each response not only induces release of gonadotropins, but also activates the storage pool for the next response. This self-priming action of GnRH requires the presence of estrogen.(43)

Because the midcycle surge of LH can be produced in the experimental monkey in the absence of a hypothalamus, and in the face of unchanging GnRH, the ovulatory surge of LH is now thought to be a response to positive feedback action of estradiol on the anterior pituitary. When the estradiol level in the circulation reaches a critical concentration and this concentration is maintained for a critical time period, the inhibitory action on LH secretion changes to a stimulatory action. The mechanism of this steroid action is not known with certainty, but experimental evidence suggests that the positive feedback action involves an increase in GnRH receptor concentration, while the negative feedback of estrogen operates through a different mechanism.(44,45)

What a logical mechanism! The midcycle surge must occur at the right time of the cycle to ovulate a ready and waiting mature follicle. What better way to achieve this extreme degree of coordination and timing than by the follicle itself, through the feedback effects of the sex steroids originating in the follicle destined to ovulate.

GnRH has been found to be increased in the peripheral blood of women and the portal blood of monkeys at midcycle. While this increase may not be absolutely necessary (as demonstrated in the monkey experiments), recent studies indicate that activity is occurring in both the hypothalamus and the pituitary. Estrogen exerts its inhibitory effects in both the hypothalamus and the anterior pituitary, decreasing both GnRH pulsatile secretion and GnRH pituitary response.(46) Therefore, while the system can operate with only an unwavering, permissive action of GnRH, fine tuning probably takes place by means of simultaneous effects on GnRH pulsatile secretion and pituitary response to GnRH.

Influencing the hypothalamic frequency of GnRH secretion can in turn influence pituitary response to GnRH. Faster or slower frequencies of GnRH pulses result in lower GnRH receptor numbers in the pituitary.(47) Thus a critical peak frequency is necessary for peak numbers of GnRH receptors and the peak midcycle response. Here is a method for the fine tuning at both the hypothalamus and the pituitary.

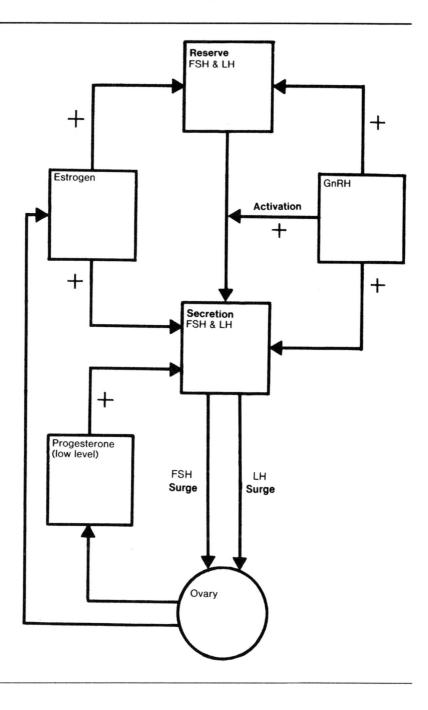

Another aspect of gonadotropin secretion is growing in significance. A disparity exists between the quantity of LH measured during the midcycle surge as determined by radioimmunoassay and bioassay. More LH is secreted at midcycle in a molecular form with greater biological activity.(48) There is a well-established relationship between the activity and half-life of glycoprotein hormones and their content of sialic acid (see Chapter 1, under ''Heterogeneity'' of tropic hormones). Estrogen enhancement of sialic acid content is an additional method for maximizing the biologic effects of the midcycle surge.

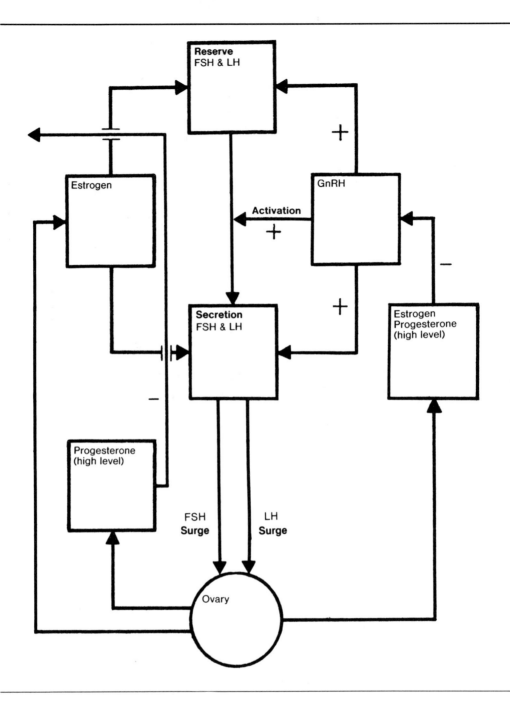

The purpose and mechanism for the midcycle surge of FSH have only recently been appreciated. A normal corpus luteum requires the induction of an adequate number of LH receptors on granulosa cells, a specific action of FSH. In addition, FSH accomplishes important intrafollicular changes necessary for the physical expulsion of the ovum. The midcycle surge of FSH, therefore, plays a critical role in ensuring ovulation and a normal corpus luteum. Emerging progesterone secretion, just prior to ovulation, is the key.

Progesterone, at low levels and in the presence of estrogen, augments the pituitary secretion of LH and is significantly responsible for the FSH surge in response to GnRH.(49-51) As the rising levels of LH produce the morphologic change of luteinization in the ovulating follicle, the granulosa layer begins to secrete progesterone directly into the bloodstream. The process of luteinization is inhibited by the presence of the oocyte, and therefore, progesterone secretion is relatively suppressed ensuring that only low levels of progesterone reach the brain.

After ovulation, rapid and full luteinization is accompanied by a marked increase in progesterone levels, which, in the presence of estrogen, exercise a profound negative feedback action to suppress gonadotropin secretion. This action of progesterone takes place in two locations.(52-54) First, there definitely is a central action to decrease GnRH. Progesterone fails to block estradiol-induced gonadotropin discharges in monkeys with hypothalamic lesions if pulsatile GnRH replacement is provided. Therefore, high levels of progesterone inhibit ovulation at the hypothalamic level. In addition, progesterone can also block estrogen-induced responses to GnRH at the pituitary level. In contrast, the facilitory action of low levels of progesterone is exerted only at the pituitary on the response to GnRH.

Summary:
Key Points

1. Pulsatile GnRH secretion must be within a critical range for frequency and concentration (amplitude).

2. GnRH has only positive actions on the anterior pituitary: synthesis and storage, activation, and secretion of gonadotropins. The gonadotropins are secreted in a pulsatile fashion in response to the similar pulsatile release of GnRH.

3. Low levels of estrogen enhance FSH and LH synthesis and storage, have little effect on LH secretion, and inhibit FSH secretion.

4. High levels of estrogen induce the LH surge at midcycle, and high steady levels of estrogen lead to sustained elevated LH secretion.

5. Low levels of progesterone acting at the level of the pituitary gland enhance the LH response to GnRH and are significantly responsible for the FSH surge at midcycle.

6. High levels of progesterone inhibit pituitary secretion of gonadotropins by inhibiting GnRH pulses at the level of the hypothalamus. In addition, high levels of progesterone antagonize pituitary response to GnRH by interfering with estrogen action.

The Pineal Gland

Although no physiologic role has been established in the human, the reproductive functions of the hypothalamus may also be under inhibitory control of the brain via the pineal gland. The pineal arises as an outgrowth of the roof of the third ventricle, but soon after birth it loses all afferent and efferent neural connections with the brain. Instead the parenchymal cells receive a new and unusual sympathetic innervation which allows the pineal gland to be an active neuroendocrine organ that responds to photic and hormonal stimuli and exhibits circadian rhythms.(55,56)

The neural pathway begins in the retina and passes through the inferior accessory optic tracts and the medial forebrain bundle to the upper cord. Preganglionic fibers terminate at the superior cervical ganglion, and postganglionic sympathetic nerves terminate directly on pineal cells. Interruption of this pathway gives the same effect as darkness, which is an increase in pineal biosynthetic activity.

Hydroxyindole-*o*-methyltransferase (HIOMT) is found mainly in pineal parenchymal cells, and its products, therefore, are essentially unique to the pineal. Norepinephrine stimulates tryptophan entry into the pineal cell and also adenylate cyclase activity in the membrane. The resulting increase in cyclic AMP leads to *N*-acetyltransferase activity, the rate-limiting step in melatonin synthesis. Thus, melatonin synthesis is controlled by norepinephrine stimulation of adenylate cyclase, and the norepinephrine is liberated by sympathetic stimulation due to the absence of light. HIOMT is also found in the retina where melatonin may serve to regulate the pigment in retinal cells, and in the intestine. However, pinealectomy completely eliminates detectable levels of melatonin in the circulation.

The association of hyperplastic pineal tumors with decreased gonadal function, and destructive tumors with precocious puberty, suggested that the pineal is the source of gonadal inhibiting substances. However, pineal mechanisms cannot be absolutely essential for gonadal function. Normal reproductive function returns to the pinealectomized rat several weeks after pinealectomy, and blind women have normal fertility.

A rat in constant light develops a small pineal with decreased HIOMT and melatonin, while the ovarian weight increases. A rat in constant dark has the opposite result, increased pineal size, HIOMT, and melatonin, with decreased ovarian weight and pituitary function. A rhythm is established in pineal HIOMT activity by the presence or absence of light. Short days and long nights result in gonadal atrophy, and this may be a mechanism governing seasonal breeding. Possible roles in humans may be to give circadian rhythmicity to other functions such as temperature and sleep. In all vertebrates tested so far, there is a daily rhythm in melatonin secretion: high values during the dark and low during light.

The pineal, therefore, serves as an interface between the environment and hypothalamic-pituitary function. In order to correctly interpret day length, animals require a daily rhythm in melatonin secretion. This coordination of temporal, environmental information is especially important in seasonal breeders. This pineal rhythm appears to require the suprachiasmatic nucleus, perhaps the site at which pineal function and light changes are coordinated.

The gonadal changes associated with melatonin are mediated via the hypothalamus and suggest a general suppressive effect on GnRH pulsatile secretion and reproductive function. In women, melatonin blood levels are highest in the prepubertal period, and they decrease with age. During the menstrual cycle, they are lowest at the time of the midcycle ovulatory surge.

Melatonin is synthesized and secreted by the pineal gland and circulates in the blood like a classical hormone. It affects distant target organs, especially the neuroendocrine centers of the central nervous system. Whether melatonin is secreted primarily into the CSF or blood is still debated, but most evidence favors blood. From the CSF, melatonin may reach the hypothalamus by way of tanycyte transport.

Pineal activity can be viewed as the net balance between hormonal and neuronal mediated influences. The pineal contains receptors for the active sex hormones, estradiol, testosterone, dihydrotestosterone, progesterone, and prolactin. Furthermore, the pineal converts testosterone and progesterone to the active 5α-reduced metabolites, and androgens are aromatized to estrogens. The pineal also appears to be unique in that a catecholamine neurotransmitter (norepinephrine), interacting with cell membrane receptors, stimulates cellular synthesis of estrogen and androgen receptors. In general, however, the sympathetic activity producing the circadian rhythm takes precedence over hormonal effects.

Despite a variety of suggestive leads, there is little evidence for a role of the pineal in humans. Nevertheless the important relationship between light exposure and circadian rhythms continues to focus attention on the pineal gland as a coordinator. A possible influence of the pineal gland may be the synchronization of menstrual cycles noted among women who spend time together. A significant increase in synchronization of cycles among roommates and among closest friends occurred in the first 4 months of residency in a dormitory of a women's college.(57)

A number of other indoles (also derivatives of tryptophan) have been identified in the pineal gland. Biologic roles for these indoles remain elusive, but one in particular has been extensively investigated. Arginine vasotocin differs from oxytocin by a single amino acid in position 8 and from vasopressin by a single amino acid in position 3. In general, arginine vasotocin has an inhibitory action on the gonads and pituitary secretion of prolactin and LH. Nevertheless a precise role continues to be evasive.

Gonadotropin Secretion through Fetal Life, Childhood, and Puberty

We have often considered the endocrine events during puberty as an awakening, a beginning. However, endocrinologically, puberty is not a beginning, but just another stage in a development which began at conception. Gonadotropin production has been documented throughout fetal life, during childhood, and into adult life (Chapter 12).(58) Remarkable levels of FSH and LH, similar to postmenopausal levels, can be measured in the fetus. GnRH is detectable in the hypothalamus by 10 weeks of gestation, and by 10-13 weeks, FSH and LH are being produced in the pituitary. The peak concentrations of FSH and LH occur at about 20 weeks of intrauterine life.

The increasing production rate of gonadotropins until midgestation reflects the growing ability of the hypothalamic-pituitary axis to perform at full capacity. Beginning at midgestation, there is an increasing sensitivity to inhibition by steroids and a resultant decrease in gonadotropin secretion. Full sensitivity to steroids is not reached until late in infancy. The rise in gonadotropins after birth reflects loss of the high levels of placental steroids. Thus, in the first year of life there is considerable follicular activity in the ovaries in contrast to later in childhood when gonadotropin secretion is suppressed.

Testicular function in the fetus can be correlated with the fetal hormonal patterns. Initial testosterone production and sexual differentiation are in response to the high fetal levels of HCG, whereas further testosterone production and masculine differentiation appear to be maintained by the fetal pituitary gonadotropins. Decreased testosterone levels in late gestation probably reflect the decrease in gonadotropin levels. In the female, the peak of oogenesis and the onset of atresia coincide with peak production and decline of pituitary gonadotropins by the fetus.

There is a sex difference in fetal gonadotropin levels. There are higher FSH and LH levels in female fetuses. The lower male levels are probably due to the higher testosterone production. In infancy, the postnatal FSH rise is more marked and more sustained in females, while LH values are not as high. After the postnatal rise, gonadotropin levels reach a nadir during early childhood (by about 6 months of age in males and 1-2 years in females) and then rise slightly between 4 and 10 years. This childhood period is characterized by low levels of gonadotropins in the pituitary and in the blood, little response of the pituitary to GnRH, and maximal hypothalamic suppression.

The precise signal which initiates the events of puberty is unknown.(59) In girls, the first steroids to rise in the blood are dehydroepiandrosterone (DHA) and its sulfate (DHAS) beginning at 6-8 years of age, at the same time that FSH begins to increase. Estrogen levels, as well as LH, do not begin to rise until 10-12 years of age. If the onset of puberty is triggered by the first hormone to increase in the circulation, then a role for adrenal steroids must be considered. However, there is no evidence to suggest that the adrenal steroids are necessary for the proper timing of puberty, and adrenarche appears to be independent, not controlled by the same mechanism which turns on the gonads.(60) Neither is there a definite relationship demonstrated between melatonin secretion and puberty. Because the studies have focused on the amount of melatonin secreted rather than the rhythm of secretion, this question remains open.

Puberty is associated with the development of episodic LH secretion associated with sleep. At the time of appearance of secondary sex characteristics, the mean LH levels are 2-4 times higher during sleep than during wakefulness. This pattern is not present before or after puberty, and is an early sign of changes taking place in the hypothalamus. This pattern can be detected in individuals who develop increasing and decreasing degrees of hypothalamic suppression (such as in individuals with worsening and improving anorexia nervosa). FSH levels plateau by midpuberty while LH and estradiol levels continue to rise until late puberty. Biologically active LH has been found to rise proportionately more than immunoactive LH with the onset of puberty.

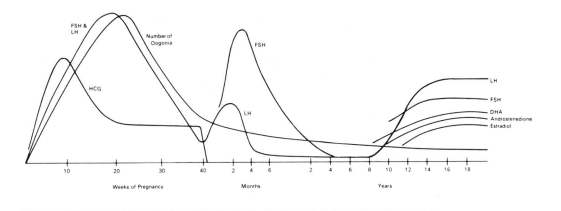

10	20	30	40			

Weeks of Pregnancy   Months   Years

The rise of gonadotropins at puberty is somewhat independent of the gonads in that the same response can be observed in patients with gonadal dysgenesis (who lack functional steroid-producing gonadal tissue). Adolescent girls with Turner's syndrome (45,X) also demonstrate augmented gonadotropin secretion during sleep.(61) Thus, maturation at puberty must involve changes in the hypothalamus which are independent of ovarian steroids.

The maturational change in the hypothalamus is followed by an orderly and predictable sequence of events. Increased GnRH secretion leads to increased pituitary responsiveness to GnRH (a combination of steroid influence on the pituitary and a frequency effect of GnRH pulses on GnRH receptor numbers), leading to increasing production and secretion of gonadotropins. Increased gonadotropins are responsible for follicular growth and development in the ovary and increased sex steroid levels. The rising estrogen contributes to achieving an adult pattern of pulsatile GnRH secretion, finally leading to cyclic menstrual patterns.

The trend toward lowering of the menarcheal age and the period of acceleration of growth appears to have halted. In a 10-year prospective study of middle class contemporary American girls, the mean age of menarche was 12.83 with a range of 9.14-17.70 years.(62) The age of onset of puberty is variable and influenced by genetic factors, socioeconomic conditions, and general health. The earlier menarche today compared to the past is undoubtedly due to improved nutrition and better health. It has been suggested that initiation of growth and menarche occur at a particular body weight (48 kg) and percent of body fat (17%).(63) It is thought that this relationship reflects a required stage of metabolism. Although this hypothesis of a critical weight is a helpful concept, the extreme variability in onset of menarche indicates that there is no particular age or size at which an individual girl should be expected to experience menarche.

In the female, the typical sequence of events is growth initiation, thelarche, pubarche, and finally menarche. This generally begins sometime between 8 and 14 years of age. The length of time involved in this evolution is usually 2-4 years. During this time-span, puberty is said to occur. Individual variation in the order of appearance of this sequence is great. For example, growth of pubic hair and breast development are not always correlated.

83

Puberty is due to the reactivation of the hypothalamic-pituitary axis, once fully active during fetal life, but now recently suppressed during childhood. If the systems are potentially responsive, what holds function in check until puberty? The hypothalamic-pituitary-gonadal system is operative prior to puberty, but extremely sensitive to steroids, and therefore suppressed. The changes at puberty are due to a gradually increasing gonadotropin secretion which takes place because of a decrease in the sensitivity of the hypothalamic centers to the negative-inhibitory action of gonadal steroids. This can be pictured as a slowly rising set point of decreased sensitivity, resulting in increasing GnRH pulsatile secretion, leading to increasing gonadotropin production and ovarian stimulation, and finally to increasing estrogen levels. The reason that FSH is the first gonadotropin to rise at puberty is that arcuate activity begins with a low frequency of GnRH pulses. This is associated with a rise in FSH and little change in LH. With acceleration of frequency, FSH and LH reach adult levels.

Negative feedback of steroids cannot be the sole explanation for the low gonadotropin levels in children. Agonadal children show the same decline in gonadotropins from age 2 to 6 as do normal children. This suggests an intrinsic CNS inhibitory mechanism independent of gonadal steroids. Therefore, the restraint of puberty can be viewed as the result of two forces:

1. A CNS inhibitory force, a mechanism suppressing GnRH pulsatile secretion.

2. A very sensitive negative feedback of gonadal steroids (6-15 times more sensitive before puberty).

Agonadal children show a rise in gonadotropins at pubertal age following suppression to a nadir during childhood. Thus, the dominant mechanism must be a CNS inhibitory force. The initial maturational change in the hypothalamus would then be a decrease in this inhibitory influence. A search for this mechanism continues.

The development of the positive feedback response to estrogen occurs later. This explains the well-known finding of anovulation in the first months (as long as 18 months) of menstruation. There are frequent exceptions, however, and ovulation can occur even at the time of menarche.

Don't think of puberty as being turned on by a controlling center in the brain, but rather as a functional summary of all the influences. This is more a concept than an actual locus of action.

The overall result of this change in the hypothalamus is the development of secondary sex characteristics, attainment of adult set point levels, and the ability to reproduce. Neoplastic and vascular disorders which alter hypothalamic sensitivity can reverse the prepubertal threshold restraint and lead to precocious puberty.

References

1. **Kendrick KM, Dixson AF,** Luteinizing hormone releasing hormone enhances proceptivity in a primate, Neuroendocrinol 41:449, 1985.

2. **Nikolics K, Mason AJ, Szonyi E, Ramachandran J, Seeburg PH,** A prolactin-inhibiting factor within the precursor for human gonadotropin-releasing hormone, Nature 316:511, 1985.

3. **Mason AJ, Pitts SL, Nikolics K, Szonyi E, Wilcox JN, Seeburg PH, Stewart TA,** The hypogonadal mouse: Reproductive functions restored by gene therapy, Science 234:1372, 1986.

4. **Barkan AL, Reame NE, Kelch RP, Marshall JC,** Idiopathic hypogonadotropic hypogonadism in men: dependence of the hormone responses to gonadotropin-releasing hormone (GnRH) on the magnitude of the endogenous GnRH secretory defect, J Clin Endocrinol Metab 61:1118, 1985.

5. **Silverman AJ, Antunes JL, Ferin M, Zimmerman EA,** The distribution of LHRH in the hypothalamus of the rhesus monkey. Light microscopic studies using immunoperoxidase technique, Endocrinology 101:134, 1977.

6. **Nakai Y, Plant TM, Hess DL, Keogh EJ, Knobil E,** On the sites of the negative and positive feedback actions of estradiol in the control of gonadotropin secretion in the rhesus monkey, Endocrinology 102:1008, 1978.

7. **Knobil E,** The neuroendocrine control of the menstrual cycle, Rec Prog Hor Res 36:53, 1980.

8. **Gross KM, Matsumoto AM, Southworth MB, Bremner WJ,** Evidence for decreased luteinizing hormone-releasing hormone frequency in men with selective elevations of follicle-stimulating hormone, J Clin Endocrinol Metab 60:197, 1985.

9. **Reame N, Sauder SE, Kelch RP, Marshall JC,** Pulsatile gonadotropin secretion during the human menstrual cycle: Evidence for altered frequency of gonadotropin-releasing hormone secretion, J Clin Endocrinol Metab 59:328, 1984.

10. **Filicori M, Santoro N, Merriam GR, Crowley WF Jr,** Characterization of the physiological pattern of epidsodic gonadotropin secretion throughout the human menstrual cycle, J Clin Endocrinol Metab 62:1136, 1986.

11. **Veldhuis JD, Evans WS, Johnson ML, Wills MR, Rogol AD,** Physiological properties of the luteinizing hormone pulse signal: Impact of intensive and extended venous sampling paradigms on its characterization in healthy men and women, J Clin Endocrinol Metab 62:881, 1986.

12. **Gambacciani M, Liu JH, Swartz WH, Tueros VS, Yen SSC, Rasmussen DD,** Intrinsic pulsatility of luteinizing hormone release from the human pituitary in vitro, Neuroendocrinology 45:402, 1987.

13. **Sameulsson B, Dahlen S-E, Lindgren JA, Rouzer CA, Serhan CN,** Leukotrienes and lipoxins: Structures, biosynthesis, and biological effects, Science 237:1171, 1987.

14. **Andersen AN, Hagen C, Lange P, Boesgaard S, Djursing H, Eldrup E, Micic S,** Dopaminergic regulation of gonadotropin levels and pulsatility in normal women, Fertil Steril 47:391, 1987.

15. **Ben-Jonathan N,** Dopamine: A prolactin-inhibiting hormone, Endocrin Rev 6:564, 1985.

16. **Rasmussen DD, Liu JH, Wolf PL, Yen SSC,** Gonadotropin-releasing hormone neurosecretion in the human hypothalamus: *In vitro* regulation by dopamine, J Clin Endocrinol Metab 62:479, 1986.

17. **Christiansen E, Veldhuis JD, Rogol AD, Stumpf P, Evans WS,** Modulating actions of estradiol on gonadotropin-releasing hormone-stimulated prolactin secretion in postmenopausal individuals, Am J Obstet Gynecol 157:320, 1987.

18. **Snyder SH,** Brain peptides as neurotransmitters, Science 209:976, 1980.

19. **Howlett TA, Rees LH,** Endogenous opioid peptides and hypothalamo-pituitary function, Ann Rev Physiol 48:527, 1986.

20. **Bacchinetti F, Petraglia F, Genazzani AR,** Localization and expression of the three opioid systems, Seminars Reprod Endocrinol 5:103, 1987.

21. **Gindoff PR, Ferin M,** Brain opioid peptides and menstrual cyclicity, Seminars Reprod Endocrinol 5:125, 1987.

22. **Shoupe D, Montz FJ, Lobo RA,** The effects of estrogen and progestin on endogenous opioid activity in oophorectomized women, J Clin Endocrinol Metab 60:178, 1985.

23. **Casper RF, Alapin-Rubilovitz S,** Progestins increase endogenous opioid peptide activity in postmenopausal women, J Clin Endocrinol Metab 60:34, 1985.

24. **Marunicic M, Casper RF,** The effect of luteal phase estrogen antagonism on luteinizing hormone pulsatility and luteal function in women, J Clin Endocrinol Metab 64:148, 1987.

25. **Petraglia F, D'Ambrogio G, Comitini G, Facchinetti F, Volpe A, Genazzani AR,** Impairment of opioid control of luteinizing hormone secretion in menstrual disorders, Fertil Steril 43:534, 1985.

26. **Khoury SA, Reame NE, Kelch RP, Marshall JC,** Diurnal patterns of pulsatile luteinizing hormone secretion in hypothalamic amenorrhea: Reproducibility and responses to opiate blockade and an α_2-adrenergic agonist, J Clin Endocrinol Metab 64:755, 1987.

27. **Suh BY, Liu JH, Berga SL, Quigley ME, Laughlin GA, Yen SS,** Hypercortisolism in patients with functional hypothalamic-amenorrhea, J Clin Endocrinol Metab 66:733, 1988.

28. **Cumming DC, Wheeler GD,** Opioids in exercise physiology, Seminars in Reprod Endocrinol 5:171, 1987.

29. **Sarkar DK, Yen SSC,** Hyperprolactinemia decreases the luteinizing hormone-releasing hormone concentration in pituitary portal plasma: A possible role for β-endorphin as a mediator, Endocrinology 116:2080, 1985.

30. **Chen CC, Chang C, Krieger DT, Bardin CW,** Expression and regulation of proopiomelanocortin-like gene in the ovary and placenta: Comparison with the testis, Endocrinology 118:2382, 1986.

31. **Petraglia F, Di Meo G, Storchi R, Segre A, Facchinetti F, Szalay S, Volpe A, Genazzani AR,** Proopiomelanocortin-related peptides and methionine enkephalin in human follicular fluid : Changes during the menstrual cycle, Am J Obstet Gynecol 157:142, 1987.

86

32. **Fishman J, Norton B,** Brain catecholestrogens: Formation and possible functions, Adv Biosci 15:123, 1975.

33. **Mais V, Kazer RR, Cetel NS, Rivier J, Vale W, Yen SSC,** The dependency of folliculogenesis and corpus luteum function on pulsatile gonadotropin secretion in cycling women using a gonadotropin-releasing hormone antagonist as a probe, J Clin Endocrinol Metab 62:1250, 1986.

34. **Dierick K, Vandesdande F,** Immunocytochemical demonstration of separate vasopressin-neurophysin and oxytocin neurophysin neurons in the human hypothalamus, Cell Tissue Res 196:203, 1979.

35. **Brownstein MJ, Russel JT, Gainer H,** Synthesis, transport, and release of posterior pituitary hormones, Science 207:373, 1980.

36. **Kasson BG, Adashi EY, Hsueh AJW,** Arginine vasopressin in the testis: An intragonadal peptide control system, Endocrin Rev 7:156, 1986.

37. **Perlow MJ, Reppert SM, Artman HA, Fisher DA, Seif SM, Robinson AG,** Oxytocin, vasopressin and estrogen-stimulated neurophsyin: Daily patterns of concentration in cerebrospinal fluid, Science 216:1416, 1983.

38. **Amico JA, Seif SM, Robinson AG,** Elevation of oxytocin and the oxytocin-associated neurophysin in the plasma of normal women during midcycle, J Clin Endocrinol Metab 53:1229, 1981.

39. **Carmichael MS, Humbert R, Dixen J, Palmisano G, Greenleaf W, Davidson JM,** Plasma oxytocin increases in the human sexual response, J Clin Endocrinol Metab 64:27, 1987.

40. **Dawood MY,. Raghavan KS, Pociask C, Fuchs F,** Oxytocin during human pregnancy and parturition, Obstet Gynecol 51:138, 1978.

41. **Ferin M, Rosenblatt H, Carmel PW, Antunes JL, Vande Wiele RL,** Estrogen-induced gonadotropin surges in female rhesus monkeys after pituitary stalk section, Endocrinology 104:50, 1979.

42. **Yen SSC, Lein A,** The apparent paradox of the negative and positive feedback control system on gonadotropin secretion, Am J Obstet Gynecol 126:942, 1976.

43. **Veldhuis JD, Evans WS, Rogol AD, Kolp L, Thorner MO, Stumpf P,** Pituitary self-priming actions of gonadotropin-releasing hormone, J Clin Invest 77:1849, 1986.

44. **Adams TE, Norman RL, Spies HG,** Gonadotropin-releasing hormone receptor binding and pituitary responsiveness in estradiol-primed monkeys, Science 213:1388, 1981.

45. **Menon M, Peegel H, Katta V,** Estradiol potentiation of gonadotropin-releasing hormone responsiveness in the anterior pituitary is mediated by an increase in gonadotropin-releasing hormone receptors, Am J Obstet Gynecol 151:534, 1985.

46. **Chappel SC, Resko JA, Norman RL, Spies HG,** Studies on rhesus monkeys on the site where estrogen inhibits gonadotropins: delivery of 17-estradiol to the hypothalamus and pituitary gland, J Clin Endocrinol Metab 52:1, 1981.

47. **Katt JA, Duncan JA, Herbon L, Barkan A, Marshall JC,** The frequency of gonadotropin-releasing hormone stimulation determines the number of pituitary gonadotropin-releasing hormone receptors, Endocrinology 116:2113, 1985.

48. **Marut EL, Williams RF, Cowan BD, Lynch A, Lerner SP, Hodgen GD,** Pulsatile pituitary gonadotropin secretion during maturation of the dominant follicle in monkeys: Estrogen positive feedback enhances the biological activity of LH, Endocrinology 109:2270, 1981.

49. **March CM, Marrs RP, Goebelsmann U, Mishell DR,** Feedback effects of estradiol and progesterone upon gonadotropin and prolactin release, Obstet Gynecol 58:10, 1981.

50. **Liu JH, Yen SSC,** Induction of midcycle gonadotropin surge by ovarian steroids in women: a critical evaluation, J Clin Endocrinol Metab 57:797, 1983.

51. **Collins RL, Hodgen GD,** Blockade of the spontaneous midcycle gonadotropin surge in monkeys by RU 486: A progesterone antagonist or agonist? J Clin Endocrinol Metab 63:1270, 1986.

52. **Wildt L, Hutchison JS, Marshall G, Pohl CR, Knobil E,** On the site of action of progesterone in the blockade of the estradiol-induced gonadotropin discharge in the rhesus monkey, Endocrinology 109:1293, 1981.

53. **Batra SK, Miller WL,** Progesterone decreases the responsiveness of ovine pituitary cultures to luteinizing hormone-releasing hormone, Endocrinology 117:1436, 1985.

54. **Araki S, Chikazawa K, Motoyama M, Ijima K, Abe N, Tamada T,** Reduction in pituitary desensitization and prolongation of gonadotropin release by estrogen during continuous administration of gonadotropin-releasing hormone in women: Its antagonism by progesterone, J Clin Endocrinol Metab 60:590, 1985.

55. **Preslock JP,** The pineal gland: Basic implications and clinical correlations, Endocrin Rev 5:282, 1984.

56. **Tamarkin L, Baird CJ, Almeida OFX,** Melatonin: A coordinating signal for mammalian reproduction? Science 227:714, 1985.

57. **McClintock MK,** Menstrual synchrony and suppression, Nature 229:244, 1971.

58. **Kaplan SL, Grumbach MM, Aubert ML,** The ontogenesis of pituitary hormones and hypothalamic factors in the human fetus: Maturation of central nervous system regulation of anterior pituitary function, Rec Prog Hor Res 32:161, 1976.

59. **Reiter EO, Grumbach MM,** Neuroendocrine control mechanisms and the onset of puberty, Ann Rev Physiol 44:595, 1982.

60. **Sklar CA, Kaplan SL, Grumbach MM,** Evidence for dissociation between adrenarche and gonadarche: Studies in patients with idiopathic precocious puberty, gonadal dysgenesis, isolated gonadotroph deficiency, and constitutionally delayed growth and adolescence, J Clin Endocrinol Metab, 51:548, 1980.

61. **Boyar RM, Ramsey J, Chapman J, Fevere M, Madden J, Marks JF,** Luteinizing hormone and follicle-stimulating hormone secretory dynamics in Turner's syndrome, J Clin Endocrinol Metab 47:1078, 1978.

62. **Zacharias L, Rand WM, Wurtman RJ,** A prospective study of sexual development and growth in American girls: The statistics of menarche, Obstet Gynecol Survey 31:325, 1976.

63. **Frisch RE,** Body fat, menarche, and reproductive ability, Seminars Reprod Endocrinol 3:45, 1985.

3 Regulation of the Menstrual Cycle

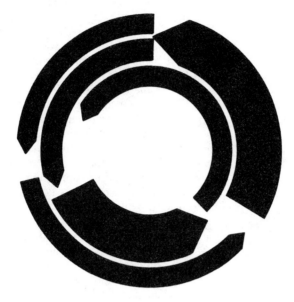

Diagnosis and management of abnormal menstrual function must be based upon an understanding of the physiological mechanisms involved in the regulation of the normal cycle. Dynamic relationships exist between the pituitary and gonadal hormones which allow for the cyclic nature of normal reproductive processes. These hormonal changes are correlated with morphological changes in the ovary, making the coordination of this system one of the most remarkable events in biology.

The menstrual cycle can be best described by dividing the cycle into 3 phases: the follicular phase, ovulation, and the luteal phase. *We will examine each of these phases, concentrating on the changes in ovarian and pituitary hormones, what governs the pattern of hormonal changes, and the effects of these hormones on the ovary, pituitary, and hypothalamus in regulating the menstrual cycle.*

Follicular Phase

During the follicular phase an orderly sequence of events takes place which ensures that the proper number of follicles is ready for ovulation. In the human ovary the end result of this follicular development is (usually) one surviving mature follicle. This process, which occurs over the space of 10-14 days, features a series of sequential actions of hormones on the follicle, leading the follicle destined to ovulate through a period of initial growth from a primordial follicle through the stages of the preantral, antral, and preovulatory follicle.

| The Primordial Follicle | The primordial follicle consists of an oocyte, arrested in the diplotene stage of meiotic prophase, surrounded by a single layer of granulosa cells. Follicular growth is a process, best described by Peters as a continuum.(1) Until their numbers are exhausted, follicles begin to grow under all physiological circumstances. Growth is not interrupted by pregnancy, ovulation, or periods of anovulation. Growth continues at all ages, including infancy and around the menopause. |

The number of follicles which starts growing each cycle appears to be dependent upon the size of the residual pool of inactive follicles. (1) Reducing the size of the pool (e.g. unilateral oophorectomy) causes the remaining follicles to redistribute their availability over time. The mechanism for determining which follicles or how many will develop during any one cycle is unknown. It is possible that the follicle which is singled out to play the leading role in a particular cycle is the beneficiary of a timely match of follicle "readiness" and appropriate tropic hormone stimulation. The first follicle able to respond to stimulation may achieve an early lead which it never relinquishes. It is now clear, however, that the follicle destined to ovulate is recruited in the first few days of the cycle.(2)

The first visible sign of follicular recruitment is when the granulosa cells become cuboidal rather than squamous in shape. At this same time, in response to follicle-stimulating hormone (FSH), small gap junctions develop between the granulosa cells and the oocyte. The gap junctions serve as the pathway for nutritional and metabolite interchange between the granulosa cells and the oocyte.

The initiation of follicular growth appears to be independent of gonadotropin stimulation. In the vast majority of instances this growth is limited and rapidly followed by atresia. The general pattern is interrupted at the beginning of the menstrual cycle when a group of follicles responds to a hormonal change and is propelled to further growth. The most important hormonal event at this time is a rise in FSH. The decline in luteal phase steroidogenesis allows the rise in FSH (accompanied by a rise in LH) which rescues a group of follicles from atresia.(3)

The Preantral Follicle

Once growth is initiated, the follicle progresses to the preantral stage as the oocyte enlarges and is surrounded by a membrane, the zona pellucida. The granulosa cells undergo a multilayer proliferation as the theca layer begins to organize from the surrounding stroma. This growth is dependent upon gonadotropins and is correlated with increasing production of estrogen.

The granulosa cells of the preantral follicle have the ability to synthesize all 3 classes of steroids; however, significantly more estrogens than either androgens or progestins are produced. An aromatase enzyme system acts to convert androgens to estrogens and appears to be a factor limiting ovarian estrogen production. Aromatization is induced or activated through the action of FSH. Specific receptors for FSH are present on preantral granulosa cells and, in the presence of FSH, the preantral follicle can aromatize limited amounts of androgens and generate its own estrogenic microenvironment.(4) Estrogen production is, therefore, also limited by FSH

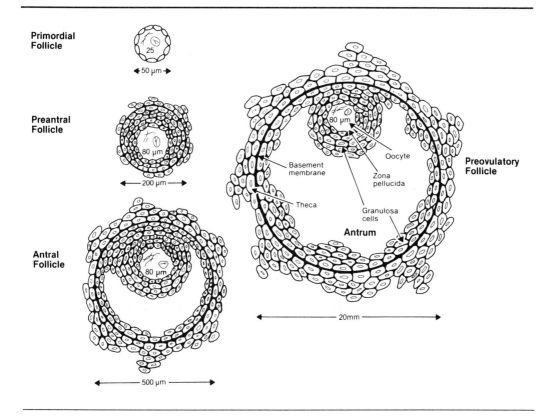

Primordial Follicle
25
50 µm

Preantral Follicle
80 µm
200 µm

Antral Follicle
80 µm
500 µm

Preovulatory Follicle
80 µm
Basement membrane
Oocyte
Zona pellucida
Theca
Granulosa cells
Antrum
20mm

receptor content. The administration of FSH will raise the concentration of its own receptor on granulosa cells both in vivo and in vitro. FSH receptors appear in the plasma membrane of granulosa cells immediately upon the initial growth of the follicle, and quickly reach a concentration of approximately 1500 receptors per granulosa cell.(5)

FSH combines with estrogen to synergistically exert a mitogenic action on granulosa cells to stimulate their proliferation. Together, FSH and estrogen promote a rapid accumulation of FSH receptors, reflecting largely the increase in the number of granulosa cells. The early appearance of estrogen within the follicle allows the follicle to respond to relatively low concentrations of FSH, an autocrine function for estrogen within the follicle. As growth proceeds, the granulosa cells differentiate into several subgroups of different cell populations. This appears to be determined by the position of the cells relative to the oocyte.

There is a system of communication which exists within follicles. Not every cell has to contain receptors for the gonadotropins. Cells with receptors can transfer a signal (presumably by gap junctions) which causes protein kinase activation in cells which lack receptors.(6) Thus, hormone-initiated action can be transmitted throughout the follicle despite the fact that only a subpopulation of cells binds the hormone.

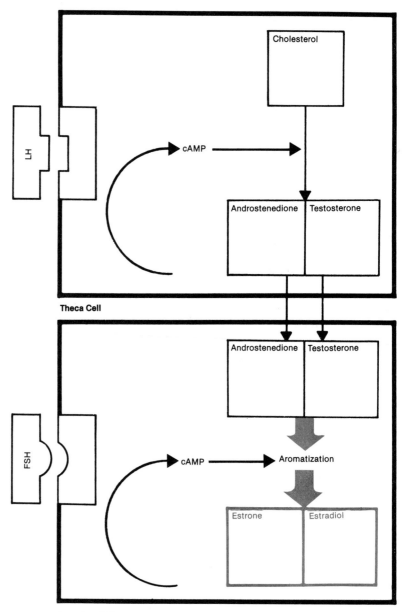

Theca Cell

Granulosa Cell

The role of androgens in early follicular development is complex. Specific androgen receptors are present in the granulosa cells. Serving not only as substrate for FSH-induced aromatization, the androgens, in low concentrations, can further enhance aromatase activity. When exposed to an androgen-rich environment, preantral granulosa cells favor the conversion of androstenedione to more potent 5α-reduced androgens rather than to estrogens.(7) These androgens cannot be converted to estrogen, and in fact, inhibit aromatase activity.(8) They also inhibit FSH induction of luteinizing hormone (LH) receptor formation, another essential step in follicular development.(9)

The fate of the preantral follicle is in delicate balance. At low concentrations, androgens enhance their own aromatization and contribute to estrogen production. At higher levels, the limited capacity of aromatization is overwhelmed, and the follicle becomes androgenic and ultimately atretic.(10) Perhaps follicles will progress in development only if emerging when FSH is elevated and LH is low. Those follicles arising at the end of the luteal phase or early in the subsequent cycle would be favored by an environment in which aromatization in the granulosa cell can prevail. *The success of a follicle depends upon its ability to convert an androgen microenvironment to an estrogen microenvironment.(11)*

Summary of events in the preantral follicle:

1. Initial follicular growth occurs independently of hormonal influence.

2. FSH stimulation propels follicles to the preantral stage.

3. FSH-induced aromatization of androgen in the granulosa results in the production of estrogen.

4. Together, FSH and estrogen increase the FSH receptor content of the follicle.

The Antral Follicle

Under the synergistic influence of estrogen and FSH there is an increase in the production of follicular fluid which accumulates in the intercellular spaces of the granulosa, eventually coalescing to form a cavity, as the follicle makes its gradual transition to the antral stage. The accumulation of follicular fluid provides a means whereby the oocyte and surrounding granulosa cells can be nurtured in a specific endocrine environment for each follicle.

In the presence of FSH, estrogen becomes the dominant substance in the follicular fluid. Conversely, in the absence of FSH, androgens predominate.(12,13) LH is not normally present in follicular fluid until the midcycle. If LH is prematurely elevated in plasma and antral fluid, mitotic activity in the granulosa decreases, degenerative changes ensue, and intrafollicular androgen levels rise. Therefore, the presence of estrogen and FSH in antral fluid is essential for sustained accumulation of granulosa cells and continued follicular growth. Antral follicles with the greatest rates of granulosa proliferation contain the highest estrogen concentrations, the lowest androgen/estrogen ratios, and are the most likely to house a healthy oocyte. An androgenic milieu antagonizes estrogen-induced granulosa proliferation and, if sustained, promotes degenerative change in the oocyte.

The Follicular Microenvironment (5)

Cycle Day	Size	Volume	Number of Granulosa Cells	FSH mIU/ml	LH mIU/ml	Prolactin	A	E₂	Prog
						ng/ml			
1	4 mm	0.0 ml	2 mill	2.5	—	60	800	100	—
4	7 mm	0.15 ml	5 mill	2.5	—	40	800	500	100
7	12 mm	0.5 ml	15 mill	3.6	2.8	20	800	1000	300
12	20 mm	6.5 ml	50 mill	3.6	6.0	5	800	2000	2000

The steroids present in follicular fluid can be found in concentrations several orders of magnitude higher than those in plasma and reflect the functional capacity of the surrounding granulosa and theca cells. The synthesis of steroid hormones is functionally compartmentalized within the follicle—the two-cell mechanism.(5,10,13,14)

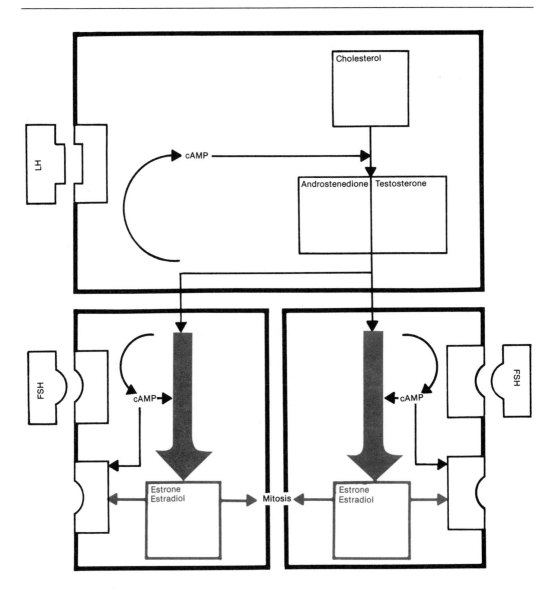

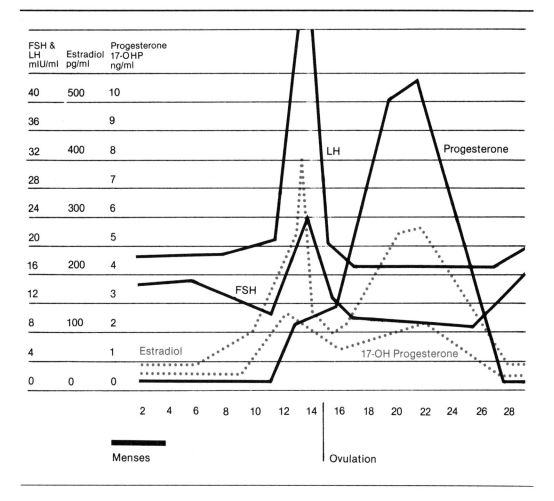

FSH & LH mIU/ml	Estradiol pg/ml	Progesterone 17-OHP ng/ml
40	500	10
36		9
32	400	8
28		7
24	300	6
20		5
16	200	4
12		3
8	100	2
4		1
0	0	0

LH

Progesterone

FSH

Estradiol

17-OH Progesterone

2 4 6 8 10 12 14 16 18 20 22 24 26 28

Menses

Ovulation

Though each compartment (theca and granulosa) retains the ability to produce progestins, androgens, and estrogens, the aromatase activity of the granulosa far exceeds that observed in the theca. In the antral follicle, LH receptors are present only on the theca cells and FSH receptors only on the granulosa cells. Theca interstitial cells, located in the theca interna, have approximately 20,000 LH receptors in their cell membranes. In response to LH, theca tissue is stimulated to produce androgens which can then be converted, through FSH-induced aromatization, to estrogens in the granulosa cells.

The interaction between the granulosa and theca compartments, with resulting accelerated estrogen production is not fully functional until later in antral development. Like preantral granulosa cells, the granulosa of small antral follicles exhibits an in vitro tendency to convert significant amounts of androgen to the more potent 5α-reduced form. In contrast, granulosa cells isolated from large antral follicles readily and preferentially metabolize androgens to estrogens. The conversion from an androgen microenvironment to an estrogen microenvironment (a conversion essential for further growth and development) is dependent upon a growing sensitivity to FSH brought about by the action of FSH and the enhancing influence of estrogen.

Selection of the Dominant Follicle. The successful conversion to an estrogen dominant follicle marks the "selection" of a follicle destined to ovulate, the process whereby, with rare exception, only a single follicle succeeds. This selection process is to a significant degree the result of two estrogen actions: 1) a local interaction between estrogen and FSH within the follicle, and 2) the effect of estrogen on pituitary secretion of FSH. While estrogen exerts a positive influence on FSH action within the maturing follicle, its negative feedback relationship with FSH at the hypothalamic-pituitary level serves to withdraw gonadotropin support from the other less developed follicles. The fall in FSH leads to a decline in FSH-dependent aromatase activity, limiting estrogen production in the less mature follicles. Even if a lesser follicle succeeds in achieving an estrogen microenvironment, decreasing FSH support would interrupt granulosa proliferation and function, promote a conversion to an androgenic microenvironment, and thereby induce irreversible atretic change. Indeed, the first event in the process of atresia is a reduction in FSH receptors in the granulosa layer.

An asymmetry in ovarian estrogen production, an expression of the emerging dominant follicle, can be detected in ovarian venous effluent on day 5 of the cycle, corresponding with the gradual fall of FSH levels observed at the midfollicular phase, and preceding the increase in diameter which marks the physical emergence of the dominant follicle.(15) This is a crucial time in the cycle. Exogenous estrogen, administered even after selection of the dominant follicle, disrupts preovulatory development and induces atresia by reducing FSH levels below the sustaining level. Because the lesser follicles have entered the process of atresia, loss of the dominant follicle during this period of time requires beginning over, with recruitment of another set of preantral follicles.(16)

The negative feedback of estrogen on FSH serves to inhibit the development of all but the dominant follicle, but the selected follicle remains dependent upon FSH and must complete its preovulatory development in the face of declining plasma levels of FSH. The dominant follicle, therefore, must escape the consequences of FSH suppression induced by its own accelerating estrogen production. The dominant follicle has a significant advantage, a greater content of FSH receptors acquired because of a rate of granulosa proliferation that surpasses that of its cohorts and enhancement of FSH action because of its high intrafollicular estrogen concentration. As a result, the stimulus for aromatization, FSH, can be maintained, while at the same time it is being withdrawn from among the less developed follicles. A wave of atresia among the lesser follicles, therefore, is seen to parallel the rise in estrogen.

The accumulation of a greater mass of granulosa cells is accompanied by advanced development of the theca vasculature. By day 9, theca vascularity in the dominant follicle is twice that of other antral follicles.(17) This may allow a preferential delivery of gonadotropins to the follicle permitting the dominant follicle to retain FSH responsiveness and sustain continued development and function despite waning gonadotropin levels.

In order to respond to the ovulatory surge and to become a successful corpus luteum, the granulosa cells must acquire LH recep-

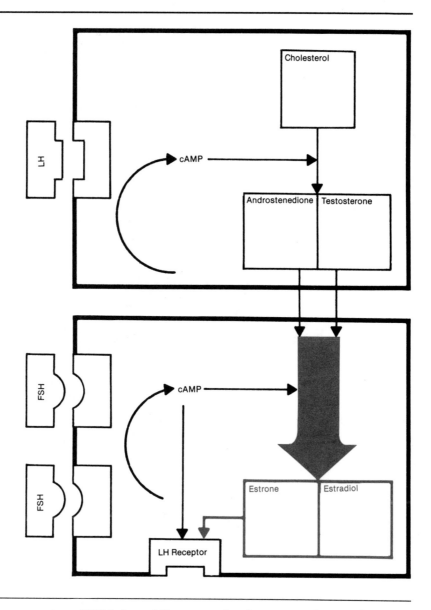

tors. FSH induces LH receptor development on the granulosa cells of the large antral follicles. Here again estrogen serves as the chief coordinator. With increasing concentrations of estrogen within the follicle, FSH changes its focus of action, from its own receptor to the LH receptor. The combination of a capacity for continued response despite declining levels of FSH and a high local estrogen environment in the dominant follicle provides optimal conditions for LH receptor development. LH can induce the formation of its own receptor in FSH-primed granulosa cells, but the primary mechanism utilizes FSH stimulation and estrogen enhancement.(18,19) The role for estrogen goes beyond synergism and enhancement; it is obligatory. Inhibition of estrogen synthesis prevents FSH-stimulated increases in LH receptors.(20)

Although prolactin is always present in follicular fluid, there is no evidence to suggest that prolactin is important during normal ovulatory cycles in the primate.

99

Growth Factors. Growth factors are polypeptides that modulate cell proliferation and differentiation, operating through binding to specific cell membrane receptors.(21) They are not classic endocrine substances; they act locally and function in paracrine and autocrine modes. There are multiple growth factors and most cells contain multiple receptors for the various growth factors.

Epidermal Growth Factor. Epidermal growth factor is a mitogen for a variety of cells, and its action is potentiated by other growth factors. Granulosa cells, in particular, respond to this growth factor, in a variety of ways related to gonadotropin stimulation.

Transforming Growth Factor. TGF-α is a structural analog of epidermal growth factor and can bind to the epidermal growth factor receptor. TGF-β utilizes a receptor distinct from the epidermal growth factor receptor. These factors are thought to be autocrine growth regulators. The follicular fluid protein, inhibin, is derived from the same gene family. TGF-β enhances FSH induction of LH receptors, an action which is opposite that of epidermal growth factor.(22)

Somatomedin-C (Insulin-like Growth Factor-I). Somatomedins are serum-derived peptides which have structural and functional similarity to insulin and mediate growth hormone action. There are specific receptors for these factors, but they also bind to insulin receptors. The granulosa cells are thought to produce somatomedin-C (IGF-I) under regulation of FSH, growth hormone, and estrogens. This factor enhances FSH stimulation of steroidogenesis and LH receptors as well as granulosa cell proliferation.

Fibroblast Growth Factor. This factor is a mitogen for a variety of cells.

Platelet-Derived Growth Factor. This growth factor modifies cyclic AMP pathways responding to FSH, especially those involved in granulosa cell differentiation. Both platelet-derived growth factor and epidermal growth factor may also modify prostaglandin production within the follicle.

Angiogenic Growth Factors. Vascularization of the follicle is influenced by peptides secreted into the follicular fluid.(23)

The Feedback System. Through its own estrogen and peptide production, the dominant follicle assumes control of its own destiny. By altering gonadotropin secretion through feedback mechanisms it optimizes its own environment to the detriment of the lesser follicles.

As reviewed in Chapter 2, gonadotropin releasing hormone (GnRH) plays largely a permissive, though obligatory, role in the control of gonadotropin secretion.(2) The pattern of gonadotropin secretion observed in the menstrual cycle is the result of feedback modulation of steroids and peptides originating in the dominant follicle, acting directly on the hypothalamus and anterior pituitary. Experimental evidence suggests that the estrogen positive feedback mechanism involves an increase in GnRH receptor concentration, while the negative feedback action operates through a different and uncertain system.(24) Estrogen exerts its inhibitory effects in both the hypothalamus and the anterior pituitary, decreasing both GnRH pulsatile secretion and GnRH pituitary response.(25) Progesterone also operates in two sites. Its inhibitory action is at the hypothalamic level, and, like estrogen, its positive action is directly on the pituitary.(26)

The secretion of FSH is very sensitive to the negative inhibitory effects of estrogen even at low levels. At higher levels, suppression of FSH is profound and sustained. In contrast, the influence of estrogen on LH release varies with concentration and duration of exposure. At low levels, estrogen commands a negative feedback relationship with LH. At higher levels, however, estrogen is capable of exerting a positive stimulatory feedback effect on LH release.

The transition from suppression to stimulation of LH release occurs as estradiol rises during the midfollicular phase. There are two critical features in this mechanism: 1) the concentration of estradiol and 2) the length of time during which the estradiol elevation is sustained. In women, the estradiol concentration necessary to achieve a positive feedback is over 200 pg/ml, and this concentration must be sustained for approximately 50 hours. The estrogen stimulus must be applied until after the surge actually begins. Otherwise, the LH surge is abbreviated or fails to occur at all.

Variation in the pattern of gonadotropin release is the result of the feedback modulation of gonadal steroids. Within the well-established monthly pattern, the gonadotropins are secreted in a pulsatile fashion with a frequency and magnitude that vary with the phase of the cycle. The pulsatile pattern is directly due to a similar pulsatile secretion of GnRH, but amplitude and frequency modulation (mean values below) is probably the consequence of steroid feedback on both hypothalamus and anterior pituitary.(27,28)

LH Pulse Frequency:

Early follicular phase: 94 minutes.

Late follicular phase: 71 minutes.

Early luteal phase: 103 minutes.

Late luteal phase: 216 minutes.

LH Pulse Amplitude:

Early follicular phase: 6.5 mIU/ml.

Midfollicular phase: 5.1 mIU/ml.

Late follicular phase: 7.2 mIU/ml.

Early luteal phase: 14.9 mIU/ml.

Midluteal phase: 12.2 mIU/ml.

Late luteal phase: 7.6 mIU/ml.

The pulsatile pattern of FSH is not easily discerned because of its relatively longer half-life compared to LH, but the experimental data indicate that FSH and LH are secreted simultaneously and that GnRH stimulates the secretion of both gonadotropins. Thus gonadotropin pulses are shorter in interval and smaller in amplitude in the follicular phase compared to the luteal phase. Only 36 hours before menses, gonadotropin secretion is characterized by infrequent LH pulses and low FSH levels typical of the late luteal phase, *but by day one of the next cycle, the early follicular characteristics are already present.(28)*

The frequency changes in the luteal phase correlate with duration of exposure to progesterone, while pulse amplitude changes appear to be influenced by changes in progesterone levels.(27) This suggests that steroids influence the hypothalamic release of GnRH for frequency changes and the pituitary for action on amplitude. The inhibitory action of luteal phase steroids may be mediated by an increase in hypothalamic endogenous opioid peptides. Both estrogen and progesterone can increase endogenous opiates, and administration of clomiphene (an estrogen antagonist) during the luteal phase increases the LH pulse frequency with no effect on amplitude.(29) Thus estrogen appears to enhance the stimulatory action of progesterone in the luteal phase on endogenous opioid peptides. The relatively high levels of endogenous opiates during the luteal phase, however, are achieved earlier in the cycle.

Plasma endorphin begins to rise in the 2 days before the LH peak, thus coinciding with the midcycle gonadotropin surge.(30) The maximal level is reached just after the LH peak, coinciding with ovulation. Levels then gradually decline until the nadir is reached during menses and the early follicular phase. Monkeys show the highest beta endorphin levels in the hypophyseal portal blood to be at midcycle.(31)

There is another, newly appreciated, action of estrogen. A disparity exists between the patterns of LH secretion as determined by radioimmunoassay and bioassay, suggesting that more biologically active LH is secreted at midcycle than at other times in the cycle.(32) This behavior, bioactivity vs immunoactivity, is determined by the molecular structure of the gonadotropin molecule, a concept referred to in Chapter 1 as heterogeneity of the tropic hormones. There is a well-established relationship between the activity and half-life of glycoprotein hormones and their sialic acid content. The feedback effects of estrogen include modulation of sialylation and the size and activity of the gonadotropins subsequently released. It certainly makes sense to intensify the gonadotropin effect at midcycle. The positive feedback action of estrogen, therefore, both increases the quantity and the quality (the bioactivity) of LH.

Follicular Fluid Substances. The follicular fluid is a veritable protein soup! It is composed of exudates from plasma and secretions from follicular cells. A variety of hormones can be found in the follicular fluid, as well as enzymes and peptides which play important roles in follicular growth and development, ovulation, and modulation of hormonal responses.

One of the more important substances is a peptide synthesized by granulosa cells in response to FSH, secreted into the follicular fluid and ovarian venous effluent, and called *inhibin* (and sometimes, folliculostatin).(33,34) Inhibin consists of two dissimilar peptides (known as alpha and beta subunits) linked by disulfide bonds. Two forms of inhibin (inhibin A and inhibin B) have been purified, each containing an identical alpha subunit and distinct but related beta subunits. Thus, there are three subunits for inhibins: alpha, beta-A, and beta-B. Each subunit is a product of different messenger RNA, therefore, there is no unique large precursor molecule.

The 2 Forms of Inhibin:

Inhibin A: Alpha-Beta$_A$

Inhibin B: Alpha-Beta$_B$

FSH stimulates the secretion of inhibin from granulosa cells, and in turn, is suppressed by inhibin—a reciprocal relationship.(35,36) The secretion of inhibin is further regulated by local paracrine control. GnRH and epidermal growth factor diminish FSH stimulation of inhibin secretion, while insulin-like growth factor-I enhances inhibin production. The inhibitory effects of GnRH and epidermal growth factor are consistent with their known ability to decrease FSH-stimulated estrogen production and LH receptor formation. The action of GnRH lends some support for an endogenous ovarian GnRH-like substance (which is found in follicular fluid) and which is involved in inhibin production.

The secretion of inhibin into the circulation is another mechanism by which an emerging follicle secures dominance, further amplifying the withdrawal of FSH from other follicles. Human plasma levels of inhibin rise in parallel with estradiol, and peak inhibin levels correlate with follicle number and the number of oocytes recovered at laparoscopy from induced cycles for in vitro fertilization.(35,36) A loss of this peptide due to old follicles of poor quality may explain the rise in FSH seen in the perimenopausal period despite the continued presence of menstrual bleeding. Furthermore, the inability to suppress gonadotropins to a normal range during estrogen replacement therapy may be due to the absence of inhibin.

There also exists a peptide which is related to inhibin but which has an opposite action (the stimulation of FSH release).(37,38) This releasing substance, called *activin*, contains two subunits which are identical to the beta subunits of inhibins A and B. Thus, when each of the beta subunits of the inhibins is combined with an alpha subunit, the resulting molecule, inhibin A or B, inhibits the release of FSH. If the beta subunits are paired together, the molecule stimulates the release of FSH, in a mechanism which is not mediated by GnRH receptors. The structure of the releasing substance is homologous to that of transforming growth factor-β, indicating that these products all come from the same gene family.(39) It is likely that more rearrangements of these gene products will be discovered.

The 3 Forms of Activin:

Beta$_A$-Beta$_A$

Beta$_A$-Beta$_B$

Beta$_B$-Beta$_B$

Follicular fluid contains concentrations of *prorenin,* the inactive precursor of renin, that are about 12 times higher than plasma levels.(40) It appears that LH stimulates its synthesis in the follicle, and there is a midcycle peak in prorenin plasma levels. The circulating levels of prorenin also increase (10-fold) during the early stages of pregnancy, the result of ovarian stimulation by the rise in HCG. These increases in prorenin from the ovary are not responsible for any significant changes in the plasma levels of the active form, renin. Possible roles for this ovarian prorenin-renin-angiotensin system include the following: stimulation of steroidogenesis to provide androgen substrate for estrogen production, regulation of calcium and prostaglandin metabolism, and stimulation of angiogenesis.(41) This system may affect vascular and tissue functions both within and outside the ovary.

Members of the proopiomelanocortin family are found in human follicular fluid.(42) Follicular levels of ACTH and β-lipotropin remain constant throughout the cycle, but β-endorphin levels peak just before ovulation. In addition, enkephalin is present in relatively unchanging concentrations.

Follicular fluid prevents resumption of meiosis until the preovulatory LH surge either overcomes or removes this inhibition. This factor is named *oocyte maturation inhibitor (OMI). Pregnancy-associated plasma protein A*, found in the placenta, is also present in follicular fluid. It may inhibit proteolytic activity within the follicle before ovulation. Another placental protein, *placental protein 12,* has also been found in follicular fluid. *FSH binding inhibitor* is found in follicles undergoing atresia, and *LH receptor binding inhibitor* has been identified in corpora lutea. *Luteinization inhibitor (LI)* prevents FSH-induced LH receptor production, and *luteinization stimulator* enhances induction of LH receptors. It is uncertain whether *GnRH-like peptides* (sometimes called gonadocrinins) have a follicular role or represent sequestered GnRH. *Oxytocin* is found in preovulatory follicles and the corpus luteum, but it is not known what it is doing there. Further modulation of gonadotropins is achieved by intrafollicular proteins which inhibit granulosa cell enzyme activity.(43) These push-pull, local and long distance feedback relationships emphasize the complexity, but also the incredible synchrony, inherent in achieving successful follicular growth, ovulation, and corpus luteum function.

Summary of events in the antral follicle:

1. Follicular phase estrogen production is explained by the two-cell, two-gonadotropin mechanism.

2. Selection of the dominant follicle is established during days 5-7, and consequently, peripheral levels of estradiol begin to rise significantly by cycle day 7.

3. Derived from the dominant follicle, estradiol levels increase steadily and, through negative feedback effects, exert progressively greater suppressive influence on FSH release.

4. While directing a decline in FSH levels, the midfollicular rise in estradiol exerts a positive feedback influence on LH.

5. The positive action of estrogen also includes modification of the gonadotropin molecule, increasing the quality (the bioactivity) as well as the quantity of LH at midcycle.

6. LH levels rise steadily during the late follicular phase, stimulating androgen production in the theca.

7. A unique responsiveness to FSH allows the dominant follicle to utilize the androgen as substrate and further accelerate estrogen production.

8. Enhanced by increasing exposure to estrogen, FSH induces the appearance of LH receptors on granulosa cells.

9. Follicular response to the gonadotropins is modulated by a variety of growth factors, including epidermal growth factor and insulin-like growth factor-I.

10. Various proteins in the follicular fluid further contribute to the synchronization of the cycle. Inhibin, secreted by the granulosa cells in reponse to FSH, directly suppresses pituitary FSH secretion.

The Preovulatory Follicle

Granulosa cells in the preovulatory follicle enlarge and acquire lipid inclusions while the theca becomes vacuolated and richly vascular, giving the preovulatory follicle a hyperemic appearance. The oocyte resumes meiosis, approaching completion of its reduction division.

Approaching maturity, the preovulatory follicle produces increasing amounts of estrogen. During the late follicular phase, estrogens rise slowly at first, then rapidly, reaching a peak approximately 24-36 hours prior to ovulation.(44) In providing the ovulatory stimulus to the selected follicle, the LH surge seals the fate of the remaining follicles with their lower estrogen and FSH content by further increasing androgen superiority.

Acting through its own receptors, LH promotes luteinization of the granulosa in the dominant follicle, resulting in the production of progesterone. An increase in progesterone can be detected in the venous effluent of the ovary bearing the preovulatory follicle as early as day 10 of the cycle.(15) This small but significant increase in the production of progesterone in the preovulatory period has immense physiological importance.

Progesterone affects the positive feedback response to estrogen in both a time and dose dependent manner. When introduced after adequate estrogen priming, progesterone facilitates the positive feedback response, and in the presence of subthreshold levels of estradiol can induce a characteristic LH surge.(45,46) Hence, the surprising onset of ovulation occasionally observed in an anovulatory, amenorrheic woman administered a progestin challenge. When administered before the estrogen stimulus, or in high doses (achieving a blood level greater than 2 ng/ml), progesterone blocks the midcycle LH surge. Appropriately low levels of progesterone derived from the maturing follicle contribute to the precise timing, the synchronization, of the midcycle surge.

In addition to its facilitory action on LH, progesterone at midcycle is significantly responsible for the FSH surge.(46) This action of progesterone can be viewed as a further step in ensuring completion of FSH action on the follicle, specifically making sure that a full complement of LH receptors is in place in the granulosa layer. In certain experimental situations, incremental estradiol alone can elicit simultaneous surges of LH and FSH, suggesting that progesterone certainly enhances the effect of estradiol but may not be obligatory.(47)

When the lesser follicles fail to achieve full maturity and undergo atresia, the theca cells return to their origin as a component of stromal tissue, retaining, however, an ability to respond to LH with steroid production. Because the products of theca tissue are androgens, the increase in stromal tissue in the late follicular phase is associated with a rise in androgen levels in the peripheral plasma at midcycle, a 15% increase in androstenedione and a 20% increase in testosterone.(48)

Androgen production at this stage in the cycle may serve two purposes: 1) a local role within the ovary to enhance the process of atresia, and 2) a systemic effect to stimulate libido.

Intraovarian androgens accelerate granulosa cell death and follicular atresia. The specific mechanism for this action is unclear, although it is attractive to suspect an interference with estrogen and its vital duties in enhancing FSH activity. Therefore, androgens may play a regulatory role in ensuring that only a dominant follicle reaches the point of ovulation.

It is well known that libido can be stimulated by androgens. If the midcycle rise in androgens affects libido, then an increase in sexual activity should coincide with this rise. Early studies failed to demonstrate a consistent pattern in coital frequency in women because of the effect of male partner initiation. If only sexual behavior initiated by women is studied, a peak in female-initiated sexual activity is seen during the ovulatory phase of the cycle, and no such peak is noted in users of birth control pills.(49) The coital frequency of married couples has also been noted to increase at the time of ovulation.(50) Therefore, the midcycle rise in androgens may serve to increase sexual activity at the time most likely to achieve pregnancy.

Summary of events in the preovulatory follicle:

1. Estrogen production becomes sufficient to achieve and maintain peripheral threshold concentrations of estradiol which are required in order to induce the LH surge.

2. Acting through its receptors, LH initiates luteinization and progesterone production in the granulosa layer.

3. The preovulatory rise in progesterone facilitates the positive feedback action of estrogen and may be required to induce the midcycle FSH peak.

4. A midcycle increase in local and peripheral androgens occurs, derived from the theca tissue of lesser, unsuccessful follicles.

Ovulation

The preovulatory follicle, through the elaboration of estradiol, provides its own ovulatory stimulus. Considerable variation in timing exists from cycle to cycle, even in the same woman. A reasonable and accurate estimate places ovulation approximately 10-12 hours after the LH peak and 24-36 hours after peak estradiol levels are attained. (44,51) The onset of the LH surge appears to be the most reliable indicator of impending ovulation, occurring 34-36 hours prior to follicle rupture.(52)

Because of the careful timing involved in in vitro fertilization programs, we have available some interesting data.(53) The LH surge tends to occur at approximately 3 AM, beginning between midnight and 7:30 AM in two-thirds of women. Ovulation occurs primarily in the morning during Spring, and primarily in the evening during Autumn and Winter. From July to February, about 90% of women ovulate between 4 and 7 PM; during Spring, half of the women ovulate between midnight and 11 AM.

The gonadotropin surge stimulates a large collection of events which ultimately leads to ovulation, the physical release of the oocyte and its cumulus mass of granulosa cells.(54) This is not an explosive event, therefore, a complex series of changes must occur which cause the final maturation of the oocyte and the decomposition of the collagenous layer of the follicular wall.

The LH surge initiates the resumption of meiosis in the oocyte, luteinization of granulosa cells, and the synthesis of prostaglandins essential for follicle rupture. Premature oocyte maturation and luteinization are prevented by local factors. LH-induced cyclic AMP activity overcomes the local inhibitory action of oocyte maturation inhibitor (OMI) and luteinization inhibitor (LI). OMI originates from the granulosa cells and its activity depends upon an intact cumulus oophorous.

With the LH surge, levels of progesterone in the follicle continue to rise up to the time of ovulation. The progressive rise in progesterone may act to terminate the LH surge as a negative feedback effect is exerted at higher concentrations. In addition to its central

107

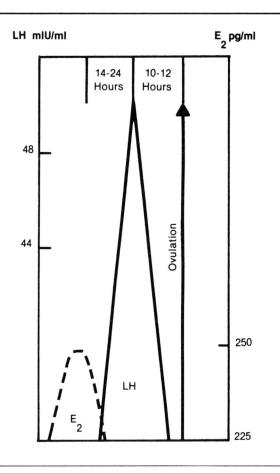

effects, progesterone increases the distensibility of the follicle wall. A change in the elastic properties of the follicular wall is necessary to explain the rapid increase in follicular fluid volume which occurs just prior to ovulation, unaccompanied by any significant change in intrafollicular pressure. The escape of the ovum is associated with degenerative changes of the collagen in the follicular wall so that just prior to ovulation the follicular wall becomes thin and stretched. LH and/or progesterone enhance the activity of proteolytic enzymes, resulting in digestion of collagen in the follicular wall and increasing its distensibility. Proteolytic enzymes such as collagenase and plasmin are present in follicular fluid and are capable of increasing follicle wall distensibility in vitro. The gonadotropin surge also releases histamine, and histamine alone can induce ovulation in some experimental models.

The proteolytic enzymes are activated in an orderly sequence.(55) The granulosa and theca cells produce plasminogen activator in response to the gonadotropin surge. The increased plasminogen activator yields increasing intrafollicular concentrations of plasmin. Plasmin (and other proteases) provoke collagenase activity which results in the degradation of the connective tissue in the wall of the follicle.

Prostaglandins of the E and F series increase markedly in the preovulatory follicular fluid, reaching a peak concentration at ovulation.(56) Inhibition of prostaglandin synthesis blocks follicle rupture without affecting the other LH-induced processes of luteinization and oocyte maturation.(57) The mechanism by which prostaglandins induce follicle rupture is unknown. They may act to free lysosomal enzymes which digest the follicular wall. Smooth muscle cells have been identified in the ovary, and prostaglandins may serve to contract this tissue, thereby aiding the extrusion of the oocyte-cumulus cell mass. This role of prostaglandins is so well demonstrated that infertility patients should be advised to avoid the use of drugs which inhibit prostaglandin synthesis.

Estradiol levels plunge as LH reaches its peak. This may be a consequence of LH down regulation of its own receptors on the follicle. Theca tissue derived from healthy antral follicles exhibits marked suppression of steroidogenesis when exposed to high levels of LH whereas exposure over a low range stimulates steroid production. The low midcycle levels of progesterone exert an inhibitory action on further granulosa cell multiplication, and the drop in estrogen may also reflect this local follicular role for progesterone.

The FSH peak, partially and perhaps totally dependent on the preovulatory rise of progesterone, has several functions. Plasminogen activator is required for conversion of plasminogen to the active proteolytic enzyme, plasmin, involved in the breakdown of the follicle wall. Its production is more sensitive to FSH than to LH. Expansion of the cumulus allows the oocyte-cumulus cell mass to become free-floating in the antral fluid just before follicle rupture.

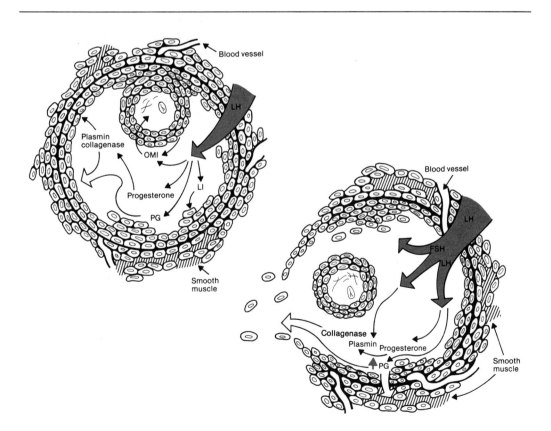

The process involves the deposition of a hyaluronic acid matrix, the synthesis of which is stimulated by FSH. Finally, an adequate FSH peak ensures an adequate complement of LH receptors on the granulosa layer. It should be noted that a shortened or inadequate luteal phase is observed in cycles when FSH levels are low or selectively suppressed at any point during the follicular phase.

The ovulatory period is also associated with a rise in plasma levels of 17α-hydroxyprogesterone. This steroid does not appear to have a role in cyclic regulation, and its appearance in the blood simply represents the secretion of an intermediate product.

The mechanism that shuts off the LH surge is unknown. Within hours after the rise in LH, there is a precipitous drop in the plasma estrogens. The decrease in LH may be due to a loss of the positive stimulating action of estradiol or to an increasing negative feedback of progesterone. The abrupt fall in LH levels may also reflect a depletion in pituitary LH content due to down regulation of GnRH receptors, either by alterations in GnRH pulse frequency or by changes in steroid levels. (58) Finally, LH may further be controlled by "short" negative feedback of LH upon the hypothalamus. Direct LH suppression of hypothalamic releasing hormone production has been demonstrated. It is likely that a combination of all of these influences contribute to the rapid decline in gonadotropin secretion.

An adequate gonadotropin surge does not ensure ovulation. The follicle must be at the appropriate stage of maturity in order for it to respond to the ovulating stimulus. In the normal cycle, gonadotropin release and final maturation of the follicle coincide because the timing of the gonadotropin surge is controlled by the level of estradiol, which in turn is a function of follicular growth and maturation. Therefore, gonadotropin release and morphological maturity are usually coordinated and coupled in time. In the majority of human cycles, the requisite feedback relationships in this system allow only one follicle to reach the point of ovulation. Non-identical multiple births may, in part, reflect the random statistical chance of more than one follicle fulfilling all the requirements for ovulation.

Summary of the ovulatory events:

1. The LH surge stimulates completion of reduction division in the oocyte, luteinization of the granulosa, and synthesis of progesterone and prostaglandins within the follicle.

2. Progesterone enhances the activity of proteolytic enzymes responsible, together with prostaglandins, for digestion and rupture of the follicular wall.

3. The progesterone-influenced midcycle rise in FSH serves to free the oocyte from follicular attachments, to convert plasminogen to the proteolytic enzyme, plasmin, and to ensure that sufficient LH receptors are present to allow an adequate normal luteal phase.

Luteal Phase

After rupture of the follicle and release of the ovum, the granulosa cells increase in size, and assume a characteristic vacuolated appearance associated with the accumulation of a yellow pigment, lutein, which lends its name to the process of luteinization and the anatomical subunit, the corpus luteum. During the first 3 days after ovulation, the granulosa cells enlarge. In addition, theca lutein cells may differentiate from the surrounding theca and stroma to become part of the corpus luteum.

Capillaries penetrate into the granulosa layer, reaching the central cavity and often filling it with blood. By day 8 or 9 after ovulation, a peak of vascularization is reached, associated with peak levels of progesterone and estradiol in the blood. The primate corpus luteum is unique in that it synthesizes all 3 classes of sex steroids, androgens, estrogens, and progestins.

Normal luteal function requires optimal preovulatory follicular development. Suppression of FSH during the follicular phase is associated with lower preovulatory estradiol levels, depressed midluteal progesterone production, and a decrease in luteal cell mass.(59) Experimental evidence supports the contention that the accumulation of LH receptors during the follicular phase predetermines the extent of luteinization and the subsequent functional capacity of the corpus luteum. The successful conversion of the avascular granulosa of the follicular phase to the vascularized luteal tissue is also of importance. Because steroid production is dependent upon low-density lipoprotein (LDL) transport of cholesterol, the vascularization of the granulosa layer is essential to allow LDL-cholesterol to reach the luteal cells. One of the important jobs for LH is to regulate LDL receptor binding, internalization, and postreceptor processing.(60)

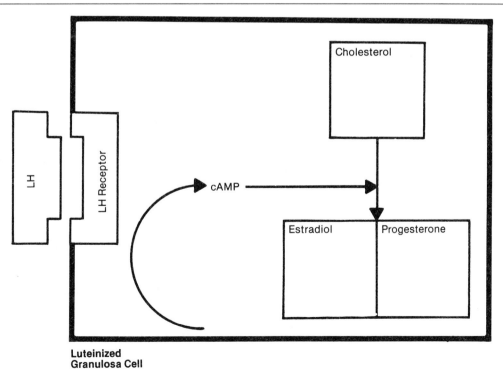

Luteinized
Granulosa Cell

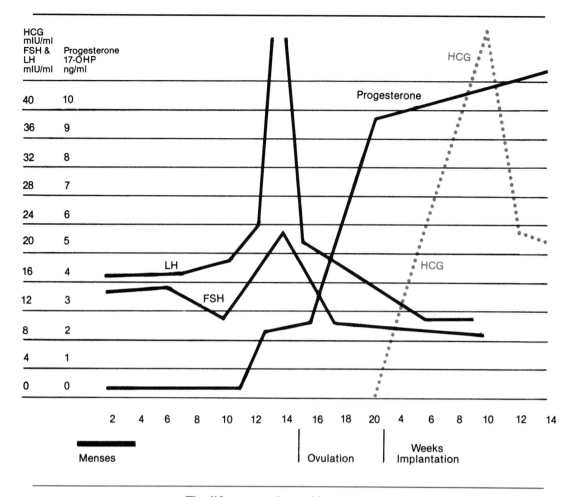

HCG mIU/ml FSH & LH mIU/ml	Progesterone 17-OHP ng/ml
40	10
36	9
32	8
28	7
24	6
20	5
16	4
12	3
8	2
4	1
0	0

HCG

Progesterone

LH

FSH

HCG

2 4 6 8 10 12 14 16 18 20 4 6 8 10 12 14

Menses

Ovulation

Weeks
Implantation

The life-span and steroidogenic capacity of the corpus luteum are dependent on continued tonic LH secretion. Studies in hypophysectomized women have clearly demonstrated that normal corpus luteum function requires the continuous presence of small amounts of LH.(61,62) There is no evidence that other luteotropic hormones, such as prolactin, play a role in the primate menstrual cycle.(63)

Progesterone levels normally rise sharply after ovulation reaching a peak approximately 8 days after the LH surge. Progesterone acts both locally and centrally to suppress new follicular growth. If progesterone concentrations are monitored in ovarian venous effluents following luteectomy in the monkey, ovulation in the subsequent cycle uniformly occurs on the side opposite the higher progesterone level and contralateral to the previous corpus luteum.(64) If circulating progesterone levels are maintained after luteectomy, the subsequent ovulation again occurs in the ovary having a lower progesterone concentration in its venous effluent.(65) Because progesterone antagonizes estrogen action (through depletion of estrogen receptors), it is not surprising that estrogen-dependent follicular mechanisms can be inhibited. Initiation of new follicular growth during the luteal phase is further inhibited by the low levels of gonadotropins due to the negative feedback actions of both estrogen and progesterone. Inhibin levels increase during the luteal phase, presumably originating in the luteinized granulosa cells, and contribute to the achievement of a luteal nadir in FSH secretion.(36) Under normal circumstances (i.e. regular, 28 day cycles), therefore, a woman may ovulate from alternate sides. (15,66) However, short-term ultrasonographic studies have failed to substantiate this.

The secretion of progesterone during the luteal phase is episodic, and the changes correlate closely with LH pulses.(27) Because of this episodic secretion, relatively low midluteal progesterone levels, which some believe are indicative of an inadequate luteal phase, can be found in the course of totally normal luteal phases.

In the normal cycle the time period from the LH midcycle surge to menses is consistently close to 14 days. For practical purposes, luteal phases lasting between 12 and 17 days can be considered normal.(67) This means that some luteal phases lasting 11 days will be normal. The incidence of short luteal phases is about 5-6%. It is well known that significant variability in cycle length among women is due to the varying number of days required for follicular growth and maturation in the follicular phase. The luteal phase cannot be extended indefinitely even with progressively increasing LH exposure, indicating that the demise of the corpus luteum is due to an active luteolytic mechanism.

The corpus luteum rapidly declines 9-11 days after ovulation, and the mechanism of the degeneration remains unknown. In certain nonprimate mammalian species, a luteolytic factor originating in the uterus (prostaglandin $F_{2\alpha}$) regulates the life-span of the corpus luteum. No definite luteolytic factor has been identified in the primate menstrual cycle and removal of the uterus in the primate does not affect the ovarian cycle; however, the morphological regression of luteal cells may be induced by the estradiol produced by the corpus luteum. There is considerable evidence to support a role for estrogen in the decline of the corpus luteum. The premature elevation of circulating estradiol levels in the early luteal phase results in a prompt fall in progesterone concentrations. Direct injections of estradiol into the ovary bearing the corpus luteum induces luteolysis while similar treatment of the contralateral ovary produces no effect. More controversial is the contention that local oxytocin or a related peptide also plays a role in luteolysis. Auletta postulates that prostaglandin $F_{2\alpha}$ produced within the ovary bearing the corpus luteum or within the corpus luteum serves as the luteolytic agent, and the production of the prostaglandin is initiated by the luteal estrogen. (68)

There is another possible role for the estrogen produced by the corpus luteum. In view of the known estrogen requirement for the synthesis of progesterone receptors, luteal phase estrogen may be necessary to allow the progesterone-induced changes in the endometrium after ovulation. Inadequate progesterone receptor content due to inadequate estrogen priming of the endometrium is an additional possible mechanism for infertility or early abortion, another form of luteal phase deficiency.

Degeneration of the corpus luteum is inevitable unless pregnancy intervenes. With pregnancy, survival of the corpus luteum is prolonged by the emergence of a new stimulus of rapidly increasing intensity, human chorionic gonadotropin (HCG). This new stimulus first appears at the peak of corpus luteum development (9-13 days after ovulation), just in time to prevent luteal regression. (69) HCG serves to maintain the vital steroidogenesis of the corpus luteum until approximately the 9th or 10th week of gestation, by which time placental steroidogenesis is well established. In some pregnancies placental steroidogenesis will be sufficiently established by the 7th week of gestation.

Summary of events in the luteal phase:

1. Normal luteal function requires optimal preovulatory follicular development (especially adequate FSH stimulation) and continued tonic LH support.

2. Progesterone acts both centrally and within the ovary to suppress new follicular growth.

3. Regression of the corpus luteum appears to involve the luteolytic action of its own estrogen production, mediated by an alteration in local prostaglandin concentrations.

4. In early pregnancy, HCG maintains luteal function until placental steroidogenesis is well established.

Key Events in the Human Menstrual Cycle

The human menstrual cycle is a recycling system dependent upon essential changes in estradiol levels at key moments in time. Estradiol plays a principal role in the following events:

1. The beginning of the cycle is initiated by a rise in FSH which occurs in response to the decline in estradiol and progesterone in the preceding luteal phase.

2. Estradiol maintains follicular sensitivity to FSH by aiding FSH in increasing the follicle's content of FSH receptors.

3. At high local concentrations estradiol enhances follicular response to LH by working synergistically with FSH to induce LH receptors.

4. Ovulation is triggered by the rapid peripheral rise in estradiol at midcycle.

5. Regression of the corpus luteum may depend upon its own estradiol production and a local luteolytic effect.

The coordination of this complex system can be understood, therefore, by an appreciation for the essential role of estrogen. The interplay between the follicle and the brain depends upon estradiol functioning as a classic hormone, i.e. to transmit the messages of negative and positive feedback, and also upon the local effect of estradiol within the follicle to ensure gonadotropin sensitivity. Events which prevent estrogen production, block estrogen action, or obtund the necessary fluctuations in circulating and local levels will interfere with the normal reproductive cycle.

References

1. **Peters H, Byskov AG, Himelstein-Graw R, Faber M,** Follicular growth: the basic event in the mouse and human ovary, J Reprod Fertil 45:559, 1975.

2. **Mais V, Kazer RR, Cetel NS, Rivier J, Vale W, Yen SSC,** The dependency of folliculogenesis and corpus luteum function on pulsatile gonadotropin secretion in cycling women using a gonadotropin-releasing hormone antagonist as a probe, J Clin Endocrinol Metab 62:1250, 1986.

3. **Vermesh M, Kletzky OA,** Longitudinal evaluation of the luteal phase and its transition into the follicular phase, J Clin Endocrinol Metab 65:653, 1987.

4. **McNatty KP, Makris A, DeGrazia C, Osathanondh R, Ryan KJ,** The production of progesterone, androgens, and estrogens by granulosa cells, thecal tissue, and stromal tissue from human ovaries in vitro. J Clin Endocrinol Metab 49:687, 1979.

5. **Erickson GF,** An analysis of follicle development and ovum maturation, Seminars Reprod Endocrinol 4:233, 1986.

6. **Fletcher WH, Greenan JRT,** Receptor mediated action without receptor occupancy, Endocrinology 116:1660, 1985.

7. **McNatty KP, Makris A, Reinhold VN, DeGrazia C, Osathanondh R, Ryan KJ,** Metabolism of androstenedione by human ovarian tissues in vitro with particular reference to reductase and aromatase activity, Steroids 34:429, 1979.

8. **Hillier SG, Van Den Boogard AMJ, Reichert LE, Van Hall EV,** Intraovarian sex steroid hormone interactions and the regulation of follicular maturation: aromatization of androgens by human granulosa cells in vitro, J Clin Endocrinol Metab 50:640, 1980.

9. **Jia XC, Kessel B, Welsh TH Jr, Hsueh AJW,** Androgen inhibition of follicle-stimulating hormone-stimulated luteinizing hormone receptor formation in cultured rat granulosa cells, Endocrinology 117:13, 1985.

10. **Erickson GF, Magoffin DA, Dyer CA, Hofeditz C,** The ovarian androgen producing cells: a review of structure/function relationships, Endocrine Rev 6:371, 1985.

11. **Chabab A, Hedon B, Arnal F, Diafouka F, Bressot N, Flandre O, Cristol P,** Follicular steroids in relation to oocyte development and human ovarian stimulation protocols, Human Reprod 1:449, 1986.

12. **McNatty KP, Smith DM, Makris A, Osathanondh R, Ryan KJ,** The microenvironment of the human antral follicle; inter-relationships among the steroid levels in antral fluid, the population of granulosa cells, and the status of the oocyte in vivo and in vitro, J Clin Endocrinol Metab 49:851, 1979.

13. **McNatty KP, Markris A, DeGrazia C, Osathanondh R, Ryan KJ,** Steroidogenesis by recombined follicular cells from the human ovary in vitro, J Clin Endocrinol Metab 51:1286, 1980.

14. **Hillier SG, Reichert LE, Van Hall EV,** Control of preovulatory follicular estrogen biosynthesis in the human ovary, J Clin Endocrinol Metab 52:847, 1981.

15. **Chikasawa K, Araki S, Tameda T,** Morphological and endocrinological studies on follicular development during the human menstrual cycle, J Clin Endocrinol Metab 62:305, 1986.

16. **Clark JR, Dierschke DJ, Wolf RC,** Hormonal regulation of ovarian folliculogenesis in rhesus monkeys: III. Atresia of the preovulatory follicle induced by exogenous steroids and subsequent follicular development, Biol Reprod 25:332, 1981.

17. **Zeleznik AJ, Schuler HM, Reichert LE,** Gonadotropin-binding sites in the rhesus monkey ovary: role of the vasculature in the selective distribution of human chorionic gonadotropin to the preovulatory follicle, Endocrinology 109:356, 1981.

18. **Jia XC, Hsueh AJW,** Homologous regulation of hormone receptors: luteinizing hormone increases its own receptors in cultured rat granulosa cells, Endocrinology 115:2433, 1984.

19. **Kessel B, Liu YX, Jia XC, Hsueh AJW,** Autocrine role of estrogens in the augmentation of luteinizing hormone receptor formation in cultured rat granulosa cells, Biol Reprod 32:1038, 1985.

20. **Knecht M, Brodie AMH, Catt KJ,** Aromatase inhibitors prevent granulosa cell differentiation: an obligatory role for estrogens in luteinizing hormone receptor expression, Endocrinology 117:1156, 1985.

21. **Adashi EY, Resnick CE, D'Ercole AJ, Svoboda ME, Van Wyk JJ,** Insulin-like growth factors as intraovarian regulators of granulosa cell growth and function, Endocrine Rev 6:400, 1985.

22. **Dodson WC, Schomberg DW,** The effect of transforming growth factor-β on follicle-stimulating hormone-induced differentiation of cultured rat granulosa cells, Endocrinology 120:512, 1987.

23. **Frederick JL, Shimanuki T, diZerega GS,** Initiation of angiogenesis by human follicular fluid, Science 224:389, 1984.

24. **Adams TE, Norman RL, Spies HG,** Gonadotropin-releasing hormone receptor binding and pituitary responsiveness in estradiol-primed monkeys, Science 213:1388, 1981.

25. **Chappel SC, Resko JA, Norman RL, Spies HG,** Studies on rhesus monkeys on the site where estrogen inhibits gonadotropins: delivery of 17β-estradiol to the hypothalamus and pituitary gland, J Clin Endocrinol Metab 52:1, 1981.

26. **Wildt L, Hutchinson JS, Marshall G, Pohl CR, Knobil E,** On the site of action of progesterone in the blockade of the estradiol-induced gonadotropin discharge in the rhesus monkey, Endocrinology 109:1293, 1981.

27. **Veldhuis JD, Christiansen E, Evans WS, Kolp LA, Rogol AD, Johnson ML,** Physiological profiles of episodic progesterone release during the midcycle phase of the human menstrual cycle: Analysis of circadian and ultradian rhythms, discreet pulse properties, and correlations with simultaneous luteinizing hormone release, J Clin Endocrinol Metab 66:414, 1988.

28. **Filicori M, Santoro N, Merriam GR, Crowley WF Jr,** Characterization of the physiological pattern of episodic gonadotropin secretion throughout the human menstrual cycle, J Clin Endocrinol Metab 62:1136, 1986.

29. **Maruncic M, Casper RF,** The effect of luteal phase estrogen antagonism on luteinizing hormone pulsatility and luteal function in women, J Clin Endocrinol Metab 64:148, 1987.

30. **Laatikainen T, Raisanen I, Tulenheimo A, Salminen K,** Plasma β-endorphin and the menstrual cycle, Fertil Steril 44:206, 1985.

31. **Wehrenberg WB, Wardlaw SL, Frantz AG, Ferin M,** β-Endorphin in hypophyseal portal blood: variations throughout the menstrual cycle, Endocrinology 111:879, 1982.

32. **Marut EL, Williams RF, Cowan BD, Lynch A, Lerner SP, Hodgen GD,** Pulsatile pituitary gonadotropin secretion during maturation of the dominant follicle in monkeys: estrogen positive feedback enhances the biological activity of LH, Endocrinology 109:2270, 1981.

33. **Rivier C, Rivier J, Vale W,** Inhibin-mediated feedback control of follicle-stimulating hormone secretion in the female rat, Science 234:205, 1986.

34. **Bicsak TA, Tucker EM, Cappel S, Vaughan J, Rivier J, Vale W, Hsueh AJW,** Hormonal regulation of granulosa cell inhibin biosynthesis, Endocrinology 119:2711, 1986.

35. **McLachlan RI, Robertson DM, Healy DL, DeKretser DM, Burger HG,** Plasma inhibin levels during gonadotropin-induced ovarian hyperstimulation for IVF: a new index of follicular function? Lancet i:1233, 1986.

36. **McLachlan RI, Robertson DM, Healy DL, Burger HG, De Kretser DM,** Circulating immunoreactive inhibin levels during the normal human menstrual cycle, J Clin Endocrinol Metab 65:954, 1987.

37. **Vale W, Rivier J, Vaughan J, McClintock R, Corrigan A, Woo W, Karr D, Spiess J,** Purification and characterization of an FSH releasing protein from porcine ovarian follicular fluid, Nature 321:776, 1986.

38. **Ling N, Ying S, Ueno N, Shimasaki S, Esch F, Hotta M, Guillemin R,** Pituitary FSH is released by a heterodimer of the β-subunits from the two forms of inhibin, Nature 321:779, 1986.

39. **Mason AJ, Hayflick JS, Ling N, Esch F, Ueno N, Ying SY, Guillemin R, Niall H, Seeburg PH,** Complementary DNA sequences of ovarian follicular fluid inhibin show precursor structure and homology with transforming growth factor-β, Nature 318:659, 1985.

40. **Sealey JE, Cholst I, Glorioso N, Troffa C, Weintraub ID, James G, Laragh JH,** Sequential changes in plasma luteinizing hormone and plasma prorenin during the menstrual cycle, J Clin Endocrinol Metab 63:1, 1987.

41. **Itskovitz J, Sealey JE,** Ovarian prorenin-renin-angiotensin system, Obstet Gynecol Survey 42:545, 1987.

42. **Petraglia F, Di Meo G, Storchi R, Segre A, Facchinetti F, Szalay S, Volpe A, Genazzani AR,** Proopiomelanocortin-related peptides and methionine enkephalin in human follicular fluid: Changes during the menstrual cycle, Am J Obstet Gynecol 157:142, 1987.

43. **Schreiber JR, diZerega GS,** Porcine follicular fluid protein(s) inhibit rat ovary granulosa cell steroidogenesis, Am J Obstet Gynecol 155:1281, 1986.

44. **Pauerstein CJ, Eddy CA, Croxatto HD, Hess R, Siler-Khodr TM, Croxatto HB,** Temporal relationships of estrogen, progesterone, and luteinizing hormone levels to ovulation in women and infrahuman primates, Am J Obstet Gynecol 130:876, 1978.

45. **Collins RL, Hodgen GD,** Blockade of the spontaneous midcycle gonadotropin surge in monkeys by RU 486: a progesterone antagonist or agonist? J Clin Endocrinol Metab 63:1270, 1986.

46. **March CM, Marrs RP, Goebelsmann U, Mishell DR,** Feedback effects of estradiol and progesterone upon gonadotropin and prolactin release, Obstet Gynecol 58:10, 1981.

47. **Liu JH, Yen SSC,** Induction of midcycle gonadotropin surge by ovarian steroids in women: a critical evaluation, J Clin Endocrinol Metab 57:797, 1983.

48. **Judd LH, Yen SSC,** Serum androstenedione and testosterone levels during the menstrual cycle, J Clin Endocrinol Metab 38:475, 1973.

49. **Adams DB, Gold AR,** Rise in female-initiated sexual activity at ovulation and its suppression by oral contraceptives, New Eng J Med 229:1145, 1978.

50. **Hedricks C, Piccinino LJ, Udry JR, Chimbira THK,** Peak coital rate coincides with onset of luteinizing hormone surge, Fertil Steril 48:234, 1987.

51. **World Health Organization Task Force Investigators,** Temporal relationships between ovulation and defined changes in the concentration of plasma estradiol-17β, luteinizing hormone, follicle stimulating hormone, and progesterone, Am J Obstet Gynecol 138:383, 1980.

52. **Hoff JD, Quigley ME, Yen SSC,** Hormonal dynamics at midcycle: a reevaluation, J Clin Endocrinol Metab 57:792, 1983.

53. **Testart J, Frydman R, Roger M,** Seasonal influence of diurnal rhythms in the onset of the plasma luteinizing hormone surge in women, J Clin Endocrinol Metab 55:374, 1982.

54. **Yoshimura Y, Wallach EE,** Studies on the mechanism(s) of mammalian ovulation, Fertil Steril 47:22, 1987.

55. **Yoshimura Y, Santulli R, Atlas SJ, Fujii S, Wallach EE,** The effects of proteolytic enzymes on in vitro ovulation in the rabbit, Am J Obstet Gynecol 157:468, 1987.

56. **Lumsden MA, Kelly RW, Templeton AA, Van Look PFA, Swanston IA, Baird DT,** Changes in the concentrations of prostaglandins in preovulatory human follicles after administration of hCG, J Reprod Fertil 77:119, 1986.

57. **O'Grady JP, Caldwell BV, Auletta FJ, Speroff L,** The effects of an inhibitor of prostaglandin synthesis (indomethacin) on ovulation, pregnancy, and pseudopregnancy in the rabbit, Prostaglandins 1:97, 1972.

58. **Katt JA, Duncan JA, Herbon L, Barkan A, Marshall JC,** The frequency of gonadotropin-releasing hormone stimulation determines the number of pituitary gonadotropin-releasing hormone receptors, Endocrinology 116:2113, 1985.

59. **Smith SK, Lenton EA, Cooke ID,** Plasma gonadotrophin and ovarian steroid concentrations in women with menstrual cycles with short luteal phase, J Reprod Fertil 75:363, 1985.

60. **Golos TG, Soto EA, Tureck RW, Strauss JF III,** Human chorionic gonadotropin and 8-bromo-adenosine 3′,5′-monophosphate stimulate [^{125}I] low density lipoprotein uptake and metabolism by luteinized human granulosa cells in culture, J Clin Endocrinol Metab 61:633, 1985.

61. **Vande Wiele RL, Bogumil J, Dyrenfurth I, Ferin M, Jewelewicz R, Warren M, Rizkallah R, Mikhail G,** Mechanisms regulating the menstrual cycle in women, Rec Prog Hor Res 26:63, 1970.

62. **Hutchison JS, Zeleznik AJ,** The corpus luteum of the primate menstrual cycle is capable of recovering from a transient withdrawal of pituitary gonadotropin support, Endocrinology 117:1043, 1985.

63. **Richardson DW, Goldsmith LT, Pohl CR, Schallenberger E, Knobil E,** The role of prolactin in the regulation of the primate corpus luteum, J Clin Endocrinol Metab 60:501, 1985.

64. **diZerega GS, Lynch A, Hodgen GD,** Initiation of asymmetrical ovarian estradiol secretion in the primate ovarian cycle after luteectomy, Endocrinology 108:1233, 1981.

65. **diZerega GS, Hodgen GD,** The interovarian progesterone gradient: a spatial and temporal regulator of folliculogenesis in the primate ovarian cycle, J Clin Endocrinol Metab 54:495, 1982.

66. **Gougeon A, Lefevre B,** Histological evidence of alternating ovulation in women, J Reprod Fertil 70:7, 1984.

67. **Lenton EA, Landgren B, Sexton L,** Normal variation in the length of the luteal phase of the menstrual cycle: identification of the short luteal phase, Brit J Obstet Gynaecol 91:685, 1984.

68. **Auletta FJ, Flint APF,** Mechanisms controlling corpus luteum function in sheep, cows, nonhuman primates, and women especially in relation to the time of luteolysis, Endocrine Rev 9:88, 1988.

69. **Catt KJ, Dufau ML, Vaitukaitis JL,** Appearance of hCG in pregnancy plasma following the initiation of implantation of the blastocyst, J Clin Endocrinol Metab 40:537, 1975.

4

The Ovary from Conception to Senescence

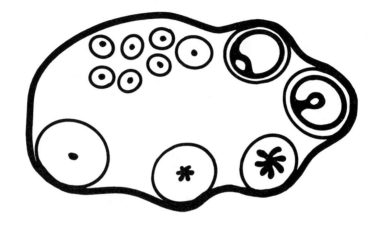

The physiologic responsibilities of the ovary are the periodic release of gametes (eggs) (oocytes) and the production of the steroid hormones, estradiol and progesterone. Both activities are integrated in the continuous repetitive process of follicle maturation, ovulation, and corpus luteum formation and regression. The ovary, therefore, cannot be viewed as a relatively static endocrine organ whose size and function expand and contract depending on the vigor of stimulating tropic hormones. Rather, the female gonad is an envelope containing subunits (follicle, corpus luteum, stroma) with different and variable biologic properties, a heterogeneous everchanging tissue whose cyclicity is measured in weeks, rather than hours. The activity of the human ovary at any given time is defined by a single subunit during the brief period of its dominance.

In this chapter, the development and differentiation of the ovary will be described with emphasis on that most critical functioning subunit of the gonad, the follicle. Events within the ovary will be traced from early embryonic formation to final senescent atrophy. Correlations of morphology with reproductive and steroidogenic functions will be emphasized. Finally, the menopause and the rationale for therapy of this physiologic state will be examined in the light of information on endogenous estrogen production and the impact of estrogen and progestational agents on nonreproductive functions of the female.

Embryology and Differentiation of the Ovary

The ovary consists of two major portions, the outer cortex and the central medulla. The follicles are located in the cortex, and thus it's not surprising that this layer becomes thinner with aging.

The outermost portion of the cortex is called the tunica albuginea, topped on its surface by a single layer of cuboidal epithelium, the germinal epithelium. During fetal life, the development of the human ovary can be traced through four stages. These are: 1) the indifferent gonadal stage, 2) the differentiation and cortical supremacy stage, 3) the period of oogonal multiplication, and finally 4) the stage of follicle formation.

Indifferent Gonadal Stage

At approximately 5 weeks of intrauterine life, the paired gonads are structurally consolidated prominences overlying the mesonephros, forming the gonadal ridge. At this point, although sexual characterization of this tissue is possible by nuclear sex chromatin studies, the gonad is morphologically indistinguishable as a primordial testis or ovary. The gonad is composed of primitive germ cells intermingled with coelomic surface epithelial cells and an inner core of medullary mesenchymal tissue. Just below this ridge lies the mesonephric duct. The germ cells originate in the primitive endoderm of the yolk sac and hindgut, and are recognizable at this site before the mesonephros is formed. They migrate to the gonadal ridge, the one and only site where they survive, in a journey which is completed by the 5th week. The germ cells are the direct precursors of sperm and ova, and by the 6th week, on completion of the indifferent state, these primordial germ cells have multiplied by mitosis to a total of 100,000.

Differentiation and Cortical Supremacy Stage

If the indifferent gonad is destined to become a testis, differentiation along this line will take place at 4-6 weeks. The absence of testicular evolution (formation of medullary primary sex cords, primitive tubules, and incorporation of germ cells) gives implicit evidence of the existence of a primitive, albeit momentarily quiescent, ovary. Despite apparent morphologic inactivity, the cortical dominance over the medulla has been asserted, and estradiol synthesis begins. Although ovarian estrogen is minor compared to the overall production by the placenta, local estrogen may be important in later ovarian differentiation. In contrast to the male, female internal and external genitalia differentiation precedes ovarian maturation. These events are related to the genetic constitution of the germ cells and the territorial receptivity of the mesenchyme. If either factor is deficient or defective, improper development occurs. As has been noted, primitive germ cells are unable to survive in locations other than the gonadal ridge. If partial or imperfect gonadal tissue is formed, the resulting abnormal non-steroidal and steroidal events have wide ranging morphologic, reproductive, and behavioral effects. In the indifferent stage, the mullerian duct system is preserved, and the wolffian potential is unrealized.

Stage of Oogonal Multiplication and Maturation

At 6-8 weeks, the first signs of ovarian differentiation are expressed by the onset of rapid mitotic multiplication of germ cells, reaching 6-7 million oogonia by 20 weeks. This represents the maximal oogonal content of the gonad. From this point in time germ cell content will irretrievably decrease until, some 50 years later, the store of oogonia will be finally exhausted. The egg depletion process by

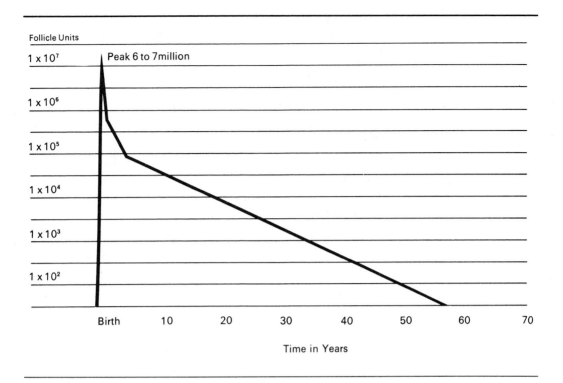

Follicle Units

1 x 10⁷ — Peak 6 to 7million

Time in Years

atresia begins at about 15 weeks of gestation when evidence of nuclear maturation is first seen. The oogonia are transformed to oocytes as they enter the first meiotic division and arrest in prophase.

Stage of Follicle Formation

When nuclear maturation within germ cells becomes noticeable, the gonad is composed of an expanded dense sheet of oogonia and oocytes in huge numbers. At 20 weeks, this highly cellular cortex is gradually perforated by vascular channels originating in the deeper medullary areas. As the finger-like vascular projections enter the cortex, the cortex takes on the appearance of secondary sex cords. As the blood vessels invade and penetrate, they divide the previously solid cortical cell mass into smaller and smaller segments. Drawn in with the blood vessels are perivascular cells which are both mesenchymal and epithelial in origin. These cells surround the oocyte in layers. The resulting unit is the primordial follicle—an oocyte arrested in prophase of meiosis enveloped by a single layer of pregranulosa (germinal epithelial) and an outer less organized matrix of mesenchymal cells (the pretheca cells). Eventually all oocytes are covered in this fashion. Residual mesenchyme not utilized in primordial follicle formation is noted in the interstices between follicles, forming the primitive ovarian stroma. The granulosa cells differentiate from mesonephric or mesenchymal precursors (their specific origin is still disputed), and like the germ cells, they must migrate to the gonadal ridge.

As soon as the oocyte is surrounded by the rosette of pregranulosa cells it may resume meiosis and the entire follicle undergoes variable degrees of maturation before arresting and becoming atretic. These events include in sequence: oocyte cytoplasmic enlargement, eccentric migration of the nucleus, and proliferation of several layers of granulosa cells by mitosis. As a result, a primary follicle is formed. Less frequently, but by no means rarely, further differentiation is expressed as more complete granulosa proliferation. Call-Exner body formation (coalescence to form an antrum) and occasionally a minor theca layer system can be seen.

Even in fetal life the cycle of follicle formation, variable ripening, and atresia occurs. Although these steps are precisely those typical of adult reproductive life, full maturity, as expressed in ovulation, does not occur. However, the ovary at birth can contain several cystic follicles of varying size, undoubtedly stimulated by the reactive gonadotropin surge accompanying the withdrawal of the neonatal hypothalamus and pituitary from negative feedback of massive fetoplacental steroids.

The initiation of follicle maturation and atresia has a profound effect on germ cell endowment. As a result of prenatal follicle differentiation, the total cortical content of germ cells falls to 2 million by birth. This huge depletion of germ cell mass (close to 4-5 million) occurrs over as short a time as 20 weeks. No similar rate of depletion will be seen again. Studies with the scanning electron microscope have indicated that the major mechanism for the loss of eggs during intrauterine life is elimination through the surface of the ovary into the peritoneal cavity.[1] Clusters of oogonia and oocytes make their way through the ovarian stroma and can be seen emerging from the ovarian surface. Due to the fixed initial endowment of germ cells, the newborn female enters life, still far from reproductive potential, having lost 80% of her oocytes.

Neonatal Ovary

At birth, the ovary is approximately 1 cm in diameter, although sizable cystic follicles can enlarge the total dimensions. Compartmentalization of the gonad into cortex and a small residual medulla has been achieved. In the cortex almost all the oocytes are involved in primordial follicle units. Varying degrees of maturation in some units can be seen as in the prenatal state.

Adult Ovary

At the onset of puberty, the germ cell mass has been reduced to 300,000 units. During the next 35-40 years of reproductive life, these units will be depleted further to a point at menopause where only a few thousand units remain. In this period of time the typical cycle of follicle maturation, including ovulation and corpus luteum formation, will be realized. This results from the complex but well-defined sequence of hypothalamic-pituitary-gonadal interactions in which follicle and corpus luteum steroid and pituitary gonadotropin production are integrated to yield ovulation. These important events are described in detail in Chapter 3. For the moment, our attention will be exclusively directed to a description of the events as the gonad is driven inexorably to final and complete exhaustion of its germ cell supply. The major feature of this reproductive period in the ovary's existence is the full maturational expression of some follicle units in ovulation and corpus luteum formation, and the accompaniment of varying steroid output of estradiol and progesterone. For every follicle which ovulates, close to 1,000 will pursue abortive growth periods of variable length.

Follicle Growth	In the adult ovary, the two stages of follicle development noted even in the prenatal period are repeated, but to a more complete degree. Initially the oocyte enlarges and the granulosa cells proliferate markedly. A solid sphere of cells encasing the oocyte is formed. At this point the theca interna is noted in initial stages of formation. The zona pellucida begins to form. In this stage of development gonadotropins must be available, but these events are not the result of an input of follicle-stimulating hormone (FSH) activity. If gonadotropin increments are available, as can be seen early in a menstrual cycle, a second gonadotropin-dependent stage of follicle maturation is seen. The number of follicles that mature is dependent on the amount of FSH and luteinizing hormone (LH) available to the gonad and the sensitivity of the follicles to the gonadotropins.

The sequence of maturation in this second phase of follicle growth proceeds in the following order: The antrum appears as a coalescence of numerous intragranulosa cavities (Call-Exner bodies). Whether this represents liquefaction or granulosa cell secretion is uncertain. At first the cavity is filled with a coagulum of cellular debris. Soon a liquor accumulates, which is essentially a transudation of blood filtered through the avascular granulosa from the theca vessels. With antral formation, the theca interna develops more fully, expressed by increased cell mass, increased vascularity, and the formation of lipid-rich cytoplasmic vacuoles within the theca cells. As the follicle expands, the surrounding stroma is compressed and is called the theca externa.

At any point in this development, individual follicles become arrested and eventually regress in the process known as atresia. At first the granulosa component begins to disrupt. The antral cavity constituents are resorbed, and the cavity collapses and obliterates. The oocyte degenerates in situ. Finally, a ribbon-like scarred streak surrounded by theca is seen. Eventually this theca mass loses its lipid and becomes indistinguishable from the growing mass of stroma. Prior to regression, the cystic follicle may be retained in the cortex for variable periods of time.

The local concentrations of estradiol within the microenvironment of the differentiating follicle exert a major influence on the possibility of its emergence as the dominant follicle destined to ovulate. Antral fluid estradiol concentrations increase as a result of interplay between theca and granulosa cells (the two-cell explanation), reviewed in detail elsewhere (Chapters 1 and 3). The relevant issue is that theca androgen is aromatized to estrogen in granulosa cells. The capacity for aromatization reflects the number of granulosa cells and the biochemical differentiation of the aromatase enzyme system of these cells. These granulosa cell reactions are FSH-induced and catalyzed by local estradiol. The more local estrogen, the more "receptivity" (more cells, more FSH receptors, more aromatase, more estrogen), and the greater likelihood of that follicle becoming dominant and avoiding atresia. Steroid and peptide concentrations found in human follicle fluid sustain this concept; as the follicle grows, androgens decrease, but FSH and estradiol increase. In anovulation, unruptured follicle cysts contain relatively high androgens and low estradiol and FSH.

Local concentrations of estrogen also have been implicated in the mechanism by which, in most cases, only a single unit is selected for the final burst of maturity expressed as ovulation. As FSH quantities diminish prior to ovulation, the most mature follicle, the most efficient estrogen producer, selectively binds available FSH better than its less successful sisters. As a result, the limited FSH supplies are directed to a single maturing follicle.

Ovulation

Of the several follicle units propelled to varying degrees of maturity, one unit will advance to ovulation if gonadotropin stimulation is adequate. Morphologically these events include distension of the antrum by increments of antral fluid, and compression of the granulosa against the limiting membrane separating the avascular granulosa and the luteinized, vascularized theca interna. In addition, the antral fluid increment gradually pinches off the cumulus oophorous, the mound of granulosa enveloping the oocyte. The mechanisms by which the thinning of the theca over the surface of the now protruding, distended follicle, the creation of an avascular area weakening the ovarian capsule, and the final acute distension of the antrum with rupture and extrusion of the oocyte in its cumulus, are not precisely known. Repeated evaluation of intrafollicular pressures has failed to indict an explosive factor in this crucial event.

As demonstrated in a variety of animal experiments, the physical expulsion of the oocyte is dependent upon a preovulatory surge in prostaglandin synthesis within the follicle. Inhibition of this prostaglandin synthesis produces a corpus luteum with an entrapped oocyte. Both prostaglandins and the midcycle surge of gonadotropins are thought to increase the concentration of local proteases, such as plasminogen conversion to plasmin. As a result of generalized tissue weakening (loss of intercellular gap junction integrity and disruption of elastic fibers), there is swift accumulation of antral fluid followed by rupture of the weakened tissue envelope surrounding the follicle.

Corpus Luteum

Shortly after ovulation profound alterations in cellular organization occur in the ruptured follicle that go well beyond simple repair. After tissue integrity and continuity are retrieved, the granulosa cells hypertrophy markedly, gradually filling in the cystic, sometimes hemorrhagic, cavity of the early corpus luteum. In addition, for the first time, the granulosa becomes markedly luteinized by incorporation of lipid-rich vacuoles within its cytoplasm. Both these properties had been the exclusive features of the theca prior to ovulation. For its part, the theca of the corpus luteum becomes less prominent, vestiges being noted eventually only in the interstices of the typical scalloping of the mature corpus luteum. As a result, a new yellow body is formed, now dominated by the enlarged, lipid-rich, fully vascularized granulosa. In the 14 days of its life, dependent on the low but important quantities of LH available in the luteal phase, this unit produces estrogen and progesterone. Failing a new enlarging source of LH-like human chorionic gonadotropin (HCG) from a successful implantation, the corpus luteum rapidly ages. Its vascularity and lipid content wane, and the sequence of scarification (albicantia) ensues.

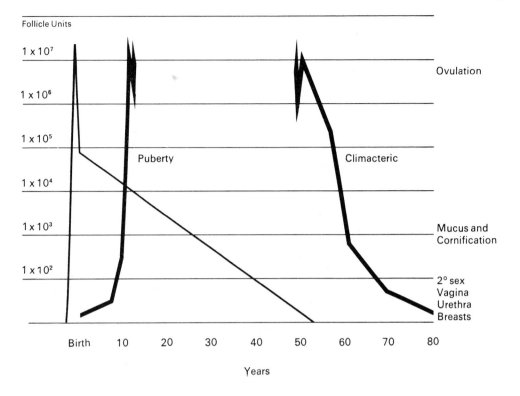

Follicle Units

1 x 10^7

1 x 10^6

1 x 10^5

1 x 10^4

1 x 10^3

1 x 10^2

Ovulation

Puberty

Climacteric

Mucus and
Cornification

2° sex
Vagina
Urethra
Breasts

Birth 10 20 30 40 50 60 70 80

Years

**Correlation of
Follicle Maturation,
Follicle Availability,
and Estrogen
Production**

If one considers the effects of increments of edogenous estrogen production on the body, certain categorical effects can be seen as varying estrogen thresholds are reached. As biologic levels of estrogen increase, the sequence of formation and maintenance of secondary sexual characteristics, cervical mucus secretion, vaginal cornification, endometrial proliferation and menses, and finally ovulation, is achieved. Each event requiring quantum increments in estrogen production is bound to the evolving, increasing maturation of the follicle units.

As we trace estrogen effects over a life-span, with increasing follicle maturation, female phenotype is asserted early, growth spurt is stimulated, and the appearance of secondary sex characteristics is also seen. As individual follicles undergo greater and greater maturity, menarche and the first ovulation are achieved in short order. For the next 30 years, estrogen production and follicle maturation work hand in hand to sustain adult reproductive efficiency via repeated (about 400) monthly ovulations. At this level of steroid production all other estrogen-dependent systems are more than sufficiently sustained.

At approximately age 38-42, ovulation becomes less frequent. It has been suggested that the residual follicle units, now only thousands in number, are the least sensitive to gonadotropin stimulation, and hence are less likely to achieve successful and complete maturation. As numbers of follicle units decrease and resistant fol-

127

licles are left behind, less and less estrogen is produced from the surviving units. Eventually estrogen is no longer sufficient to proliferate endometrium to yield menstruation, and menopause ensues. Further retreat in estrogen production then affects all of those tissues which are estrogen dependent.

At one point during pubescence, enough follicle maturation has yielded sufficient estrogen to cause the first period (menarche). In this respect, menarche is only one point on a curve of ascending estrogen production. Similarly, the climacteric defines a more prolonged period of estrogen withdrawal, starting with the first decrease in frequency of ovulation, and ending in atrophy of secondary sex characteristics. A single point in that curve, when insufficient follicle maturity results in inadequate estrogen and no menses, is the menopause.

Hormone Production After Follicle Exhaustion

Shortly after the menopause, one can safely say that there are no remaining follicles.(2) Prior to menopause, the remaining follicles begin to perform less well. During the perimenopausal period, women who are having regular periods can have lower estradiol levels and higher levels of FSH, and the cycle begins to change, mainly because of a shortening of the follicular phase. (3) This is a time period during which postmenopausal levels of FSH (greater than 40 mIU/ml) can be seen despite continued menstrual bleeding, while LH levels usually still remain in the normal range. It is likely that the elevated FSH levels reflect a declining regulation by the negative feedback action of a nonsteroidal substance produced by the granulosa cells, a peptide called inhibin. Occasionally corpus luteum formation and function occur, and the perimenopausal woman is not totally safe from the threat of an unplanned and unexpected pregnancy until elevated levels of both FSH and LH can be demonstrated.

As cycles become irregular, vaginal bleeding occurs at the end of an inadequate luteal phase or after a peak of estradiol without subsequent ovulation or corpus luteum formation. Eventually there is a 10-20-fold increase in FSH and approximately a 3-fold increase in LH, reaching a maximal level 1-3 years after menopause, after which there is a gradual, but slight, decline in both gonadotropins. Elevated levels of both FSH and LH at this time in life are conclusive evidence of ovarian failure. FSH levels are higher than LH because LH is cleared from the blood so much faster (half-lives are about 30 minutes for LH and 4 hours for FSH).

After menopause, the circulating level of androstenedione is about one half that seen prior to menopause.(4) Most of this postmenopausal androstenedione is derived from the adrenal gland, with only a small amount secreted from the ovary. Testosterone levels do not fall appreciably, and, in fact, the postmenopausal ovary in most women, but not all, secretes more testosterone than the premenopausal ovary. With the disappearance of follicles and estrogen, the elevated gonadotropins probably drive the remaining stromal tissue in the ovary to a level of increased testosterone secretion. The total amount of testosterone produced, however, is decreased because the amount of the primary source, peripheral conversion of androstenedione, is reduced.

The circulating estradiol level after menopause is approximately 10-20 pg/ml, most of which is derived from peripheral conversion of estrone.(4,5) The circulating level of estrone in postmenopausal women is higher than that of estradiol, the mean level being approximately 30-70 pg/ml. The average production rate of estrogen is approximately 45 μg/24 hours; almost all, if not all, being estrogen derived from the peripheral conversion of androstenedione. With increasing age, a decrease can be measured in the circulating levels of dehydroepiandrosterone (DHA) and its sulfate (DHAS), whereas the circulating postmenopausal levels of androstenedione, testosterone, and estrogen remain relatively constant.

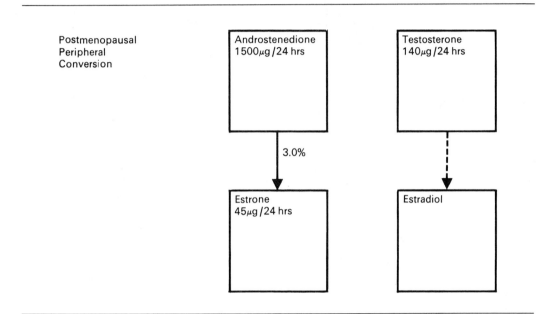

The percent conversion of androstenedione to estrogen correlates with body weight. Increased production of estrogen from androstenedione with increasing body weight is probably due to the ability of fat to aromatize androgens. This fact and a decrease in the levels of sex hormone binding globulin (which results in increased free estrogen concentrations) are the basis for the well-known association between obesity and the development of endometrial cancer. Body weight, therefore, has a positive correlation with the circulating levels of estrone and estradiol. Aromatization of androgens to estrogens is not limited to adipose tissue, however, as almost every tissue tested has shown this activity.

Estrogen production by the ovaries does not continue beyond the menopause; however, estrogen levels in postmenopausal women can be significant, principally due to the extraglandular conversion of androstenedione and testosterone to estrogen. The clinical impact of this estrogen will vary from one postmenopausal woman to another, depending upon the degree of extraglandular production, modified by a variety of factors.

Two major influences are:

1. An increase in substrate (e.g. stress-induced increase in adrenal production of androstenedione).

2. An increase in the percent conversion of androgens to estrogens (a positive correlation exists with body weight and probably with age as well).

Estrogen derived from extraglandular production may be sufficient to sustain breasts and estrogen-stimulated surfaces such as urethra and vagina.

From this review of the physiology of the perimenopause, particularly with respect to mechanisms of hormone production during this period, the physician gains appreciation for mechanisms involved in the clinical diversity of symptomatology seen in practice. Among these are the mechanisms whereby:

—Postmenopausal women may not display signs of progessive genital atrophy.
—Thin women are more likely to have estrogen deprivation symptoms than obese women.
—Obese women are more prone to dysfunctional uterine bleeding, endometrial hyperplasia, and neoplasia.
—Hot flushes and elevated gonadotropins may appear before true menopause (and even on rare occasions be followed by an ovulatory cycle).
—Stress (acute and chronic) may induce a menstrual flow in postmenopausal women.
—Hirsutism may recur or appear for the first time after the menopause.
—Endometrial hyperplasia and carcinoma can occur in untreated, oophorectomized women.

Eventually, the ovarian stroma is exhausted and, despite huge reactive increments in FSH and LH, no further steroidogenesis of importance results from gonadal activity. With increasing age, the adrenal contribution of precursors for estrogen production proves inadequate. In this final stage of estrogen availability, levels are insufficient to sustain secondary sex tissues.

Problems during the Reproductive Years

The Premenstrual Syndrome. It is commonly recognized that behavioral changes may be associated with the menstrual cycle. Indeed, this has been recognized throughout recorded history; this is not a condition which has been ignored. Despite this long period of awareness and attention, however, little progress has been made in clarifying a menstrually-related syndrome.

The simplest definition is a common sense one: the cyclic appearance of a large collection of symptoms, occurring to such a degree that lifestyle or work are affected, and followed by a period of time entirely free of symptoms. The most frequently encountered symptoms include the following: abdominal bloating, anxiety, breast tenderness, crying spells, depression, fatigue, irritability, thirst and appetite changes, and variable degrees of edema of the extremities—all occurring in the last 7 to 10 days of the cycle. The exact constellation of symptoms in an individual is irrelevant; the diagnosis is made by prospectively and accurately charting the cyclic nature of the symptoms.

It is estimated that 20-40% of women report significant problems related to their cycles, and about 20% of that group report a degree of impact on work or lifestyle. The exact prevalence, however, is difficult to ascertain. The symptoms are variable and difficult to quantitate. A further problem which complicates the evaluation of published studies as well as dealing with individual cases, is that behavior is usually related to menstruation in a retrospective fashion. This is prone to considerable subjective bias.(6) For example, studies in the literature point out that some women do not actually experience problems in relation to menstruation, but believe they do.(7) It is argued, rather convincingly, that men and women in our culture have been conditioned to expect symptoms in a woman's premenstrual phase and have been taught to expect fluid retention, pain, and emotional reactions. These sterotypic expectations are precisely what are reported when retrospective charting is utilized. Most importantly, carefully constructed studies (prospective with appropriate statistical analyses) show no significant variation associated with the cycle for cognitive, motor, or social behavior.(8)

Efforts to isolate a specific pathophysiologic mechanism have failed to demonstrate differences between women with and without symptoms for steroid levels throughout the menstrual cycle, or weight gain and measurements of substances involved in fluid regulation, such as aldosterone. Various methods of treatment have been proposed, each championing a presumed etiology. All of the following have failed to demonstrate any clear-cut benefits over placebo: oral contraceptives, vitamin B6, bromocriptine, monomine oxidase inhibitors, and synthetic progestational agents. There has been significant publicity given to the use of progesterone treatment by injection or suppository, long proposed and promoted by Dalton.(9) It is disappointing that this proponent of progesterone treatment has not offered us any scientific evidence to support her claims over 30 years. Very recent appropriately designed and controlled studies have been unable to demonstrate any benefit for progesterone treatment.(10)

Is PMS due to an individual pathologic problem or is it due to cultural beliefs, beliefs that lead to the menstrual cycle being associated with a variety of negative reactions? Throughout our recorded history, we find evidence of menstrual taboos, and the scientific study of menstruation has been hampered by the overpowering influence of traditions, and social and cultural beliefs. What if our societies and cultures had celebrated menstruation as a time of pleasure (and even public joy) rather than something private (to be hidden) and negative? Would we have PMS today? The answer may lie in the unraveling of what role our shared beliefs about menstruation play in our society, rather than the functioning of those beliefs in individuals. To assume that menstrual beliefs and taboos are the creation of men and directed toward women is only an admission of our lack of historical and cultural understanding. However, it is not enough to demonstrate the reality of negative attitudes towards menstruation; it is still an assumption, yet to be proven, that this has etiologic influence on premenstrual experiences.

Where scientists have failed to provide proof, practitioners have seldom failed to provide theories. The list of biological theories is impressive:

Low progesterone levels
High estrogen levels
Falling estrogen levels
Changes in estrogen/progesterone ratios
Increased aldosterone activity
Increased renin-angiotensin activity
Increased adrenal activity
Endogenous endorphin withdrawal
Subclinical hypoglycemia
Central changes in catecholamines
Response to prostaglandins
Vitamin deficiencies
Excess prolactin secretion

But to this date, no firm evidence exists substantiating one or more of these biological theories, and not a single agent can be identified with proven therapeutic efficacy.(11,12)

We offer a modern perspective on this syndrome, suggesting that it is not a single disorder, but rather a collection of different problems. If the practitioner and the patient are convinced of the cyclic nature of a problem (by a prospective record of at least 3 months' duration), try to isolate the specific symptoms and treat with a specific therapy. If fluid retention is perceived by the patient as a principal problem, offer diuretic therapy with spironolactone. If dysmenorrhea is a component of the symptom complex, try one of the inhibitors of prostaglandin synthetase.

A failure to identify a specific disorder with a specific mechanism suggests that premenstrual syndrome represents a variety of psychological manifestations triggered by normal, physiologic hormonal changes. This latter process can be either physiologic in nature or psychosocial and deeply rooted in our cultural history. For that reason, it makes some sense to completely eliminate endogenous sex steroid variability. This can be achieved with medroxyprogesterone acetate, 10-30 mg daily. On occasion, we have induced beneficial and gratifying results in patients with incapacitating emotional swings. But in view of the vague and subjective nature of this syndrome, any such empiric therapeutic treatment must be pursued in a fully informed fashion. If a patient is willing to undergo an empiric trial, we are willing. In doing so, however, neither partner in this contract should be deceived; we must remember that the placebo response may be the underlying basis for any positive response.

Dysmenorrhea. Primary dysmenorrhea, a condition associated with ovulatory cycles and affecting over 50% of menstruating women, is due to myometrial contractions induced by prostaglandins originating in secretory endometrium, while secondary dysmenorrhea is associated with a variety of pathological conditons.(13) Other symptoms associated with menstrual flow, such as headache, nausea and vomiting, backache, and diarrhea, can be explained by entry of the prostaglandins and prostaglandin metabolites into the systemic circulation. There is a 3-fold increase in prostaglandin levels in the endometrium from the follicular phase to the luteal phase, with a further increase during menstruation. Women with primary dysmenorrhea have greater endometrial production of prostaglandins compared to asymptomatic women. Most of the release of prostaglandins during menstruation occurs during the first 48 hours, which coincides with the greatest intensity of the symptoms.

Prostaglandin $F_{2\alpha}$ ($PGF_{2\alpha}$) is the agent responsible for dysmenorrhea. It always stimulates uterine contractions, while the E prostaglandins inhibit contractions in the nonpregnant uterus. Uterine muscle from both normal and dysmenorrheic women is sensitive to $PGF_{2\alpha}$, but the amount of $PGF_{2\alpha}$ produced is the major differentiating factor.

The clinical benefit derived from the pharmacological use of inhibitors of prostaglandin synthesis depends upon a significant decrease in prostaglandin production in the endometrium. An additional role may be attributed to decreased prostaglandins from the platelets participating in the clotting of menstrual blood. The best explanation for the benefit seen with oral contraceptives is decreased prostaglandin synthesis associated with the atrophic decidualized endometrium.

Family	Agents	Dosage
Indoleacetic acid	Indomethacin	25 mg 3–6 times/day
Fenamates	Flufenamic acid	100–200 mg tid
	Mefenamic acid	250–500 mg qid
	Tolfenamic acid	133 mg tid
Arylpropionic acid	Ibuprofen	400 mg qid
	Naproxen	275 mg qid
	Ketoprofen	500 mg tid

The findings in 51 clinical trials of prostaglandin synthetase inhibitors indicate that the fenamates are most effective for relieving pain.(14) The fenamates, in addition to inhibiting prostaglandin synthesis, also have an antagonistic action, competing for prostaglandin binding sites. Side effects associated with these agents are minimal, but can include blurred vision, headaches, dizziness, and gastrointestinal discomfort. The latter can be reduced by taking the medication with milk or food. All of these agents are more potent than aspirin, because the uterus is relatively insensitive to aspirin. Indomethacin has a higher incidence of gastrointestinal side effects. The major contraindications to the use of these agents include gastrointestinal ulcers and hypersensitivity to aspirin and similar agents.

About 80% of dysmenorrheic women are relieved by prostaglandin inhibitors. Improvement is noted in a constellation of symptoms associated with menses, specifically cramping, backache, nausea, vomiting, dizziness, leg pain, insomnia, and headache. A trial of up to 6 months is warranted, with necessary changes in dosage and inhibitors, before abandoning this therapy. Initially it was felt that better relief was achieved if treatment was started 2-3 days before menses in order to lower the tissue level of prostaglandins before breakdown of the endometrium. Fortunately, studies have indicated that treatment is just as effective if begun at the sign of first bleeding, thus decreasing the possibility of taking one of these agents early in pregnancy. Another benefit of prostaglandin inhibition is a reduction in the amount of blood lost with periods. Indeed the agents may be used to treat idiopathic menorrhagia, or the excess flow associated with an intrauterine device (IUD). Most women do not need to take the medication more than 2-3 days.

If dysmenorrhea is not relieved by one of the nonsteroidal, anti-inflammatory analgesics, laparoscopy should be seriously considered to determine the cause of the symptoms.

Climacteric (Menopause and Postmenopause): Clinical Implications and Rationale for Estrogen-Progestin Replacement Therapy

At approximately 40 years of age, the frequency of ovulation decreases. This initiates a period of waning ovarian function called the climacteric, which will last as long as 20 years, and will carry a woman through decreased fertility, menopause, and manifestations of progressive tissue atrophy and aging. The major factor in this evolving picture is the decrease in estrogen production associated with this period of life. A single point in time is the menopause, when insufficient ovarian follicle maturation results in inadequate estrogen and no menses.

Menopause occurs in American women between the ages 48 and 55, with the median age being approximately 50.(15) An earlier menopause is associated with cigarette smoking and living at high altitudes.(16) There is reason to believe that premature ovarian failure occurs in women who have previously undergone abdominal hysterectomy, presumably because ovarian vasculature has been compromised.(17) About 1% of women will experience menopause before the age of 40. In contrast to a decline in the age of menarche during modern times, a review of medieval sources has indicated that the age of menopause has not changed significantly since early Greek days.(18)

The population of postmenopausal women is increasing. Current American census figures indicate that in the 1990's we will approach a figure of 50 million women over 50 years of age. An American woman at the age of 50 can expect to live another 30 years; therefore, women in our country now live approximately one-third of their lives after ovarian failure. The problems of the postmenopausal period, by virtue of the older population size alone, have achieved the status of a major public health concern.

There is a concern at the individual level as well. For some women, menopause signals the beginning of an era of aging with its connotations of diminishing abilities and competence. The menopause, however, should and can mark the beginning of a new and promising period of life, relatively free from previous obligations, ready

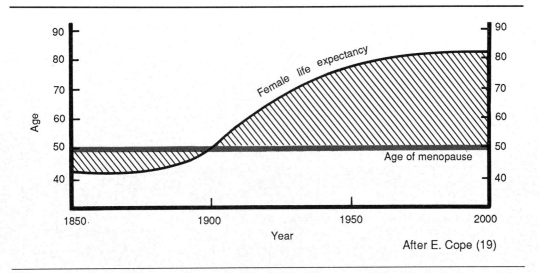

Age

90
80
70
60
50
40

Female life expectancy

Age of menopause

90
80
70
60
50
40

1850   1900   1950   2000

Year

After E. Cope (19)

for new career choices, more education, and new ventures. Good medical practice dictates that the concerned physician should support patients in a positive outlook for this period of time, a period of time which is growing in length and should be increasingly productive and rewarding.

In this section, the clinical implications of estrogen withdrawal will be reviewed. A policy supporting replacement hormonal therapy, consistent with cautious medical practice and based on supporting data, will be offered. The standard hormonal replacement program now includes the combination of estrogen with a progestational agent. The reason for this combined estrogen-progestin approach is the need to prevent the increased risk of endometrial cancer associated with exposure to unopposed estrogen. In our consideration of the risks and benefits of this approach, attention must be directed to the impact of the progestational agent on the important health issues of the postmenopausal years.

Clinical Implications of Progressive Estrogen Withdrawal

Although estrogen does not wane in a straight line function, its progressive diminution over time leads to a sequential loss of estrogen-dependent functions: ovulation, menstrual function, vaginal and vulvar tissue strength, and finally, generalized atrophy of all estrogen-sensitive tissues.

This estrogen loss is due to the continued attrition in the numbers of residual follicle units in the 5th decade of life. Because fewer follicles are available, less and less estrogen production is possible. It must be remembered that these oldest follicle units have perhaps remained in the ovary unstimulated by gonadotropins not entirely by chance, but possibly due to their inherent refractoriness to otherwise appropriate gonadotropin stimulation. When these are finally activated, the degree of differentiation each is likely to experience is limited. Thus each follicle growth period will be increasingly blunted, with less estrogen produced. Eventually even the older and sluggish follicles are exhausted, and estrogen production is now at a low level, resulting almost entirely from indirect resources, the peripheral conversion in nonendocrine tissue sites of ovarian and adrenal precursors to active estrogen.

135

Finally, the gonadal resource becomes defunct, and the ovary shrivels to an atrophic mass of fibrous tissue. Estrogenicity, now at marginally sustaining levels, depends upon adrenal activity. As peripheral tissues age (now in the 7th, 8th, and 9th decades) even these low levels wane still further.

The symptoms frequently seen and related to estrogen loss in this protracted climacteric are:

1. Disturbances in menstrual pattern, including anovulation and reduced fertility, decreased flow or hypermenorrhea, and irregular frequency of menses.

2. Vasomotor instability (hot flushes and sweats). Hot flushes are not well understood, but apparently are the result of instability between the hypothalamus and the autonomic nervous system, brought about by a decline in estrogen. They are especially disturbing at night, perhaps because the hypothalamus is relatively unoccupied.

3. Psychological symptoms, including anxiety, increased tension, mood depression, and irritability, although a direct cause and effect relationship between these symptoms and estrogen is hard to establish.

4. Atrophic conditions: atrophy of vaginal epithelium, formation of urethral caruncles, dyspareunia and pruritus due to vulvar, introital, and vaginal atrophy, general skin atrophy, urinary difficulties such as urgency and abacterial urethritis and cystitis.

5. A variety of complaints such as headaches, insomnia, myalgia, and changes in libido.

6. Health problems secondary to long-term deprivation of estrogen: the consequences of osteoporosis and cardiovascular disease.

A precise understanding of the symptom complex the individual patient may display is often difficult to achieve. Some patients will experience severe multiple reactions that may be disabling. Others will show no reactions, or minimal reactions, which go unnoticed until careful medical evaluation. The majority of women (50-60%) require medical assistance and support for intermittent difficulties of moderate severity.

It appears that 3 factors are at work in all climacteric women. The symptomatic reaction is the sum of the impact of these 3 components:

1. The amount of estrogen depletion and the rate at which estrogen is withdrawn.

2. The collective inherited and acquired propensities to succumb or withstand the impositions of the overall aging process.

3. The psychologic impact of aging and the individual's reaction to the emotional implications of ''a change of life.''

We have found it helpful to classify the hormonal problems in 3 categories:

1. Those associated with *estrogen deprivation* such as flushes, atrophic vaginitis, urethritis, and osteoporosis.

2. Those associated with relative *estrogen excess* such as dysfunctional uterine bleeding, edometrial hyperplasia, and endometrial cancer.

3. Those associated with *estrogen-progestin replacement* therapy.

The Problems of Estrogen Deprivation

Altered Menstrual Function. Oligomenorrhea followed by amenorrhea is usually the first clinical evidence of the female climacteric, although fertility has declined since age 30, and many premenopausal women note the transient presence of hot flushes prior to the cessation of menses. The diagnosis of permanent loss of menses requires sufficient follow-up time for retrospective confirmation. Usually 6-12 months of amenorrhea in a woman over 45 years of age is the commonly accepted rule of thumb for diagnosis of menopause. Only rarely will vaginal bleeding reappear; when it does, organic pathology must be ruled out. Many women will insist that pregnancy be ruled out and confirmation of postmenopausal status be obtained by measurement of FSH and LH levels.

Vasomotor Symptoms. The vasomotor flush is viewed as the hallmark of the female climacteric, experienced to some degree by at least 85% of postmenopausal women. The term "hot flush" is descriptive of a sudden onset of reddening of the skin over the head, neck and chest, accompanied by a feeling of intense body heat and concluded by sometimes profuse perspiration. Their duration varies from a few seconds to several minutes, and rarely for an hour. Their frequency may be rare to recurrent every 10-30 minutes. Finally, flushes are more frequent and severe at night (when a woman is often awakened from sleep) or during times of stress. Although the flush can occur in the premenopause, it is a major feature of postmenopause, lasting in most women for 1-2 years, but, in some (as many as 25-50%) for longer than 5 years.

Although the hot flush is the most common problem of the postmenopause, it presents no inherent health hazard. The flush coincides with a surge of LH (not FSH) and is preceded by a subjective prodromal awareness that a flush is beginning.(20) This aura is followed by measurable increased heat over the entire body surface. Core temperature falls. In short, the flush is not a release of accumulated body heat but is a sudden inappropriate excitation of heat release mechanisms. Its relationship to the LH surge and temperature change within the brain is not understood. The observation that flushes occur after hypophysectomy indicates that the mechanism is not dependent or due directly to LH release. In other words, the same hypothalamic event that causes flushes also stimulates gonadotropin releasing hormone (GnRH) secretion and elevates LH.

The correlation between the onset of flushes and estrogen reduction is clinically supported by the effectiveness of estrogen replacement therapy and the absence of flushes in hypoestrogen states, such as gonadal dysgenesis. Only after estrogen is administered and with-

137

drawn do hypogonadal women experience the hot flush. Curiously, control of this symptom can require estrogen doses in excess of premenopausal physiologic levels. Although the clinical impression that premenopausal surgical castrates suffer more severe vasomotor reactions is widely held, this is not borne out in objective study.(21)

Osteoporosis. Osteoporosis, a change of bone structure characterized by a reduction in quantity rather than chemical composition, results in mechanical fragility with subsequent fracture. Bones get their strength from a structure of protein fibers combined with hard calcium phosphate crystals. A reduction of both bone protein and calcium results in osteoporosis.

The osteoporotic disabilities sustained by the castrate or postmenopausal woman include back pain, decreased height and mobility, and fractures of the vertebral body, humerus, upper femur, distal forearm, and ribs. Loss of mineral content of bone happens in all aging individuals; however, white and oriental women start losing bone earlier and at a more rapid rate than black women. Thus, not only a sexual but also a racial difference exists. Epidemiologic studies have revealed the following:

1. Spinal (vertebral) compression fracture: Symptomatic spinal osteoporosis causing pain, loss of height, postural deformities with consequent pulmonary, gastrointestinal, and bladder dysfunction, is 5 times more common in white women than men. Approximately one-third of women over 65 years of age have spinal compression fractures. The average non-treated postmenopausal white woman can expect to shrink 2.5 inches.

2. Colles fractures: There is a 10-fold increase in distal forearm fractures in white women as they progress from age 35 to 60 years.

3. Head of femur fractures: The incidence of hip fractures also increases with age in white women, rising from 0.3/1000 to 20/1000 from 45 to 85 years. Eighty percent of all hip fractures are associated with osteoporosis. This fracture carries a heavy risk of morbidity and mortality. Between 15-20% of patients with hip fracture die due to the fracture or its complications (surgical, embolic, cardiopulmonary) within 3 months, and Beals found that only half of hip fracture victims in Portland, Oregon, survived for 1 year.(22) In addition, the survivors are frequently severely disabled and may become permanent invalids.

Loss of estrogen is a major factor affecting the risk of osteoporosis for postmenopausal women; 75% or more of the bone loss which occurs in women during the first 20 years after menopause is attributable to estrogen deficiency rather than to aging itself.(23,24) Vertebral bone is especially vulnerable, beginning to decline as early as 20 years of age.(25) Vertebral bone mass can be found to be significantly decreased in perimenopausal and early postmenopausal women who have rising FSH and decreasing estrogen levels, while bone loss from the radius is not found until at least a year out from the menopause.(26) This early loss of axial skeleton bone suggests that the hypoestrogenic postmenopausal state is not the only cause of vertebral osteoporosis.(27) The obvious suspect is a decline in dietary intake of calcium, nevertheless menopause and the loss of estrogen remain as the major contributors to bone loss. The risk of fracture depends upon 2 factors: the bone mass achieved at maturity and the subsequent rate of bone loss. The bone density which is the threshold for vertebral fractures is only slightly below the lower limit of normal for premenopausal women. (28)

There is an epidemic of fractures in older people in the parts of the world with a high standard of living.(29) The incidence in Oslo, Norway, was 5 times greater in 1982 than in 1950.(30) This increase is greater than can be explained by the increasing number of elderly people. A favored explanation is the change in dietary practices in affluent societies, notably the elimination of dairy products. Other possibilities include decreasing parity and the loss of a protective effect from the high steroid levels of pregnancy, and an earlier and greater loss of bone because of the impact of smoking.

Unquestionably, exercise and diet have a beneficial effect on bone integrity. Equally impressive is the accumulating evidence that an appropriate estrogen replacement program can have a major impact on the risk of fractures. One can expect a 50 to 60% decrease in fractures of the arm and hip (31-33), and when estrogen is supplemented with calcium, an 80% reduction in vertebral compression fractures can be observed.(34) It should be noted that the addition of vitamin D, or its active metabolite, has no impact on the fracture rate, and some women develop hypercalcemia with a risk of renal stone formation.(34,35) The addition of fluoride, a potent stimulator of bone formation, does offer some benefit; however a high rate of side effects (40%) is encountered, including joint and tendon inflammation, anemia, and gastrointestinal disturbances. Therefore, the optimal regimen is a combination of sex steroids and calcium.

An analysis of aging women's calcium needs indicated a greater requirement than previously appreciated.(36) In order to remain in zero calcium balance, women on estrogen replacement require a total of 1,000 mg elemental calcium per day. Since the average woman receives only 500 mg of calcium in her diet, the minimal daily supplement equals an additional 500 mg. Women not on estrogen replacement require a daily supplement of at least 1,000 mg. Unfortunately in the absence of estrogen, there is significant impairment of calcium absorption. Even with the commonly used therapeutic intake doses, nearly 40% of postmenopausal women will have inefficient absorption.(37) Therefore estrogen improves calcium absorption and makes it possible to utilize supplemental calcium in effective doses without the side effects associated with higher doses (constipation and flatulence) which diminish compliance.

Despite the important role for calcium, a woman cannot totally substitute for the effectiveness of estrogen by compensatory increases in calcium supplementation. In the absence of estrogen, calcium, even in supplemental doses of 2000 mg/day, has only a little impact on trabecular bone, and a minor impact on compact bone.(38,39) This makes one think that the action of estrogen, besides its effect on calcium absorption, must include a direct protective mechanism on the bone. Bone resorption is regulated by osteoclasts whereas osteoblasts form bone. Estrogen receptors have now been identified in osteoblasts.

**Calcium requirement
for zero balance (36)**

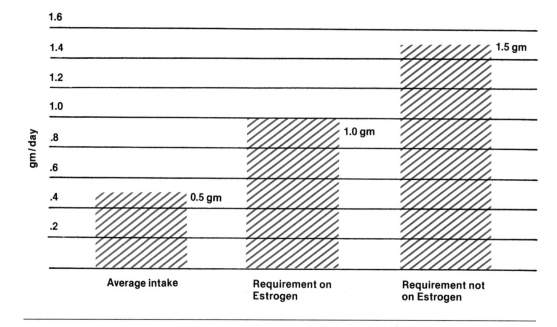

Because progestational agents are anti-estrogenic, it is not illogical to question whether the addition of a progestin to an estrogen program counters the beneficial impact of estrogen on the bone. Fortunately progestational agents independently, in a manner similar to estrogen, reduce bone resorption, but when added to estrogen, progestins actually lead to an increase in bone formation, associated with a positive balance of calcium. (40-42) This positive calcium balance has been documented to last for at least 3 years in early postmenopausal women, and for at least 1 year in 70 year old women. This is a strong argument in favor of treating very old women who have never been on estrogen. Estrogen use between the ages of 65 and 74 has been documented to protect against hip fractures.(33)

The precise mechanism of action for sex steroid protection of bones remains unknown. It is apparent that the beneficial impact is achieved without significant changes in the blood levels of the various calcium regulating hormones. In addition, recent data do not support a role for calcitonin in postmenopausal osteoporosis.(43) Increased efficiency of calcium absorption and a still to be determined role for the estrogen receptors in the osteoblasts are likely important factors.

The protection of estrogen is maintained only while women are maintained on the replacement hormone. In the 3 to 5 year period following loss of estrogen, whether after menopause or after cessation of estrogen therapy, there is an accelerated loss of bone.(44,45) While this was not confirmed in one study (46), a careful analysis points out that bone mineral must be measured in the same exact sites because of differences in composition. When this is done an effect of estrogen is seen only in current users, and prior users have a prevalence rate of vertebral osteoporosis similar to women who have never taken estrogen.(47) For the greatest impact on fractures, it is vital that estrogen-progestin replacement be initiated as close to the menopause as possible, and it must be maintained long-term, if not life long.

Cigarette smoking is associated with an earlier menopause and an increased risk of osteoporosis. Because estrogen blood levels are lower in smokers who are on estrogen when compared to non-smokers, it is concluded that smoking increases liver metabolism of estrogen.(48) Others have documented that smoking induces 2-hydroxylation of estradiol; the metabolic products, 2-hydroxyestrogens, have minimal estrogenic activity and are cleared rapidly from the circulation.(49) In addition, constituents of cigarette smoke inhibit granulosa cell aromatase, providing a further explanation for an earlier menopause in smokers.(50) Lower blood levels of estrogen in smokers have been correlated with a reduced bone density, and therefore, estrogen replacement does not totally counteract the predisposition of smoking towards osteoporosis.

Patients who already have osteoporosis should be treated more vigorously. In addition to hormone replacement, treatment should include the active metabolite of vitamin D, and either fluoride or calcitonin or both, depending upon the severity of the condition. Patients with apparent osteoporosis should also be screened for other conditions which lead to osteoporosis:

1. Serum parathyroid hormone, calcium, phosphorous, and alkaline phosphatase—for primary hyperparathyroidism.

2. Renal function tests—for secondary hyperparathyroidism with chronic renal failure.

3. Blood count and smear, and sedimentation rate—for multiple myeloma, leukemia, or lymphoma.

4. Thyroid function tests—for thyrotoxicosis.

5. Careful history and, when indicated, appropriate laboratory studies to rule out hypercortisolism.

The prevention of osteoporosis in aging women now constitutes a major public health problem. By virtue of the large number of women living a significant postmenopausal time-span, a major reduction in the clinical manifestations of osteoporosis will have a very large impact on our health care system and our patients in terms of quality of life, mortality, and money saved.

An aggressive approach is necessary for two reasons. First, therapy is more effective the closer it is initiated to menopause, and second, once significant amounts of bone have been lost, complete retrieval can never be achieved.

Finally, we would be remiss if we did not promote the benefits of exercise. Physical activity (weight-bearing), as little as 30 minutes a day for 3 days a week, will increase the bone mineral content of bone in older women.(51) The exercise need not be extreme. Walking and ordinary calisthenics will suffice. The impact of exercise on vertebral trabecular bone is significantly less, however, and women require the full combination of hormone replacement, calcium supplementation, and exercise in order to fully minimize the risk of vertebral compression fractures.

Cardiovascular Effects. In the United States, diseases of the heart and the circulation are now the leading causes of death.

Relative Risks of Conditions Affected by Estrogen (52)	
Condition	*Cumulative Mortality Ages 50–75 per 100,000*
Ischemic heart disease	10,500
Breast cancer	1,875
Osteoporotic fractures	938
Endometrial cancer	188
Gallbladder disease	3

A protective effect of replacement estrogen on heart disease, if real, would be a significant benefit of therapy. A review of the literature finds overwhelming support for a reduced risk of cardiovascular disease in estrogen users. In 8 case-control studies, only one failed to show a decreased relative risk of cardiovascular disease, a study which included only 17 cases, most of whom were smokers and all under age 50. (53-60)

In 8 cohort studies, 5 showed a reduced risk of ischemic heart disease in estrogen users; the 3 others produced conflicting data.(61-68) The Walnut Creek Study (64) had only 26 women with infarctions, and only 9 were estrogen users.

The Framingham Study presented data in 1978, and in 1985, which argued that there was a 50% increased risk for cardiovascular disease among estrogen users, although there was no difference in fatality rates between users and non-users.(63,67) Because of the respect the Framingham Study carries, especially in the circles of Internal Medicine, its impact is significant. There are, however, 2 major criticisms of the Framingham report. First, the patient numbers are relatively small (302 postmenopausal women on estrogen) in comparison to the patient numbers in other studies on this particular issue. Furthermore, the effect of dose and duration of treatment cannot be ascertained; they were not recorded. Finally and most conclusively, a subsequent reanalysis of the Framingham data by the authors of the study reversed their conclusion.(69) The early reports from the Framingham Study, therefore, stand in lonely opposition to overwhelming evidence that appropriately low doses of estrogen protect postmenopausal women against cardiovascular disease.

The Nurses' Health Study surveyed 121,964 nurses; 32,317 postmenopausal women were free of coronary heart disease when initially evaluated, and subsequently 90 had either nonfatal or fatal disease.(68) The age-adjusted relative risk of coronary disease in ever users showed a 50% reduction, and current users showed a 70% reduction!

The Lipid Research Clinics Follow-Up Study (a prospective 8.5 year follow-up of 2270 women) has demonstrated a 63% reduction in the relative risk of fatal cardiovascular disease in current estrogen users, including a protective effect in current and exsmokers.(65) A prospective study in a retirement community (under relatively controlled and accurate conditions), begun in 1981, had, by 1986, demonstrated a 16% decrease in death from all causes in estrogen users, and a 46% decrease in death from acute myocardial infarctions.(52)

Sophisticated assessment and analysis (using the methods of information synthesis and meta-analysis) indicate that the effect of estrogen on heart disease is not controversial or ambiguous, but there clearly exists a protective benefit.(70) The public health importance of the impact of estrogen on cardiovascular disease is very significant, outranking even osteoporosis.

Estimated Mortality Changes Induced by Estrogen (52)		
Condition	Relative Risk	Cumulative Change in Mortality Ages 50–75 per 100,000
Ischemic heart disease	0.5 RR	−5,250
Osteoporotic fractures	0.4 RR	−563
Endometrial cancer	2.0 RR	+63
Gallbladder disease	1.5 RR	+2

The bulk of evidence, when controlled for age and cigarette smoking, indicates that women who undergo a natural menopause do not have an appreciable increase in the risk of coronary heart disease as compared with premenopausal women.(71) In contrast, bilateral oophorectomy, especially relatively early in life, does increase the risk of heart disease. These findings strongly suggest that the beneficial impact of estrogen replacement on heart disease cannot be explained by presuming that the premenopausal state is restored. Rather this effect of estrogen must be achieved by specific pharmacologic consequences. Approximately 75% of the overall reduction in mortality in estrogen ever-users is due to protection against heart disease. The mechanism of this protection appears to be due in significant part to a pharmacologic effect of estrogen on lipoprotein levels.(65)

The lipoproteins which carry cholesterol in the blood affect the risk of cardiovascular disease. The low-density lipoprotein carrier of cholesterol (LDL-cholesterol) is the fraction which is most atherogenic. Particularly in older age people, an inverse relationship exists between the high-density lipoprotein (HDL-cholesterol) and coronary mortality. The mechanism of change due to sex steroids involves a plasma enzyme, hepatic lipase, which catalyzes the hydrolysis of phospholipids on the surface of the lipoproteins, allowing the lipoproteins to be irreversibly degraded. Androgens increase this enzyme activity, and estrogen decreases it.(72) Thus the elevated levels of HDL-cholesterol associated with estrogen replacement, and protection against heart disease, consist of the subfraction of HDL-cholesterol which is most strongly associated with both estrogen and risk of cardiovascular disease. The small increase in triglyceride often seen with estrogen is of no consequence except in individuals with genetic disorders of triglyceride metabolism.

The impact of estrogen therapy on the lipid profile is maintained as long as women remain on the estrogen. A higher HDL-cholesterol and lower LDL-cholesterol have been documented to persist through at least 10 years of postmenopausal treatment.(73) Here too is another argument in favor of physical exercise. There is a significant positive relationship between HDL-cholesterol levels and physical activity in postmenopausal women.(74)

Because the public health benefit of estrogen replacement on cardiovascular disease is of such enormous impact, it is vital that we know whether the addition of monthly progestin has an adverse effect on the lipid profile, and ultimately on cardiovascular disease. A review of the literature on this question suggests a dose-response relationship.(75-82)

A decrease in HDL-cholesterol has been noted with 10 day monthly treatment with norethindrone (5 mg), megestrol acetate (5 mg), levonorgestrel (250 μg), and even medroxyprogesterone acetate (10 mg). No significant change was noted with micronized progesterone (200 mg). It is probable that there is a dose-response relationship between progestins and their effect on the lipoproteins. The lack of an effect noted with micronized progesterone was observed with a dose (200 mg daily) which yields a normal luteal phase blood level of progesterone. A similar "physiologic" dose of synthetic progestins may be free of an adverse impact on HDL-cholesterol. In at least one study, a small amount of synthetic progestin (30 μg levonorgestrel) had no effect on LDL-cholesterol and HDL-cholesterol.(81) It is imperative that clinical studies determine the long-term relationship between various progestins and the lipoproteins as soon as possible. This underscores the need to determine the lowest progestational dose which safely maintains endometrial protection (and perhaps the breast) as well. One 3 year study of the usual sequential program with the utilization of 10 mg medroxyprogesterone acetate for 10 days every month concluded that a favorable lipoprotein profile was maintained.(83)

Hypertension is both a risk factor for cardiovascular mortality and a common problem in older people. It is important, therefore, to know that no relationship has been established between hypertension and the doses of estrogen used for replacement therapy. Studies have either shown no effect or a small, but statistically significant, decrease in blood pressure due to estrogen treatment.(84-87) This has been the case in both normotensive and hypertensive women. The rare cases of increased blood pressure due to estrogen replacement therapy truly represent idiosyncratic reactions. Because of the protective impact of appropriate estrogen replacement on the risk of cardiovascular disease, it can be argued that a woman with controlled hypertension is in need of that specific benefit of estrogen.

The blood pressure impact of the addition of a progestational agent to an estrogen replacement program is yet unknown. Here again, until this information is available, there is no reason to change the current practice or to withhold an estrogen-progestin program from women with controlled hypertension; however, close monitoring of the blood pressure makes good clinical sense.

Finally, when estrogen replacement therapy is administered in the usual dosage to postmenopausal women, there is no increase observed in stroke, thromboembolism, or myocardial infarction. This reinforces the dose-response relationship between estrogen and thrombosis (also discussed in Chapter 15), and it is not surprising that relatively physiologic doses of estrogen are free of thrombotic side effects.

Atrophic Change. With extremely low estrogen production in the late postmenopausal age, or many years after castration, atrophy of all mucosal surfaces takes place, accompanied by vaginitis, pruritus, dyspareunia, and stenosis. Genitourinary atrophy leads to a variety of symptoms which affect the ease and quality of living. Urethritis with dysuria, urgency incontinence, and urinary frequency are further results of mucosal thinning, in this instance, of the urethra. Vaginal relaxation with cystocele, rectocele, and uterine prolapse, and vulvar dystrophies are not a consequence of estrogen deprivation. Genuine stress incontinence will not be affected by treatment with estrogen.(88)

Unless dermatologic conditions exist masquerading as menopausal atrophy, estrogen replacement is invariably successful in reversing these atrophic problems. Relief from these problems often results in significant improvements in general well-being.

Dyspareunia seldom brings older women to our offices. A basic reluctance to discuss sexual behavior still permeates our society, especially among older patients and physicians. Gentle questioning may lead to estrogen treatment of atrophy and enhancement of sexual enjoyment. Objective measurements have demonstrated that vaginal factors which influence the enjoyment of sexual intercourse can be maintained by appropriate doses of estrogen.(89) Both patient and physician should be aware that a significant response can be expected by one month but it takes a long time to fully restore the genitourinary tract (6-12 months), and physicians and patients should not be discouraged by an apparent lack of immediate response. Furthermore sexual activity by itself supports the circulatory response of the vaginal tissues and enhances the therapeutic effects of estrogen. Therefore sexually active older women will have less atrophy of the vagina even without estrogen replacement.

One of the features of aging in men and women is a steady reduction in muscular strength. Many factors affect this decline, including height, weight, and level of physical activity. However, women currently using estrogen replacement do not demonstrate this age-related decline in muscular competence (as measured by handgrip strength).(90) This can be viewed as another substantial benefit of estrogen replacement, with potential protective consequences against fractures, as well as a benefit due to the ability to maintain vigorous physical exercise. In addition, there is evidence from the Netherlands, that estrogen replacement before the onset of joint disease is associated with protection against rheumatoid arthritis.(91)

Menopausal Syndrome. There are additional problems encountered in the early postmenopause that are seen frequently, but their causal relation with estrogen is uncertain. Called the menopausal syndrome, these problems include: fatigue, nervousness, headaches, insomnia, depression, irritability, joint and muscle pain, dizziness, and palpitations. Attempts to study the effects of estrogen on these problems have been hampered by the subjectivity of the complaints (high placebo responses) and the "domino effect" of what reduction of hot flushes does to the frequency of the symptoms. Using a double-blind crossover prospective study format, Campbell and Whitehead (92) have concluded that many symptomatic "improvements" ascribed to estrogen therapy result from relief of hot flushes—a domino effect. On the other hand, a tonic effect (improvement in memory and reduction of anxiety) was also noted in these observations. Fatigue, irritability, headache, and depression are not thought to be estrogen-related phenomena.

Emotional stability during the perimenopausal period, may be disrupted by poor sleep patterns. Estrogen therapy improves the quality of sleep, decreasing the time to onset of sleep, and increasing the rapid eye movement (REM) sleep time.(93) Perhaps flushing may be insufficient to awaken a woman, but sufficient to affect the quality of sleep, thereby diminishing the ability to handle the next day's problems and stresses.

There is a general clinical consensus that certain physical changes (redistribution of fat deposits and loss of elastic tissue of the skin with wrinkling) are due to aging rather than to estrogen deprivation.

Problems of Excess Estrogen

Not all climacteric women experience symptoms or signs of estrogen deprivation. Some actually manifest estrogen excess via the presence of uterine bleeding, dysfunctional uterine bleeding.

Throughout the usual period of life identified with perimenopause (ages 40-60), there is a significant incidence of dysfunctional uterine bleeding. Although the greatest concern provoked by this symptom is endometrial neoplasia, the usual finding is non-neoplastic tissue displaying estrogen effects unopposed by progesterone. This results from anovulation in the premenopausal women and from extragonadal endogenous estrogen production or estrogen administration in the postmenopausal woman.

There are 4 mechanisms which could result in increased endogenous estrogen levels:

1. Increased precursor androgen (functional and nonfunctional endocrine tumors, liver disease, stress).

2. Increased aromatization (obesity, hyperthyroidism, liver disease).

3. Increased direct secretion of estrogen (ovarian tumors).

4. Decreased levels of SHBG (sex hormone binding globulin) leading to increased levels of free estrogen.

In all women, whether premenopausal or postmenopausal, whether on or off hormone therapy, specific organic causes (intrauterine tumor, carcinoma, complications of unexpected pregnancy, or bleeding from extrauterine sites) must be ruled out. In addition to careful history and physical examination, dysfunctional uterine bleeding should be evaluated by aspiration endometrial biopsy. If the uterus is normal to examination, for reasons of both accuracy and cost effectiveness, the method of biopsy should be an office aspiration curettage, NOT the traditional, more costly and risky, in hospital dilatation and curettage.(94)

In the absence of organic disease, appropriate management is dependent upon the age of the woman and endometrial tissue findings. In the perimenopausal woman with dysfunctional uterine bleeding associated with proliferative or hyperplastic endometrium (uncomplicated by atypia or dysplastic constituents), periodic oral progestin therapy is mandatory, such as 10 mg medroxyprogesterone acetate given daily the first 10 days of each month. If hyperplasia is present, follow-up aspiration curettage is required, and if progestin is ineffective and histological regression is not observed, formal curettage is an essential preliminary to alternate therapeutic surgical choices.

When monthly progestin therapy reverses hyperplastic changes (which it does in 95-98% of cases) and controls irregular bleeding, treatment should be continued until withdrawal bleeding ceases. This is a reliable sign (in effect, a bioassay) indicating the onset of estrogen deprivation and the need for the addition of estrogen. If vasomotor disturbances begin before the cessation of menstrual bleeding, the combined estrogen-progestin program can be initiated as needed to control the flushes.

Problems of Estrogen-Progestin Therapy

General and Metabolic. The increased incidence of thromboembolic disease, hypertension, and altered carbohydrate metabolism during oral contraceptive usage is well documented. Because of the lower dosage in a hormone replacement program, these metabolic effects are not seen in postmenopausal therapy. Postmenopausal women on estrogen therapy are NOT at risk for myocardial infarction, thromboembolism, or breast tumors. As with oral contraception, however, estrogen replacement therapy may carry a 1.5-2.0-fold increased risk of gallbladder disease. The routine, periodic use of blood chemistries is not cost effective, and careful monitoring for the appearance of the symptoms and signs of biliary tract disease will suffice.

Patients with high risk factors need special attention when a decision for estrogen therapy is debated. Metabolic contraindications to estrogen replacement therapy include: chronically impaired liver function, acute vascular thrombosis (with or without emboli), and neurophthalmologic vascular disease. Estrogens may have adverse effects on some patients with seizure disorders, familial hyperlipidemias, and migraine headaches. The risk in women with a past history of thromboembolism is not known, and a careful assessment of the risk-benefit balance may justify treatment of such patients.

147

Endometrial Neoplasia. Estrogen normally promotes mitotic growth of the endometrium. Abnormal progression of growth through cystic hyperplasia, adenomatous hyperplasia, atypia, and early carcinoma has been associated with unopposed estrogen activity. Some 10% of women with adenomatous hyperplasia progress to frank cancer, and adenomatous hyperplasia is observed to antedate adenocarcinoma in 25-30% of cases. Retrospective studies have estimated that the risk of endometrial cancer in women on estrogen replacement therapy (unopposed by a progestational agent) is increased by a factor of 4 to 8 times the normal incidence of 1 per 1,000 postmenopausal women per year. The risk increases with duration of exposure and dose of estrogen, lingers for up to 10 years after estrogen is discontinued, and the risk of cancer that has already spread beyond the uterus is increased 3-fold in women who have used estrogen a year or longer.(95)

It is now apparent, however, that this risk can be reduced by the addition of a progestational agent to the program. Whereas estrogen promotes the growth of endometrium, progestins inhibit that growth. This counter effect is accomplished by progestin reduction in cellular receptors for estrogen, and by induction of target cell enzymes that convert estradiol to an excreted metabolite, estrone sulfate. As a result, the number of estrogen receptor complexes that are retained in the endometrial nuclei is decreased, as is the overall intracellular availability of the powerful estradiol.

Reports of the clinical impact of adding progestin in sequence with estrogen include both the reversal of hyperplasia and a diminished incidence of endometrial cancer.(96-98) The protective action of progestational agents operates via a mechanism which requires time in order to reach its maximal effect. For that reason, the duration of exposure to the progestin each month is critical. The optimal number of days for progestin administration remains somewhat controversial. While the standard method has incorporated the addition of a progestational agent for the last 10 days of estrogen exposure, some have argued in favor of 12 or 14 days. Clinical data to resolve this debate are not available, however, a study from London is noteworthy.(99) A total of 398 women are being treated with a variety of estrogens and progestins, with a duration of progestin exposure that varies from 7 to 21 days per month. These women have received an endometrial curettage under general anesthesia every year since 1976. By 1985, not one woman who received 10 or more days of progestin had developed hyperplasia, and there have been no cases of adenomatous hyperplasia or cancer. About 2% of the women developed cystic hyperplasia when progestin was administered for only 7 days. Until new data argue to the contrary, it is appropriate to adhere to the standard of 10 days as a minimal requirement for monthly progestational exposure.

It is likely that the daily dose of the progestational agent is associated with a threshold level below which endometrial protection can be insufficient. Currently, the standard program utilizes 10 mg of medroxyprogesterone acetate. Although lower doses of progestational agents are effective in achieving target tissue responses (such as reducing the nuclear concentration of estrogen receptors), the long-term impact on endometrial histology has not yet been firmly established. The question of dose is an issue of major importance, especially in terms of the cardiovascular system.

Although adenocarcinoma of the endometrium is an estrogen-dependent neoplasm, experience in providing estrogen replacement to women who have completed therapy for all grades of Stage I disease does not show an increased risk of recurrence.(100) Prudent judgment would strongly suggest that combined treatment with a progestational agent is the method of choice.

Breast Cancer. The possibility that estrogen use increases the risk of breast cancer must be intensively scrutinized. The epidemiologic data on the scope of human female breast cancer are astonishing: 1 of every 10 women will develop breast cancer in her lifetime. In America, breast cancer is the leading type of cancer in women (28%) and now second to lung cancer as the leading cause of cancer death in women (18%), about 10 times the number of deaths from endometrial cancer. The mortality rate from breast cancer has not changed in 50 years.

Unlike endometrial cancer, the incidence of breast cancer continues to rise progressively throughout life. Factors which increase the relative risk of breast cancer have a common theme: prolonged accumulated exposure to unopposed estrogen. These factors include: low parity, first childbirth after age 30, obesity, anovulation, early menarche, and late menopause. Early studies on estrogen use and breast cancer indicated higher risks in special subcategories, such as women with benign breast disease or natural vs. surgical menopause. Two definitive case-control studies are now available, and they do not show an increased risk for breast cancer associated with the postmenopausal use of estrogen.(101,102) These studies are large enough to have reliable results in the various subcategories, and an absence of an effect was evident in all of the following designations: parity, age at first pregnancy, early or late menopause, menopause by hysterectomy or oophorectomy, family history of breast cancer, presence of benign breast disease, use for many years, and use of high doses.

There is a growing story that exposure to progestational agents offers protection against breast cancer.(103,104) Although this remains to be definitely demonstrated, its probability leads to the recommendation that the combined estrogen-progestin program be utilized even in the absence of a uterus. It is logical to expect that the same mechanism of estrogen receptor depletion should operate in both the endometrium and the breast, and that protection against abnormal mitotic activity should exist in both target tissues. The unique progestin-induced breast neoplasia observed in the beagle dog (discussed in Chapter 15) is not seen in women.

Postmenopausal Estrogen-Progestin Replacement Therapy

In view of the above considerations, our opinion is as follows: There is little question that women who suffer from hot flushes or atrophy of reproductive tract tissues can and should be relieved of their problems by use of estrogens. It also is now definite that the long-term disabilities of osteoporosis can be largely prevented by therapy with estrogen and progestin. It is very probable that appropriate doses of estrogen have a beneficial impact on the lipid profile and the risk of cardiovascular disease. We suggest treatment with estrogen for all women showing any stigmata of hormone deprivation, and advocate hormonal prophylaxis against osteoporosis and cardiovascular disease. The lowest dose of estrogen that reverses the deficiency should be used, and the addition of a progestin is mandatory. In practice, we exclude from therapy those patients in whom estrogen is specifically contraindicated (estrogen dependent tumors, impaired liver metabolism, and sometimes, in a difficult manner of clinical judgment, patients with previous thromboembolic problems or conditions predisposing to thromboembolism). The decision to use or not to use estrogen belongs to the patient, and it should be based upon the information available in this chapter. The recommendation that replacement therapy be given for the shortest period of time appears to be shortsighted in view of the impressive evidence that therapy has a profound impact on osteoporosis and cardiovascular disease, and that there are more beneficial than potentially harmful effects.

Women Under the Age of 40 (Castrates and Women with Gonadal Dysgenesis)

In these women, the duration of estrogen deprivation is prolonged and the loss of estrogen acute. The cyclic use of estrogen is recommended for short-term reduction of vasomotor symptoms and for long-term prophylaxis against cardiovascular disease, osteoporosis, and target organ atrophy. In many young patients, 0.625 mg conjugated estrogens are insufficient to allow menstrual bleeding. Because women of this age ordinarily are exposed to estrogen levels which stimulate endometrial growth and withdrawal bleeding, and for psychological reasons, a higher dose should be used to maintain withdrawal bleeding until the menopausal time of life. Progestin for 10 days monthly is always added. In those patients castrated because of endometriosis, recurrence of endometriosis has very rarely been a problem with estrogen replacement, but because endometrial cancer has been reported to occur in remaining endometriosis exposed to unopposed estrogen, the estrogen and progestin daily combination is recommended.

Perimenopausal Dysfunctional Uterine Bleeding

After exclusion of other gynecologic causes, dysfunctional bleeding is treated by progestin therapy, and if necessary, biopsy surveillance. Vasomotor reactions appearing in women despite the presence of menstrual bleeding (presumably the flushes are due to a relative decrease in estrogen) can be treated by the usual estrogen-progestin regimen.

The Early Postmenopause

Progestin therapy is administered periodically (every month) until withdrawal bleeding does not occur. If vasomotor reactions begin, then estrogen is added regardless of the presence of menstrual bleeding. The long-term postmenopausal use of hormone therapy depends heavily upon a woman's own informed assessment, a process which should occur at this point in life. An understanding of hormone replacement is an important component in any preventive health program directed towards the postmenopausal years. At the low doses of estrogen recommended for replacement, increased growth of uterine fibroids, endometriosis, and breast reactions are rarely seen.

As a result of immediate responses in early climacteric symptoms, the patient enters the climacteric more confident of herself emotionally, sexually, and physically. In our view, this establishes or cements good patient-physician interchange and relations. The follow-up of the patient on effective estrogen-progestin replacement is more secure and certain. The practitioner offering estrogen-progestin replacement has a better and more reliable opportunity to act as primary physician for these aging women. All monitoring of health systems will be improved as a result of this single involvement.

The Late
Postmenopause

Atrophic conditions can be effectively treated with local or oral therapy in low maintenance doses. If there is no apparent basis for osteoporosis other than aging and ovarian failure, estrogen-progestin therapy and calcium supplementation are advisable even for very old women. Further loss of bone can be slowed, and the risk of fractures reduced. In these older women, a higher dose of estrogen (1.25 mg conjugated estrogens or equivalent) may be necessary; an assessment of progress can be obtained by measuring bone density, using either photon absorptiometry or CT scanning.

Method of
Management

Which Drug Should Be Used? There currently is no evidence that one form of estrogen is superior to another. The specific estrogen is not as important as the duration, dose, and the presence or absence of a progestin. Which estrogen is administered is not as important as the method with which it is used.

The dose of estrogen which is effective in maintaining the axial and peripheral bone mass is equivalent to 0.625 mg conjugated estrogens.(105,106) The relative potencies of commercially available estrogens become of great importance when prescribing estrogen.

Relative Estrogen Potencies (107,108)

Estrogen	FSH Levels	Liver Proteins	Bone Density
Piperazine estrone sulfate	1.0 mg	2.0 mg	—
Micronized estradiol	1.0 mg	1.0 mg	1.0 mg
Conjugated estrogens	1.0 mg	0.625 mg	0.625 mg
Ethinyl estradiol	5.0 μg	2–10 μg	5–10 μg

The dose-response effect of ethinyl estradiol on bone has not been sufficiently studied, and it is probable that the dose equivalent to 0.625 mg conjugated estrogens approximates 5-10 μg. The 17α-ethinyl group of ethinyl estradiol appears to be responsible for a specific hepatic effect, for no matter by which route it is administered, liver metabolism is affected.(109) The same is true for conjugated equine estrogens. Contrary to the case with estradiol, the liver appears to preferentially extract ethinyl estradiol and conjugated equine estrogens no matter what the route of administration.

Thus the route of administration appears to influence the metabolic responses only in the case of specific estrogens, most notably estradiol.

At one point in time, the consequence of the first pass through the liver of estrogens other than ethinyl estradiol and conjugated equine estrogens was thought to be of great importance in terms of HDL-cholesterol. Initial reports of transdermal application, subdermal implants, and cutaneous administration of estradiol all demonstrated profound impacts on hot flushes and vaginal cytology, but only a limited impact on lipoproteins. (110-113) These were short-term studies, however, and while oral therapy is associated with an immediate impact on the lipoprotein profile, percutaneous administration achieves significant changes in lipids and lipoproteins only after 6 months of treatment. After 12 months of percutaneous *high dose* estrogen therapy, there is a significant reduction in the serum levels of total cholesterol and LDL-cholesterol, and after 24 months, HDL cholesterol levels are increased by percutaneous estrogen combined with cyclic micronized progesterone.(114) The blood level of estradiol achieved in this study was significantly elevated (3-5 fold those associated with transdermal estradiol), and the standard dose required to produce a favorable lipoprotein profile remains to be established for each method of administration other than the oral route. It is likely that the dose administered is more critical than "first pass" through the liver.

One would not expect the route of administration to influence the effect on postmenopausal bone loss, and indeed this may be the case. Percutaneous as well as oral estrogen therapy offers effective protection against osteoporosis.(115) But once again effective dosage for long-term protection against osteoporosis is established only for the oral route of administration. Until dose response studies are available indicating the range which without question provides the desired benefits for vaginal, parenteral, and transdermal types of administration, the oral program must be followed in the interests of patient safety and health.

The Classic Sequential Method of Treatment. Estrogens are administered on a cyclic basis, from the 1st through the 25th of each month, as a convenient aid to remembering the routine. For the last 10 days of estrogen administration, a daily dose of 10 mg of medroxyprogesterone acetate is added. Some patients develop unwanted reactions to this dose of progestin: weight gain, fluid retention, breast tenderness, and/or depression. A lower dose (5 mg) usually solves this problem. The lowest effective dose of medroxyprogesterone acetate has not been established, and for this reason, the starting dose remains at 10 mg. Studies with endometrium, however, indicate that lower doses are effective in reducing the target tissue content of estrogen receptors.(116) Future studies may reveal that lower doses protect the endometrium (and perhaps the breast) and maintain the advantage of elevated HDL-cholesterol levels. Unfortunately, the great majority of women (80%) on this regimen experience withdrawal menstrual bleeding.

In the absence of a uterus, some do not see the need to use cyclic administration of a progestin. However, in view of a possible impact on the breast, it seems best to adhere to a cyclic schedule including the terminal use of a progestin.

There are no clinical studies to guide us in dealing with a woman who is symptomatic during the days off of medication. Clinical judgment has led us to combine daily estrogen (every day through the month) with progestin daily for the first 14 days each month.

The dose of estrogen utilized is that which will provide sufficient estrogen to sustain physiologic functions. For early climacteric where there is still considerable endogenous estrogen present, the usual effective dose is 0.625 mg conjugated estrogens per day. In late climacteric where endogenous estrogen is very low, a higher dose, 1.25 mg, may be necessary. Unfortunately, there are no studies available which have utilized very old women. For optimal protection against osteoporosis, the hormonal regimen is supplemented with 500 mg calcium daily.

The New Continuous/Combined Method of Treatment. Manipulation of the standard sequential regimen was often necessary in order to maintain patient compliance in the presence of bleeding and other symptoms. One approach for the problem of bleeding has been to reduce the daily dose of estrogen. It is useful to note that bone density remains stable with a daily dose of 0.3 mg conjugated estrogens if the daily calcium supplementation is increased to 1,500 mg, although this response may also be dependent upon the inclusion of monthly exposure to a progestational agent as well.(39)

More recently we and others have advocated the continuous daily use of an estrogen-progestin combination.(79,117-121) We have used combinations of the following estrogens and progestins:

Daily Estrogen: 0.625 mg conjugated estrogen, or
1.0 mg micronized estradol

Daily Progestin: 2.5-5.0 mg medroxyprogesterone acetate, or
0.35-0.7 mg norethindrone

After 4 months of such continuous treatment, bleeding usually ceases and essentially all biopsies show atrophic endometrium. While one study has reported a decrease in HDL-cholesterol, another demonstrated a favorable impact on the cholesterol-lipoprotein profile.(79,119) In our own experience, this continuous approach maintains a beneficial lipoprotein pattern and increases the bone density in the spinal column. Also of note, we have encountered no adverse effects on blood pressure.

Clinical trials are essential to ascertain the effects of various doses and formulations on the lipoprotein profile and the risk of cardiovascular disease, beyond the obvious need for a safe impact on bones and the endometrium. Until such data are available, annual assessment of the lipoprotein profile is worthwhile to detect any adverse affects. While a nonfasting sample can be used to screen the serum cholesterol, reliable assessment of the lipoprotein profile requires a 12 hour (overnight) fast.

Heart Disease Risk Based on Cholesterol/HDL Ratio		
Lowest risk	—	Less than 2.5
Below average risk	—	2.5–3.7
Average risk	—	3.8–5.6
High risk	—	5.7–8.3
Dangerous	—	Greater than 8.3

Dietary modifications are indicated for all patients with total cholesterol levels above 200 mg/dl, and intensive effort should be directed to patients with levels above 240 mg/dl. The goal for the cholesterol/HDL ratio should be 3.7 or below. The HDL cholesterol level should be at least 35 mg/dl. Regardless of the values for total and HDL cholesterol levels, a strict dietary program is also recommended if the LDL cholesterol is greater than 130 mg/dl and triglyceride is greater than 250 mg/dl. Because of the variability involved, cholesterol levels above 200 should be confirmed by repeat testing. Hisk risk individuals merit drug therapy. An excellent review of the detection, evaluation, and treatment of this problem is available. (122)

When Estrogen is Contraindicated. Oral medroxyprogesterone acetate (10-20 mg daily) is effective in relieving vasomotor symptoms, and there is a beneficial impact on calcium balance, consistent with an inhibition of bone resorption. When estrogen administration is not possible, however, calcium should be supplemented at the rate of 1,000 mg per day. Unfortunately vaginal atrophy is not improved with progestin treatment, and dyspareunia due to dryness can even be intensified. In addition, this approach is probably associated with a decrease in HDL cholesterol, and surveillance of the lipoprotein profile is indicated.

Other Considerations. Calcium supplementation can unmask asymptomatic hyperparathyroidism. Women receiving calcium supplementation should have their blood levels of calcium and phosphorous measured yearly for the first 2 years. If normal, no further surveillance is necessary.

A striking and consistent finding in most studies dealing with menopause and hormonal replacement is a marked placebo response in a variety of symptoms including flushing. A significant clinical problem encountered in our referral practice is the following scenario: A woman will occasionally undergo an apparent beneficial response to estrogen, only to have the response wear off in several months. This leads to a sequence of periodic visits to the physician and ever-increasing doses of estrogen therapy. When a patient reaches a point of requiring large doses of estrogen (2.5 mg conjugated estrogens), a careful inquiry must be undertaken for a basic psychoneurotic problem.

Clonidine has been found to reduce the frequency of flushes, but it is less effective than either estrogen or progestin, and the dose required is associated with a high rate of side effects. Propranolol and similar agents are ineffective.

Hormonal treatment for decreased libido should be discouraged. Psychosocial reasons are usually to blame. However, we have found that occasionally the addition of androgen (methyltestosterone, up to 5 mg daily), in addition to the estrogen, may provide an increased sense of well-being, along with an increase in libido, and this has been supported by well-designed, controlled studies.(123) A commercial preparation is available in the U.S. (Estratest), containing 0.625 mg esterified estrogens and 1.25 mg methyltestosterone. The patient should be cautioned that hirsutism can develop. The long-term effect on the lipid profile is unknown, and the lipoprotein profile should be monitored. In addition, the estrogen-androgen combination does not prevent endometrial hyperplasia, and the addition of a progestational agent is still necessary.

We find no need to monitor dosage by any means other than symptoms and bleeding; assessing vaginal cytology is not useful.

We believe that the benefits of estrogen-progestin replacement therapy make it worthwhile to offer this preventive health care program to almost all women. It is not cost effective to attempt to select a high risk group (e.g. bone density measurements to select those at high risk for osteoporosis).(124) Such efforts are useful only when an individual woman requires the information in order to make an informed decision regarding hormone replacement. The method of choice, in terms of accuracy and sensitivity, is either dual-photon absorptiometry or a quantitative CT scan of the metabolically active trabecular bone in the spine.

When To Biopsy? The cost effectiveness of routine endometrial biopsies can be argued. It has been estimated that over 3,000 biopsies are necessary in order to detect a single case of an atypical lesion in an asymptomatic woman. A reasonable economic moderation would be to limit biopsies to patients at higher risk for endometrial changes: those women with conditions associated with chronic estrogen exposure (obesity, dysfunctional uterine bleeding, anovulation and infertility, hirsutism, high alcohol intake, hepatic disease, metabolic problems such as diabetes mellitus and hypothyroidism) and those women in whom irregular bleeding occurs while on estrogen-progestin therapy. In the absence of abnormal bleeding, a certain amount of trust in the protective effects of the progestin is justified, and routine, periodic biopsies are not necessary.

Conclusion. No one can hope to stay young forever, and hormones certainly will not prevent aging. There should be no misconception here. Some of the difficulties of menopause, however, can be softened with estrogen-progestin therapy, and several potentially disabling problems avoided. Unanswered questions remain. Controlled clinical studies are necessary in order to determine what schedule of administration is best, and most importantly, the safety and dosage of the progestational agent. Until these questions are answered, close clinical surveillance of our patients is necessary.

References

1. **Bonilla-Musoles F, Renau J, Hernandez-Yago J, Torres YJ,** How do oocytes disappear? Arch Gynaekol 218:233, 1975.

2. **Gosden RG,** Follicular status at menopause, Human Reprod 2:617, 1987.

3. **Sherman BM, West JH, Korenman SG,** The menopausal transition: analysis of LH, FSH, estradiol, and progesterone concentrations during menstrual cycles of older women, J Clin Endocrinol Metab 42:629, 1976.

4. **Meldrum DR, Davidson BJ, Tataryn IV, Judd HL,** Changes in circulating steroids with aging in postmenopausal women, Obstet Gynecol 57:624, 1981.

5. **Judd HL, Shamonki IM, Frumar AM, Lagasse LD,** Origin of serum estradiol in postmenopausal women, Obstet Gynecol 59:680, 1982.

6. **Endicott J, Halbreich U,** Retrospective report of premenstrual depressive changes: factors affecting confirmation by daily ratings, Psychopharm Bull 18:109, 1983.

7. **Rubinow DR, Roy-Byrne P,** Premenstrual syndromes: Overview from a methodologic perspective, Am J Psych 141:2, 1984.

8. **Sommer B,** The effect of menstruation on cognitive and perceptual-motor behavior: A review, Psychosom Med 35:515, 1973.

9. **Dalton K,** *The Premenstrual Syndrome and Progesterone Therapy,* Year Book Medical Publishers, Inc., Chicago, 2nd edition, 1984.

10. **Maddocks SE, Hahn P, Moller F, Reid RL,** A double-blind placebo-controlled trial of progesterone vaginal suppositories in the treatment of premenstrual syndrome, Am J Obstet Gynecol 154:573, 1986.

11. **Bancroft J, Backstrom T,** Premenstrual syndrome, Clin Endocrinol 22:313, 1985.

12. **Rubinow DR, Hoban MC, Grover GN, Galloway DS, Roy-Byrne P, Andersen R, Merriam GR,** Changes in plasma hormones across the menstrual cycle in patients with menstrually related mood disorder and in control subjects, Am J Obstet Gynecol 158:5, 1988.

13. **Dawood MY,** editor, *Dysmenorrhea,* Williams & Wilkins, Baltimore, 1981.

14. **Owens PR,** Prostaglandin synthetase inhibitors in the treatment of primary dysmenorrhea: Outcome trials reviewed, Am J Obstet Gynecol 148:96, 1984.

15. **Krailo MD, Pike MC,** Estimation of the distribution of age at natural menopause from prevalence data, Am J Epidemiol 117:356, 1983.

16. **McKinlay SM, Bifano NL, McKinlay JB,** Smoking and age at menopause in women, Ann Int Med 103:350, 1985.

17. **Siddle N, Sarrel P, Whitehead M,** The effect of hysterectomy on the age at ovarian failure: identification of a subgroup of women with premature loss of ovarian function and literature review, Fertil Steril 47:94, 1987.

18. **Amundsen DW, Diers CJ,** The age of menopause in medieval Europe, Hum Biol 45:605, 1973.

19. **Cope E,** Physical changes associated with the post-menopausal years, in Campbell S, editor, *The Management of the Menopause & Post-Menopausal Years,* University Park Press, Baltimore, 1976, p. 33.

20. **Meldrum DR,** The pathophysiology of postmenopausal symptoms, Seminars Reprod Endocrinol 1:11, 1983.

21. **Aksel S, Schomberg DW, Tyrey L, Hammond CB,** Vasomotor symptoms, serum estrogens and gonadotropin levels in surgical menopause, Am J Obstet Gynecol 126:165, 1976.

22. **Beals RK,** Survival following hip fracture: long term follow-up of 607 patients, J Chronic Dis 25:235, 1972.

23. **Richelson LS, Wahner HW, Melton LJ III, Riggs BL,** Relative contributions of aging and estrogen deficiency to postmenopausal bone loss, New Eng J Med 311:1273, 1984.

24. **Nilas L, Christiansen C,** Bone mass and its relationship to age and the menopause, J Clin Endocrinol Metab 65:697, 1987.

25. **Avioli LV,** Calcium and osteoporosis, Ann Rev Nutr 4:471, 1984.

26. **Johnston CC Jr, Hui SL, Witt RM, Appledorn R, Baker RS, Longcope C,** Early menopausal changes in bone mass and sex steroids, J Clin Endocrinol Metab 61:905, 1985.

27. **Riggs BL, Wahner HW, Melton LJ III, Richelson LS, Judd HL, Offord KP,** Rates of bone loss in the appendicular and axial skeletons of women, J Clin Invest 77:1487, 1986.

28. **Riggs BL, Wahner HW, Dunn WL, Mazess RB, Offord KP, Melton LJ III,** Differential changes in bone mineral density of the appendicular and axial skeleton with aging: Relationship to spinal osteoporosis, J Clin Invest 67:328, 1981.

29. **Lindsay R, Herrington BS,** Estrogens and osteoporosis, Seminars Reprod Endocrinol 1:55, 1983.

30. **Falch JA, Ilebekk A, Slungaard U,** Epidemiology of hip fractures in Norway, Acta Orthoped Scand 56:12, 1985.

31. **Weiss NC, Ure CL, Ballard JH, Williams AR, Daling JR,** Estimated incidence of fractures of the lower forearm and hip in postmenopausal women, New Eng J Med 303:1195, 1980.

32. **Ettinger B, Genant HK, Cann CE,** Long-term estrogen replacement therapy prevents bone loss and fractures, Ann Int Med 102:319, 1985.

33. **Kiel DP, Felson DT, Anderson JJ, Wilson PWF, Moskowitz MA,** Hip fracture and the use of estrogens in postmenopausal women: The Framingham Study, New Eng J Med 317:1169, 1987.

34. **Riggs BL, Seeman E, Hodgson SF, Taves DR, O'Fallon WM,** Effect of the fluoride/calcium regimen on vertebral fracture occurrence in postmenopausal osteoporosis, New Eng J Med 306:446, 1982.

35. **Jensen GF, Christiansen C, Transbol I,** Treatment of postmenopausal osteoporosis. A controlled therapeutic trial comparing oestrogen/gestagen, 1,25-dihydroxy-vitamin D3, and calcium, Clin Endocrinol 16:515, 1982.

36. **Heaney RP, Recker RR, Saville PD,** Menopausal changes in calcium balance performance, Lab Clin Med 92:953, 1978.

37. **Heaney RP, Recker RR,** Distribution of calcium absorption in middle-aged women, Am J Clin Nutrition 43:299, 1986.

38. **Riis B, Thomsen K, Christiansen C,** Does calcium supplementation prevent postmenopausal bone loss? New Eng J Med 316:173, 1987.

39. **Ettinger B, Genant HK, Cann CE,** Postmenopausal bone loss is prevented by treatment with low-dosage estrogen with calcium, Ann Int Med 106:40, 1987.

40. **Abdalla HI, Hart DM, Lindsay R, Leggate I, Hooke A,** Prevention of bone mineral loss in postmenopausal women by norethisterone, Obstet Gynecol 66:789, 1985.

41. **Selby PL, Peacock M, Barkworth SA, Brown WB, Taylor GA,** Early effects of ethinyl oestradiol and norethisterone treatment in postmenopausal women on bone resorption and calcium regulating hormones, Clin Sci 69:265, 1985.

42. **Christiansen C, Nilas L, Riis BJ, Rodbro P, Deftos L,** Uncoupling of bone formation and resorption by combined oestrogen and progestagen therapy in postmenopausal osteoporosis, Lancet ii:800, 1985.

43. **Tiegs RD, Body JJ, Wahner HW, Barta J, Riggs BL, Heath H,** Calcitonin secretion in postmenopausal osteoporosis, New Eng J Med 312:1097, 1985.

44. **Lindsay R, MacLean A, Kraszewski A, Clark AC, Garwood J,** Bone response to termination of estrogen treatment, Lancet i:1325, 1978.

45. **Horsman A, Nordin BEC, Crilly RG,** Effect on bone of withdrawal of estrogen therapy, Lancet ii:33, 1979.

46. **Christiansen C, Christiansen MS, Transbol IB,** Bone mass in postmenopausal women after withdrawal of oestrogen/gestagen replacement therapy, Lancet i:459, 1981.

47. **Wasnich R, Yano K, Vogel J,** Postmenopausal bone loss at multiple skeletal sites: Relationship to estrogen use, J Chron Dis 36:781, 1983.

48. **Jensen J, Christiansen C, Rodbro P,** Cigarette smoking, serum estrogens, and bone loss during hormone replacement therapy early after menopause, New Eng J Med 313:973, 1985.

49. **Michnovicz JJ, Hershcopf RJ, Naganuma H, Bradlow HL, Fishman J,** Increased 2-hydroxylation of estradiol as a possible mechanism for the anti-estrogenic effect of cigarette smoking, New Eng J Med 315:1305, 1986.

50. **Barbieri RL, McShane PM, Ryan KJ,** Constituents of cigarette smoke inhibit human granulosa cell aromatase, Fertil Steril 46:232, 1986.

51. **Chow RK, Harrison JE, Brown CF, Hajek V,** Physical fitness effect on bone mass in postmenopausal women, Arch Phys Med Rehabil 67:231, 1986.

158

52. **Henderson BE, Ross RK, Paganini-Hill A, Mack TM,** Estrogen use and cardiovascular disease, Am J Obstet Gynecol 154:1181, 1986.

53. **Rosenberg L, Armstrong B, Jick H,** Myocardial infarction and estrogen therapy in postmenopausal women, New Eng J Med 294:1256, 1976.

54. **Pfeffer RI, Whipple GH, Kurosake TT, Chapman JM,** Coronary risk and estrogen use in postmenopausal women, Am J Epidemiol 107:479, 1978.

55. **Jick H, Dinan B, Rothman KJ,** Noncontraceptive estrogens and non-fatal myocardial infarction, JAMA 239:1407, 1978.

56. **Rosenberg L, Sloane D, Shapiro S, Kaufman D, Stolley PD, Miethinen OS,** Noncontraceptive estrogens and myocardial infarction in young women, JAMA 224:339, 1980.

57. **Ross RK, Paganini-Hill A, Mack TM, Arthur M, Henderson BE,** Menopausal oestrogen therapy and protection from death from ischaemic heart disease, Lancet i:585, 1981.

58. **Bain C, Willett W, Hennekens CH, Rosner B, Belanger C, Speizer FE,** Use of postmenopausal hormones and risk of myocardial infarction, Circulation 64:42, 1981.

59. **Adam S, Williams V, Vessey MP,** Cardiovascular disease and hormone replacement treatment: A pilot case-control study, Brit Med J 282:1277, 1981.

60. **Szklo M, Tonascia J, Gordis L, Bloom I,** Estrogen use and myocardial infarction risk: A case-control study, Prevent Med 13:510, 1984.

61. **Burch JC, Byrd BF, Vaughn WK,** The effects of long-term estrogen on hysterectomized women, Am J Obstet Gynecol 118:778, 1974.

62. **Hammond CB, Jelovsek FR, Lee KL, Creasman WT, Parker RT,** Effects of long-term estrogen replacement therapy: I. Metabolic effects, Am J Obstet Gynecol 133:525, 1979.

63. **Gordon T, Kannel WB, Hjortland MC, McNamara PM,** Menopause and coronary heart disease: The Framingham Study, Ann Int Med 89:157, 1978.

64. **Petitti DB, Wingerd J, Pellegrin F, Ramcharan S,** Risk of vascular disease in women: smoking, oral contraceptives, non-contraceptive estrogens, and other factors, JAMA 242:1150, 1979.

65. **Bush TL, Barrett-Connor E, Cowan DK, Criqui MH, Wallace RB, Suchindran CM, Tyroler HA, Rifkind BM,** Cardiovascular mortality and noncontraceptive use of estrogen in women: results from the Lipid Research Clinics Program Follow-up Study, Circulation 75:1102, 1987.

66. **Lafferty FW, Helmuth DO,** Postmenopausal estrogen replacement: The prevention of osteoporosis and systemic effects, Maturitas 7:147, 1985.

67. **Wilson PWF, Garrison RJ, Castelli WP,** Postmenopausal estrogen use, cigarette smoking, and cardiovascular morbidity in women over 50. The Framingham Study, New Eng J Med 313:1038, 1985.

68. **Stampfer MJ, Willett WC, Colditz GA, Rosner B, Speizer FE, Hennekens CH,** A prospective study of postmenopausal estrogen therapy and coronary heart disease, New Eng J Med 313:1044, 1985.

69. **Eaker ED, Castelli WP,** Differential risk for coronary heart disease among women in the Framingham study, Proceedings of the Workshop on Coronary Heart Disease in Women, Bethesda, Md. January 26-28, 1986.

70. **Speroff T, Dawson N, Speroff L,** Is postmenopausal estrogen use risky? Results from a methodologic review and information synthesis, Clin Res 35:362A, 1987.

71. **Colditz GA, Willett WC, Stampfer MJ, Rosner B, Speizer FE, Hennekens CG,** Menopause and the risk of coronary heart disease in women, New Eng J Med 316:1105, 1987.

72. **Sorva R, Kuusi T, Dunkel L, Taskinen M-R,** Effects of endogenous sex steroids on serum lipoproteins and postheparin plasma lipolytic enzymes, J Clin Endocrinol Metab 66:408, 1988.

73. **Hart DM, Farish E, Fletcher DC, Howie C, Kitchener H,** Ten years postmenopausal hormone replacement therapy—effect on lipoproteins, Maturitas 5:271, 1984.

74. **Cauley JA, La Porte RE, Sandler RB, Orchard TJ, Slemenda CW, Petrini AM,** The relationship of physical activity to high density lipoprotein cholesterol in postmenopausal women, J Chron Dis 39:687, 1986.

75. **Hirvonen E, Malkonen M, Manninen V,** Effects of different progestogens on lipoproteins during postmenopausal therapy, New Eng J Med 304:560, 1981.

76. **Mattsson L, Cullberg LG, Samsioe G,** Influence of esterified estrogens and medroxyprogesterone on lipid metabolism and sex steroids. A study in oophorectomized women, Hormone Metab Res 14:602, 1982.

77. **Silferstolpe G, Gustafsson A, Samsioe G, Syanborg A,** Lipid metabolic studies in oophorectomized women: effects on serum lipids and lipoproteins of three synthetic progestogens, Maturitas 4:103, 1983.

78. **Ylostalo P, Kauppila A, Kivinen S, Tuimala R, Vihkoo R,** Endocrine and metabolic effects of low-dose estrogen-progestin treatment in climacteric women, Obstet Gynecol 62:682, 1983.

79. **Mattsson L, Cullberg G, Samsioe G,** A continuous estrogen-progestogen regimen for climacteric complaints, Acta Obstet Gynecol Scand 63:673, 1984.

80. **Ottosson UB, Carlstrom K, Damber JE, von Schoultz B,** Serum levels of progesterone and some of its metabolites including deoxycorticosterone after oral and parenteral administration, Brit J Obstet Gynecol 91:1111, 1984.

81. **Wren B, Garrett D,** The effect of low-dose piperazine oestrogen sulphate and low-dose levonorgestrel on blood lipid levels in postmenopausal women, Maturitas 7:141, 1985.

82. **Ottosson UB, Johansson BG, von Schoultz B,** Subfractions of high-density lipoprotein cholesterol during estrogen replacement therapy: A comparison between progestogens and natural progesterone, Am J Obstet Gynecol 151:746, 1985.

83. **Ravnikar V, Murin V, Nutkik J, Ryan KJ, Schiff I,** Blood lipid levels in postmenopausal women on hormone replacement therapy, 35th Annual Meeting, Soc Gynecol Invest, Abstract No. 422, 1988.

84. **Lind T, Cameron EC, Hunter WM, Leon C, Moran PF, Oxley A, Gerrard J, Lind UCG,** A prospective, controlled trial of six forms of hormone replacement therapy given to postmenopausal women, Brit J Obstet Gynaecol (Suppl 3) 86:1, 1979.

85. **Pfeffer RI, Kurosaki TT, Charlton SK,** Estrogen use and blood pressure in later life, Am J Epidemiol 110:469, 1979.

86. **Lutola H,** Blood pressure and hemodynamics in postmenopausal women during estradiol-17β substitution, Ann Clin Res (Suppl 38) 15:9, 1983.

87. **Wren BG, Routledge AD,** The effect of type and dose of oestrogen on the blood pressure of postmenopausal women, Maturitas 5:135, 1983.

88. **Wilson PD, Faragher B, Butler B, Bullock D, Robinson EL, Brown ADG,** Treatment with oral piperazine oestrone sulphate for genuine stress incontinence in postmenopausal women, Brit J Obstet Gynaecol 94:568, 1987.

89. **Semmens JP, Wagner G,** Effects of estrogen therapy on vaginal physiology during menopause, Obstet Gynecol 66:15, 1985.

90. **Cauley JA, Petrini AM, LaPorte RE, Sandler RB, Bayles CM, Robertson RJ, Slemenda CW,** The decline of grip strength in the menopause: relationship to physical activity, estrogen use and anthropometric factors, J Chron Dis 40:115, 1987.

91. **Vandenbroucke JP, Witteman JCM, Valkenburg HA, Boersma JW, Cats A, Festen JJM, Hartman AP, Huber-Bruning O, Rasker JJ, Weber J,** Noncontraceptive hormones and rheumatoid arthritis in perimenopausal and postmenopausal women, JAMA 255:1299, 1986.

92. **Campbell S, Whitehead M,** Estrogen therapy and the menopausal syndrome, Clin Obstet Gynecol 4:31, 1977.

93. **Schiff I, Regestein Q, Tulchinsky D, Ryan KJ,** Effects of estrogens on sleep and psychological state of hypogonadal women, JAMA 242:2405, 1979.

94. **Grimes DA,** Diagnostic dilation and curettage: A reappraisal, Am J Obstet Gynecol 142:1, 1982.

95. **Shapiro S, Kelly JP, Rosenberg L, Kaufman DW, Helmrich SP, Rosenshein NB, Lewis JL Jr, Knapp RC, Stolley PD, Schottenfeld D,** Risk of localized and widespread endometrial cancer in relation to recent and discontinued use of conjugated estrogens, New Eng J Med 313:969, 1985.

96. **Thom MH, White PJ, Williams RM, Sturdee PW, Paterson MEL, Wade-Evans T, Studd JWW,** Prevention and treatment of endometrial disease in climacteric women receiving estrogen, Lancet ii:455, 1979.

97. **Whitehead MI, Townsend PT, Pryse-Davies J, Ryder TA, King RJB,** Effects of estrogen and progestins on the biochemistry and morphology of the postmenopausal endometrium, New Eng J Med 305:1599, 1981.

98. **Gambrell RD Jr, Babgnell CA, Greenblatt RB,** Role of estrogens and progesterone in the etiology and prevention of endometrial cancer: A review, Am J Obstet Gynecol 146:696, 1983.

99. **Varma TR,** Effect of long-term therapy with estrogen and progesterone on the endometrium of postmenopausal women, Acta Obstet Gynecol Scand 64:41, 1985.

100. **Creasman WT, Henderson D, Hinshaw W, Clarke-Pearson DL,** Estrogen replacment therapy in the patient treated for endometrial cancer, Obstet Gynecol 67:326, 1986.

101. **Kaufman DW, Miller DR, Rosenberg L, Helmrich SP, Stolley P, Schottenfeld D, Shapiro S,** Noncontraceptive estrogen use and the risk of breast cancer, JAMA 252:63, 1984.

102. **Wingo PA, Layde PM, Lee NC, Rubin G, Ory HW,** The risk of breast cancer in postmenopausal women who have used estrogen replacement therapy, JAMA 257:209, 1987.

103. **Gambrell RD Jr, Maier R, Sancers BI,** Decreased incidence of breast cancer in postmenopausal estrogen-progestogen users, Obstet Gynecol 62:435, 1983.

104. **W.H.O. collaborative study of neoplasia and steroid contraceptives.** Breast cancer, cervical cancer, and medroxyprogesterone acetate, Lancet ii:1207, 1984.

105. **Genant HK, Cann CE, Ettinger B, Gordan GS,** Quantitative computed tomography of vertebral spongiosa: A sensitive method for detecting early bone loss after oophorectomy, Ann Int Med 97:699, 1982.

106. **Lindsay R, Hart M, Clark DM,** The minimum effective dose of estrogen for prevention of postmenopausal bone loss, Obstet Gynecol 63:759, 1984.

107. **Mashchak CA, Lobo RA, Dozono-Takano R, Eggena P, Nakamura RM, Brenner PF, Mishell DR Jr,** Comparison of pharmacodynamic properties of various estrogen formulations, Am J Obstet Gynecol 144:511, 1982.

108. **Horsman A, Jones M, Francis R, Nordin C,** The effect of estrogen dose on postmenopausal bone loss, New Eng J Med 309:1405, 1983.

109. **Goebelsmann U, Mashchak CA, Mishell DR Jr,** Comparison of hepatic impact of oral and vaginal administration of ethinyl estradiol, Am J Obstet Gynecol 151:868, 1985.

110. **Laufer LR, DeFazio JL, Lu JKH, Meldrum DR, Eggena P, Sambhi MP, Hershman JM, Judd HL,** Estrogen replacement therapy by transdermal estradiol administration, Am J Obstet Gynecol 146:533, 1983.

111. **Fahraeus L, Larsson-Cohn U, Wallentin L,** Lipoproteins during oral and cutaneous administration of oestradiol-17β to menopausal women, Acta Endocrinol 101:597, 1982.

112. **Fahraeus L, Wallentin L,** High density lipoprotein subfraction during oral and cutaneous administration of 17β-estradiol to menopausal women, J Clin Endocrinol Metab 56:797, 1983.

162

113. **Fletcher CD, Farish E, Hart DM, Barlow DH, Gray CE, Conaghan CJ,** Long-term hormone implant therapy—effects on lipoproteins and steroid levels in post-menopausal women, Acta Endocrinol 111:419, 1986.

114. **Jensen J, Riis BJ, Strom V, Nilas L, Christiansen C,** Long-term effects of percutaneous estrogens and oral progesterone on serum lipoproteins in postmenopausal women, Am J Obstet Gynecol 156:66, 1987.

115. **Riis BJ, Thomsen K, Strom V, Christiansen, C,** The effect of percutaneous estradiol and natural progesterone on postmenopausal bone loss, Am J Obstet Gynecol 156:61, 1987.

116. **Gibbons WE, Moyer DL, Lobo RA, Roy S, Mishell DR Jr,** Biochemical and histologic effects of sequential estrogen/progestin therapy on the endometrium of postmenopausal women, Am J Obstet Gynecol 154:456, 1986.

117. **Mattsson L, Cullberg G, Samsioe G,** Evaluation of a continuous oestrogen-progestogen regimen for climacteric complaints, Maturitas 4:95, 1982.

118. **Magos AL, Brincat M, Studd JWW, Wardle P, Schlesinger P, O'Dowd T,** Amenorrhea and endometrial atrophy with continuous oral estrogen and progestogen therapy in postmenopausal women, Obstet Gynecol 65:496, 1985.

119. **Jensen J, Riis BJ, Strom V, Christiansen C,** Continuous oestrogen-progestogen treatment and serum lipoproteins in postmenopausal women, Brit J Obstet Gynaecol 94:130, 1987.

120. **Prough SG, Aksel S, Wiebe RH, Shepherd J,** Continuous estrogen/progestin therapy in menopause, Am J Obstet Gynecol 157:1449, 1987.

121. **Williams SR, Frenchek B, Speroff L,** A continuous combination hormone replacement therapy vs. standard sequential therapy: effects on bone density in a high risk population, 35th Annual Meeting, Soc Gynecol Invest, Abstract No. 424, 1988.

122. **The National Cholesterol Education Program, National Heart, Lung, and Blood Institute,** Report of the national cholesterol education program expert panel on detection, evaluation, and treatment of high blood cholesterol in adults, Arch Int Med 148:36, 1988.

123. **Sherwin BB, Gelfand MM, Brender W,** Androgen enhances sexual motivation in females: a prospective, crossover study of sex steroid administration in the surgical menopause, Psychosom Med 47:339, 1985.

124. **Hall FM, Davis MA, Baran DT,** Bone mineral screening for osteoporosis, New Eng J Med 316:212, 1987.

5   Amenorrhea

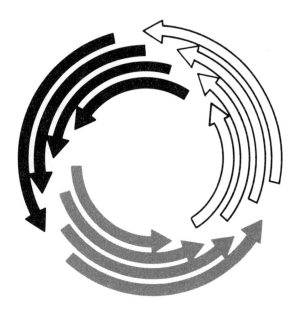

Few problems in gynecologic endocrinology are as challenging or taxing to the clinician as amenorrhea. The physician must be concerned with an array of potential diseases and disorders involving, in many instances, unfamiliar organ systems, some carrying morbid and even lethal consequences for the patient. Not infrequently, the otherwise confident and experienced physician dismisses the problem as too complex for his/her busy practice and refers the patient to a "specialist" in the field. In doing so, the nonavailability of sophisticated laboratory techniques is often cited as necessitating the costly and frequently inconvenient transfer of the patient.

The intent of this chapter is to provide a simple mechanism for differential diagnosis of amenorrhea of all types and chronology, utilizing procedures available to all physicians. Strict adherence to this design will unerringly pinpoint the organ system locus of disorder leading to the presenting symptom of amenorrhea. Once this is accomplished, the detailed evidence confirming the diagnosis can be sought and the assistance of appropriate specialists (neurosurgeon, internist, endocrinologist, psychiatrist) confidently chosen. In the end, the patient receives the most reliable diagnosis and therapy at minimal cost and optimal convenience. The majority of patients with amenorrhea have relatively simple problems which can be managed easily by the patients' primary care physicians.

The "workup" to be described is not new. With minor modifications, it has been continuously and successfully applied for several decades. Before presenting the diagnostic workup in detail, it is necessary to provide a definition of amenorrhea, designating the appropriate selection of patients. In addition, a brief review of the physiologic mechanisms by which a menstrual flow is produced is

165

presented to clarify the logic of the various steps in the diagnostic procedures.

Definition of Amenorrhea

Any patient fulfilling the following criteria should be evaluated as having the clinical problem of amenorrhea:

1. No period by age 14 in the absence of growth or development of secondary sexual characteristics.

2. No period by age 16 regardless of the presence of normal growth and development with the appearance of secondary sexual characteristics.

3. In a woman who has been menstruating, the absence of periods for a length of time equivalent to a total of at least 3 of the previous cycle intervals, or 6 months of amenorrhea.

Having affirmed the traditional criteria, let us now point out that strict adherence to these criteria can result in improper management of individual cases. There is no reason to defer the evaluation of a young girl who presents with the obvious stigmata of Turner's syndrome. Similarly, the 14 year old girl with an absent vagina who is otherwise completely normal should not be told to return in 2 years. A patient deserves a considerate evaluation whenever her anxieties, or those of her parents, bring her to a physician. Finally, the possibility of pregnancy should always be considered.

Another tradition has been to categorize amenorrhea as primary or secondary in nature. While these stipulations are inherent in the definitions noted above, experience has shown that premature categorization of this sort leads to diagnostic omission in certain instances, and frequently, unnecessary and expensive diagnostic procedures. Because the prescribed workup to be detailed here applies comprehensively to all amenorrheas, the classic definitions are not retained.

Basic Principles in Menstrual Function

The clinical demonstration of menstrual function depends on visible external evidence of the menstrual discharge. This requires an intact outflow tract which connects the internal genital source of flow with the outside. As such, the outflow tract requires patency and continuity of the vaginal orifice, the vaginal canal, and the endocervix with the uterine cavity. The presence of a menstrual flow depends on the existence and development of the endometrium lining the uterine cavity. This tissue is stimulated and regulated by the proper quantity and sequence of the steroid hormones, estrogen and progesterone. The secretion of these hormones originates in the ovary, but more specifically in the evolving spectrum of follicle development, ovulation, and corpus luteum function. This essential maturation of the follicular apparatus is guided by the stimuli provided by the sequence and magnitude of the gonadotropins, follicle-stimulating hormone (FSH) and luteinizing hormone (LH), originating in the anterior pituitary. The secretion of these hormones is in turn dependent upon gonadotropin releasing hormone (GnRH), the specific peptide releasing hormone produced in the basal hypothalamus and blood borne via the portal vessels of the stalk to receptive cells within the anterior pituitary. The entire system is regulated by a complex mechanism which integrates biophysical and biochemical information comprised of interactive levels of hormonal signals and target cell receptor function in the uterus, ovary, pituitary, hypothalamus, and other CNS sources (feedback levels of ovarian steroids and pituitary gonadotropins as well as neurohumors derived from higher hypothalamic and other CNS resources).

The basic principles underlying the physiology of menstrual function permit formulation of several discrete compartmental systems on which proper menstruation depends. It is useful to employ a diagnostic evaluation which segregates causes of amenorrhea into the following compartments:

Compartment I:
Disorders of outflow tract or uterine target organ.

Compartment II:
Disorders of the ovary.

Compartment III:
Disorders of the anterior pituitary.

Compartment IV:
Disorders of CNS (hypothalamic) factors.

Evaluation of Amenorrhea

A careful history and physical examination should seek the following: evidence for psychological dysfunction or emotional stress, family history of apparent genetic anomalies, signs of a physical problem with a focus on nutritional status, abnormal growth and development, the presence of a normal reproductive tract, and evidence for CNS disease. A patient with amenorrhea is then exposed to a combined therapeutic and laboratory dissection according to the depicted flow diagrams. Because a significant number of patients with amenorrhea also have galactorrhea, and there are similarities in the evaluation of these two conditions, the workup as described is appropriate for patients who have amenorrhea or galactorrhea, or both. Galactorrhea is also considered in Chapter 9.

Amenorrhea and galactorrhea need be the sole pertinent initial items of information. Although additional data are undoubtedly available at this time, derived from history and physical examination and evaluation of other endocrine glands such as the thyroid and adrenal, these items should not be utilized for diagnostic purposes until the entire workup is completed. Experience has shown that premature diagnostic bias at this point, while frequently accurate, not uncommonly leads to erroneous judgments as well as inappropriate, costly, and useless testing.

Step 1

The initial step in the workup of the amenorrheic patient after excluding pregnancy begins with a measurement of thyroid stimulating hormone (TSH), a prolactin level, and a progestational challenge. The initial step in the patient presenting with galactorrhea, regardless of menstrual history, also includes TSH and prolactin measurement, but adds a coned-down, lateral x-ray view of the sella turcica.

167

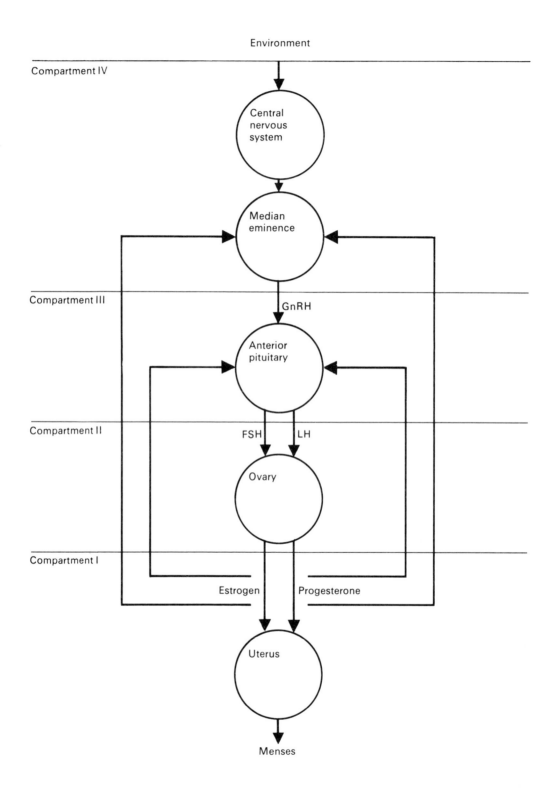

Environment

Compartment IV

Central
nervous
system

Median
eminence

Compartment III

GnRH

Anterior
pituitary

Compartment II

FSH   LH

Ovary

Compartment I

Estrogen   Progesterone

Uterus

Menses

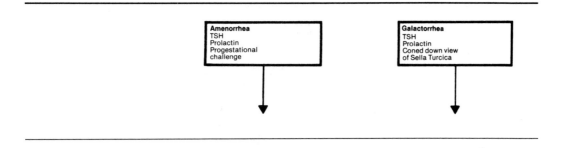

Only a few patients presenting with amenorrhea and/or galactorrhea will have hypothyroidism which is not clinically apparent. Although it seems rather extravagant to measure TSH in such a large number of patients for such a small return, treatment for hypothyroidism is so simple and is rewarded by such a prompt return of ovulatory cycles, and if galactorrhea is present, by a disappearance of the breast secretions (a slower process which can take several months), TSH measurement is warranted.

It is not sufficient to measure the routine thyroid function tests. A patient may be in a compensated state with normal thyroxine (T_4) levels achieved by increased TSH secretion. With regard to the mechanism of the galactorrhea, the duration of the hypothyroidism is important; the longer the duration the higher the incidence of galactorrhea and the higher the prolactin levels.(1) This is thought to be associated with declining hypothalamic content of dopamine with on-going hypothyroidism. This would lead to an unopposed TRH stimulatory effect on the pituitary cells which secrete prolactin. In our experience, prolactin levels associated with primary hypothyroidism have always been less than 100 ng/ml.

The constant stimulation by hypothalamic releasing hormones results in hypertrophy or hyperplasia of the pituitary. The x-ray picture of a tumor, distortion, expansion, or erosion of the sella turcica, can be seen, therefore, with primary hypothyroidism, and in patients with elevated GnRH and gonadotropin secretion due to premature ovarian failure.(2) Patients with primary hypothyroidism and hyperprolactinemia can present with either primary or secondary amenorrhea.(3)

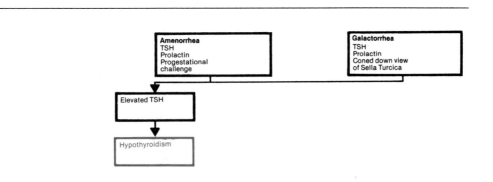

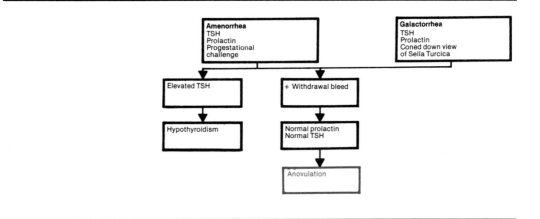

The purpose of the progestational challenge is to assess the level of endogenous estrogen and the competence of the outflow tract. A course of a progestational agent totally devoid of estrogenic activity is administered. There are two choices: parenteral progesterone in oil (200 mg) or orally active medroxyprogesterone acetate, 10 mg daily for 5 days. The use of an orally active agent avoids an unpleasant intramuscular injection (although this might be necessary when compliance is a concern). Other hormonal preparations, such as birth control pills, are not appropriate since they do not exert a purely progestational effect.

Within 2-7 days after the conclusion of progestational medication, the patient will either bleed or not bleed. If the patient bleeds, a diagnosis of anovulation has been reliably and securely established. The presence of a functional outflow tract and a uterus lined by reactive endometrium sufficiently prepared by endogenous estrogen is confirmed. With this demonstration of the presence of estrogen, minimal function of the ovary, pituitary, and CNS is established. In the absence of galactorrhea, with a normal prolactin level, and a normal TSH, further evaluation is unnecessary.

All anovulatory patients require therapeutic management, and with this minimal evaluation, therapy can be planned immediately. Because of the short latent period in the progression from normal endometrial tissue to atypia to cancer, clinicians are sensitive to the issue of endometrial cancer. But all too often, the clinician believes that this is a problem limited to older age. The critical feature is the duration of exposure to constant, unopposed estrogen. Therefore even young women, anovulatory for relatively long periods of time, can develop endometrial cancer. If there is any concern, evaluation of the endometrium (with aspiration curettage) is in order.

On the other hand, the latent phase for breast cancer is long, perhaps as long as 20 years. It is only recently that data have emerged indicating that women who are anovulatory when they are young have an increased risk of breast cancer when they are postmenopausal.(4) While the evidence is not conclusive, there is support for the contention that periodic exposure to a progestational agent not only protects the endometrium, but also the breast.

170

Minimal therapy of anovulatory women requires the monthly administration of a progestational agent. An easily remembered program is to prescribe 10 mg medroxyprogesterone acetate daily for the first 10 days of each month. Experience with the endometrium in estrogen replacement programs has established the importance of a time period of at least 10 days to provide adequate protection against the growth promoting effects of constant estrogen. When reliable contraception is essential, the use of low dose oral contraceptive pills in the usual cyclic fashion is appropriate. Attempts to demonstrate a relationship between pill use and subsequent postpill amenorrhea have not been successful. Anovulation with amenorrhea or oligomenorrhea should not be viewed as a contraindication to the use of oral contraception.

If, at any time, an anovulatory patient fails to have withdrawal bleeding on a monthly progestin program, this is a sign (providing the patient is not pregnant) that she has moved to the negative withdrawal bleed category, and the remainder of the workup must be pursued. The progestational challenge will occasionally trigger an ovulation in an anovulatory patient. The tip-off will be a later withdrawal bleed, 14 days after the progestational challenge!

In the absence of galactorrhea, if the serum prolactin level is normal (less than 20 ng/ml in most laboratories), further evaluation for the presence of a pituitary tumor is unnecessary when the patient has undergone a withdrawal bleed. Random single samples for prolactin are sufficient, as variations in the amplitude of the spikes of secretion and the sleep-related and food-related increases appear to be attenuated in both functional and tumor hyperprolactinemic states. If the prolactin is elevated, x-ray evaluation of the sella turcica by a coned-down view is essential (as discussed below). Likewise the presence of galactorrhea, regardless of the bleeding pattern or the prolactin level, requires a coned-down view. At this point in the workup, the following statement is a useful clinical rule of thumb: *A positive withdrawal bleeding response to progestational medication, the absence of galactorrhea, and a normal prolactin level together effectively rule out the presence of a significant pituitary tumor.*

How much bleeding constitutes a positive withdrawal response? The appearance of only a few blood spots following progestational medication implies marginal levels of endogenous estrogen. Such patients should be followed closely and periodically re-evaluated, since the marginally positive response may progress to a clearly negative response, placing the patient in a new diagnostic category. Bleeding in any amount beyond a few spots is considered a positive withdrawal response.

There are two rare situations associated with a negative withdrawal response despite the presence of adequate levels of endogenous estrogen. In both situations, the endometrium is decidualized, and therefore, it will not be shed following the withdrawal of exogenous progestin. The first condition finds the endometrium decidualized in response to high androgen levels, for example due to the anovulatory state (with polycystic ovaries). In the second unusual clinical situation, the endometrium is decidualized by high progesterone levels associated with a specific adrenal enzyme deficiency.

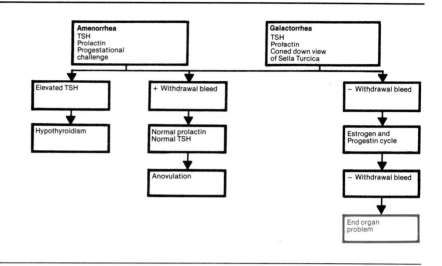

Step 2

If the course of progestational medication does not produce withdrawal flow, either the target organ outflow tract is inoperative or preliminary estrogen proliferation of the endometrium has not occurred. Step 2 is designed to clarify this situation. Orally active estrogen is administered in quantity and duration certain to stimulate endometrial proliferation and withdrawal bleeding provided that a completely reactive uterus and patent outflow tract exist. An appropriate dose is 2.5 mg conjugated estrogens daily for 21 days. The terminal addition of an orally active progestational agent (medroxyprogesterone acetate 10 mg daily for the last 5 days) is necessary to achieve withdrawal. In this way the capacity of Compartment I is challenged by exogenous estrogen. In the absence of withdrawal flow, a validating second course of estrogen is a wise precaution.

As a result of the pharmacologic test of Step 2, the patient with amenorrhea will either bleed or not bleed. If there is no withdrawal flow, the diagnosis of a defect in the Compartment I systems (endometrium, outflow tract) can be made with confidence. If withdrawal bleeding does occur, one can assume that Compartment I systems have normal functional abilities if properly stimulated by estrogen.

In a patient with normal external and internal genitalia by pelvic examination, and in the absence of a history of infection or trauma (such as curettage), Step 2 can be safely omitted. Abnormalities in the systems of Compartment I are not commonly encountered.

Step 3

With the elucidation of the amenorrheic patient's inability to provide adequate stimulatory amounts of estrogen, the physiologic mechanisms responsible for the elaboration of this steroid must be tested. In order to produce estrogen, ovaries containing a normal follicular apparatus and sufficient pituitary gonadotropins to stimulate that apparatus are required. Step 3 is designed to determine which of these two crucial components (gonadotropins or follicular activity) is functioning improperly.

172

Clinical State	Serum FSH	Serum LH
Normal adult female	5–30 mIU/ml, with the ovulatory midcycle peak about 2 times the base level	5–20 mIU/ml with the ovulatory midcycle peak about 3 times the base level
Hypogonadotropic state: Prepubertal, Hypothalamic and Pituitary Dysfunction	Less than 5 mIU/ml	Less than 5 mIU/ml
Hypergonadotropic state: Postmenopausal, Castrate and Ovarian Failure	Greater than 40 mIU/ml	Greater than 25 mIU/ml

This step involves an assay of the level of gonadotropins in the patient. Because Step 2 involved administration of exogenous estrogen, endogenous gonadotropin levels may be artificially and temporarily altered from their true baseline concentrations. Hence, a delay of 2 weeks following Step 2 must ensue before doing Step 3, the gonadotropin assay. One should keep in mind that the midcycle surge of LH is approximately 3 times the baseline level. Therefore, if the patient does not bleed 2 weeks after the blood sample was obtained, a high level can be safely interpreted as abnormal.

Step 3 is designed to determine whether the lack of estrogen is due to a fault in the follicle (Compartment II) or in the CNS-pituitary axis (Compartments III and IV). The result of the gonadotropin assay in the amenorrheic woman who does not bleed following a progestational agent will be abnormally high, abnormally low, or in the normal range.

High Gonadotropins

The association between castrate or postmenopausal levels of gonadotropins and ovarian failure is very reliable. However, there are several rare situations in which high gonadotropins can be accompanied by ovaries that contain follicles.

1. On rare occasions, tumors can produce gonadotropins. This situation is usually associated with lung cancer and is so infrequent, that with a normal history and physical examination, routine chest x-ray is not warranted in amenorrheic patients.

2. There have been a handful of reports of a single gonadotropin deficiency. The importance of measuring both FSH and LH can be appreciated since a high level of one and a baseline level of the other would reveal this rare condition. A high FSH and a low LH should make one suspect a gonadotropin-secreting pituitary adenoma. Most, if not all, of these uncommon tumors are FSH-secreting, and are associated with hypogonadism due to the low LH.(5) Furthermore, most of the reported cases have been in men.

173

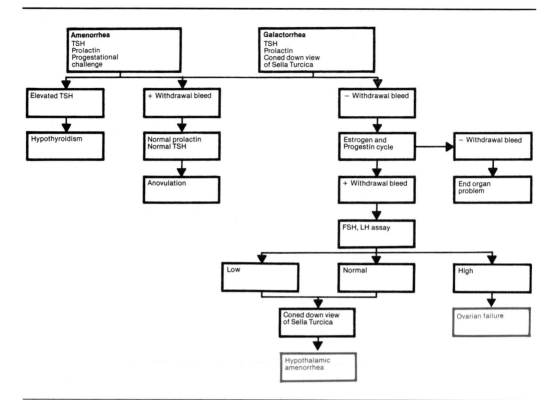

3. During the perimenopausal period it is normal for FSH levels to begin to rise even before bleeding has ceased. (6) This is true whether the perimenopausal period is premature at age 25-35 or at the usual time. It is believed that FSH is partly under the negative feedback control of a peptide (inhibin) produced by granulosa cells. During the perimenopausal period the remaining follicles may be viewed as the least sensitive of all follicles because they have remained in place and failed to respond to gonadotropins for many years. As these remaining follicles begin to respond to the rising gonadotropin levels during the perimenopause, the production of the peptide responsible for the negative feedback may be inadequate, and the patient can have elevated levels of FSH despite continued bleeding or a very recent onset of amenorrhea. Attention must be paid to this situation because a period of postmenopausal levels of FSH can be followed by a pregnancy. The value of measuring both FSH and LH is again emphasized in that this special perimenopausal condition is usually associated with a high FSH, but a normal LH.

4. In the resistant or insensitive ovary syndrome the patient with amenorrhea has elevated gonadotropins despite the presence of ovarian follicles. It is believed that this condition represents an absence of gonadotropin receptors on the follicles, or a postreceptor defect.(7) In these cases laparotomy is the only definitive way to evaluate the ovaries, because follicles are contained deep within the ovary, yielding only to a full thickness biopsy.(8) Because this condition is very rare, and the chance of achieving pregnancy is probably impossible even with large doses of exogenous gonadotropins, laparotomy is *not* recommended for every patient with amenorrhea and high gonadotropins. One might consider the use of ultrasonography—if follicles can be definitely outlined by the ultrasonographer, exogenous gonadotropin stimulation can be considered.

5. Secondary amenorrhea due to premature ovarian failure can be due to autoimmune disease.(9) The ovaries contain normal-appearing primordial follicles, but developing follicles contain lymphocytes and plasma cells in the theca cell and granulosa cell layers. Most commonly, evidence of abnormal thyroid function is detected, and therefore, complete thyroid testing (with antibodies) is necessary in all patients with premature ovarian failure. The extensive polyglandular syndrome which includes hypoparathyroidism, adrenal insufficiency, thyroiditis, and moniliasis is rare. Other rare conditions associated with premature ovarian failure include: myasthenia gravis, idiopathic thrombocytopenic purpura, rheumatoid arthritis, vitiligo, and autoimmune hemolytic anemia. Classically premature ovarian failure precedes adrenal failure, and thus a case can be made for continuing adrenal surveillance. Only one pregnancy has been reported in women with ovarian failure and autoimmune disease, although ovulation has been restored temporarily with corticosteroid treatment, and at least one patient had a temporary spontaneous return of menstrual ovarian activity.(10) Pregnancy is therefore extremely unlikely.

6. The final rare clinical situations associated with high gonadotropins and normal ovarian follicles include galactosemia and an enzymatic deficiency in both ovaries and the adrenal glands, the 17-hydroxylase deficiency. In patients with galactosemia, an abnormal carbohydrate component of the gonadotropin molecules may render FSH and LH inactive. On the other hand, the problem in patients with galactosemia may be primarily gonadal; fewer oogonia may be the result of a direct effect of galactose on germ cell migration to the genital ridge. (11) A patient with a deficiency of 17-hydroxylase is readily detectable because she would present with absent secondary sexual development (sex steroids cannot be produced due to the enzyme block in the adrenal glands and the ovaries), and this patient would also be hypertensive and have high blood levels of progesterone.

The Need for
Chromosome
Evaluation

All patients under the age of 30 who have been assigned the diagnosis of ovarian failure on the basis of elevated gonadotropins must have a karyotype determination. The presence of mosaicism with a Y chromosome requires laparotomy and excision of the gonadal areas because the presence of any testicular component within the gonad carries with it a 25% chance of malignant tumor formation. These are highly malignant secondary tumors from germ cells: gonadoblastomas, dysgerminomas, yolk sac tumors, and choriocarcinoma. Approximately 30% of patients with a Y chromosome will not develop signs of virilization. Therefore, even the normal appearing adult woman with elevated gonadotropin levels must be karyotyped. Even if the karyotype is normal, as an added precaution all patients with ovarian failure should have an annual pelvic examination. Such preventive care is also indicated because these patients will be on hormone replacement therapy. Over the age of 30, amenorrhea with high gonadotropins is best labeled premature menopause. Genetic evaluation is unnecessary because it is essentially unheard of to have a gonadal tumor appear in these patients after the age of 30.

Patients with elevated gonadotropin levels can be reliably diagnosed as having ovarian failure and considered sterile. In the past this was a diagnosis made with great confidence, and careful explanation was given to the patient indicating that future pregnancy was impossible. In recent years, however, rare cases have been reported of patients presenting with secondary amenorrhea and elevated gonadotropins who several months later demonstrated resumption of normal function.(12,13) This has commonly been associated with the use of estrogen replacement therapy, suggesting that the estrogen may activate receptor formation on follicles, and the high gonadotropins may thus stimulate follicular growth and development. In some patients, return of normal ovarian function with pregnancy has occurred spontaneously. While resumption of normal function is extremely rare, it is now necessary to tell patients who fit into this category that there is a very remote possibility of future pregnancy. In addition the feasibility of pregnancy with the transfer of a fertilized donated ovum should be presented as a possible option. (Chapter 21)

Because a number of cases of ovarian failure have been reported with autoimmune disorders, a reasonable approach is to perform a few selected blood tests for autoimmune disease:

Calcium
Phosphorus
A.M. cortisol
Free T_4
TSH
Thyroid antibodies
Complete blood count and sedimentation rate
Total protein, albumin/globulin ratio
Rheumatoid factor
Antinuclear antibody

The percentage of T lymphocytes expressing the immune-associated antigen will be increased, and this test, which may be more available than measuring antiovarian antibodies, more accurately correlates with remission and exacerbation.(14) Testing for ACTH reserve (with metyrapone, see Chapter 22) seems debatable if clinical appearance and other laboratory tests are normal. Periodic surveillance for adrenal failure is in order because ovarian failure usually precedes adrenal failure.

It has been suggested that blood gonadotropins and estradiol should be measured weekly on 4 occasions.(12) If FSH is not higher than LH (an FSH/LH ratio less than 1.0), and if estradiol is not in the postmenopausal range (greater than 50 pg/ml), induction of ovulation can be considered. Prior to treatment with exogenous gonadotropins, there may be some advantage to first bring the elevated gonadotropins down to normal range with administration of estrogen. It seems appropriate to offer the patient a choice between a full thickness ovarian biopsy and empirical treatment. In our view, empirical treatment appears to outweigh the cost and risk of laparotomy, since only a very rare woman with hypergonadotropic amenorrhea can be expected to conceive. In other words, even if there is some gonadotropic and estradiol evidence of follicular activity, the response to exogenous gonadotropin stimulation has been very disappointing.

Normal Gonadotropins

Why is it that hypoestrogenic (negative progestational withdrawal) patients will frequently have normal circulating levels of FSH and LH as measured by the radioimmunoassay? If normal gonadotropins were truly present in the circulation, follicular growth should be maintained and estrogen levels would be adequate to provide a positive withdrawal bleed. The answer to this paradox lies in the heterogeneity of the glycoprotein hormones.

The molecules of gonadotropins produced by these amenorrheic patients have increased amounts of sialic acid in the carbohydrate portion. Therefore, the molecules are qualitatively altered and biologically inactive. The antibodies in the radioimmunoassay, however, are able to recognize a sufficient portion of the molecule to return a normal answer. Another very rare possibility is an inherited disorder of gonadotropin synthesis leading to the production of immunologically active, but biologically inactive hormones.(15)

The significant clinical point is the following: FSH and LH levels in the normal range in a patient with a negative progestational withdrawal test are consistent with pituitary-CNS failure. Indeed, this is the most commonly encountered clinical situation. Extremely low or nondetectable gonadotropins are seldom found, and usually only with large pituitary tumors or in patients with anorexia nervosa. Further evaluation, therefore, is in order, and follows the recommendations for low gonadotropins.

Low Gonadotropins

If the gonadotropin assay is abnormally low, or in the normal range, one final localization is required to distinguish between a pituitary (Compartment III) or CNS-hypothalamic (Compartment IV) cause for the amenorrhea. This is achieved by an x-ray evaluation of the sella turcica for signs of abnormal change.

X-ray Evaluation of the Sella Turcica. In recent years, the radiologic evaluation of the pituitary area has undergone rapid change. There now is no argument that the diagnostic modality of choice is thin section coronal computerized tomography (CT scan) with intravenous contrast enhancement. The most modern CT scan (capable of high resolution 1 mm cuts) is able to evaluate the contents of the sella turcica as well as the suprasellar area. Magnetic resonance imaging is even more sensitive than the CT scan, but it is also even more expensive, and it requires a lengthy period of time to obtain the images. The intention of this workup is to be conscious of cost and to isolate those few patients who require the sophisticated, but expensive, CT scan.

There has been growing conservatism in the management of small prolactin-secreting pituitary tumors because of an appreciation that the majority of these tumors never change. We have adopted the conservative approach of close surveillance, recommending bromocriptine treatment for those tumors that display rapid growth, or those tumors which are already large, and reserving surgery only for those tumors that are unresponsive to bromocriptine. This means that small tumors (microadenomas are less than 1 cm in diameter) need not be treated at all. Hence, the initial x-ray evaluation for

177

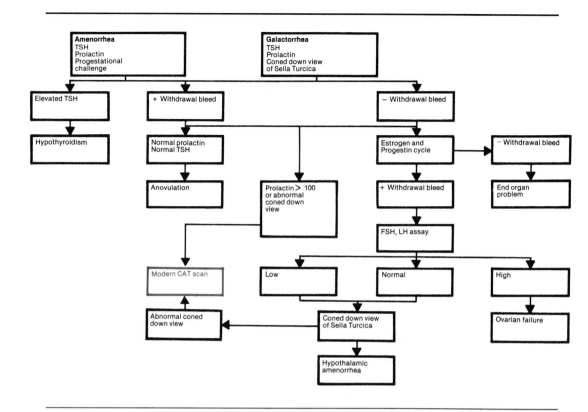

amenorrheic patients with or without galactorrhea is the coned-down view of the sella turcica. This will detect the presence of a large tumor, although an incredibly rare suprasellar extension might escape this method. Combining this screening technique with the prolactin assay, we are able to select those few patients who require the modern CT scan. If the prolactin level is greater than 100 ng/ml, or if the coned-down view of the sella turcica is abnormal, we recommend CT scan evaluation. *A double floor of the sella is often seen on the coned-down view and, in absence of enlargement and/or demineralization, is interpreted as a normal variation rather than asymmetrical depression of the sellar floor by a tumor.*

The presence of visual problems and/or headaches should also encourage CT scan evaluation. Headaches are definitely correlated with the presence of a pituitary adenoma.(16) Although they are usually bifrontal, retroorbital, or bitemporal, no locations or features are specific for pituitary tumors.

If the CT scan rules out an empty sella syndrome, or a suprasellar problem, treatment is dictated by the patient's desires, the size of the tumor, and the rapidity of growth of the tumor.

The prolactin level of 100 ng/ml for determining a more aggressive approach has been empirically chosen. Both in our own experience, and that of others, large tumors are most frequently associated with prolactin levels greater than 100.

The above approach to the problem of pituitary tumors implies that patients with prolactin levels less than 100 ng/ml and with normal coned-down views of the sella turcica can be offered a choice between treatment and surveillance. An annual prolactin level and an annual coned-down view are indicated for continued observation to detect an emerging and slow-growing tumor. Bromocriptine therapy is recommended for patients wishing to achieve pregnancy, and for those patients who have galactorrhea to the point of discomfort. Thus far, long term therapy with bromocriptine has not been proven to be successful in producing a complete reversal of the problem (with either permanent suppression of elevated prolactin levels or evidence of elimination of small tumors).

Evaluation of the Abnormal Sella Turcica and/or High Prolactin. The high incidence of pituitary tumors in patients with amenorrhea has prompted a search for a reliable method of diagnosing the condition. Expectations for the utilization of endocrine testing to discriminate between disorders of the hypothalamus and the anterior pituitary have not been realized. These endocrine maneuvers include GnRH stimulation, TRH stimulation, and other steps to alter prolactin, growth hormone, and ACTH secretion. TRH stimulation of the prolactin response is the most consistently abnormal response (a blunter response of prolactin), but some patients with tumors respond normally. Variability in response to all maneuvers is the rule.

Frankly, the endocrine maneuvers yield no more useful information than the two major screening procedures, the blood prolactin and the coned-down view of the sella turcica. Visual field examination is not useful in screening for pituitary tumors because abnormalities are seen only with large tumors which are evident by prolactin, x-ray evaluation, and/or visual symptoms and headaches.

If the coned-down view is abnormal and/or the prolactin level is over 100, further evaluation and treatment require consultation with expert endocrine resources. These patients are rare, and accumulated experience which can provide the necessary clinical judgment can be found only with the referral resource. On the other hand, our workup easily deals with the vast majority of patients, and the few who require a multidisciplinary team approach are readily identified.

Hypogonadotropic Hypogonadism. Patients with amenorrhea and without galactorrhea who have reached this point in the workup and have normal x-rays are classified as *hypothalamic amenorrhea*. The mechanism of the amenorrhea is suppression of pulsatile GnRH secretion below its critical range. This is a diagnosis by exclusion because we can identify probable causes (e.g. anorexia and weight loss) but we cannot test, manipulate, or measure the hypothalamus to prove our diagnosis.

Specific Disorders within Compartments

With only modest effort, expense, and time the problem of amenorrhea has been dissected into compartments of dysfunction which positively correlate with specific organ systems. At this point, with the specific anatomic locus of the defect defined, the clinician can now undertake steps to elucidate the specific disorder leading to amenorrhea. Congenital abnormalities are limited to amenorrhea which presents in the pubertal period of life. In a collection of 262 patients with secondary amenorrhea of adult onset, the following diagnostic frequencies were most often observed: (17)

Compartment I:

    Asherman's Syndrome   — 7.0%

Compartment II:

    Abnormal chromosomes   — 0.5%
    Normal chromosomes   —10.0%

Compartment III:

    Prolactin tumors   — 7.5%

Compartment IV:

    Anovulation   —28.0%
    Weight loss/anorexia   —10.0%
    Hypothalamic suppression —10.0%
    Hypothyroidism   — 1.0%

Compartment I

Asherman's Syndrome. Secondary amenorrhea follows destruction of the endometrium (Asherman's Syndrome). (18) This condition generally is the result of an overzealous postpartum curettage resulting in intrauterine scarification. A typical pattern of multiple synechiae is seen on a hysterogram. In the presence of normal ovarian function, the basal body temperature will be biphasic. The adhesions may partially or completely obliterate the endometrial cavity, the internal cervical os, or the cervical canal, or combinations of these areas. Surprisingly, despite stenosis or atresia of the internal os, hematometra does not inevitably occur. The endometrium, perhaps in response to a buildup of pressure, becomes refractory and simple cervical dilatation cures the problem. Asherman's Syndrome also can occur following uterine surgery, including cesarean section, myomectomy, or metroplasty. Very severe adhesions have been noted following postpartum curettage and postpartum hypogonadism, e.g. in Sheehan's Syndrome.

Patients with Asherman's Syndrome may present with other problems besides amenorrhea, including abortions, dysmenorrhea, or hypomenorrhea. They may even have normal menses. Infertility can be present with mild adhesions, an association not readily explainable. Patients with repeated abortions, infertility, or pregnancy wastage should have investigation of the endometrial cavity by hysterogram or hysteroscopy.

Impairment of the endometrium resulting in amenorrhea can be caused by tuberculosis, a condition that is rare in the United States. Diagnosis is made by culture of the menstrual discharge or tissue obtained by endometrial biopsy. Uterine schistosomiasis is another rare cause of end organ failure, and eggs may be found in urine, feces, rectal scrapings, menstrual discharge, or endometrium. In recent years, we have seen the syndrome following intrauterine device (IUD)-related infections, and severe, generalized pelvic infections.

Asherman's Syndrome can be treated with a dilatation and curettage to break up the synechiae, and if necessary an on-the-table hysterogram to ensure a free uterine cavity. Advocates of the hysteroscope claim that direct lysis of adhesions yields better results than the "blind" dilatation and curettage. Following operation, a method should be utilized to prevent the sides of the uterine cavity from adhering. Previously an IUD was used for this purpose; however, a pediatric Foley catheter appears to be a better option. The bag is filled with 3 ml of fluid; the catheter is removed after 7 days. A broad-spectrum antibiotic is started preoperatively and maintained for 10 days. An inhibitor of prostaglandin synthesis can be used if uterine cramping is a problem. The patient is treated for 2 months with high stimulatory doses of estrogen (e.g. conjugated estrogens 2.5 mg daily 3 weeks out of 4 with medroxyprogesterone acetate 10 mg daily added during the 3rd week). When the initial attempt fails to re-establish menstrual flow, repeated attempts are worthwhile. Persistent treatment with repeated procedures may be necessary to regain reproductive potential. Approximately 70-80% of patients with this condition have achieved a successful pregnancy. Pregnancy, however, is frequently complicated by premature labor, placenta accreta, placenta previa, and/or postpartum hemorrhage.

Müllerian Anomalies. In primary amenorrheas, discontinuity by segmental disruptions of the müllerian tube should be ruled out. Thus, imperforate hymen, obliteration of the vaginal orifice, and lapses in continuity of the vaginal canal must be ruled out by direct observation. The cervix or the entire uterus may be absent. Far less common, the uterus may be present, but the cavity absent, or, in the presence of a cavity, the endometrium may be congenitally lacking. With the exception of the latter abnormalities, the clinical problem of amenorrhea due to obstruction is compounded by the painful distention of hematocolpos, hematometra, or hematoperitoneum. In all instances an effort must be made to incise and drain from below at the points of closure of the müllerian tube. Even in complicated circumstances re-establishment of müllerian duct continuity usually can be achieved surgically. The unfortunate consequences of operative extirpation of painful masses from above with damage to bladder, ureter, and rectum, as well as irretrievable loss of distended but otherwise healthy, reproductive organs are rare but well-remembered.

Knowing what to expect prior to attempting surgical correction is a great advantage. Recently, magnetic resonance imaging (MRI) has been utilized to accurately delineate the anatomical abnormality.(19) A correct preoperative diagnosis will certainly facilitate the planning and execution of surgery.

Müllerian Agenesis. Lack of müllerian development *(MAYER-ROKITANSKY-KUSTER-HAUSER SYNDROME)* is the diagnosis for the individual with primary amenorrhea and no apparent vagina.(20) This is a relatively common cause of primary amenorrhea, more frequent than testicular feminization, and second only to gonadal dysgenesis. These patients have an absence or hypoplasia of the vagina. The uterus may be normal, but lacking a conduit to the introitus, or there may only be rudimentary, bicornuate cords present. If a partial endometrial cavity is present, cyclic abdominal pain may be a complaint. Because of the similarity to some types of male pseudohermaphroditism, it is worthwhile to demonstrate the normal female karyotype. Ovarian function is normal and can be documented with basal body temperatures or peripheral levels of progesterone. Growth and development are normal. Although usually sporadic, occasional occurrence may be noted within a family.

Further evaluation should include radiologic studies. Approximately one-third of patients have urinary tract abnormalities and 12% or more have skeletal anomalies, most involving the spine. Renal tract abnormalities include ectopic kidney, renal agenesis, horseshoe kidney, and abnormal collecting ducts. When the presence of a uterine structure is suspected on examination, ultrasound can be utilized to depict the size and symmetry of the structure. Laparoscopic visualization of the pelvis is not necessary, and extirpation of the müllerian remnants is certainly not necessary unless they are causing a problem such as uterine fibroid growth, hematometra, endometriosis, or symptomatic herniation into the inguinal canal.

Because of the difficulties and complications experienced in surgical series, we favor, when possible, an alternative to the surgical construction of an artificial vagina. Instead, we encourage the use of progressive dilatation as initially described by Frank (21) and later by Wabrek et al. (22) Beginning first in a posterior direction, and then after 2 weeks changing upward to the usual line of the vaginal axis, pressure with commercially available vaginal dilators is carried out for 20 min daily to the point of modest discomfort. Utilizing increasingly larger dilators, a functional vagina can be created in approximately 6-12 weeks. *Plastic syringe covers can be used instead of the expensive commercial glass dilators.* Operative treatment should be reserved for those women in whom the Frank method is unacceptable, or fails, or when a well-formed uterus is present and fertility might be preserved. The symptoms of retained menstruation should identify these patients. A modern approach for this problem recommends an initial laparotomy to evaluate the cervical canal; if the cervix is atretic, the uterus should be removed.(23) Unless it is the relatively simple problem of an imperforate hymen or a transverse vaginal septum, some have recommended against trying to preserve fertility in the presence of complete vaginal agenesis. The morbidity subsequent to surgery argues for removal of the müllerian structures at the time of construction of a neovagina. Patients with a transverse vaginal septum, which is a failure of canalization of the distal third of the vagina, usually present with symptoms of obstruction and urinary frequency. A transverse septum can be differentiated from an imperforate hymen by a lack of distention at the introitus with Valsalva's maneuver.

Distal obstruction of the genital tract is the only condition in this category which can be considered an emergency. Delay in surgical treatment can lead to infertility due to inflammatory changes and endometriosis. Definitive surgery should be accomplished as soon as possible. Diagnostic needling should be avoided because a hematocolpos can be converted into a pyocolpos.

Reassurance and support are necessary to carry a patient through these procedures. Problems with body image and sexual enjoyment can be avoided, and, although infertile, a full and normal life as a woman can be achieved.

Testicular Feminization. Testicular feminization is the likely diagnosis when a blind vaginal canal is encountered and the uterus is absent. The patient with testicular feminization is a male pseudohermaphrodite. The adjective male refers to the gonadal sex; thus, the individual has testes and an XY karyotype. Pseudohermaphrodite means that the genitalia are opposite of the gonads; thus, the individual is phenotypically female, but with absent or meager pubic and axillary hair.

The male pseudohermaphrodite is a genetic and gonadal male with failure of virilization. Failures in male development can be considered as a spectrum with incomplete forms of testicular feminization being represented by some androgen response. Transmission of this disorder is by means of an X-linked recessive gene that is responsible for the androgen intracellular receptor. Clinically the diagnosis should be considered in:

1. A female child with inguinal hernias, since the testes are frequently partially descended;

2. A patient with primary amenorrhea and an absent uterus;

3. A patient with absent body hair.

These patients appear normal at birth except for the possible presence of an inguinal hernia, and most patients are not seen by a physician until puberty. Growth and development are normal, although overall height is usually greater than average, and there may be an eunuchoidal tendency (long arms, big hands and feet). The breasts, although large, are abnormal; actual glandular tissue is not abundant, nipples are small, and the areolae are pale. More than 50% have an inguinal hernia; the labia minora are usually underdeveloped, and the blind vagina is less deep than normal. Rudimentary fallopian tubes are composed of fibromuscular tissue with only occasional epithelial lining.

Perhaps urological evaluation in these patients has been inadequately pursued. Horseshoe kidneys have been reported.

The testes may be intra-abdominal, but often are in a hernia. They are similar to any cryptorchid testis except that they may be nodular. After puberty, the testis displays immature tubular development, and tubules are lined by immature germ cells and Sertoli cells. There is no spermatogenesis. The incidence of neoplasia in these gonads is high. In 50 reported cases, there were 11 malignancies, 15 adenomas, and 10 benign cysts: a 22% incidence of malignancy and a 52% incidence of neoplasia.(24) Therefore, once full development is attained after puberty, the gonads should be removed and the patient placed on hormonal replacement therapy. *This is the only exception to the rule that gonads with a Y chromosome should be removed prior to puberty.* There are two reasons: first, the development achieved with hormonal replacement does not seem to match the smooth pubertal changes due to endogenous hormones, and second, gonadal tumors in these patients have not been encountered prior to puberty.

When testicular feminization was first studied, it was found that the urinary 17-ketosteroids were normal, and it was suggested that there might be a resistance to androgen action rather than an absence of androgens—a congenital androgen insensitivity. Indeed, the plasma levels of testosterone are in the normal to high male range, and the plasma clearance and metabolism of testosterone are normal. Thus, these patients produce testosterone, but they do not respond to androgens, either their own or those given locally or systemically. Therefore, the critical steps in sexual differentiation which require androgens fail to take place, and development is totally female.

Appropriately this condition is now referred to as the *CONGENITAL ANDROGEN INSENSITIVITY SYNDROME*. It is marked by a unique combination:

1. Normal female phenotype.

2. Normal male karyotype, 46,XY.

3. Normal or slightly elevated male blood testosterone levels.

Cases of *INCOMPLETE TESTICULAR FEMINIZATION* represent individuals with some androgen effect. These individuals may have clitoral enlargement, or a phallus may even be present. Axillary and pubic hair develop along with breast growth. Gonadectomy should not be deferred in such cases, because it will obviate unwanted further virilization. Patients with a deficit in testicular 17-dehydrogenase activity will have impaired testosterone production and present clinically as incomplete testicular feminization. Since treatment (gonadectomy) is the same, precise diagnosis is not essential.

Conventional wisdom warns against unthinking and needless disclosure of the gonadal and chromosomal sex to a patient with testicular feminization. Although infertile, these patients are certainly completely female in their gender identity, and this should be reinforced rather than challenged. There are exceptions to every rule, however, and certain situations may call for a more straightforward, accurate discussion. One example in our own practice was a student nurse who pointed out that she would much rather have learned the facts from her parents and physician than from the textbooks she was reading in school.

184

Differences between Müllerian Agenesis and Testicular Feminization		
	Müllerian Agenesis	Testicular Feminization
Karyotype	46,XX	46,XY
Heredity	Not known	Maternal X-linked recessive; 25% risk of affected child, 25% risk of carrier
Sexual hair	Normal female	Absent to sparse
Testosterone level	Normal female	Normal to slightly elevated male
Other anomalies	Frequent	Rare
Gonadal neoplasia	Normal incidence	25% incidence of malignant tumors

Compartment II

Problems in gonadal development can present with either primary or secondary amenorrhea. 30-40% of primary amenorrhea cases have gonadal streaks due to abnormal development: gonadal dysgenesis. These patients can be grouped according to the following karyotypes:

50% — 45,X
25% — Mosaics
25% — 46,XX

Women with gonadal dysgenesis can also present with secondary amenorrhea. The karyotypes associated with this presentation are, in order of decreasing frequency:

46,XX (most common)
Mosaics (e.g. 45,X/46,XX)
Deletions of X short and long arms
47,XXX
45,X

The finding of a normal karyotype, the most common situation, is most perplexing. Simpson suggests that maldevelopment is the result of an autosomal recessive defect in meiosis, a failure of synapses, an event which is very common in plants and animals.(25) Gonadal dysgenesis associated with a normal karyotype is also linked to neurosensory deafness. Auditory evaluation should be considered in all 46,XX gonadal dysgenesis cases.

Turner's Syndrome. Turner's Syndrome (45,X) is a well-known and thoroughly studied entity. The characteristics of short stature, webbed neck, shield chest, and increased carrying angle at the elbow, combined with hypergonadotropic hypoestrogenic amenorrhea, make a diagnosis possible on the most superficial evaluation. However, special attention must be given to the less common variations of this syndrome. Coarctation of the aorta and various renal collecting system anomalies must be ruled out. A karyotype should be performed on all patients with elevated gonadotropins, despite the appearance of a typical case of Turner's syndrome. The presence of a pure syndrome, 45,X chromosome single cell line, should

185

be confirmed. This expensive test cannot be viewed just as a step toward academic perfection.

Mosaicism. The presence of mosaicism (multiple cell lines of varying sex chromosome composition) must be ruled out for a very important reason. The presence of a Y chromosome in the karyotype requires laparotomy and excision of the gonadal areas because the presence of any medullary (testicular) component within the gonad is a predisposing factor to tumor formation and to heterosexual development (virilization). Only in the patient with the complete form of testicular feminization can laparotomy be deferred until after puberty, because the individual is resistant to androgens. In all other patients with a Y chromosome, gonadectomy should be performed before puberty to avoid virilization and early tumor formation. One should be aware that approximately 30% of patients with a Y chromosome will not develop signs of virilization. Therefore, even the normal appearing adult patient with elevated serum levels of gonadotropins must be karyotyped to detect a silent Y chromosome, so that prophylactic gonadectomy can be performed before neoplastic changes occur. Assays for the H-Y antigen are neither generally available nor totally reliable. The fully stained and banded karyotype continues to be the best method to detect the presence of testicular tissue or other mosaic combinations.

The impact of mosaicism, even in the absence of a Y-containing line, is significant. With an XX component (e.g. XX/XO), functional cortical (ovarian) tissue can be found within the gonad, leading to a variety of responses, including some degree of female development, and, on occasion, even menses and reproduction. These individuals may appear normal, attaining normal stature before premature menopause is experienced. More commonly, these patients are short. Most patients with missing sex chromosome material are less than 63 inches in height. The menopause is early, presumably because the functioning follicles undergo an accelerated rate of atresia.

This complex array of gonadal dysgenesis variations, from the typical pure form to an otherwise normal appearing and functioning woman with premature menopause, is the result of a variety of mosaicism which produces a complex mixture of cortical and medullary gonadal tissue. The clinical importance of this information justifies obtaining karyotypes in all cases of elevated gonadotropins in women under age 30. All patients with absent ovarian function and quantitative alterations in the sex chromosomes are categorized as having *GONADAL DYSGENESIS*.

XY Gonadal Dysgenesis. A Patient with an XY karyotype who has a palpable müllerian system, normal female testosterone levels, and lack of sexual development has *SWYER'S SYNDROME*. Tumor transformation in the gonadal ridge can occur at any age, and extirpation of the gonadal streaks should be performed as soon as the diagnosis is made.

Gonadal Agenesis. No complicated clinical problems accompany the gonadal failure due to agenesis. Without precise information, only conjecture as to the causes of absent development can be made.

Thus, viral and metabolic influences in early gestation are suspected. Nevertheless, the final result is irretrievable—hypergonadotropic hypogonadism.

The Resistant Ovary Syndrome. There is a rare patient with amenorrhea who has elevated gonadotropins despite the presence of ovarian follicles, and there is no evidence of autoimmune disease. Laparotomy is necessary to arrive at a correct diagnosis by obtaining adequate histological evaluation of the ovaries. This can demonstrate not only the presence of follicles, but the absence of the lymphocytic infiltration seen with autoimmune disease. Because of the rarity of this condition, and the very low chance of achieving pregnancy even with high doses of exogenous gonadotropins, we do not feel it is worthwhile to perform a laparotomy for the purpose of ovarian biopsy on every patient with amenorrhea, high gonadotropins, and a normal karyotype.

Premature Ovarian Failure. The etiology of premature ovarian failure is unknown in many cases. It is useful to explain to the patient that it is probably a genetic disorder with an increased rate of follicle disappearance. Often, specific sex chromosome anomalies can be identified.(26) The most common abnormalities are 45,X and 47,XXY, followed by mosaicism and specific structural abnormalities on the sex chromosomes. Accelerated atresia is most likely as even 45,X (Turner's Syndrome) patients begin with a full complement of germ cells. In addition, premature ovarian failure can be due to an autoimmune process, or perhaps to destruction of follicles by infections such as mumps oophoritis or a physical insult such as irradiation or chemotherapy.

The problem can present at varying ages depending upon the number of follicles left. It is useful to view the various presentations as representing a stage in the process of perimenopausal change, no matter what the chronological age of the patient. If loss of follicles has been rapid, then primary amenorrhea and lack of sexual development will be present. If loss of follicles takes place during or after puberty then the extent of adult phenotypic development and the time of onset of secondary amenorrhea will vary accordingly.

In view of the increasing number of case reports documenting resumption of normal function, we cannot be certain that these patients will be sterile forever. On the other hand, laparotomy and full thickness ovarian biopsy surely are not necessary for all of these patients. We believe that a minimal approach, with a survey for autoimmune disease and an assessment of ovarian-pituitary activity, is sufficient.

The Effect of Radiation and Chemotherapy. The effect of radiation is dependent upon age and the x-ray dose. (27) Steroid levels begin to fall and gonadotropins rise within 2 weeks after irradiation to the ovaries. The higher number of oocytes in younger age is responsible for the resistance to total castration in young women exposed to intense radiation. Function can resume after many years of amenorrhea. If pregnancy does occur, the risk of congenital abnormalities is no greater than normal. Gonads are not in danger in the kitchen; microwave ovens utilize wavelengths with low tissue penetrating power. The following table indicates the risk of sterilization according to dose: (27)

Ovarian Dose	Sterilization Effect
60 rads	No effect
150 rads	Some risk over age 40.
250–500 rads	Ages 15–40: 60% sterilized.
500–800 rads	Ages 15–40: 60–70% sterilized.
over 800 rads	100% permanently sterilized.

Alkylating agents are very toxic to the gonads. As with radiation, there is an inverse relationship between the dose required for ovarian failure and age at the start of therapy. Other chemotherapeutic agents have the potential for ovarian damage, but they have been less well studied. Resumption of menses and pregnancy can occur, but there is no way to predict which patient will reacquire ovulatory function.

Compartment III

Disorders of the hypothalamic-pituitary axis must first focus on the problem of the pituitary tumor. Through the appearance of amenorrhea, the patient with a slowly growing pituitary tumor can present years before the tumor becomes evident by standard radiologic techniques. Fortunately, malignant tumors are almost never encountered (through 1985, there were 3 reported cases of prolactin cell metastatic carcinomas [28]), but growth of a benign tumor can cause problems because it expands in a confined space. The tumor grows upward, compressing the optic chiasm and producing the classic findings of bitemporal hemianopsia. With small tumors, however, abnormal visual fields are rarely encountered. In contrast, other tumors of this region (e.g. craniopharyngioma, usually marked by calcifications on x-ray) may be associated with the early development of blurring of vision and visual field defects because of their close proximity to the optic chiasm.

Sometimes the suspicion of a pituitary tumor is increased because of clinical signs of acromegaly due to excessive secretion of growth hormone, or Cushing's disease due to excessive secretion of ACTH. Amenorrhea and/or galactorrhea may precede the eventual full clinical expression of a tumor which secretes ACTH or growth hormone. If clinical criteria suggest Cushing's disease, ACTH levels and the 24-hour urinary levels of free cortisol should be measured, and the rapid suppression test (Chapter 7) should be utilized. If acromegaly is suspected, growth hormone should be measured in the fasting state and during an oral glucose tolerance test. Though usually a problem in adult life, prolactin secreting tumors can be seen in preadolescent and adolescent children, and thus be a cause of failure of growth and development or primary amenorrhea.

Not all intrasellar masses are neoplastic. Gummas, tuberculomas, and fat deposits have been reported as causes of pituitary compression leading to hypogonadotropic amenorrhea. Nearby lesions such as internal carotid artery aneurysms and obstruction of the aqueduct of Sylvius can also cause amenorrhea. Pituitary insufficiency can be secondary to ischemia and infarction and appear as a late sequela to obstetrical hemorrhage—the well-known Sheehan's syndrome. These problems as well as genetic disorders, such as Laurence-Moon-Biedl and Prader-Willi syndromes, are so rarely encountered that consultation with textbooks and colleagues is necessary.

Pituitary Prolactin-Secreting Adenomas

Prolactin-secreting adenomas are the most common tumors. Tumors less than 1 cm in diameter are referred to as microadenomas, those greater than 1 cm, macroadenomas. Classically pituitary adenomas have been grouped according to their staining ability as eosinophilic, basophilic, or chromophobic. This classification is misleading and of no clinical usefulness. Pituitary adenomas should be classified according to their function, e.g. prolactin-secreting adenoma.

With the utilization of the serum prolactin assay and the increased sensitivity of the new x-ray techniques, the association of amenorrhea and small pituitary tumors has become recognized as a relatively common problem. This is not a new phenomenon, rather it reflects more sensitive diagnostic techniques. Attempts to link the problem to oral contraceptive use have proved negative. (29)

The exact incidence of this clinical problem is unknown. In autopsy series the number of pituitary glands found to contain adenomas ranged from 9 to 27%. (30-34) The age distribution ranged from 2 to 86, with the greatest incidence in the 6th decade of life. The sex distribution was equal. However, clinical manifestations, mainly a disruption of the reproductive mechanism, occur almost exclusively in women, and are probably due to estrogen-induced activity of the pituitary lactotrophs.

A high prolactin level is encountered in about one-third of women with no obvious cause of amenorrhea.(35) Only one-third of women with high prolactin levels will have galactorrhea, probably because the low estrogen environment associated with the amenorrhea prevents a normal response to prolactin. Another possible explanation again focuses on the heterogeneity of peptide hormones. Prolactin is secreted in various forms (different sizes known as little prolactin, big prolactin, and big big prolactin) with varying bioactivity (manifested by galactorrhea) and immunoactivity (recognition by radioimmunoassay). The predominant variant is little prolactin (80-85%) which also has more biological activity compared to the larger sized variants. Therefore it is not surprising that big prolactins compose the major form of circulating prolactin in women with normal menses and minimal galactorrhea.(36) This is not always the case, however, as a high blood level (350-400 ng/ml) of prolactin composed predominantly of high molecular weight prolactin has been reported in a woman with oligomenorrhea and galactorrhea but with no evidence of a pituitary tumor. (37) Explanations for clinically illogical situations can be found in the variable molecular heterogeneity of the peptide hormones.

About one-third of women with galactorrhea have normal menses. As the prolactin concentration increases, a women can progress sequentially from normal ovulation to an inadequate luteal phase to intermittent anovulation to total anovulation to complete suppression and amenorrhea.

189

Probably as many as one-third of patients with secondary amenorrhea will have a pituitary adenoma, and if galactorrhea is also present, half will have an abnormal sella turcica.(35) The clinical symptoms do not always correlate with the prolactin level, and patients with normal prolactins can have pituitary tumors.(38) The highest prolactin levels, however, are associated with amenorrhea, with or without galactorrhea.

The amenorrhea associated with elevated prolactin levels appears to be due to prolactin inhibition of the pulsatile secretion of GnRH. The pituitary glands in these patients respond normally to GnRH, or in augmented fashion (perhaps due to increased stores of gonadotropins), thus indicating that the mechanism of the amenorrhea is a decrease in GnRH.(39,40) This inhibition may be mediated by increased opioid activity.(41) Regardless of the mechanism, treatment which lowers the circulating levels of prolactin restores ovarian responsiveness and menstrual function. This is true whether the treatment consists of removal of a prolactin-secreting tumor or suppression of prolactin secretion.

The increased ability to detect pituitary tumors has been accompanied by the development of a surgical technique which effectively removes the small tumors with a high margin of safety. Utilizing the operating microscope, the transsphenoidal technique approaches via a sublabial incision (under the upper lip), with dissection under the nasal mucosa, removal of the nasal septum to expose the sphenoidal sinus, and resection of the floor of the sphenoid sinus to expose the sella turcica. Tumor tissue is usually distinguishable from the yellow-orange, firm tissue of the normal anterior pituitary. However, because pituitary adenomas do not have a capsule, the borderline between tumor and normal tissue is often vague. The ideal time for excision is when the adenoma is a small nodule. When enlarged it becomes more difficult to distinguish normal from pathological tissue. Once the adenoma grows beyond the sella, total removal is essentially impossible.

The development of transsphenoidal surgery was paralleled by the availability and clinical application of the drug, bromocriptine, which specifically suppresses prolactin secretion. Initially, appropriate decisions between the surgical approach and medical treatment were difficult to make. With increasing experience, clinical perspective has been achieved, and reasonable judgments are now possible. Let us first consider results with surgery, then examine bromocriptine.

Results with Surgery

Transsphenoidal neurosurgery achieves complete resolution of hyperprolactinemia with resumption of cyclic menses in about 40% of patients with macroadenomas and 80% of patients with microadenomas. Besides an inability to achieve a complete cure, surgery may be followed by recurrence of tumor (long-term cure rate is about 50% overall, ranging from 70% for microadenomas to 10% for macroadenomas) and a still unknown but significant percentage (perhaps as high as 10-30% after surgery for macroadenomas) of development of panhypopituitarism. (42,43) Other complications of surgery include: cerebrospinal fluid leaks, an occasional case of meningitis, and the frequent postoperative problem of diabetes insipidus. The diabetes insipidus is a transient problem, rarely lasting as long as 6 months. While initial follow-up reports of the results of transsphenoidal adenomectomy were discouraging (high recurrence rates), other authors have argued that surgical techniques have improved with time, and recurrent hyperprolactinemia is relatively low.(44)

There are 3 possible explanations for the recurrence or persistence of hyperprolactinemia after surgery.

1. The prolactin producing tumor looks like the surrounding normal pituitary, and it is difficult to resect completely.

2. The tumor may be multifocal in origin.

3. There may be a continuing abnormality of the hypothalamus giving rise to chronic stimulation of the lactotrophs. In other words, this is a problem of recurrent hyperplasia, not adenomas.

We recommend the following surveillance for those patients who have had surgery:

1. If cyclic menses return: periodic evaluation for the problem of anovulation.

2. If amenorrhea or oligomenorrhea and hyperprolactinemia persist or recur: prolactin levels every 6 months and a limited (2 selected views) CT scan yearly for 2 years, then a coned-down view every few years. If tumor growth becomes evident, control of growth should be achieved with bromocriptine treatment. In addition, bromocriptine can be used to induce ovulation if pregnancy is desired.

Results with radiation therapy are less satisfactory than with surgery. In addition, response is very slow; prolactin concentrations may take several years to fall. After radiation, panhypopituitarism can occur as long as 10 years after treatment. Patients who have been treated with radiation should be followed for a long time, and any symptoms suggestive of pituitary failure require investigation.

Bromocriptine

Bromocriptine is a lysergic acid derivative with a bromine substitute at position 2.(45) It is available as the methane-sulfonate (mesylate) in 2.5 mg tablets. It is a dopamine agonist, binding to dopamine receptors, and, therefore, directly mimicking dopamine inhibition of pituitary prolactin secretion. Absorption from the gastrointestinal tract is rapid and complete, therefore, the side effect of vomiting is due to a central rather than a local effect. Bromocriptine is metabolized into at least 30 excretory products. Excretion is mainly biliary, and more than 90% appears in the feces over 5 days after a single dose of 2.5 mg. A small part, 6-7%, is excreted unchanged or as metabolites in the urine.

Nausea, headache, and faintness are the usual initial problems. The faintness is due to orthostatic hypotension which can be attributed to relaxation of smooth muscle in the splanchnic and renal beds, as well as inhibition of transmitter release at noradrenergic nerve endings and central inhibition of sympathetic activity. Neuropsychiatric symptoms, occasionally with hallucinations, occur in less than 1% of patients. This may be due to hydrolysis of the lysergic acid part

191

of the molecule. Other side effects include dizziness, fatigue, nasal congestion, vomiting, and abdominal cramps.

Side effects can be minimized by slowly building tolerance toward the usual dose, 2.5 mg b.i.d. Treatment should be started with an initial dose of 2.5 mg given at bedtime. The peak level is achieved 2 hours after ingestion, and the biological half-life is about 3 hours. If intolerance occurs with this initial dose, then the tablet should be cut in half, and an even slower program should be followed. Usually a week after the initial dose, the second 2.5 mg dose can be added at breakfast or lunch. Patients who are extremely sensitive to the drug should be instructed to divide the tablets and to devise their own schedule of increasing dosage in order to achieve tolerance. A very small percentage of patients cannot tolerate any dosage.

The dose that suppresses prolactin is 10 times lower than that which improves the symptoms of Parkinson's disease. For some patients, one pill a day (or half a pill b.i.d. for a more consistent suppression) will be effective. On the other hand, an occasional patient will require 7.5 mg or 10 mg daily in order to suppress adenoma secretion of prolactin.

Results of Treatment. In 22 clinical trials, 80% of patients with amenorrhea/galactorrhea, associated with hyperprolactinemia but no demonstrable tumors, had menses restored.(46) The average treatment time to the initiation of menses was 5.7 weeks. Complete cessation of galactorrhea occurred in 50-60% of patients, in an average time of 12.7 weeks, and a 75% reduction of breast secretions was achieved in 6.4 weeks. *It is important to advise patients that the loss of galactorrhea is a slower and less certain response compared to restoration of ovulation and menses.* Amenorrhea recurred in 41% of the patients within an average of 4.4 weeks of discontinuing treatment; galactorrhea recurred in 69% at an average of 6.0 weeks. About 5% of patients terminated treatment because of adverse reactions.

There are two bromocriptine treatment methods to follow in those patients seeking pregnancy. The first is simply daily administration of 2.5 mg b.i.d. until the patient is pregnant as judged by the basal body temperature chart. In the second method, bromocriptine is administered during the follicular phase, and the drug is stopped when a basal body temperature rise indicates that ovulation has occurred, thus avoiding high drug levels early in pregnancy. The drug is resumed at menses when it is apparent the patient is not pregnant. No comparative study has been performed to tell us whether the follicular phase only method is as effective as the daily method. Furthermore, there has been no evidence that bromocriptine ingestion during early pregnancy is harmful to the fetus.

Regression of Tumors with Bromocriptine

There is no question that macroadenomas will regress with bromocriptine treatment.(45,47) In some there is prompt shrinkage with low dose treatment (5-7.5 mg daily); in others, prolonged treatment is required with higher doses. Visual improvement may be noted within several days. Reduction in tumor size can take place in several days to 6 weeks, but in some cases it is not observed until 6 months or more. Very high prolactin levels, greater than 2000-3000 ng/ml, are probably the result of invasion of the cavernous sinuses with release directly into the bloodstream. Even these cases show remarkable resolution with bromocriptine treatment. While tumor shrinkage is always preceded by a decrease in prolactin levels, the overall response cannot be predicted by the basal prolactin level, the absolute or relative fall in prolactin, or even the attainment of normal prolactin levels.

The response of macroadenomas to bromocriptine is impressive, and a most compelling reason in favor of its use is that it has been successful when previous surgery or radiation has failed. The problem, however, is that it probably must be taken indefinitely, as there is yet to be a convincing report of complete disappearance and resolution of tumor which can be attributed to drug therapy and not spontaneous resolution. Light and electron microscopic, immunohistochemical, and morphometric analyses all indicate that bromocriptine causes not only a reduction in the size of individual cells, but also necrosis of the cells with replacement fibrosis.(48) Nevertheless, prolactin levels generally return to an elevated state after discontinuation of the drug. There are cases of improvement in sellar x-rays; however, the occurrence of spontaneous regression of prolactin-secreting tumors makes it impossible to attribute "cures" to bromocriptine. Recurrence of hyperprolactinemia has been observed following as many as 4-8 years of treatment.

New Drugs

Other ergoline derivatives with dopaminergic activity are available throughout the world. Pergolide is the most widely used. It is more potent, longer-lasting, and better tolerated by some patients than bromocriptine. Pergolide is given in a single daily dose of 50-150 μg, and it may be effective in bromocriptine-resistant patients.(49,50) New long-acting derivatives are being examined which can be administered on a weekly basis.

Summary: Therapy of Pituitary Tumors

Macroadenomas. Currently bromocriptine treatment is advocated, utilizing as low a dose as possible. Shrinkage of a tumor may require 5-20 mg bromocriptine daily, but once shrinkage has occurred, the daily dose should be progressively reduced until the lowest maintenance dose is achieved. The serum prolactin level can be utilized as a marker. In many (but not all) patients, control of tumor growth correlates with maintenance of a baseline prolactin level, and can be achieved in some patients with as little as one-quarter a tablet (0.625 mg) daily.(51) Withdrawal of the drug is usually associated with re-growth or re-expansion of the tumor, and therefore, treatment must be long-term if not indefinite. Some patients will prefer surgery, and it is certainly a legitimate option. In view of better results claimed in more recent times, this choice should be presented to the patient. Short-term treatment (several weeks) with bromocriptine can make surgery easier due to a reduction in size; however, long-term treatment is associated with fibrosis which makes complete surgical removal more difficult and more likely to be associated with the sacrifice of other pituitary hormonal function. Furthermore, even though prolactin levels usually increase when bromocriptine treatment is discontinued after several years, the majority of tumors do not regrow.(52) Pregnancy should be deferred until repeat CT scan confirms shrinkage of the macroadenoma.

193

Microadenomas. The treatment of microadenomas should be directed to alleviating one of two problems: infertility or breast discomfort. Bromocriptine is the method of choice. Again, some patients, deliberately and understandably, choose the surgical approach in hopes of achieving a cure and avoiding the worry and annoyance of continuing surveillance.

The major therapeutic dilemma can be expressed by the following question: should chronic bromocriptine treatment be utilized to retrieve ovarian function in those patients with hypoestrogenic amenorrhea, or should estrogen replacement be offered? Until a clear-cut benefit is demonstrated by clinical studies, we cannot advocate widespread bromocriptine therapy for those patients not interested in becoming pregnant. This conservative approach is supported by documentation of a benign clinical course with spontaneous resolution in many patients.(53,54) Patients with hypoestrogenic amenorrhea are encouraged to be on an estrogen replacement program to maintain the health of their bones and the vascular system. *Estrogen-induced tumor expansion or growth has not been a problem.*

Long-Term Follow-Up. Because these tumors grow slowly, it is appropriate in the absence of symptoms to evaluate patients with microadenomas annually. The evaluation consists of a measurement of the prolactin level and coned-down view of the sella turcica. If the course is unchanged, x-ray evaluation can be spaced out to every 2-3 years. CT scan evaluation is reserved for patients with a change in the coned-down x-ray view, an increasing prolactin, or the development of headaches and/or visual complaints. It should be noted that progressively increasing prolactin levels have been observed *without* associated tumor growth of a microadenoma.(55) Patients with macroadenomas deserve an initial period of follow-up every 6 months. If the adenoma appears to be clinically stable, yearly prolactin measurement and coned-down x-ray views are appropriate. Again the CT scan is reserved for situations suggestive of tumor expansion.

Pregnancy and Pituitary Adenomas

Approximately 80% of hyperprolactinemic women achieve pregnancy with bromocriptine treatment.(56) *Breast feeding, if desired, can be carried out normally without fear of stimulating tumor growth.* Interestingly, some women resume cyclic menses after pregnancy. This spontaneous improvement may be due to tumor infarction brought about by the expansion and shrinkage during and after pregnancy, or there may be a correction of a hypothalamic dysfunction followed by a disappearance of the associated pituitary hyperplasia.

A very small percentage (less than 2%) of women with hyperprolactinemia and microadenomas will develop signs or symptoms suggestive of tumor growth during pregnancy. (56) About 5% of these patients will develop asymptomatic tumor enlargement (determined by radiologic techniques), and essentially none will ever require surgical intervention. The risk is higher with macroadenomas, approximately 15%. Headaches usually precede visual disturbances, and both may occur in any trimester. There is no characteristic headache; they are variable in intensity, location, and character. Bitemporal hemianopsia is the classic visual field finding, but other defects can occur. It has been argued in the past that a desire for pregnancy was a reason for the surgical approach. This argument hinged on the risk of tumor enlargement during pregnancy due to the well-known stimulatory effects of estrogen on the pituitary lactotrophs. As noted above, however, experience with this risk has indicated that very few patients develop problems.

It is impossible to identify which patient is at risk for symptomatic expansion during pregnancy. Other than a very large tumor, the size is not critical in that both microadenomas and macroadenomas can undergo uneventful pregnancies. There is no increase in abortions, or perinatal mortality or morbidity. It is virtually unheard of to develop a problem that results in perinatal damage or serious maternal sequelae.

Surveillance during pregnancy at first consisted of monthly visual field and prolactin measurements. With experience, this has proven to be unnecessary. The patient and the clinician can be guided by the development of symptoms. Assessment of visual fields, prolactin, and the sella turcica by limited CT scanning can await the onset of headaches or visual disturbances.

Definite evidence of tumor expansion, as well as the symptoms of headaches and visual changes, promptly regress with bromocriptine treatment. Termination of pregnancy or neurosurgery, therefore, should rarely, if ever, be necessary. Although bromocriptine treatment profoundly lowers both maternal and fetal blood levels of prolactin, no adverse effects on the pregnancy or the newborn have been noted.(56-59) Fortunately, amniotic fluid prolactin (and its presumed action on regulation of amniotic fluid water and electrolytes) is derived from decidual tissue, and its secretion is controlled by estrogen and progesterone, not dopamine. Therefore, it is not surprising that bromocriptine does not affect amniotic fluid levels of prolactin.

The Empty Sella Syndrome

A patient may have an abnormal sella turcica, but rather than a tumor, she may have the empty sella syndrome. In this condition there is a congenital incompleteness of the sellar diaphragm, allowing an extension of the subarachnoid space into the pituitary fossa. The pituitary gland is separated from the hypothalamus and is flattened. The sella floor may be demineralized due to pressure from the cerebrospinal fluid, and the x-ray picture on coned-down views will be similar to a tumor. The empty sella syndrome can also occur secondary to surgery or radiotherapy.

An empty sella is found in approximately 5% of autopsies, and approximately 85% are in women, previously thought to be concentrated in middle aged and obese women.(60) A closer look at the sella turcica, brought about by our pursuit of elevated prolactin levels, has revealed an incidence of empty sellas in 4-16% of patients who present with amenorrhea/galactorrhea.(35,38) Galactorrhea and elevated prolactins can be seen with an empty sella, and there may be a coexisting prolactin-secreting adenoma. This suggests that the empty sella in these patients may have arisen because of tumor infarction.

This condition is benign; it does not progress to pituitary failure. The chief hazard to the patient is inadvertent treatment for a pituitary tumor. Even though enlargement of the sella turcica with a normal shape is more likely associated with an empty sella than a tumor, all patients should have examination by CT scan for confirmation.

Because of the possibility of a coexisting adenoma, patients with elevated prolactins or galactorrhea and an empty sella should undergo annual surveillance (prolactin assay and coned-down view) for a few years to detect tumor growth. It is totally safe and appropriate to offer hormone replacement or induction of ovulation.

Compartment IV

Hypothalamic Amenorrhea. Hypothalamic problems are usually diagnosed by exclusion of pituitary lesions and are the most common category of hypogonadotropic amenorrhea. Frequently there is an association with a stressful situation, such as in business or in school. There is also a higher proportion of underweight women and a higher occurrence of previous menstrual irregularity. Nevertheless, the clinician is obliged to go through the process of exclusion prior to prescribing hormone replacement therapy, or attempting induction of ovulation to achieve pregnancy.

These patients are categorized by low or normal gonadotropins, normal prolactin levels, a normal x-ray evaluation of the sella turcica, and a failure to demonstrate withdrawal bleeding. A good practice is to evaluate such patients annually. This annual surveillance should include a prolactin assay and the coned-down view of the sella turcica. After several years with no change, the x-ray is necessary only every 2-3 years. In the only long-term follow-up of a large group of women with secondary amenorrhea, it was noted that amenorrhea associated with psychological stress or weight loss demonstrated a spontaneous recovery after 6 years in 72% of the women.(61) This still leaves a significant percentage of women who require on-going surveillance.

Experimental evidence in the monkey indicates that corticotropin-releasing hormone (CRH) inhibits gonadotropin secretion, perhaps by augmenting endogenous opioid secretion.(62) This could be the pathway by which stress interrupts reproductive function.

Even though a patient may not be currently interested in pursuing pregnancy, it is important to assure these patients that at the appropriate time treatment for the induction of ovulation will be available, and that fertility can be achieved. Concern with potential fertility is often an unspoken fear, especially in the younger patients, even teenagers. On the other hand, induction of ovulation should be carried out only for the purpose of producing a pregnancy. There is no evidence that cyclic hormone administration or induction of ovulation will stimulate the return of normal function.

Weight Loss, Anorexia and Bulimia

A special example of hypothalamic amenorrhea is that associated with weight loss. It is true that obesity can be associated with amenorrhea, but amenorrhea in an obese patient is usually due to anovulation, and a hypogonadotropic state is not encountered unless the patient also has a severe emotional disorder. Acute weight loss, on the other hand, in some unknown way, can lead to the hypogonadotropic state. Again, the clinician must pursue the presence of a pituitary tumor, and the diagnosis of hypothalamic amenorrhea is made by exclusion.

Clinically a spectrum is encountered which ranges from a limited period of amenorrhea associated with a crash diet, to the severely ill patient with the life-threatening attrition of anorexia nervosa. It is a common experience for a physician to be the first to recognize anorexia nervosa in a patient presenting with the complaint of amenorrhea. It is also not infrequent that a physician will evaluate and manage an infertility problem due to hypogonadotropism and not be aware of a developing case of anorexia. Because the mortality rate associated with this syndrome is significant (5-15%), it is important that attention be directed to this condition.

Diagnosis of Anorexia Nervosa

1. Onset between ages 10 and 30.

2. Weight loss of 25%, or weight 15% below normal for age and height.

3. Special attitudes:
   —Denial,
   —Distorted body image,
   —Unusual hoarding or handling of food.

4. At least one of the following:
   —Lanugo,
   —Bradycardia,
   —Overactivity,
   —Episodes of overeating (bulimia),
   —Vomiting, which may be self-induced.

5. Amenorrhea.

6. No known medical illness.

7. No other psychiatric disorder.

8. Other characteristics:
   —Constipation,
   —Low blood pressure,
   —Hypercarotenemia,
   —Diabetes insipidus.

Anorexia nervosa occurs almost exclusively in young white middle to upper class females under age 25. The families of anorectics are success-achievement-appearance oriented. Serious problems may be present within the family, but the parents make every effort to

197

maintain an apparent marital harmony, glossing over or denying conflicts. In one psychiatric interpretation, each parent, in secret dissatisfaction with the other, expects affection from their "perfect" child. Anorexia begins when the role of the perfect child becomes too difficult. The pattern usually starts with a voluntary diet to control weight. This brings a sense of power and accomplishment, soon followed by a fear that weight cannot be controlled if discipline is allowed to relax. A reasonable view is to consider anorexia as a mechanism which identifies a generally disturbed family.

At puberty, the normal weight gain may be interpreted as excessive, and this can trip the teenager over into true anorexia nervosa. Excessive physical activity can be the earliest sign of incipient anorexia nervosa. The children are characteristically overachievers and strivers. They seldom give any trouble, but are judgmental and demand that others live up to their rigid value system, often resulting in social isolation.

The cultural value our society places on thinness definitely plays a role in eating disorders. Both occupational and recreational environments that stress thinness put women at greater risk for anorexia nervosa and bulimia. But basically, an eating disorder is a method being utilized to solve a psychological dilemma.

Besides amenorrhea, constipation is a common symptom, often severe and accompanied by abdominal pain. The preoccupation with food may manifest itself by large intakes of lettuce, raw vegetables, and low calorie foods. Hypotension, hypothermia, rough dry skin, soft lanugo-type hair on the back and buttocks, bradycardia, and edema are the most commonly encountered signs. Long-term diuretic and laxative abuse may produce significant hypokalemia. An elevation of the serum carotene is not always associated with a large intake of yellow vegetables, suggesting that a defect in vitamin A utilization is present. The yellowish coloration of the skin is usually seen on the palms.

Bulimia is a syndrome marked by episodic and secretive binge eating followed by self-induced vomiting, fasting, or the use of laxatives and diuretics.(63) It appears to be a growing problem among young women, however a careful study indicates that while bulimic behaviors may be relatively common, clinically significant bulimia is not (approximately 1.0% of female students and 0.1% of male students in a college sample).(64) Bulimic behavior is frequently seen in patients with anorexia nervosa (about half), but not in all. Patients with bulimia have a high incidence of depressive symptoms, and a problem with shoplifting (usually food). Little is known about the long-term outcome. There is a growing tendency to divide patients with anorexia nervosa into bulimic anorectics and dieters. Bulimic anorectics are older, less isolated socially, and have a higher incidence of family problems. Body weight in a "pure" bulimic fluctuates but it does not fall to the low levels seen in anorectics.

The serious case of anorexia nervosa is seen more often by an internist. However, the borderline anorectic frequently presents to a gynecologist, pediatrician, or family physician as a teenager who has low body weight, amenorrhea, and hyperactivity (excellent grades and many extracurricular activities). The amenorrhea can precede, follow, or appear coincidentally with the weight loss.

The various problems associated with anorexia represent dysfunction of the body mechanisms regulated by the hypothalamus: appetite, thirst and water conservation, temperature, sleep, autonomic balance, and endocrine secretion.(65) Endocrine studies can be summarized as follows: FSH and LH levels are low, cortisol levels are elevated due to decreased clearance in the face of a normal production rate, prolactin levels are normal, TSH and thyroxine (T_4) levels are normal, but the 3,5,3'-triiodothyronine (T_3) level is low and reverse T_3 is high. Indeed many of the symptoms can be explained by relative hypothyroidism (constipation, cold intolerance, bradycardia, hypotension, dry skin, low metabolic rates, hypercarotenemia). There appears to be a compensation to the state of undernourishment, with diversion from formation of the active T_3 to the inactive metabolite, reverse T_3. With weight gain, all of the metabolic changes revert to normal. Even though normal gonadotropin secretion may be restored with weight gain, 30% of patients remain amenorrheic.(65)

This is one of the rare conditions in which gonadotropins may be undetectable (large pituitary tumors and genetic deficiencies being the others). If necessary, a high plasma cortisol can differentiate this condition from pituitary insufficiency.

The central origin for the amenorrhea is suggested by the demonstration that the response to GnRH is regained at approximately 15% below the ideal weight, and this return to normal responsiveness occurs before the resumption of menses.(66) Patients with anorexia nervosa have persistent low levels of gonadotropins similar to prepubertal children. With weight gain, sleep-associated episodic secretion of LH appears, similar to the early pubertal child. With full recovery the 24-hour pattern is similar to that of an adult, marked by fluctuating peaks. This sequence of changes with increasing and decreasing weight is explained by increasing and decreasing pulsatile secretion of GnRH.

Extensive laboratory testing in these patients is not necessary. Adherence to our scheme for the evaluation of amenorrhea is indicated to rule out other pathological processes. Further endocrine assessment, however, is not essential for patient management.

A careful and gentle revelation to the patient of the relationship between the amenorrhea and the low body weight is often all that is necessary to stimulate the patient to return to normal weight and normal menstrual function. Occasionally it is necessary to see the patient frequently and become involved in a program of daily calorie counting (a minimal intake of 2600 calories) in order to break the patient's established eating habits. If progress is slow, hormone replacement therapy should be initiated. In an adult weighing less than 100 pounds, continued weight loss requires psychiatric consultation. Some would argue that any patient with an eating disorder requires psychiatric intervention.

Going away to school or the development of a relationship with a male friend often are turning points for young women with mild to moderate anorexia. This is also true of pregnancy, and once pregnancy is achieved, its course is not influenced by the past history of anorexia. A failure to respond to these life changes is relatively ominous, predicting a severe problem with a protracted course.

It is disappointing that despite the impressive studies on anorexia there is no specific or new therapy available. This only serves to emphasize the need for early recognition to allow psychologic intervention before the syndrome is entrenched in its full severity. Physicians (and parents) should pay particular attention to weight and diet in young women with amenorrhea.

Exercise and Amenorrhea

Soranus of Ephesus in the 1st century AD observed in his famous treatise "On the Diseases of Women," that amenorrhea is frequently observed in the youthful, the aged, the pregnant, in singers, and in those who take much exercise. In the 20th century, there has been a new awareness that competitive female athletes, as well as women engaged in strenuous recreational exercise and women engaged in other forms of demanding activity such as ballet and modern dance, have a significant incidence of menstrual irregularity and amenorrhea, in the pattern called hypothalamic suppression. The extent of this problem has perhaps been underestimated because of a lack of attention to anovulatory cycles. As many as two-thirds of runners who have menstrual periods have short luteal phases or are anovulatory.(67) When training starts before menarche, menarche can be delayed by as much as 3 years, and the subsequent incidence of menstrual irregularity is higher.

There appear to be two critical influences: a critical level of body fat and the effect of stress itself. Young women who weigh less than 115 pounds and lose more than 10 pounds while exercising are the women most likely to develop the problem, (68) an association which supports the critical weight concept of Frisch.(69)

The critical weight hypothesis states that the onset and regularity of menstrual function necessitate maintaining weight above a critical level, and therefore, above a critical amount of body fat. In dealing with patients, it is helpful to use the nomogram derived from Frisch, which is based on the calculation of the amount of total body water as a percentage of body weight. This relates to the percentage of body fat, and therefore, is an index of fatness. The 10th percentile at age 16 is equivalent to about 22% body fat, the minimal weight for height necessary for sustaining menstruation, and the 10th percentile at age 13 is equivalent to 17% body fat, the minimum for initiating menarche. A loss of body weight in the range of 10-15% of normal weight for height represents a loss of about one-third of the body fat, which will result in a drop below the 22% line and may result in amenorrhea.

Although the nomogram is useful to show these relationships to patients, individual variation is such that the nomogram cannot be utilized to predict without fail the return of menses for an individual patient. Indeed, the accuracy of the nomogram has been challenged. (70) The fat criteria were derived from the indirect estima-

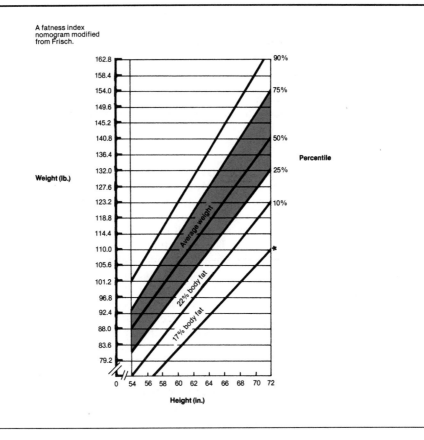

A fatness index nomogram modified from Frisch.

tion of body fat from predicted total body water, using a regression equation which employs height and weight. There is no question that the most reliable and accurate method for estimating body fatness is hydrostatic weighing of body density. But one can hardly maintain a small pool for this purpose in a clinical office. Granted that the nomogram, and specifically the 22% body fat criterion, are not absolutely accurate, nevertheless the concept is valid, and the nomogram remains useful to illustrate the concept to patients.

The competitive female athlete has about 50% less body fat than the noncompetitor. The mean is very much under the 10th percentile for secondary amenorrhea (the 22% body fat line). This change in body fat can occur with no discernible change in total body weight, as fat is converted to lean muscle mass.

In addition to the role of body fat, stress and energy expenditure appear to play an independent role. Warren has pointed out that dancers will have a return of menses during intervals of rest, despite no change in body weight or percent body fat.(71) High energy output and stress, therefore, may act independently, as well as additively to low body fat, in suppressing reproductive function. It is not surprising that a woman with low body weight who is engaged in competitive activity (athletic or aesthetic) is highly susceptible to anovulation and amenorrhea.

201

Running in the dark is even more risky. Studies indicate that ovarian activity can be affected independently by strenuous activity and seasonal variation.(72) Decreased ovarian activity in Autumn could be related to a greater dark photoperiod with increased pineal secretion of melatonin. Indeed, the conception rate of women living in northern Scandinavia is higher during the summer than in the winter. The practical conclusion is that serious runners can expect to encounter more problems with menstrual function in Autumn and Winter.

This menstrual disruption is similar to the hypothalamic dysfunction which is more marked in the classic cases of anorexia nervosa. Acute exercise decreases gonadotropins and increases prolactin, growth hormone, testosterone, ACTH, the adrenal steroids, and endorphins, as a result of both enhanced secretion and reduced clearance.(73) The prolactin increase is in contrast to the absence of prolactin changes in undernourished women. The prolactin increases are variable, small in amplitude, and exceedingly short in duration. Thus it is unlikely that the prolactin increase is responsible for the suppression of the menstrual cycle. Most importantly, insignificant differences occur in prolactin when amenorrheic runners are compared to eumenorrheic runners or non-runners.(74)

It has been suggested that a suboptimal amount of body fat adversely affects estrogen metabolism, specifically leading to an increased conversion of biologically active estrogens to relatively inactive catecholestrogens. There is no evidence to support this theory, although body fat does affect the rate of catecholestrogen production.

In running circles, there is frequent talk about the runner's "high," the feeling of euphoria and exhilaration after competition or an extensive workout. It is still not clear whether this is a psychologic reaction or whether it is due to an increase in endogenous opiates. The site of GnRH secretion, the arcuate nucleus area in the hypothalamus, is rich in opioid receptors and endorphin production. There is considerable evidence indicating that endogenous opiates inhibit gonadotropin secretion by suppressing hypothalamic GnRH. Women studied during a period of endurance conditioning demonstrated a steadily increasing endorphin output after exercise.(75-77) This link of endorphins to the menstrual suppression associated with exercise is very plausible, but yet unproven. How this suppression is further intensified or activated by a state of low body fat is unknown.

Whatever the mechanism, the final pathway is suppression of GnRH.(78) Even in runners with regular menstrual patterns, LH pulsatile frequency and amplitude are significantly reduced.(79) A central inhibition of GnRH can be discerned even before there is perceptible evidence of menstrual irregularity.

In the subculture of exercise and amenorrhea, the characteristics strikingly remind one of anorexia nervosa: significant physical exercise, a necessity for control of the body, striving for artistic and technical proficiency, and the consequent preoccupation with the body—together with the stressful pressures of performing and competition.(80) Individuals in this lifestyle are prone to develop what can be called the anorectic reaction. Fries (81) has described four stages of dieting behavior which can form a continuum:

1. Dieting for cosmetic reasons.

2. Dieting due to neurotic fixation on food intake and weight.

3. The anorectic reaction.

4. True anorexia nervosa.

There are several important distinctions between the anorectic reaction and true anorexia nervosa. Psychologically the patient with true anorexia nervosa has a misperception of reality and a lack of insight into the disease and her problem. She does not consider herself underweight and displays an impressive lack of concern over her dreadful physical condition and appearance. The doctor-patient relationship is difficult with no visible emotional involvement and a great deal of mistrust. Patients with the anorectic reaction have the capability for self-criticism. They can see the problem and describe it with insight and an absence of denial. The exercising woman and the competing athlete or dancer can develop an anorectic reaction. The anorectic reaction develops consciously and voluntarily just as in anorexia nervosa, as the exercising woman deliberately makes an effort to decrease body weight. A clinician may be the first to be aware of the problem having encountered the patient because of the present complaint of either amenorrhea or now uncontrolled weight loss. Early recognition, concentrated counseling, and confidential support may intercept and prevent a progressive problem.

Prognosis is excellent with early recognition, and simple weight gain may reverse the state of amenorrhea. The degree of reversibility is unknown, although general experience indicates that the majority of women regain ovulation when stress and exercise diminish or cease. (82,83) However, these patients are often unwilling to give up their routines of exercise, and a sensitive clinician can perceive that the exercise is an important means for coping with daily life. Hormone replacement therapy is therefore encouraged for these hypoestrogenic patients. It is now apparent that the exercise is not sufficient to balance the loss of estrogen protection against osteoporosis.(84-86) The amenorrheic exerciser should be made aware that the hypoestrogenic state is associated with a greater risk of injury (e.g stress fractures).(87-89) When pregnancy is desired, a reduction in the amount of exercise and a gain in weight should be recommended, or induction of ovulation must be pursued.

Amenorrhea and Anosmia. A rare condition in females is the syndrome of hypogonadotropic hypogonadism associated with anosmia. A similar syndrome in the male is hereditary and known as Kallmann's syndrome. There is a chronology of eponyms assigning credit for original descriptions of this syndrome, but with all due respect to the physicians who first recognized this association, it is far easier to remember it in a descriptive way, as a syndrome of amenorrhea and anosmia.(90-93) In the female, this problem is characterized by primary amenorrhea, infantile sexual development. low gonadotropins, a normal female karyotype, and the inability to perceive odors, e.g. coffee grounds or perfume. The gonads can respond to gonadotropins, therefore induction of ovulation with exogenous gonadotropins is successful. However, clomiphene is ineffective.

Kallmann's syndrome is associated with a specific anatomic defect. Magnetic resonance imaging (as well as post mortem examination) demonstrates hypoplastic or absent olfactory sulci in the rhinencephalon.(94) A similar developmental defect probably centers on the hypothalamic production site for GnRH.

Postpill Amenorrhea. In the past it was assumed that secondary amenorrhea reflected persistent suppressive effects of oral contraceptive medication or the use of the intramuscular depot form of medroxyprogesterone acetate (Depo-Provera). It is now recognized that the fertility rate is normal following discontinuance of either of these forms of contraception (Chapter 15), and attempts to identify a cause-effect relationship in case-control studies have failed. Therefore, amenorrhea following the use of steroids for contraception requires investigation as described in order to avoid missing a significant problem. This investigation should be pursued if a patient is amenorrheic 6 months after discontinuing oral contraception or 12 months after the last injection of Depo-Provera.

Hormone Replacement Therapy

The patient who is hypoestrogenic and who is not a candidate for induction of ovulation deserves hormone replacement therapy. This includes patients appropriately evaluated and diagnosed as having gonadal failure, patients with hypothalamic amenorrhea, and postgonadectomy patients. The long-term impact of the hypoestrogenic state in terms of cardiovascular disease has long been recognized, and it is now appreciated that the bone density in women is dependent upon normal reproductive age levels of estrogen. The same arguments that apply to hormone replacement in older women (Chapter 4) can be convincingly used to encourage these younger women to replace the estrogen they are lacking. It should be noted that bone loss in amenorrheic women shows the same pattern over time as seen in postmenopausal women.(95) The loss is most rapid in the first few years, emphasizing the need for early treatment.

Several reports have indicated that patients with hyperprolactinemia are at risk for osteoporosis. At first this appeared not to be related to estrogen status, suggesting an independent effect of prolactin. Results have been confusing for several reasons. Controls in various studies were matched in different fashions, e.g. only for age, ignoring height and weight. Photon absorptiometry, the method of study in some reports, has a reduced sensitivity and significant variation when used to assess the axial skeleton. And finally, the estrogen status of the hyperprolactinemic patients was not always carefully quantified. It is most likely that the bone density changes observed in hyperprolactinemic amenorrheic women are due to the hypoestrogenic state.

The standard program for estrogen replacement should be used. A good schedule is the following: on days 1 through 25 of each month, take 0.625 mg conjugated estrogens; on days 16 through 25, add 10 mg medroxyprogesterone acetate. Beginning medication on the first of every month establishes an easily remembered routine. If the progestational agent is responsible for side effects, the daily dose can be decreased to 5 mg. In a few individuals, the estrogen dosage may have to be increased to 1.25 mg in order to achieve menstrual bleeding. Whether a flow-provoking dose of estrogen is necessary for optimal protection of the bones has not been addressed in a clinical study.

Menstruation generally occurs 3 days after the last medication, the 28th day of each month. Bleeding which occurs at any time other than the usual expected time may be a sign that endogenous function has returned. The hormone replacement program should be discontinued and the patient monitored for the resumption of ovulation.

The importance of monthly menstruation to a young woman cannot be overemphasized. Regular and visible menstrual bleeding is often a gratifying experience in the young patient with gonadal dysgenesis and serves to reinforce her identification with the feminine gender role. On the other hand, serious exercisers (such as athletes and dancers) may wish to avoid menstrual bleeding. One can provide hormonal replacement to these women utilizing the daily combination approach: 0.625 mg conjugated estrogens and 5.0 mg medroxyprogesterone acetate given together every day without a break.

In individuals who have not developed secondary sexual characteristics, it is not necessary to start with higher doses of estrogen. Normal breast and feminine development will occur with these replacement doses. If for some reason, a hypoestrogenic woman refuses hormone replacement, supplemental calcium (1000-1500 mg daily) should be strongly encouraged. High calcium intake when combined with a high level of exercise is more effective in protecting the vertebral bone density than either exercise or calcium alone.

Patients with hypothalamic amenorrhea must be cautioned that replacement therapy will not protect against pregnancy in the event that normal function unknowingly returns. In the occasional patient who must have the most effective contraception possible, it is reasonable to utilize a low dose oral contraceptive to provide the missing estrogen.

References

1. **Contreras P, Generini G, Michelson H, Pumarino H, Campino C,** Hyperprolactinemia and galactorrhea: spontaneous versus iatrogenic hypothyroidism, J Clin Endocrinol Metab 53:1036, 1981.

2. **Danziger J, Wallace S, Handel S, Samaan NG,** The sella turcica in primary end organ failure, Radiology 131:111, 1979.

3. **Poretsky L, Garber J, Kleefield J,** Primary amenorrhea and pseudoprolactinoma in a patient with primary hypothyroidism, Am J Med 81:180, 1986.

4. **Coulam CB, Annegers JF, Kraz JC,** Chronic anovulation syndrome and associated neoplasia, Obstet Gynecol 61:403, 1983.

5. **Whitaker MD, Prior JC, Scheithauer B, Dolman L, Durity F, Pudek MR,** Gonadotropin-secreting pituitary tumour: report and review, Clin Endocrinol 22:43, 1985.

6. **Sherman BM, Korenman SG,** Hormonal characteristics of the human menstrual cycle throughout reproductive life, J Clin Invest 55:699, 1975.

7. **Talbert LM, Raj MHG, Hammond MG, Greer T,** Endocrine and immunologic studies in a patient with resistant ovary syndrome, Fertil Steril 442:741, 1984.

8. **Sutton C,** The limitations of laparoscopic ovarian biopsy, J Obstet Gynecol Brit Commonwlth 81:317, 1974.

9. **Alper MM, Garner PR,** Premature ovarian failure: its relationship to autoimmune disease, Obstet Gynecol 66:27, 1985.

10. **Cowchock FS, McCabe JL, Montgomery BB,** Pregnancy after corticosteroid administration in premature ovarian failure (polyglandular endorinopaty syndrome), Am J Obstet Gynecol 158:118, 1988.

11. **Robinson ACR, Dockeray CJ, Cullen MJ, Sweeney EC,** Hypergonadotrophic hypogonadism in classical galactosaemia: evidence for defective oogenesis: case report, Brit J Obstet Gynaecol 91:199, 1984.

12. **Rebar RW, Erickson GF, Yen SSC,** Idiopathic premature ovarian failure: clinical and endocrine characteristics, Fertil Steril 37:35, 1982.

13. **Aiman J, Smentek C,** Premature ovarian failure, Obstet Gynecol 66:9, 1985.

14. **Rabinowe SL, Berger MJ, Welch WR, Dluhy RO,** Lymphocyte dysfunction in autoimmune oophoritis: Resumption of menses with corticosteroids, Am J Med 81:347, 1986.

15. **Axelrod L, Neer RM, Kliman B,** Hypogonadism in a male with immunologically active, biologically inactive luteinizing hormone: an exception to a venerable rule, J Clin Endocrinol Metab 48:279, 1979.

16. **Strebel PM, Zacur HA, Gold EB,** Headache, hyperprolactinemia, and prolactinomas, Obstet Gynecol 68:195, 1986.

17. **Reindollar RH, Novak M, Tho SPT, McDonough PG,** Adult-onset amenorrhea: a study of 262 patients, Am J Obstet Gynecol 155:531, 1986.

18. **Schenker JG, Margalioth EJ,** Intrauterine adhesions: an updated appraisal, Fertil Steril 37:593, 1982.

19. **Markham SM, Parmley TH, Murphy AA, Huggins GR, Rock JA,** Cervical agenesis combined with vaginal agenesis diagnosed by magnetic resonance imaging, Fertil Steril 48:143, 1987.

20. **Griffin JE, Edwards C, Ladden JD, Harrod MJ, Wilson JD,** Congential absence of the vagina, Ann Intern Med 85:224, 1976.

21. **Frank RT,** Formation of artificial vagina without operation, Am J Obstet Gynecol 35:1053, 1938.

22. **Wabrek AJ, Millard PR, Wilson WB Jr, Pion RJ,** Creation of a neovagina by the Frank nonoperative method, Obstet Gynecol 37:408, 1971.

23. **Bates GW, Wiser WL,** A technique for uterine conservation in adolescents with vaginal agenesis and a functional uterus, Obstet Gynecol 66:290, 1985.

24. **Morris JM, Mahesh VB,** Further observations on the syndrome "testicular feminization," Am J Obstet Gynecol 87:731, 1963.

25. **Simpson JL,** Genetic forms of gonadal dysgenesis in 46,XX and 46,XY individuals, Seminars Reprod Endocrinol 1:93, 1983.

26. **Dewald GW, Spurbeck JL,** Sex chromosome anomalies associated with premature gonadal failure, Seminars Reprod Endocrinol 1:79, 1983.

27. **Asch P,** The influence of radiation on fertility in man, Brit J Radiol 53:271, 1980.

28. **Schelthauer BW, Randall RV, Laws ER Jr, Kovacs KT, Horvath E, Whitaker MD,** Prolactin cell carcinoma of the pituitary, Cancer 55:598, 1985.

29. **Pituitary Adenoma Study Group,** Pituitary adenomas and oral contraceptives: a multicenter case-control study, Fertil Steril 39:753, 1983.

30. **Costello RT,** Subclinical adenoma of the pituitary gland, Am J Pathol 12:191, 1936.

31. **Kraus HE,** Neoplastic diseases of the human hypophysis, Arch Pathol 39:343, 1945.

32. **McCormick WF, Halmi NS,** Absence of chromophobe adenomas from a large series of pituitary tumors, Arch Pathol 92:231, 1971.

33. **Sheline GE,** Untreated and recurrent chromophobe adenomas of the pituitary, Radiology 112:768, 1971.

34. **Burrow GN, Wortzman G, Rewcastle NB, Holgate RC, Kovacs K,** Microadenomas of the pituitary and abnormal sellar tomograms in an unselected autopsy series, New Eng J Med 304:156, 1981.

35. **Schlechte J, Sherman B, Halmi N, Van Gilder J, Chapler FK, Dolan K, Granner D, Duello T, Harris C,** Prolactin-secreting pituitary tumors, Endocrin Rev 1:295, 1980.

36. **Jackson RD, Wortsman J, Malarkey WB,** Characterization of a large molecular weight prolactin in women with idiopathic hyperprolactinemia and normal menses, J Clin Endocrinol Metab 61:258, 1985.

37. **Jackson RD, Wortsman J, Malarkey WB,** Macroprolactinemia presenting like a pituitary tumor, Am J Med 78:346, 1985.

38. **Speroff L, Levin RM, Haning RV Jr, Kase NG,** A practical approach for the evaluation of women with abnormal polytomography or elevated prolactin levels, Am J Obstet Gynecol 135:896, 1979.

39. **Monroe SE, Levine L, Chang RJ, Keye WR Jr, Yamamoto M, Jaffe RB,** Prolactin-secreting pituitary adenomas: V. Increased gonadotropin responsivity in hyperprolactinemic women with pituitary adenomas, J Clin Endocrinol Metab 52:1171, 1981.

40. **Sauder SE, Frager M, Case GD, Kelch RP, Marshall JC,** Abnormal patterns of pulsatile luteinizing hormone secretion in women with hyperprolactinemia and amenorrhea: Responses to bromocriptine, J Clin Endocrinol Metab 59:941, 1984.

41. **Petraglia F, De Leo V, Nappi C, Facchinetti F, Montemagno U, Brambilla F, Genazzani AR,** Differences in the opioid control of luteinizing hormone secretion between pathological and iatrogenic hyperprolactinemic states, J Clin Endocrinol Metab 64:508, 1987.

42. **Schlechte JA, Sherman BM, Chapler FK, VanGilder J,** Long term follow-up of women with surgically treated prolactin-secreting pituitary tumors, J Clin Endocrinol Metab 62:1296, 1986.

43. **Parl FF, Cruz VE, Cobb CA, Bradley CA, Aleshire SL,** Late recurrence of surgically removed prolactinomas, Cancer 57:2422, 1986.

44. **Thomson JA, Teasdale GM, Gordon D, McCruden DC, Davies DL,** Treatment of presumed prolactinoma by transsphenoidal operation: early and late results, Brit Med J 291:1550, 1985.

45. **Vance ML, Evans WS, Thorner MO,** Bromocriptine, Ann Int Med 100:78, 1984.

46. **Cuellar FG,** Bromocriptine mesylate (Parlodel) in the management of amenorrhea/galactorrhea associated with hyperprolactinemia, Obstet Gynecol 55:278, 1980.

47. **Sieck JO, Niles NL, Jinkins JR, Al-Mefty O, El-Akkad S, Woodhouse N,** Extrasellar prolactinomas: successful management of 24 patients using bromocriptine, Hor Res 23:167, 1986.

48. **Mori H, Mori S, Saitoh Y, Arita N, Aono T, Uozumi T, Mogami H, Matsumoto K,** Effects of bromocriptine on prolactin-secreting pituitary adenomas, Cancer 56:230, 1985.

49. **Kletzky OA, Borenstein R, Mileikowsky GN,** Pergolide and bromocriptine for the treatment of patients with hyperprolactinemia, Am J Obstet Gynecol 154:431, 1986.

50. **Ahmed SR, Shalet SM,** Discordant responses of prolactinoma to two different dopamine agonists, Clin Endocrinol 24:421, 1986.

51. **Liuzzi A, Dallabonzana D, Oppizzi G, Verde GG, Cozzi R, Chiodini P, Luccarelli G,** Low doses of dopamine agonists in the long-term treatment of macroprolactinomas, New Eng J Med 313:656, 1985.

52. **Johnston DG Hall K, Kendall-Taylor P, Patrick D, Watson MJ, Cook DB,** Effect of dopamine agonist withdrawal after long-term therapy in prolactinomas. Studies with high-definition computerized tomography, Lancet ii:187, 1984.

53. **Koppelman MCS, Jaffe MJ, Rieth KG, Caruso RC, Loriaux DL,** Hyperprolactinemia, amenorrhea, and galactorrhea: a retrospective assessment of twenty-five cases, Ann Int Med 100:115, 1984.

54. **Martin TL, Kim M, Malarkey WB,** The natural history of idiopathic hyperprolactinemia, J Clin Endocrinol Metab 60:855, 1985.

55. **Sisam DA, Sheehan JP, Schumacher OP,** Lack of demonstrable tumor growth in progressive hyperprolactinemia, Am J Med 80:279, 1986.

56. **Molitch ME,** Pregnancy and the hyperprolactinemic woman, New Eng J Med 312:1362, 1985.

57. **De Wit W, Coelingh Bennink HJT, Gerards LJ,** Prophylactic bromocriptine treatment during pregnancy in women with macroprolactinomas: report of 13 pregnancies, Brit J Obstet Gynaecol 91:1059, 1984.

58. **Ruiz-Velasco V, Tolis G,** Pregnancy in hyperprolactinemic women, Fertil Steril 41:793, 1984.

59. **Holmgren U, Bergstrand G, Hagenfeldt K, Werner S,** Women with prolactinoma-effect of pregnancy and lactation on serum prolactin and on tumour growth, Acta Endocrinol 111:452, 1986.

60. **Hodgson SF, Randall RV, Holman CB, MacCarty CS,** Empty sella syndrome, Med Clin North Am 56:897, 1972.

61. **Hirvonen E,** Etiology, clinical features and prognosis in secondary amenorrhea, Int J Fertil 22:69, 1977.

62. **Olster DH, Ferin M,** Corticotropin-releasing hormone inhibits gonadotropin secretion in the ovariectomized Rhesus monkey, J Clin Endocrinol Metab 65:262, 1987.

63. **Herzog DB, Coopeland PM,** Eating disorders, New Eng J Med 313:295, 1985.

64. **Schotte DE, Stunkard AJ,** Bulimia vs bulimic behaviors on a college campus, JAMA 258:1213, 1987.

65. **Warren MP, Vande Wiele RL,** Clinical and metabolic features of anorexia nervosa, Am J Obstet Gynecol 117:435, 1973.

66. **Warren MP, Jewelewicz R, Dyrenfurth I, Ans R, Khalaf S, Vande Wiele RL,** The significance of weight loss in the evaluation of pituitary response to LH-RH in women with secondary amenorrhea, J Clin Endocrinol Metab 40:601, 1975.

67. **Prior JC,** Luteal phase defects and anovulation: adaptive alterations occurring with conditioning exercise, Seminars Reprod Endocrinol 3:27, 1985.

68. **Speroff L, Redwine DB,** Exercise and menstrual function, Physician Sportsmed 8:42, 1980.

69. **Frisch RE,** Body fat, menarche, and reproductive ability, Seminars Reprod Endocrinol 3:45, 1985.

70. **Loucks AB, Horvath SM, Freeedson PS,** Menstrual status and validation of body fat prediction in athletes, Human Biol 56:383, 1984.

71. **Warren MP,** Effect of exercise and physical training on menarche, Seminars Reprod Endocrinol 3:17, 1985.

72. **Ronkainen H, Pakarinen A, Kirkinen P, Kauppila A,** Physical exercise-induced changes and season-associated differences in the pituitary-ovarian function of runners and joggers, J Clin Endocrinol Metab 60:416, 1985.

73. **Cumming DC, Rebar RW,** Hormonal changes with acute exercise and with training in women, Seminars Reprod Endocrinol 3:55, 1985.

74. **Chang FE, Richards SR, Kim MH, Malarkey WB,** Twenty-four prolactin profiles and prolactin responses to dopamine in long distance runners, J Clin Endocrinol Metab 59:631, 1984.

75. **Howlett TA, Tomlin S, Hgahfoong L, ReesLH, Bullen BA, Skrinar GS, McArthur JW,** Release of beta-endorphin and met-enkephalin during exercise in normal women: response to training, Brit Med J 288:1950, 1984.

76. **Russell JB, Mitchell DE, Musey PI, Collins DC,** The role of beta-endorphins and catechol estrogens on the hypothalamic-pituitary axis in female athletes, Fertil Steril 42:690, 1984.

77. **Laatikainen T, Virtanen T, Apter D,** Plasma immunoreactive beta-endorphin in exercise-associated amenorrhea, Am J Obstet Gynecol 154:94, 1986.

78. **Veldhuis JD, Evans WS, Demers LM, Thorner MO, Wakat D, Rogol AD,** Altered neuroendocrine regulation of gonadotropin secretion in women distance runners, J Clin Endocrinol Metab 61:557, 1985.

79. **Cumming DC, Vickovic MM, Wall SR, Fluker MR,** Defects in pulsatile LH release in normally menstruating runners, J Clin Endocrinol Metab 60:810, 1985.

80. **Smith NJ,** Excessive weight loss and food aversion in athletes simulating anorexia nervosa, Pediatrics 66:139, 1980.

81. **Fries H,** Secondary amenorrhea, self-induced weight reduction and anorexia nervosa, Acta Psychiatr Scand, Suppl 248, 1974.

82. **Bullen BA, Skriinar GS, Beitins IZ, von Mering G, Turnbull BA, McArthur JW,** Induction of menstrual disorders by strenuous exercise in untrained women, New Eng J Med 312:1349, 1985.

83. **Stager JM, Ritchie-Flanagan RB, Robertshaw D,** Reversibility of amenorrhea in athletes, New Eng J Med 310:51, 1984.

84. **Drinkwater BL, Nilson K, Chestnut CH, Bremmer WJ, Shainholtz S, Southworth MB,** Bone mineral content of amenorrheic and eumenorrheic athletes, New Eng J Med 311:277, 1984.

85. **Drinkwater BL, Nilson K, Ott S, Chestnut CH III,** Bone mineral density after resumption of menses in amenorrheic athletes, JAMA 256:380, 1986.

86. **Fisher EC, Nelson ME, Frontera WR, Turksoy RN, Evans WJ,** Bone mineral content and levels of gonadotropins and estrogens in amenorrheic running women, J Clin Endocrinol Metab 62:1232, 1986.

87. **Lindberg JS, Fears WB, Hunt MM, Powell MR, Boll D, Wade CE,** Exercise-induced amenorrhea and bone density, Ann Int Med 101:647, 1984.

88. **Marcus R, Cann CE, Madvig P, Minkoff J, Goddard M, Bayer M, Martin M, Gaudiani L, Haskell W, Genant H,** Menstrual function and bone mass in elite women distance runners, Ann Int Med 102:158, 1985.

89. **Lloyd T, Triantafyllou SJ, Baker ER, Houts PS, Whiteside JA, Kalenak A, Stumpf PG,** Women athletes with menstrual irregularity have increased musculoskeletal injuries, Med Sci Sports Exerc 18:374, 1986.

90. **Maestre de San Juan A,** Falta total de los nervious olfaatorios con anosmia en un individuo en quien existia una atrofia congenita de los testiculos y meiembro viril, El Siglo Medico 131:211, 1856.

91. **Kallmann FJ, Schoenfeld WA, Barrera SE,** The genetic aspects of primary eunuchoidism, Am J Ment Defic 48:203, 1944.

92. **De Morsier G, Gauthier G,** La dysplasie olfacto genitale, Pathol Biol 11:1267, 1963.

93. **Tagatz G, Fialkow PJ, Smith D, Spadoni L,** Hypogonadotropic hypogonadism associated with anosmia in the female, New Eng J Med 282:1326, 1970.

94. **Klingmuller D, Dewes W, Krahe T, Brecht G, Schweikert H,** Magnetic resonance imaging of the brain in patients with anosmia and hypothalamic hypogonadism (Kallmann's Syndrome), J Clin Endocrinol Metab 65:581, 1987.

95. **Cann CE, Martin MC, Jaffe RB,** Duration of amenorrhea affects rate of bone loss in women runners: implications of therapy, Med Sci Sports Ex 17:214, 1985.

6   Anovulation

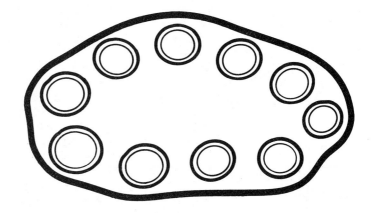

Anovulation is a very common problem which presents in a variety of clinical manifestations, including amenorrhea, irregular menses, and hirsutism. Serious consequences of chronic anovulation are infertility and a greater risk for developing carcinoma of the endometrium and the breast. The physician must appreciate the clinical impact of anovulation and undertake therapeutic management of all anovulatory patients to avoid these unwanted consequences.

Normal ovulation requires coordination of the menstrual system at all levels: the central hypothalamic-pituitary axis, the feedback signals, and local responses within the ovary. The loss of ovulation may be due to any one of an assortment of factors operating at each of these levels. The end result is a dysfunctional state: anovulation. *In this chapter, we will discuss the variety of mechanisms by which dysfunction of the ovulatory cycle can occur and how the clinical expressions of the resulting abnormal menstrual function are produced.*

Pathogenesis of Anovulation

During menses, escape from the negative feedback of estrogen and progesterone results in increased follicle-stimulating hormone (FSH) secretion by the anterior pituitary. This initial increase in FSH is essential for follicular growth and steroidogenesis. With continued growth of the follicle, estradiol production within the follicle maintains follicular sensitivity to FSH allowing conversion from a microenvironment dominated by androgens to one dominated by estrogen, a change necessary for a complete and successful follicular life-span. Continuing and combined action of FSH and estradiol leads to the appearance of luteinizing hormone (LH) receptors on the granulosa cells, a prerequisite for luteinization and ovulation. Ovulation is triggered by the rapid rise in circulating levels of estradiol. A positive feedback response at the level of the anterior pituitary (and perhaps at the hypothalamus as well) results in the midcycle surge of LH necessary for expulsion of the egg and formation of the corpus luteum. A rise in progesterone follows ovulation along with a second rise in estradiol, producing the 14-day

213

luteal phase characterized by low FSH and LH levels. The demise of the corpus luteum, concomitant with a fall in hormone levels, allows FSH to increase again, thus initiating a new cycle.

This recycling mechanism is regulated largely by estradiol. The negative feedback relationship between estradiol and FSH results in the critical initial rise in that gonadotropin during menses, and the positive feedback relationship between estradiol and LH is the ovulatory stimulus. Within the ovary, estradiol induces follicular receptor responses necessary for growth and function. Estradiol is, therefore, properly viewed as the critical agent for appropriate hypothalamic-pituitary-ovarian responses. Dysfunction in the cycle may be due to an abnormality in one of the various roles for estradiol, or an inability to respond to estradiol signals. Problems in normal function may be conveniently organized into central defects, abnormalities in the feedback signals, and abnormal function within the ovary itself.

Central Defects

The hypothalamic-pituitary axis may be unable to respond, even if given adequate and appropriately timed feedback signals. A pituitary tumor represents an obvious example of a central defect in menstrual function, and is discussed in Chapter 5, "Amenorrhea."

Although difficult to demonstrate definitively, malfunction within the hypothalamus is both a likely, as well as a favorite, explanation for ovulatory failure. Normal pituitary ovulatory response to the follicle's steroid signals requires the presence of gonadotropin releasing hormone (GnRH) pulsatile secretion within a critical range. The teenager between menarche and the onset of ovulation cannot generate a normal cycle until full GnRH pulsatile secretion is achieved. Increasing intensity of GnRH suppression is associated with increasing dysfunction and a changing clinical presentation. A variety of problems, such as stress and anxiety, borderline anorexia nervosa, and acute weight loss after a crash diet are thought to inhibit normal GnRH pulsatile secretion so that the gonadotropin surge is not possible and only homeostatic pituitary-ovarian function is maintained.

At least one specific clinical syndrome of central anovulatory dysfunction has been recognized: hyperprolactinemia. Increasing levels of prolactin can cause a woman to progress through a spectrum, beginning with an inadequate luteal phase to anovulation to the amenorrhea associated with complete GnRH suppression. A search for galactorrhea and measurement of the prolactin level are important screening procedures for all women who are not ovulating normally. The presence of galactorrhea or elevated prolactin levels dictates a choice of bromocriptine for the induction of ovulation. In the absence of evidence for elevated prolactin secretion, however, bromocriptine fails to alter FSH and LH levels or response to GnRH.[1,2]

Normal Prolactin	Increasing Hyperprolactinemia ⟶		
Normal Ovulation	Inadequate Luteal Phase	Anovulation	Amenorrhea

Anovulatory women have a higher LH (and presumably GnRH) pulse frequency and amplitude when compared to the midfollicular phase.(3) Central opioid tone appears to be normal as there is no difference in response to naloxone.(4) Interaction at the dopamine-endorphin sites, however, may be altered as pretreatment with a dopamine precursor leads to a naloxone-induced increase in LH in anovulatory women compared to controls. There is increased pituitary activity, marked by increased LH, β-endorphin, and β-lipoprotein secretion.(5) How all this fits together is yet unknown.

Abnormal Feedback Signals

Abnormal cycles can be due to failures within the system, or due to the introduction of confounding factors. It is instructive to focus on the blood estradiol concentration as the critical signal for the machinery of the ovulatory cycle. In order to achieve the appropriate changes within the cycle, estradiol levels must rise and fall in synchrony with morphologic events. Therefore, two possible signal failures may occur: 1) estradiol levels may not fall low enough to allow sufficient FSH response for the initial growth stimulus, and 2) levels of estradiol may be inadequate to produce the positive stimulatory effects necessary to induce the ovulatory surge of LH.

1. **Loss of FSH Stimulation.** In order to achieve recycling, a nadir in blood sex steroid levels must occur so that the initial event in the cycle, the rise in FSH, can take place. Sustained estrogen at such a key moment would not permit FSH stimulation of follicular growth and maturation, and recycling would be thwarted. The necessary decline in blood estrogen requires reduction of secretion, appropriate clearance and metabolism, and the absence of a significant contribution of estrogen to the circulation by extragonadal sources.

   Persistent Estrogen Secretion. The most common clinical example of anovulation associated with continued secretion of estrogen is pregnancy. Persistent and elevated secretion of estrogen can be encountered rarely with an ovarian or adrenal tumor. In such a case, anovulation or amenorrhea may bring the patient to a physician's attention.

   Abnormal Estrogen Clearance and Metabolism. The clearance and metabolism of estrogen can be impaired by other pathologic conditions, such as thyroid or hepatic disease. It is for this reason that a careful history and physical examination are important elements in the differential diagnosis of anovulation. Both hyperthyroidism and hypothyroidism can cause persistent anovulation by altering not only metabolic clearance, but also the peripheral conversion rates among the various steroids. The subtle presence of hypothyroidism, which may be associated with elevated prolactin levels, demands screening of anovulatory and amenorrheic women with a thyroid stimulating hormone (TSH) level.

215

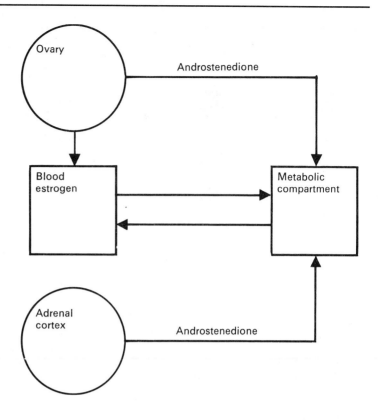

Extraglandular Estrogen Production. Extragonadal contribution to
the blood estrogen level can reach significant proportions. While
the adrenal gland does not secrete appreciable amounts of estrogen
into the circulation, it indirectly contributes to the total estrogen
level. This is accomplished by the extragonadal peripheral conversion of C-19 androgenic precursors, mainly androstenedione, to estrogen. In this manner psychologic or physical stress may increase
the adrenal contribution of estrogenic precursor, and subsequent
conversion to estrogen may sustain the blood level of estrogen at a
time when a decline is necessary for successful recycling of the
menstrual cycle. Adipose tissue is capable of converting androstenedione to estrogen; hence, the percent conversion increases with
increasing body weight.(6) This is at least one mechanism for the
well-known association between obesity and anovulation.

2. **Loss of LH Stimulation.** A failure in gonadal production of estrogen need not be absolute. Obviously the patient with gonadal dysgenesis and ovarian failure will present with amenorrhea and infertility because of a total lack of estrogen secretion. More commonly,
the clinician is concerned with the patient who has gonadotropin
and estrogen production, but does not ovulate. The failure to achieve
a critical midcycle level of estradiol necessary to trigger the gonadotropin surge may be due to a relative deficiency in steroid production. The perimenopausal woman undergoes a terminal period of
anovulation which may represent a steroidogenic refractoriness within
the remaining elderly follicles. This inadequacy may be due to intrinsic follicular weaknesses or an impairment in the follicular-go-
nadotropin interaction. In any case, the end result is the same—a

216

failure to achieve critical signal levels of estradiol at the appropriate time in midcycle.

Local Ovarian
Conditions

An understanding of the critical role for estradiol within the follicle indicates possible points of failure which may lead to anovulation. Estradiol prevents atresia despite declining FSH levels by enhancing the action of FSH in increasing the number of FSH receptors within the follicle, thus increasing follicular sensitivity to FSH. In addition, estradiol enhances the induction of LH receptors by FSH, making it possible for the follicle to respond to the LH surge at midcycle. A follicle can fail to grow and ovulate either because of inadequate estradiol production within the follicle, or because of interference with the action of estradiol.

The factors which control follicular production of estradiol are now understood in terms of the two-cell explanation described in Chapter 1 and Chapter 3. A very precise coordination is necessary between morphologic development and hormonal stimulation. Pertubations may arise from an infectious process, from the presence of endometriosis, by abnormal qualitative or quantitative changes in tropic hormone receptors (ovarian insensitivity), or the necessary biologic effects may be blocked by an improper molecular constitution of the gonadotropins (heterogeneity of the glycopeptide hormones).

Local ovarian androgens induce follicular atresia. Whereas this action in the normal cycle may be important in ensuring that only one follicle reaches the point of ovulation, an excessive concentration of androgens can prevent normal cycling. This effect of androgens can be mediated by interference with the key actions of estradiol. Thus, the important effects of estradiol on gonadotropin receptors will be impeded, leading to chronic anovulation. This may be another mechanism by which obesity leads to persistent anovulation.

Obese women depress their sex hormone binding globulin (SHBG) levels out of proportion to changes in estrogen or testosterone when compared to normal weight patients. (7,8) This change also has been noted in men, but the mechanism is unknown, although the SHBG level is inversely proportional to the dietary lipid intake.(9) Thus, obesity itself would increase free sex steroid levels, and the resulting increase in free testosterone could serve as the factor which acts locally within the ovary to prevent normal follicular growth and ovulation.

Obesity, therefore, is associated with 3 alterations which interfere with normal ovulation, and weight loss improves all 3:

1. Increased peripheral aromatization of androgens to estrogens.

2. Decreased levels of SHBG resulting in increased levels of free estradiol and testosterone.

3. Increased insulin levels which may stimulate ovarian stromal tissue production of androgens.

217

The Insulin Resistance Story. There is now a well-recognized association between increased insulin resistance and polycystic ovaries. A positive correlation exists between insulin secretion and androgen levels, independent of body weight in anovulatory, hyperandrogenized women.(10) The greater the insulin response during an oral glucose tolerance test, the greater an increase in androgen levels. In other words, the utilization of sugar in these women causes an increase in androgen secretion.

Because obesity itself is associated with insulin resistance, it is important to note that this correlation of increased androgen secretion and insulin resistance has been reported in both obese and non-obese anovulatory women.(11,12) Turning off the ovary with a GnRH agonist does not change the hyperinsulinemia or insulin resistance, suggesting that disordered insulin action precedes the increase in androgens.(13)

To further pursue the relationship between obesity and insulin resistance, it is interesting to note that localization of body fat to the upper body (android obesity, see Chapter 14) is specifically associated with diminished hepatic insulin extraction, which adds to the hyperinsulinemia of obesity. Upper body fat localization and the accompanying decline in hepatic insulin extraction along with a decrease in peripheral insulin action are partly mediated by a hyperandrogenic state. (14) Thus there is growing evidence for a relationship between androgen levels and insulin and glucose homeostasis. The mechanism for this relationship is unclear, but it does not involve direct androgen stimulation of pancreatic insulin secretion.

Because insulin (and insulin-like growth factor-I) can stimulate in vitro androgen secretion by ovarian stromal and theca tissue, this raises the possibility of a special subgroup of women who create the cycle of anovulation, polycystic ovaries, and hyperandrogenism through the pathway of abnormal insulin secretion. (15,16) One subgroup may create this picture initially by excessive weight gain, as the insulin resistance in some women increases with weight gain.(17) Another subgroup may be mediated by the increased androgen secretion.(12)

Finally, another syndrome is encountered: hyperandrogenism, insulin resistance, and acanthosis nigricans.(18) Acanthosis nigricans is a brown velvety, sometimes verrucous, discoloration of the skin, usually at the neck and axillae, which appears to be a marker for insulin resistance. In this case, the severe insulin resistance is out of proportion to any associated hyperandrogenism or obesity, and the acanthosis nigricans skin lesions are thought to be due to the hyperinsulinemia.(19) There is good evidence to indicate that the insulin resistance is not caused by the elevated androgens.(20)

Precise Etiology

The normal ovulatory function of the menstrual system relies on a dynamic coordination of complex actions. Abnormal function may represent discordance at all of the levels reviewed in the above paragraphs. Thus, a minor deficiency in the estradiol signal will be associated with a subnormal central response, and an impaired or inappropriate degree of follicular growth and function. Dysfunction is sustained by the internal feedback mechanisms within the system, and anovulation may become a persistent problem.

It is usually impossible to reduce the issue of etiology to a single factor of abnormal menstrual function, except in severe disease states such as pituitary tumors, anorexia nervosa, gonadal dysgenesis, and perhaps hyperprolactinemia and obesity. Not only is it often impossible, but it is also often unnecessary to define the precise etiology. Regardless of the nature of the initial cause of the problem, the final clinical statement of the dysfunction is predictable, and easily diagnosed and managed. In patients who have abnormal or absent menstrual function, but are otherwise medically normal, the diagnosis will fall into one of three categories:

1. **Ovarian Failure.** Hypergonadotropic hypogonadism, the inability of the ovary to respond to any gonadotropic stimulation, usually due to the absence of follicular tissue on a genetic basis (discussed in Chapter 5).

2. **Central Failure.** Hypogonadotropic hypogonadism, hypothalamic or pituitary suppression as expressed in abnormally low or normal serum gonadotropins (discussed in Chapter 5).

3. **Anovulatory Dysfunction.** The patient who has asynchronous gonadotropin and estrogen production and does not ovulate presents with a variety of clinical manifestations. The associated clinical signs and symptoms depend upon the level of gonadal function preserved, and are represented by the following principal problems:

Endometrial hyperplasia and cancer (Chapter 4),

Amenorrhea (Chapter 5),

Hirsutism (Chapter 7),

Dysfunctional uterine bleeding (Chapter 8),

Breast disease (Chapter 9),

Infertility and induction of ovulation (Chapter 20),

The polycystic ovary (this chapter).

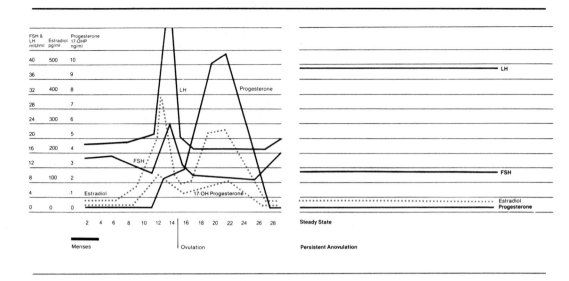

			LH	
			Progesterone	
	FSH			
	Estradiol		17-OH Progesterone	
Menses		Ovulation		Persistent Anovulation

Steady State

The Polycystic Ovary

In 1935 Stein and Leventhal first described a symptom complex due to anovulation. Acceptance of this syndrome as a singular clinical entity led to a rather rigid approach to this problem for many years. Only those women qualified who had a history of oligomenorrhea, hirsutism, and obesity, together with a demonstration of enlarged, polycystic ovaries. It is far more useful clinically to avoid the use of eponyms and even the term polycystic ovary syndrome or disease. It is better to consider this problem as one of persistent anovulation with a spectrum of etiologies and clinical manifestations.

A question which has puzzled gynecologists and endocrinologists for many years is what causes polycystic ovaries. The answer is now apparent. The characteristic polycystic ovary emerges when a state of anovulation persists for any length of time. Because there are many causes of anovulation, there are many causes of polycystic ovaries. A similar clinical picture and ovarian condition may reflect any of the dysfunctional states discussed above. In other words, the polycystic ovary is the result of a functional derangement, not a specific central or local defect.

In contrast to the characteristic picture of fluctuating hormone levels in the normal cycle, a "steady state" of gonadotropins and sex steroids can be depicted in association with persistent anovulation. This steady state is only relative, and is being exaggerated here to present a concept of this clinical problem.

In patients with persistent anovulation, the average daily production of estrogen and androgens is both increased and dependent upon LH stimulation.(21,22) This is reflected in higher circulating levels of testosterone, androstenedione, dehydroepiandrosterone (DHA), dehydroepiandrosterone sulfate (DHAS), 17-hydroxyprogesterone (17-OHP), and estrone.(23,24) The testosterone, androstenedione, and DHA are secreted directly by the ovary while the DHAS is almost exclusively an adrenal contribution.(24)

Treatment of women with polycystic ovaries with a GnRH agonist is associated with the following helpful observations:(21)

1. The increases in androstenedione and testosterone are almost exclusively from the ovary.

2. The increase in 17-OHP is also from the ovary.

3. Secretion of DHA, DHAS, and cortisol are not influenced by GnRH agonist treatment, and presumably adrenal secretion of these substances is independent of the ovary. However, GnRH agonist treatment for 4 weeks may be insufficient to change adrenal secretion; DHAS changes are notoriously slow, taking months to occur.

The ovary does not secrete increased amounts of estrogen, and estradiol levels are equivalent to early follicular phase concentrations. The increased total estrogen is due to peripheral conversion of the increased amounts of androstenedione to estrone. That is not to say that there is no ovarian secretion of estrogen. Both estrone and estradiol continue to be secreted in significant although low amounts.(25)

The levels of SHBG are controlled by a balance of hormonal influences on its synthesis in the liver; testosterone is inhibitory, estrogen and thyroxine are stimulatory. Due to the increased levels of testosterone in anovulatory patients, there is an approximate 50% reduction in SHBG. Indeed, in hirsute females the mean SHBG concentration is similar to that of males.(26)

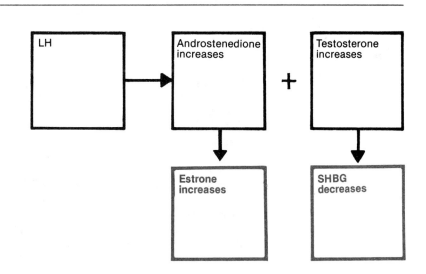

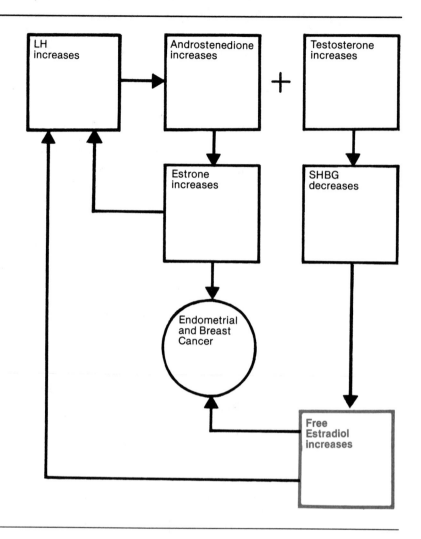

When compared to levels found in normal women, patients with persistent anovulation have higher mean concentrations of LH, but low or low-normal levels of FSH.(23,27-29) The elevated levels of LH can be in the range of the midcycle surge or equivalent to post-menopausal values. Early evidence (an augmented response to GnRH) indicated that the elevated LH levels were due to an increased sensitivity of the pituitary to releasing hormone stimulation (not a central change in GnRH release), manifested primarily by an increase in LH pulse amplitude rather than increased pulse frequency. (30) This is consistent with the concepts discussed in Chapter 2, linking a high estrogen environment with anterior pituitary secretion of LH and suppression of FSH. It is noteworthy that this high level of LH is characterized by an increased level of LH bioactivity. (22)

On the other hand, the gonadotropin pattern (high LH and low FSH) may represent partial desensitization of the pituitary due to increased frequency of GnRH secretion. (31) This is associated with an increase in amplitude and frequency of LH secretion which is correlated with the level of circulating estrogen. Previous reports which failed to detect an increased frequency sampled the circulating levels less intensively. It is likely that this increased activity is taking place at both hypothalamic and pituitary sites.

The increased pituitary and hypothalamic sensitivity can be attributed to the increased estrone levels,(32) but a newly appreciated factor is the impact of the decreased SHBG concentration. Despite no increase in estradiol secretion, free estradiol levels are increased because of the significant decrease in SHBG. The increased LH secretion as expressed by the LH:FSH ratio is positively correlated with the increased free estradiol.(31,33) The lower FSH levels represent the sensitivity of the FSH negative feedback system to the elevated estrogen, both free estradiol and the estrone formed from peripheral conversion of androstenedione. In addition, polycystic ovaries produce higher levels of inhibin, which may contribute to the FSH suppression,(34) and finally, the altered pattern of GnRH secretion can contribute to this characteristic LH:FSH ratio.(31) The clinical consequences of uninterrupted estrogen stimulation (endometrial and breast cancer) as well as the increased LH are the result of the two estrogenic influences (estrone and free estradiol).

Because the FSH levels are not totally depressed, new follicular growth is continuously stimulated, but not to the point of full maturation and ovulation. Despite the fact that full growth potential is not realized, follicular life-span may extend several months in the form of multiple follicular cysts, 2-6 mm in diameter. These follicles are surrounded by hyperplastic theca cells, often luteinized in response to the high LH levels. The accumulation of follicular tissue in various stages of development allows an increased and relatively constant production of steroids in response to the gonadotropin stimulation. This condition is self-sustaining. As various follicles undergo atresia, they are immediately replaced by new follicles of similar limited growth potential.

The tissue derived from follicular atresia is also sustained by the steady state, and now contributes to the stromal compartment of the ovary. In terms of the two-cell explanation of follicular steroidogenesis, atresia is associated with a degenerating granulosa, leaving the theca cells to contribute to the stromal compartment of the ovary. It is not surprising, therefore, that this functioning stromal tissue secretes significant amounts of androstenedione and testosterone, the usual products of theca cells. In response to the elevated LH levels, the androgen production rate is increased. In turn, in a vicious cycle, the elevated androgen levels compound the problem through the process of extraglandular conversion as well as the suppression of SHBG synthesis, resulting in elevated estrogen levels. In addition, the decrease in SHBG is associated with a twofold increase in free testosterone.

The elevated androgens contribute to the morphologic effect within the ovary by blocking the actions of estradiol on the granulosa cells, preventing normal follicular development and inducing premature atresia. Indeed, in another aspect of the vicious cycle, the local androgen block appears to be a major obstacle which maintains the steady state of persistent anovulation. A sustained reduction in androgen levels following surgical wedge resection of the ovaries precedes the return of ovulatory cycles, indicating that the intraovarian androgen effect is the principal factor in preventing normal cycling.(35-37) In addition, testosterone can have a direct inhibitory action on the hypothalamic-pituitary axis.(38)

In this manner the classic picture of the polycystic ovary is attained, displaying numerous follicles in the early stages of development and atresia, and dense stromal tissue. The loss of recycling has resulted in a hormonal steady state causing persistent anovulation which may be associated with the increased production of androgens.

The polycystic ovary is the result of a "vicious cycle" which can be initiated at any one of many entry points. Altered function at any point in the cycle leads to the same result: the polycystic ovary. Recent studies, in an effort to be accurate, have usually included only patients fulfilling strict criteria. Thus only certain subgroups of a large heterogeneous clinical problem have been characterized. *Don't lose sight of the fact that the polycystic ovary is a sign, not a disease.*

The polycystic ovary is usually enlarged and is characterized by a smooth pearly white capsule. For years, it was erroneously believed that the thick sclerotic capsule acted as a mechanical barrier to ovulation. A more accurate concept is that the polycystic ovary is a consequence of the loss of ovulation and the achievement of the steady state of persistent anovulation. The characteristics of the ovary reflect this dysfunctional state:(39)

1. The surface area is doubled, giving an average volume increase of 2.8 times.

2. The same number of primordial follicles is present, but the number of growing and atretic follicles (up to the secondary follicle stage) is doubled. Each ovary may contain 20-100 cystic follicles.

3. The thickness of the tunica is increased by 50%.

4. A one-third increase in cortical stromal thickness and a 5-fold increase in subcortical stroma are noted. The increased stroma is due both to hyperplasia and to increased formation subsequent to the excessive follicular maturation and atresia.

5. There are 4 times more ovarian hilus cell nests (hyperplasia).

Hyperthecosis refers to patches of luteinized theca-like cells scattered throughout the ovarian stroma. It is characterized by the same histologic findings as seen in polycystic ovaries.(40) The clinical picture of more intense androgenization is a result of greater androgen production. This condition is associated with lower LH levels, which is a likely consequence of the higher testosterone levels blocking estrogen action at the pituitary level.(40,41) It seems appropriate to view hyperthecosis as a manifestation of the same process, persistent anovulation, but with greater intensity. A greater degree of insulin resistance is correlated with the degree of hyperthecosis.(42)

The typical histologic changes of the polycystic ovary can be encountered with any size ovary. There is a spectrum of time involved in the development of this condition, and it is useful to view the attainment of high LH levels and large ovaries as a stage of maximal effect of persistent anovulation. Increased size of the ova-

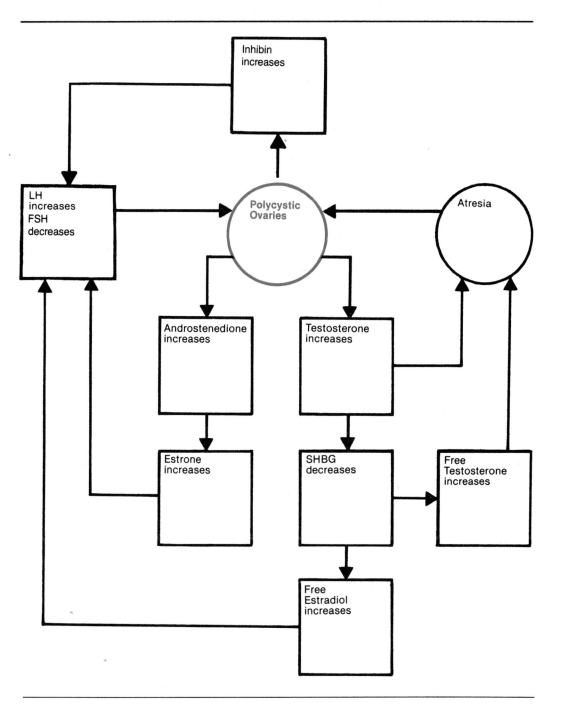

ries is not a critical feature, nor is it necessary for diagnosis. The key to understanding this clinical problem is an appreciation for the disruption in ovulatory recycling function.

There is no specific pathophysiologic defect. The hypothalamic-pituitary response is entirely appropriate, a response to chronically elevated estrogen feedback. The changes are a functional derangement brought about by accumulated and increased androgen due to a failure of ovulation, whatever the reason. Hence, the polycystic ovary may be associated with extragonadal sources of androgens (43,44) or with ovarian androgen-producing tumors.(45,46)

The functional problem can be understood in terms of the two-cell explanation of steroidogenesis (Chapter 3). The follicles are unable to successfully change their microenvironment from androgen dominance to estrogen dominance, the change that is essential for continued follicular growth and development.(47) The functional picture that emerges (incompetent granulosa cells and very active theca cells) corresponds to the morphologic histology of underdeveloped granulosa and hyperplastic and luteinized theca. Granulosa cells obtained from the small follicles of polycystic ovaries produce negligible amounts of estradiol, but show a dramatic increase in estrogen production when FSH is added.(48) In terms of the two-cell explanation, this behavior is consistent with deficient FSH receptors and granulosa function, not an intrinsic steroid synthesis enzyme defect. Successful treatment depends, therefore, on altering the ratio of FSH to androgens; either increasing FSH (with clomiphene) or decreasing androgens (wedge resection) to overcome the androgen block at the granulosa level. This permits development of aromatization to bring about conversion of the microenvironment to estrogen dominance. Because anovulation with polycystic ovaries is a functional derangement, it is not surprising that these patients occasionally may ovulate spontaneously. Indeed, ovulation is unpredictable and contraception may be necessary.

At least one group of patients with this condition inherits the disorder, possibly by means of an X-linked dominant transmission. There is a two-fold higher incidence of hirsutism and oligomenorrhea with paternal transmission, but with marked variability of phenotypic expression.(49)

The adrenal gland is involved in this problem. Higher circulating levels of DHAS, almost exclusively an adrenal product, testify to adrenal participation. The mechanism and the clinical importance of this involvement will be discussed in Chapter 7, "Hirsutism."

Clinical Consequences

Anovulation is the key feature of this condition and presents as amenorrhea in approximately 55% of cases, and with irregular, heavy bleeding in 28%.(50) True virilization is rare, but 70% of anovulatory patients complain of cosmetically disturbing hirsutism. The development of hirsutism depends not only on the concentration of androgens in the blood, but on the genetic sensitivity of hair follicles to androgens. Obesity has been classically regarded as an important feature, but in view of the concept of persistent anovulation arising from many causes, its presence is extremely variable and has no diagnostic value.

While an elevated LH value in the presence of a low or low-normal FSH may be diagnostic, the diagnosis is easily made by the clinical presentation alone. Indeed, the androgen impact may be such that the estrogen-induced LH secretion is suppressed. About 10-20% of patients with this condition do not have elevated LH levels with reversal of the LH:FSH ratio. We do not routinely measure FSH and LH levels in anovulatory patients.

The symptoms are a consequence of the loss of ovulation: dysfunctional bleeding, amenorrhea, hirsutism, and infertility. Each requires a specific diagnostic and therapeutic approach, as discussed in separate chapters in this book.

226

There are potentially severe clinical consequences of the steady state of hormone secretion. Besides the problems of bleeding, amenorrhea, hirsutism, and infertility, the effect of the unopposed and uninterrupted estrogen is to place the patient in considerable risk for cancer of the endometrium and cancer of the breast.(51,52) The risk of endometrial cancer is increased threefold, while chronic anovulation during the reproductive years is associated with a 3-4 times increased risk of breast cancer appearing in the postmenopausal years.

If left unattended, patients with persistent anovulation develop clinical problems, and therefore, appropriate therapeutic management is essential for all anovulatory patients. The typical patient presents with anovulation and irregular menses, or amenorrhea with withdrawal bleeding after a progestational challenge. If there is no hirsutism or virilism, evaluation of androgen production is not necessary. There is no need for urinary 17-ketosteroids, blood testosterone, blood DHAS, or any other laboratory procedures. In the patient who has long-standing anovulation, an endometrial biopsy (with extensive sampling) is a wise precaution. The well-known association between this syndrome and abnormal endometrial changes must be kept in mind. Documentation of anovulation is usually unnecessary, especially in view of menstrual irregularity with periods of amenorrhea.

Therapy of most anovulatory patients can be planned at the first visit. If the patient desires pregnancy, she is a candidate for the medical induction of ovulation. (Chapter 20). If the patient presents with amenorrhea, an investigation must be pursued as outlined in Chapter 5. The management of significant dysfunctional uterine bleeding is discussed in Chapter 8, and hirsutism in Chapter 7.

For the patient who does not wish to become pregnant and does not complain of hirsutism, but is anovulatory and has irregular bleeding, therapy is directed toward interruption of the steady state effect on the endometrium and breast. The use of medroxyprogesterone acetate (10 mg daily for the first 10 days of every month) is favored to ensure complete withdrawal bleeding, and to prevent endometrial hyperplasia and atypia. The monthly 10 day duration has been shown to be essential to protect the endometrium from cancer in women on estrogen replacement therapy. Until specific clinical data are available, it seems logical that young, anovulatory women also require 10 days of progestational exposure every month. The patient will be aware of the onset of ovulatory cycles because bleeding will occur at a time other than the expected withdrawal bleed. The use of oral contraceptive medication for therapy in these patients requires individual patient judgment. In our opinion, when reliable contraception is essential, the use of low dose combination oral contraception in the usual cyclic fashion is appropriate.

There is another argument in favor of continuous suppression rather than periodic progestational interruption. The lipoprotein profile in androgenized women with polycystic ovaries is similar to the male pattern.(8) The long-term impact on cardiovascular disease is unknown, but it makes sense to be concerned about this health problem. Monthly treatment with a progestational agent has no significant effect on the androgen production by polycystic ovaries. Thus, assessment of the lipoprotein profile is a reasonable clinical response, and in the presence of a male pattern, serious consideration should be given to suppression with birth control pills.

Overweight, hyperandrogenic, anovulatory women must be cautioned regarding diabetes mellitus. The long-term consequences of the documented hyperinsulinism and insulin resistance are also not known, but this should be a further inducement for dietary control.

References

1. **Steingold KA, Lobo RA, Judd HL, Lu JKH, Chang RJ,** The effect of bromocriptine on gonadotropin and steroid secretion in polycystic ovarian disease, J Clin Endocrinol Metab 62:1048, 1986.

2. **Buvat J, Buvat-Herbaut M, Marcolin G, Racadot A, Fourlinnie JC, Beuscart R, Fossati P,** A double blind controlled study of the hormonal and clinical effects of bromocriptine in the polycystic ovary syndrome, J Clin Endocrinol Metab 63:119, 1986.

3. **Burger CW, Korsen T, van Kessel H, van Dop PA, Caron JM, Schoemaker J,** Pulsatile luteinizing hormone patterns in the follicular phase of the menstrual cycle, polycystic ovarian disease (PCOD) and non-PCOD secondary amenorrhea, J Clin Endocrinol Metab 61:1126, 1985.

4. **Barnes RB, Lobo RA,** Central opioid activity in polycystic ovary syndrome with and without dopaminergic modulation, J Clin Endocrinol Metab 61:779, 1985.

5. **Barnes RB, Lobo RA,** Endogenous opioids in polycystic ovary syndrome, Seminars Reprod Endocrinol 5:185, 1987.

6. **Siiteri PK, MacDonald PC,** Role of extraglandular estrogen in human endocrinology, in *Handbook of Physiology, Section 7, Endocrinology,* Geyer SR, Astwood EB, Greep RO, editors, American Physiology Society, Washington DC, 1973, pp 615-629.

7. **Plymate SR, Fariss BL, Bassett ML, Matej L,** Obesity and its role in polycystic ovary syndrome, J Clin Endocrinol Metab 52:1246, 1981.

8. **Wild RA, Painter PC, Coulson PB, Carruth KB, Ranney GB,** Lipoprotein lipid concentrations and cardiovascular risk in women with polycystic ovary syndrome, J Clin Endocrinol Metab 61:946, 1985.

9. **Reed MJ, Cheng RW, Simmonds m, Richmond W, James VHT,** Dietary lipids: An additional regulator of plasma levels of sex hormone binding globulin, J Clin Endocrinol Metab 64:1083, 1987.

10. **Smith S, Ravnikar VA, Barbieri RL,** Androgen and insulin response to an oral glucose challenge in hyperandrogenic women, Fertil Steril 48:72, 1987.

11. **Chang RJ, Nakamura RM, Judd HL, Kaplan SA,** Insulin resistance in non-obese patients with polycystic ovarian disease, J Clin Endocrinol Metab 57:356, 1983.

12. **Jialal I, Naiker P, Reddi K, Moodley J, Joubert SM,** Evidence for insulin resistance in nonobese patients with polycystic ovarian disease, J Clin Endocrinol Metab 64:1066, 1987.

13. **Geffner ME, Kaplan SA, Bersch N, Golde DW, Landaw EM, Chang RJ,** Persistence of insulin resistance in polycystic ovarian disease after inhibition of ovarian steroid secretion, Fertil Steril 45:327, 1986.

14. **Peiris AN, Mueller RA, Struve MF, Smith GA, Kissebah AH,** Relationship of androgenic activity to splanchnic insulin metabolism and peripheral glucose utilization in premenopausal women, J Clin Endocrinol Metab 64:162, 1987.

15. **Barbieri RL, Makris A, Ryan KJ,** Insulin stimulates androgen accumulation in incubations of human ovarian stroma and theca, Obstet Gynecol 64:73S, 1984.

16. **Barbieri RL, Makris A, Randall RW, Daniels G, Kistner RW, Ryan KJ,** Insulin stimulates androgen accumulation in incubations of ovarian stroma obtained from women with hyperandrogenism, J Clin Endocrinol Metab 62:904, 1986.

17. **Pasquali R, Fabbri R, Venturoli S, Paradisi R, Antenucci D, Melchionda N,** Effect of weight loss and antiandrogenic therapy on sex hormone blood levels and insulin resistance in obese patients with polycystic ovaries, Am J Obstet Gynecol 154:139, 1986.

18. **Barbieri RL, Ryan KJ,** Hyperandrogenism, insulin resistance and acanthosis nigricans: A common endocrinopathy with distinct pathophysiologic features, Am J Obstet Gynecol 147:90, 1983.

19. **Stuart CA, Peters EJ, Prince MJ, Richards G, Cavallo A, Meyer WJ III,** Insulin resistance with acanthosis nigricans: The roles of obesity and androgen excess, Metabolism 35:197, 1986.

20. **Pepper GM, Poretsky L, Gabrilove JL, Ariton MM,** Ketoconazole reverses hyperandrogenism in a patient with insulin resistance and acanthosis nigricans, J Clin Endocrinol Metab 65:1047, 1987.

21. **Chang RJ,** Ovarian steroid secretion in polycystic ovarian disease, Seminars Reprod Endocrinol 2:244, 1984.

22. **Calogero AE, Macchi M, Montanini V, Mongioi A, Maugeri G, Vicari E, Coniglione F, Sipione C, D'Agata R,** Dynamics of plasma gonadotropin and sex steroid release in polycystic ovarian disease after pituitary-ovarian inhibition with an analog of gonadotropin-releasing hormone, J Clin Endocrinol Metab 64:980, 1987.

23. **DeVane GW, Czekala NM, Judd HL, Yen SSC,** Circulating gonadotropins, estrogen and androgens in polycystic ovarian disease, Am J Obstet Gynecol 121:496, 1975.

24. **Laatikainen TJ, Apter DL, Paavonen JA, Wahlstrom TR,** Steroids in ovarian and peripheral venous blood in polycystic ovarian disease, Clin Endocrinol 13:125, 1980.

25. **Wajchenberg BL, Achando SS, Mathor MM, Czeresnia CE, Neto DG, Kirschner MA,** The source(s) of estrogen production in hirsute women with polycystic ovarian disease as determined by simultaneous adrenal and ovarian venous catheterization, Fertil Steril 49:56, 1988.

26. **Moll GW Jr, Rosenfield RL, Helke JH,** Estradiol-testosterone binding interactions and free plasma estradiol under physiological conditions, J Clin Endocrinol Metab 52:868, 1981.

27. **Kletzky OA, Davajan V, Nakamura RM, Thorneycroft IH, Mishell DR Jr,** Clinical categorization of patients with secondary amenorrhea using progesterone induced uterine bleeding and measurement of serum gonadotropin levels, Am J Obstet Gynecol 121:695, 1975.

28. **Rebar R, Judd HL, Yen SSC, Rakoff J, Vandenberg G, Naftolin F,** Characterization of the inappropriate gonadotropin secretion in polycystic ovary syndrome, J Clin Invest 57:1320, 1976.

29. **Rebar RW,** Gonadotropin secretion in polycystic ovary disease, Seminars Reprod Endocrinol 2:223, 1984.

30. **Kazer RR, Kessel B, Yen SSC,** Circulating luteinizing hormone pulse frequency in women with polycystic ovary syndrome, J Clin Endocrinol Metab 65:233, 1987.

31. **Waldstreicher J, Santoro NF, Hall JE, Filicori M, Crowley WF Jr,** Hyperfunction of the hypothalamic-pituitary axis in women with polycystic ovarian disease: Indirect evidence for partial gonadotroph desensitization, J Clin Endocrinol Metab 66:165, 1988.

32. **Chang RJ, Mandel FP, Lu JK, Judd HL,** Enhanced disparity of gonadotropin secretion by estrone in women with polycystic ovarian disease, J Clin Endocrinol Metab 54:490, 1982.

33. **Lobo RA, Granger L, Goebelsmann U, Mishell DR Jr,** Elevations in unbound serum estradiol as a possible mechanism for inappropriate gonadotropin secretion in women with PCO, J Clin Endocrinol Metab 52:156, 1981.

34. **Tanabe K, Gagliano P, Channing CP, et al,** Levels of inhibin-F activity and steroids from human follicular fluid from normal women and women with polycystic ovary disease, J Clin Endocrinol Metab 57:24, 1983.

35. **Judd HL, Rigg LA, Anderson DC, Yen SSC,** The effects of ovarian wedge resection on circulating gonadotropin and ovarian steroid levels in patients with polycystic ovary syndrome, J Clin Endocrinol Metab 43:347, 1976.

36. **Mahesh VB, Bratlid D, Lindabeck T,** Hormone levels following wedge resection in polycystic ovary syndrome, Obstet Gynecol 51:64, 1978.

37. **Katz M, Carr PJ, Cohen BM, Milhin RP,** Hormonal effects of wedge resection of polycystic ovaries, Obstet Gynecol 51:437, 1978.

38. **Serafini P, Silva PD, Paulson RJ, Elind-Hirsch K, Hernandez M, Lobo RA,** Acute modulaton of the hypothalamic-pituitary axis by intravenous testosterone in normal women, Am J Obstet Gynecol 155:1288, 1986.

39. **Hughesdon PE,** Morphology and morphogenesis of the Stein-Leventhal ovary and of so-called "hyperthecosis," Obstet Gynecol Surv 37:59, 1982.

40. **Judd HL, Scully RE, Herbst AL, Yen SSC, Ingersol FM, Kliman B,** Familial hyperthecosis: comparison of endocrinologic and histologic findings with polycystic ovarian disease, Am J Obstet Gynecol 117:979, 1973.

41. **Nagamani M, Lingold JC, Gomez LG, Barza JR,** Clinical and hormonal studies in hyperthecosis of the ovaries, Fertil Steril 36:326, 1981.

42. **Nagamani M, Dinh TV, Kelver ME,** Hyperinsulinemia in hyperthecosis of the ovaries, Am J Obstet Gynecol 154:384, 1986.

43. **Kase N, Kowal J, Perloff W, Soffer LJ,** In vitro production of androgens by a virilizing adenoma and associated polycystic ovaries, Acta Endocrinol 44:15, 1963.

44. **Amerikia H, Savoy-Moore RT, Sundareson AS, Moghissi KS,** The effects of long-term androgen treatment on the ovary, Fertil Steril 45:202, 1986.

45. **Zourlas PA, Jones HW Jr,** Stein-Leventhal syndrome with masculinizing ovarian tumors, Obstet Gynecol 34:861, 1969.

46. **Dunaif A, Scully RE, Andersen RN, Chapin DS, Crowley WF Jr,** The effects of continuous androgen secretion on the hypothalamic-pituitary axis in women: Evidence from a luteinized thecoma of the ovary, J Clin Endocrinol Metab 59:389, 1984.

47. **McNatty KP, Smith DM, Makris A, DeGrazia C, Tulchinsky D, Osathanondh R, Schiff I, Ryan KJ,** The intraovarian sites of androgen and estrogen formation in women with normal and hyperandrogenic ovaries as judged by in vitro experiments, J Clin Endocrinol Metab 50:755, 1980.

48. **Erickson GF, Hsueh AJN, Quigley ME, Rebar R, Yen SSC,** Functional studies of aromatase activity in human granulosa cells from normal and polycystic ovaries, J Clin Endocrinol Metab 49:514, 1979.

49. **Givens JR,** Hirsutism and hyperandrogenism, Adv Intern Med 21:221, 1976.

50. **Prunty FTG,** Hirsutism, virilism, and apparent virilism, and their gonadal relationships, J Endocrinol 38:203, 1967.

51. **Coulam CB, Annegers JF,** Breast cancer and chronic anovulation syndrome, Surgical Forum 33:474, 1982.

52. **Coulam CB, Annegers JF, Kranz JS,** Chronic anovulation syndrome and associated neoplasia, Obstet Gynecol 61:403, 1983.

7 Hirsutism

Excessive facial and body hair usually is associated with loss of cyclic menstrual function due to excess androgen production by anovulatory ovaries. The more severe states of virilism (clitoromegaly, deepening of the voice, balding, and changes in body habitus) are rarely seen and usually are secondary to adrenal hyperplasia or androgen-producing tumors of adrenal or ovarian origin. Although these are rare, diagnostic evaluation is required. Furthermore, a concerned and sympathetic approach must be offered to the patient. The responsible physician must view hirsutism both as an endocrine problem and as a cosmetic problem. To the affected woman, hair growth over the face, abdomen, or breasts is disturbing on several levels: Is there disease? Is sexuality changing? Is social acceptance altered? Is fertility impaired?

This chapter will review the biology of hair growth and the endocrine causes that can yield hirsutism. An uncomplicated, effective program for diagnostic evaluation and therapeutic management will be offered.

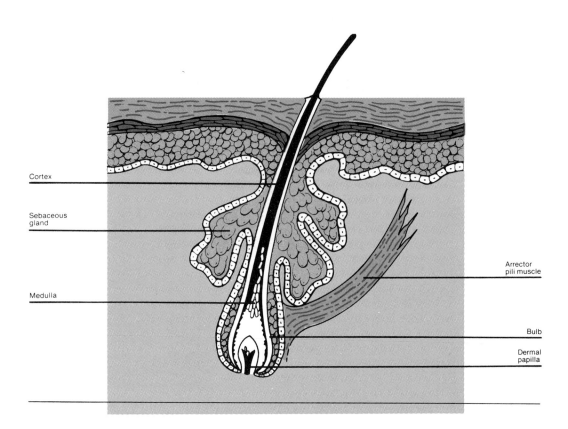

Cortex

Sebaceous gland

Medulla

Arrector pili muscle

Bulb

Dermal papilla

Biology of Hair Growth

Embryology

Each hair follicle develops at about 8 weeks of gestation as a derivative of the epidermis. It is composed initially of a solid column of cells which proliferates from the basal layers of the epidermis and protrudes downward into the dermis. As the column elongates it encounters a cluster of mesodermal cells (the dermal papilla) which it envelops at its bulbous tip (bulb). The solid epithelial column then hollows out to form a hair canal, and the polisebaceous apparatus is laid down.

Hair growth begins with proliferation of the epithelial cells at the base of the column in contact with the dermal papilla. The *lanugo hair* present at this stage is lightly pigmented, thin in diameter, short in length, and fragile in attachment. Important to note here is the fact that the total endowment of hair follicles is made at an early gestational stage, and that no new hair follicles will be produced de novo. The concentration of hair follicles laid down per unit area of facial skin does not differ materially between sexes but does differ between races and ethnic groups (Caucasian > Oriental; Mediterranean > Nordic). The natural pattern of hair growth is genetically predetermined.

| Structure and Growth | Hair does not grow continuously, but rather in a cyclic fashion with alternating phases of activity and inactivity. The cycles are referred to by the following terms: |

Anagen - the growing phase.
Catagen - rapid involution phase.
Telogen - quiescent phase.

In the resting phase (telogen), the hair is short and loosely attached to the base of the epithelial canal. The bulb is formed around the dermal papilla. As growth begins (anagen), epithelial matrix cells at the base begin to proliferate and extend downward into the dermis. The bulb is reformed and the epithelial column elongates some 4-6 times from the resting state. Once downward extension is completed, continued rapid growth of the matrix cells pushes upward to the skin surface. The tenuous contact of the previous hair is broken, and that hair is shed. The superficial matrix cells differentiate forming a keratinized column. Growth continues as long as active mitoses persist in the basal matrix cells. When finished (catagen), the column shrinks, the bulb shrivels, and the resting state is reachieved (telogen).

The length of hair is primarily determined by duration of the growth phase (anagen). Scalp hair remains in anagen for 3 years and has only a relatively short resting phase. Elsewhere (forearm) a short anagen and long telogen will lead to short hair of stable nongrowing length. The appearance of continuous growth (or periodic shedding) is determined by the degree to which individual hair follicles act asynchronously with their neighbors. Scalp hair is asynchronous and therefore always seems to be growing. The resting phase that some hairs (10-15%) are in is not apparent. If marked synchrony is achieved, then all hairs may undergo telogen at the same time leading to the appearance of shedding. Occasionally, women will complain of marked hair loss from the scalp, but this time period of shedding is usually limited (6-8 months), and normal growth resumes.

Factors which
Influence Hair Growth

The dermal papilla is the director of the events which control hair growth. Despite major injury to the epithelial component of the follicle (such as freezing, x-rays, or a skin graft), if the dermal papilla survives, the hair follicle will regenerate and regrow hair. Injury to, or degeneration of, the dermal papilla is the crucial factor in permanent hair loss.

Sexual hair can be defined as that hair which responds to the sex steroids. Sexual hair grows on the face, lower abdomen, anterior thighs, the chest, the breasts, the pubic area and in the axillae. Once androgen influences hair follicles in sexual areas and larger, longer, more pigmented hair is induced, these final hair characteristics recur in typical cycles, even in the absence of sustaining androgen.

From animal studies and human disease patterns, the following list of hormonal effects can be compiled:

1. Androgens, particularly testosterone, initiate growth, increase the diameter and pigmentation of the keratin column, and probably increase the rate of matrix cell mitoses, in all but scalp hair.

2. Estrogens act essentially opposite from androgens, retarding the rate and initiation of growth, and leading to finer, less pigmented and slower growing hair.

3. Progestins have minimal direct effect on hair.

4. Pregnancy (high estrogen and progesterone) may increase the synchrony of hair growth, leading to periods of growth or shedding.

An important clinical characteristic of hair growth can be understood from studies of the effects of castration. If castration occurs before puberty, the male will not grow a beard. If castration occurs after puberty with beard and sexual hair distribution fully developed, then these hairs continue to grow albeit more slowly and with finer caliber. Clearly androgen stimulates sexual hair follicle conversion from lanugo to terminal adult hair growth patterns, but *once established, these patterns persist despite withdrawal of androgen.* Hypertrichosis is a generalized increase in hair of the fetal lanugo type, associated with the use of drugs or malignancy. *Vellus hair* is the downy hair associated with the prepubertal years. *Terminal hair* is the coarse hair which grows on various parts of the body during the adult years. Hirsutism implies a vellus to terminal hair transformation.

Sexual and nonsexual hair growth can be affected by endocrine problems. In hypopituitarism, there is marked reduction of hair growth. Acromegaly will be associated with hirsutism in 10-15% of patients. While the impact of thyroid hormone is not clear, hypothyroid individuals sometimes display less axillary, pubic, and, curiously, lateral eyebrow hair.

Hair growth may be influenced by nonhormonal factors, such as local skin temperature, blood flow, and edema. Hair grows faster in the summer than in the winter. Hair growth may be seen with CNS problems such as encephalitis, cranial trauma, multiple sclerosis, and with drugs. Plucking hair, but not shaving, induces hair regrowth.

Androgen Production

The production rate of testosterone in the normal female is 0.2 to 0.3 mg/day. Approximately 50% of testosterone arises from peripheral conversion of androstendione, while the adrenal gland and ovary contribute approximately equal amounts (25%) to the circulating levels of testosterone, except at midcycle when the ovarian contribution increases by 10-15%. Dehydroepiandrosterone sulfate (DHAS) arises almost exclusively from the adrenal gland, while 90% of dehydroepiandrosterone (DHA) is from the adrenal.

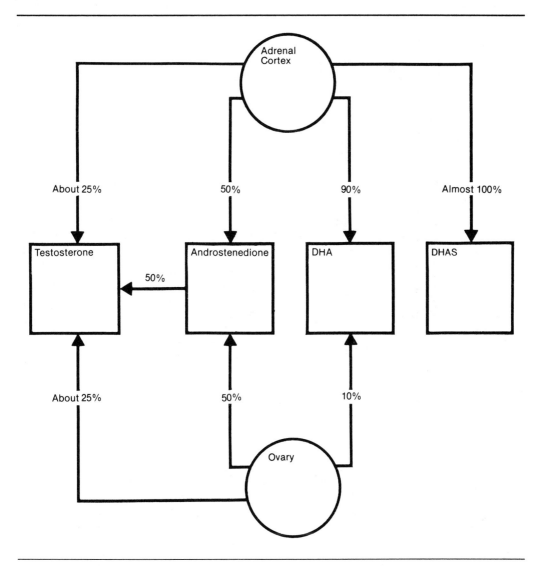

About 80% of circulating testosterone is bound to a beta-globulin known as sex steroid hormone binding globulin (SHBG). Approximately 19% is loosely bound to albumin, leaving about 1% unbound. Androgenicity is dependent mainly upon the unbound fraction and partly upon the fraction associated with albumin. DHA, DHAS, and androstenedione are not significantly protein bound, and routine radioimmunoassay reflects their biologically available hormone activity. This is not the case with testosterone, for routine assays measure the total testosterone concentration, bound and unbound.

SHBG production in the liver is decreased by androgens. Hence, the binding capacity in men is lower than in normal women, and 2-3% of testosterone circulates in the free, active form in a man. SHBG is increased by estrogens and thyroid hormone. Therefore, binding capacity is increased in women, in hyperthyroidism, in pregnancy, and by estrogen-containing medication. In a hirsute woman, the SHBG level is depressed by the excess androgen, and the percent free and active testosterone is elevated as is the metabolic clearance rate of testosterone. The total testosterone concen-

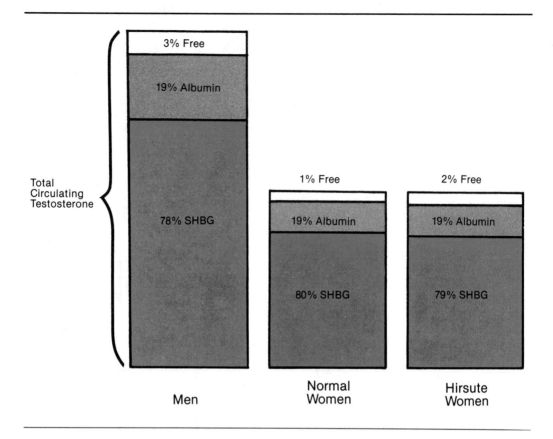

Men

Normal Women

Hirsute Women

- 3% Free
- 19% Albumin
- 78% SHBG

Total Circulating Testosterone

- 1% Free
- 19% Albumin
- 80% SHBG

- 2% Free
- 19% Albumin
- 79% SHBG

tration, therefore, may be in the normal range in a woman who is hirsute. There is no clinical need for a specific assay for the free portion of testosterone. The very presence of hirsutism or masculinization indicates increased androgen effects. One can reliably interpret a normal testosterone level in these circumstances as compatible with decreased binding capacity and increased free testosterone.

In hirsute women, only 25% of the circulating testosterone arises from peripheral conversion, and most is due to direct tissue secretion. Indeed, data overwhelmingly indicate that the ovary is the major source of increased testosterone and androstenedione in hirsute women.[1] The most common cause of hirsutism in women is anovulation and excessive androgen production by the ovaries. Adrenal causes are most uncommon.

3α-Androstanediol Glucuronide. While testosterone is the major circulating androgen, it is clear that dihydrotestosterone (DHT) is the major nuclear androgen in many sensitive tissues, including the hair follicles. 3α-Androstanediol is the peripheral tissue metabolite of DHT, and its glucuronide, 3α-androstanediol glucuronide (3α-AG), has been utilized as a marker of target tissue cellular action.[2,3] There is an excellent correlation between the serum levels of 3α-AG and the clinical manifestatons of androgens. Specifically, 3α-AG correlates with the level of 5α-reductase activity (testosterone and androstenedione to dihydrotestosterone) in the skin.

Thus there are 3 principal laboratory measurements of potential clinical use for the evaluation of androgen excess:

1. Testosterone—a measure of ovarian and tumor activity.

2. DHAS—a measure of adrenal gland activity.

3. 3α-AG—a measure of peripheral target tissue activity.

Hirsutism is not a disorder of hair, rather it reflects increased 5α-reductase activity which produces more DHT leading to the stimulation of hair growth. This enzyme activity is increased by an increased availability of precursor (therefore the circulating testosterone level is a primary factor) or by still unknown local tissue mechanisms. Measurement of 3α-AG has revealed that true idiopathic hirsutism may not exist (or at least it is very rare). In the presence of other laboratory measurements which are normal, increased levels of 3α-AG indicate an increased activity of 5α-reductase in the peripheral compartment.(4)

There are 2 reasons why the measurement of 3α-AG is not part of the routine clinical approach to the problem of hirsutism. First, it is not an absolute measurement. Values in hirsute women overlap the normal range by about 20%. Second, and most importantly, the ultimate diagnosis and therapy of the problem are not affected by this test.

Evaluation of Hirsutism

Cosmetically disfiguring hirsutism is the end result of a number of factors:

1. The number of hair follicles present (Japanese women bearing androgen-producing tumors rarely are hirsute because of the low concentration of hair follicles per unit skin area).

2. The degree to which androgen has converted resting lanugo hair to terminal adult hair.

3. The ratio of the growth to resting phases in affected hair follicles.

4. The asynchrony of growth cycles in aggregates of hair follicles.

5. The thickness and degree of pigmentation of individual hairs.

The primary factor is an increase in androgen levels (primarily testosterone) which produces an initial growth stimulus and then acts to sustain continued growth. Essentially every woman with hirsutism will be found to have an increased production rate of testosterone and androstenedione if studied with sophisticated techniques. (5)

The most sensitive marker for increased androgen production is hirsutism. This is followed in order by acne and increased oiliness of the skin, menstrual irregularity, increased libido, clitoromegaly, and finally, masculinization. Masculinization and virilization are terms reserved for extreme androgen effects (usually, but not always, associated with a tumor) leading to the development of a male hair pattern, clitoromegaly, deepening of the voice, increased muscle mass, and general male body habitus.

The most common clinical problem is the hirsute woman with irregular menses, with the onset of hirsutism during teenage years or in the early 20s, and a long, gradual worsening of the condition. About 70% of anovulatory women develop hirsutism. The picture is so characteristic that a careful history may be sufficient for the diagnosis.

A good history may reveal some of the rare causes of hirsutism: environmental factors producing chronic irritation or reactive hyperemia of the skin, the use of drugs, changes associated with Cushing's syndrome or acromegaly, or even the presence of pregnancy (indicating the possibility of a luteoma). Hair-stimulating drugs include methyltestosterone, anabolic agents such as Nilevar or Anavar, Dilantin, and danazol. The 19-nortestosterones in the current low dosage birth control pills rarely (if ever) cause acne or hirsutism. Especially important in the history is the rapidity of development. A woman who develops hirsutism after the age of 25 and demonstrates very rapid progression of masculinization over several months usually has an androgen-producing tumor.

Adrenal hyperplasia due to an enzymatic deficiency presenting in adult life is also rare. Congenital adrenal hyperplasia which may lead to hirsutism is usually diagnosed and treated prior to puberty. Hirsutism in childhood is usually caused by congenital adrenal hyperplasia or androgen-producing tumors. Genetic problems, such as Y-containing mosaics or incomplete testicular feminization, will produce signs of androgen stimulation at puberty.

Virilization during pregnancy raises the suspicion of a luteoma, not a true tumor, but an exaggerated reaction of the ovarian stroma to chorionic gonadotropin.(6) The solid luteoma is usually unilateral and associated with a normal pregnancy, in contrast to the bilateral theca-lutein cysts seen with trophoblastic disease. Virilization due to theca-lutein cysts can also be seen with the high human chorionic gonadotropin (HCG) titers associated with multiple gestation. Since a luteoma regresses postpartum, the only risk is masculinization of a female fetus. Subsequent pregnancies are normal.

Hirsutism, therefore, is usually associated with persistent anovulation. Although anovulatory ovaries are usually the source for excess androgens, a minimal workup is necessary, dedicated to ruling out the adrenal sources and tumors. It should be emphasized that hospitalization for extensive evaluation of hirsutism is required only rarely.

| **The Diagnostic Workup** | For years, the mainstay of the diagnostic workup was a 24-hour urine collection for measurement of 17-ketosteroids and 17-hydroxysteroids. With the general availability of radioimmunoassays for blood steroids, these old faithful urine measurements have been retired for screening purposes. Currently, the initial laboratory evaluation of hirsutism consists of the radioimmunoassay for the blood levels of testosterone, DHAS, and 17-hydroxyprogesterone (17-OHP). In addition, as part of the evaluation for anovulation, prolactin levels and thyroid function should be measured, and a suction endometrial biopsy should be considered. Patients with intense androgen action may be amenorrheic due to endometrial suppression and may not demonstrate withdrawal bleeding after a progestational challenge. |

Cushing's syndrome may present with hirsutism, and later masculinization. Remember that one of the most common referral diagnoses is Cushing's syndrome, but this is one of the least common final diagnoses. When clinical suspicion is high, a screen for Cushing's syndrome is indicated.

The Screen for Cushing's Syndrome

Cushing's syndrome, the persistent oversecretion of cortisol, can develop in 3 different ways: ACTH overproduction (Cushing's disease), ectopic ACTH overproduction by tumors, or autonomous cortisol-secreting adrenal, or very rarely, ovarian tumors. A clinician must first make the diagnosis of Cushing's syndrome before determining the etiology.

The most useful measurements in the basal state to detect Cushing's syndrome are the 24-hour urinary free cortisol excretion (20-90 μg) and the late evening plasma cortisol level (<15 μg/dl). The urinary excretion of 17-ketosteroids and 17-hydroxysteroids and measurement of morning and afternoon plasma cortisol levels are less reliable because of a significant overlap between normal and abnormal patients.

The single dose overnight dexamethasone test is excellent because of the very low incidence of false results. Dexamethasone (1 mg) is given orally at bedtime, and a plasma cortisol is drawn at 8:00 the next morning. A value less than 6 μg/dl rules out Cushing's syndrome. Cushing's syndrome is unlikely with intermediate values between 6 and 10 μg/dl, while a value higher than 10 μg/dl is diagnostic of adrenal hyperfunction. The number of patients with Cushing's syndrome who show a normal suppression in the single dose overnight test is negligible (less than 2%) and normal patients have a very low incidence of false positive results (less than 1%). (7) Obese patients, however, have a false positive rate up to 13%.

If the single dose overnight test is abnormal, go to the 2 mg low dose suppression test. Dexamethasone (0.5 mg every 6 hours) is administered for 2 consecutive days after 2 days of baseline urinary 17-hydroxysteroid measurements. Patients with Cushing's syndrome will not suppress their urine 17-hydroxysteroids below 4.0 mg/day. Combining the low dose test with the 24-hour urinary free cortisol and the 10 PM plasma cortisol should definitely provide the diagnosis of Cushing's syndrome.

The etiology of Cushing's syndrome can be established by combining an 8 mg high dose dexamethasone suppression test with measurement of the basal state blood ACTH level. Dexamethasone (2 mg every 6 hours) is administered for 2 days, and the urinary 17-hydroxysteroids on the 2nd day are compared with basal levels. If basal ACTH is undetectable, and the urinary steroids do not decrease by at least 40%, an adrenal tumor is likely. When ACTH is measurable in the blood, an ectopic ACTH producing tumor is unlikely if the 17-hydroxysteroids decrease by at least 40%. Cushing's disease is present when the blood ACTH level is in the normal range, a chest x-ray is normal, and CT scanning detects an abnormal sella turcica. A level of plasma ACTH greater than 500 pg/ml suggests ectopic ACTH release; a level less than 20 pg/ml suggests an autonomous cortisol-secreting tumor.

CT scanning is very accurate and reliable in detecting adrenal tumors (as small as 1.5 by 2.5 cm).(8) In addition, it reliably predicts which patients have an ectopic ACTH-producing tumor by detecting bilateral adrenal enlargement in such patients. The CT scan can differentiate between an adenoma (well rounded and circumscribed) and a carcinoma (irregular or lobulated with signs of infiltration into adjacent structures).

Finally, a very rare cause of Cushing's syndrome is the autonomous production of cortisol by an ovarian tumor. (9)

The DHAS Level

DHAS is the only blood assay which can be substituted for urinary 17-ketosteroids in the evaluation of hirsutism. A random sample is sufficient, needing no corrections for body weight, creatinine excretion, or random variation. Variations are minimized because of its high circulating concentration and its long half-life. A slow turn-over rate results in a large and stable pool in the blood with insignificant variation.

DHAS circulates in higher concentration than any other steroid, and is derived almost exclusively from the adrenal gland. It is, therefore, a direct measure of adrenal androgen activity, correlating clinically with the urinary 17-ketosteroids.(10) The upper limit of normal in most laboratories is 250 μg/dl, but may be substantially higher in some labs. As with urinary 17-ketosteroids, aging is associated with a decrease in the blood concentration of DHAS; the decrease accelerates after menopause and DHAS is almost undetectable after age 70.(11) This decline is 4 times greater than the age-related decline in cortisol, which is further support for the contention that there is an agent besides ACTH which controls DHAS secretion. Although there is rapid decline associated with the menopause, the same decline has been observed in women over 65 and on estrogen replacement. Either a lack of estrogen is not responsible for the decline, or replacement estrogen does not mimic the estrogen milieu of the reproductive years.

Both 17-ketosteroids and circulating levels of DHAS are elevated in association with hyperprolactinemia.(12,13) The mechanism is unknown, but both return to normal with prolactin suppression by bromocriptine. In addition, increased free testosterone levels associated with decreased SHBG are found in hyperprolactinemic women.

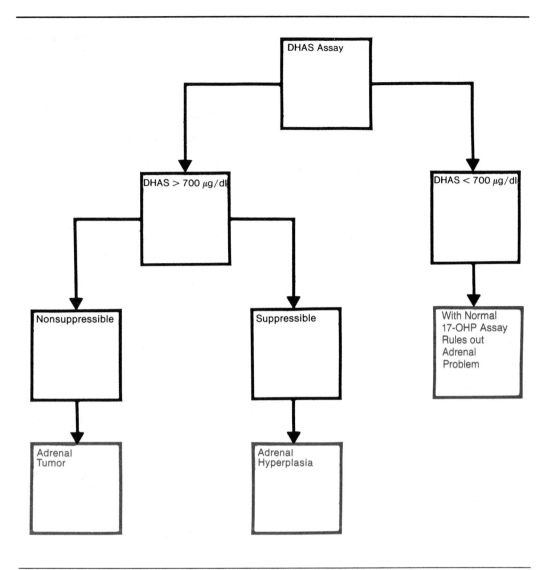

(14,15) This underscores the need to search for galactorrhea and to obtain a prolactin in all anovulatory women. The androgen changes are probably secondary to the persistent anovulatory state induced by the elevated prolactin, although direct prolactin effects on the adrenal, ovary, or SHBG are possible.

When the DHAS level is normal, adrenal disease is most unlikely, and the diagnosis of excess androgen production by the ovaries is likely. There are only rare cases of adrenal tumors with normal 17-ketosteroids and normal DHAS levels,(16) and further evaluation of such cases would be indicated by the presence of markedly elevated blood levels of testosterone. These rare tumors are responsive to luteinizing hormone (LH), suggesting that they are derived from embryonic rest cells. Late-onset adrenal hyperplasia commonly is not associated with an increased level of DHAS as discussed below. This condition relies on the measurement of 17-OHP for screening.

243

The clinical problem with DHAS measurement in the evaluation of hirsutism is the common finding of a moderately elevated DHAS level in anovulatory patients with polycystic ovaries. This is similar to the moderate elevations of 17-ketosteroids encountered in these patients. If the 17-OHP level is normal, we believe that it is not worthwhile to subject these patients to a search for an adrenal enzyme defect. Clinical experience has established that a DHAS level of 700 μg/dl or below does not require further evaluation.

When the rare patient with a DHAS over 700 μg/dl is encountered, adrenal function must be suppressed with dexamethasone to reveal the nature and extent of the adrenal androgen contribution. Adequate adrenal androgen suppression requires a minimum of 4 days, and suppression can be carried out on an outpatient basis with 2.0 mg dexamethasone q.i.d. for 5 days.(17) On the last day of suppression a repeat DHAS determination is obtained. A lack of adrenal suppression is consistent with an autonomously functioning adrenal tumor. CT scan evaluation of the adrenal gland should be obtained.

Late-Onset Adrenal Hyperplasia

Congenital adrenal hyperplasia is due to an enzyme defect leading to excessive androgen production. This severe condition, with its prenatal onset, is inherited in an autosomal recessive fashion, now referred to as the classical form of the disease (discussed in Chapter 12). In recent years, a more mild form of the disease, appearing later in life, has been designated by a variety of adjectives, including late-onset, partial, nonclassical, attenuated, and acquired adrenal hyperplasia.(18,19) An asymptomatic form, cryptic adrenal hyperplasia, is revealed only on biochemical testing.

Although each of the enzymatic steps from cholesterol to cortisol can be expressed in specific clinical disease, the most common enzymes to be deficient are 21-hydroxylase, 11β-hydroxylase, and 3β-hydroxysteroid dehydrogenase. The discovery of a linkage between 21-hydroxylase and the human leukocyte antigen (HLA) loci on the short arm of chromosome 6 has allowed an in depth study of this particular enzyme defect.

The 21-Hydroxylase Defect. The HLA complex codes for a large number of leukocyte surface antigens. It includes several closely linked loci, four of which can be defined by serologic testing: HLA-A, HLA-B, HLA-C, HLA-D/DR. Each locus has been further divided according to the specific tissue antigen produced by each of their multiple alleles (e.g. B14). One allele from each of the HLA loci constitutes a "haplotype." Each individual inherits one haplotype from the father and one from the mother. The 21-hydroxylase deficiency gene segregates with HLA-B, and thus is genetically linked with this locus.(20)

A particular HLA-coded antigen occurs more frequently in patients with 21-hydroxylase deficiency than in the general population (for classical 21-hydroxylase deficiency—HLA-Bw47;DR7, for late-onset 21-hydroxylase deficiency—HLA-B14;DR1). It is estimated that about two-thirds of HLA-B14 positive individuals are heterozygote carriers for 21-hydroxylase deficiency. Because this condition is inherited by an autosomal recessive gene, parents are obligate heterozygotes, and ACTH stimulation can reveal mild compromises in enzyme function. Women with late-onset adrenal hyperplasia respond to ACTH in a moderate fashion, between the classical homozygote response and the mild heterozygote reaction. (See 17-OHP nomogram)

The severity of the clinical presentation is explained by a concept of allelic variants.[21] It is proposed that there are 3 alleles for 21-hydroxylase deficiency:

1. 21-hydroxylase deficiency[normal].

2. 21-hydroxylase deficiency[mild].

3. 21-hydroxylase deficiency[severe].

Classical disease results when an individual is homozygous for the severe allele. All of the recent terms (late-onset, attenuated, acquired, nonclassical, including the cryptic form) refer to individuals who are either homozygous for the mild allele or carry one mild and one severe allele.

This condition is now recognized to be the most common autosomal recessive disorder, surpassing cystic fibrosis and sickle cell anemia.[22] An unusually high incidence of classical congenital adrenal hyperplasia is seen in the Yupik Eskimos of Alaska. The late-onset form is found in high frequency in Ashkenazic Jews (1 in 30), Hispanics (1 in 40), Yugoslavs (1 in 50), and Italians (1 in 300).

The clinical presentation is extremely variable, and the symptoms may appear and disappear over time. Therefore the diagnosis requires laboratory evaluation as discussed under "The 17-OHP Level." There are at least 3 reasons which make it worthwhile to seek the correct diagnosis:

1. Therapy should be accurately applied because it must be long-term.

2. Pregnant couples with this condition require genetic counseling for the prenatal diagnosis and possible treatment of the congenital form of the disease as well as HLA typing and ACTH stimulation of asymptomatic offspring.

3. Theoretically, these patients might be subject to cortisol deficiency during severe stress.

Other Enzyme Defects. The 3β-hydroxysteroid dehydrogenase deficiency exists in both the ovaries and the adrenals. This defect precludes significant androgen production; however, this enzyme activity appears to remain intact in peripheral tissues. Therefore, hirsutism seen with this deficiency is probably due to target tissue conversion of the increased levels of precursors. Unlike 21-hydroxylase deficiency, no genetic markers are currently available. The 11β-hydroxylase deficiency is quite rare, and it is usually diagnosed at a younger age (Chapter 12).

The 17-OHP Level   Somewhere from 1 to 5% of women who complain of hirsutism display a biochemical response which is consistent with the less severe form of adrenal hyperplasia.(23-25) This relative frequency of late-onset adrenal hyperplasia dictates routine 17-OHP screening of women who complain of hirsutism. On the other hand, the routine use of the ACTH stimulation test is not warranted.(23) Besides using the 17-OHP screen to make a cost effective decision regarding ACTH stimulation, one can be swayed by pertinent clinical findings.(26) A strong family history of androgen excess suggests the presence of an inherited disorder. Hirsutism due to an adrenal enzyme defect usually is more severe and begins at a young age, typically at puberty. Short stature and very high blood levels of androgens also signify a more severe problem. Finally, it's worth considering the following: with normal baseline steroid levels, even if a woman has a subtle enzyme defect, the management of the problem may not require its discovery.

17-OHP must be measured first thing in the morning to avoid later elevations due to the diurnal pattern of ACTH secretion. The baseline 17-OHP level should be less than 300 ng/dl. Levels greater than 300 ng/dl, but less than 800 ng/dl, require ACTH testing. Levels over 800 ng/dl are virtually diagnostic of the 21-hydroxylase deficiency. The DHAS level is usually normal. The hallmarks of late-onset adrenal hyperplasia are elevated levels of 17-OHP and a dramatic increase after ACTH stimulation.(24) However, the elevated levels of 17-OHP are often not impressive (e.g. overlapping with those found in women with polycystic ovaries due to anovulation), and a simple ACTH stimulation test must be utilized.

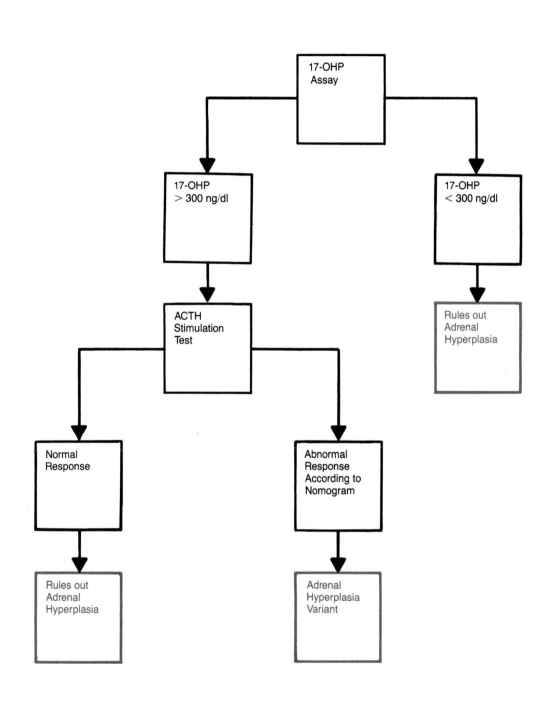

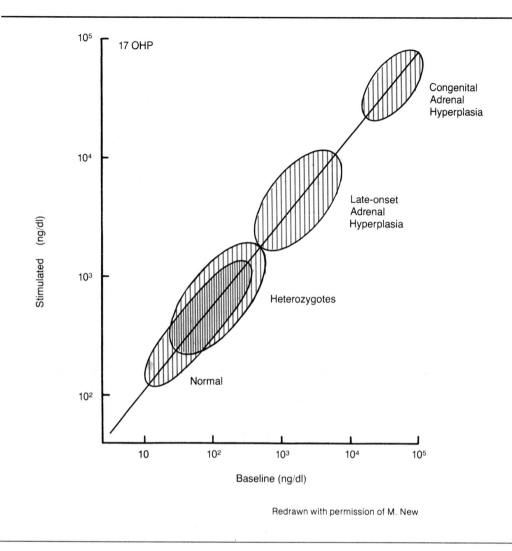

Redrawn with permission of M. New

The ACTH Stimulation Test. Synthetic ACTH (Cortrosyn) is administered intravenously in a dose of 0.25 mg. Blood samples for the measurement of 17-OHP are obtained at time 0 and again at 1 hour. The testing must be performed in the morning (8 AM), but it can be scheduled at any time during the menstrual cycle. The 1 hour value can be plotted on a nomogram which predicts the genotype of homozygote and heterozygote forms of the 21-hydroxylase deficiency.(27) Dexamethasone pretreatment the night before testing is not necessary.(28)

For the diagnosis of the 3β-hydroxysteroid dehydrogenase deficiency, the same ACTH stimulation test is utilized, measuring 17-OHP and 17-hydroxypregnenolone. An abnormal 17-OH pregnenolone/17-OHP ratio is usually greater than 6.0.(29) This deficiency is also usually marked by a significant elevation of DHAS in the face of normal or mildly elevated testosterone levels. In the 11β-hydroxylase deficiency, the level of 11-desoxycortisol will be increased (it is normal with the 21-hydroxylase defect).

248

The Adrenal Gland and Anovulation

Adrenal involvement in the syndrome of anovulation and hirsutism has long been recognized. Adrenal suppression, for example, will induce regular menses and ovulation in some patients, and empiric treatment with glucocorticoid has been advocated in the past.

Late-onset adrenal hyperplasia does not explain every anovulatory woman encountered with a moderate elevation in DHAS. The important clincal question is the following: Is excessive androgen secretion by the adrenal gland a primary disorder in these women, or is it a secondary reaction to the hormonal milieu associated with anovulation?

One possibility is that the adrenal hyperactivity (as indicated by elevated DHAS levels) is due to an estrogen-induced 3β-hydroxysteroid dehydrogenase insufficiency. Considerable effort has been devoted to demonstrating an estrogen influence on adrenal androgen secretion. Unfortunately there is no clear-cut conclusion, with both positive (30-34) and negative (35-38) results reported.

This picture is similar to that of the fetal adrenal gland. Studies have demonstrated that the low level of 3β-hydroxysteroid dehydrogenase activity and high secretion of DHA by the fetal adrenal cortex are due to estrogen.(39) Inconsistent with this explanation is the fact that ACTH levels in adult anovulatory women are not elevated.(26,40) A recent kinetics study of the 3β-hydroxysteroid dehydrogenase enzyme activity strongly suggests that this enzyme is inhibited by steroids (both androgens and estrogens) in concentrations to be expected within the adrenal gland (and difficult to achieve with exogenous administration); and changes in adrenal secretion, therefore, reflect varying action of steroids, especially estrone and estradiol, in different layers of the adrenal cortex without changes in ACTH.(41) In another study, testosterone administration was associated with circulating steroid level changes consistent with subtle inhibition of 21-hydroxylase or 11β-hydroxylase.(42) Thus it remains attractive to explain adrenal hyperactivity seen in anovulatory women as a secondary reaction induced and maintained either by the constant estrogen state associated with persistent anovulation or by the increased androgens.

The inconclusiveness of this situation and the rarity of a true adrenal enzyme deficiency in the adult make a cost-effective argument against routine endocrine testing. Accordingly, we have adopted a blood DHAS level of 700 μg/dl and a 17-OHP level of 300 ng/dl, below which we ordinarily do not pursue the possibility of a primary adrenal enzyme problem.

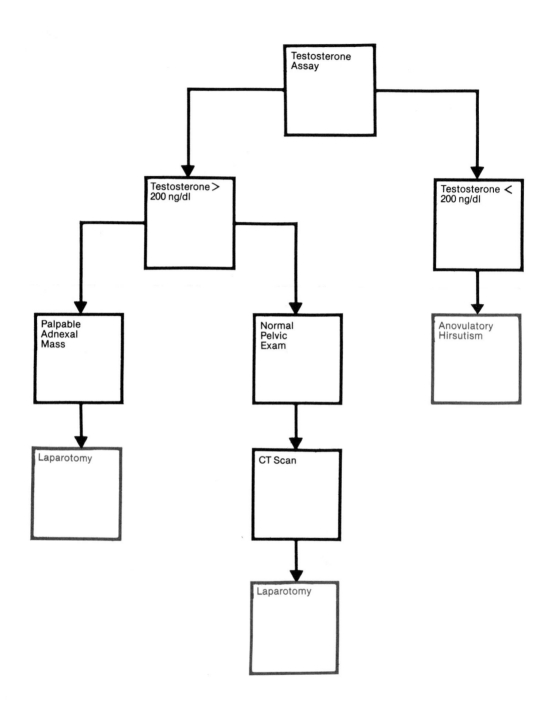

The Testosterone Level	Plasma testosterone levels (normal 20-80 ng/dl) are elevated in the majority of women (70%) with anovulation and hirsutism. Individual variation is great, however, largely due to the changes in the testosterone binding capacity of the sex hormone binding globulin in the blood. Because the binding globulin levels are depressed by androgens, the total testosterone concentration can be in the normal range in a woman who is hirsute even though the percent unbound and active testosterone is elevated. Indeed, the unbound or free testosterone is approximately twice normal (an increase from 1% to 2%) in women with anovulation and polycystic ovaries.(43) Therefore a normal testosterone level in a hirsute woman is still consistent with elevated androgen production rates.

It is not necessary to measure the free testosterone (a technically difficult and expensive assay) because a routine total testosterone assay adequately serves the purpose of screening for testosterone-secreting tumors. Such tumors are associated with testosterone levels in the male range,(44,45) and therefore the fine discrimination of the free testosterone level is unnecessary. *If the testosterone level exceeds 200 ng/dl, an androgen-producing tumor must be suspected.* This arbitrary cut off point has been challenged because variations in secretion can yield misleading values.(46) It is recommended that at least 3 daily samples must reach a level 2.5 times greater than the upper limit of normal for a given laboratory.

Androgen-Producing Tumors

There are two findings which should stimulate the clinician to suspect the presence of an androgen-producing tumor. One is a history of rapidly progressive masculinization. Hirsutism associated with anovulation is generally slow to develop, usually covering a time period of at least several years. Tumors are associated with a short time course, measured in months. Occasionally, virilization is encountered with a nonfunctional tumor due to tumor stimulation of androgen secretion in the surrounding stromal tissue. The second finding which should arouse suspicion is a testosterone level greater than 200 ng/dl.

In our view, androgen-producing tumors are one of medicine's vastly overrated problems. First, they are incredibly rare, and yet they attract an inordinate amount of attention at our meetings, and a disproportionate number of printed pages in texts and journals. Second, there is an endocrine mystique surrounding the functioning tumor. Actually it is a straightforward problem.

Functioning ovarian tumors are almost all palpable, and like any ovarian mass, rapid laparotomy and surgical removal are in order. The only diagnostic dilemma is when to explore a patient in whom a mass is not palpable. Suppression and stimulation tests, popular for many years, have been known to falsely lead to oophorectomy in the presence of a virilizing adrenocortical adenoma.(45) In addition, it is now recognized that suppression and stimulation methods do not specifically isolate ovarian or adrenal function.(47,48) Selective angiography is not without problems. It is technically difficult to achieve bilateral catheterization of the ovaries, steroid secretion is episodic (especially by the adrenal gland), and the technique is not without risk.

When an androgen-producing tumor is suspected, an adnexal mass is not palpable, and the DHAS level is normal, CT scanning of the adrenal glands and the ovaries should be obtained. CT scanning of the adrenal has proven to be a sensitive diagnostic technique for small tumors producing Cushing's syndrome (8) as well as for virilizing adrenal adenomas.(45) There is still insufficient experience to date to assess the accuracy of CT scanning in diagnosing the rare functioning ovarian tumors.

The use of CT scanning of the abdomen will lead to the incidental discovery of adrenal masses. Masses larger than 6 cm are rarely benign, and therefore, solid masses 6 cm or greater in diameter should be removed. (49) If a large mass (no matter what the diameter) is cystic, clear fluid on puncture can be assumed to indicate a benign lesion. If the mass is less than 6 cm in diameter, removal is indicated only if biochemical activity is present. When following a mass, CT scans should be performed at 2, 6, and 18 months. Any mass which is stable after 18 months can be left in place.

Selective angiography should be reserved for those patients with negative CT scans. We believe that angiography should be limited to the adrenal gland, relying upon surgical exploration and bivalving of the ovaries if adrenal angiography is negative. In postmenopausal women with hyperandrogenism, it is appropriate to be more aggressive surgically. Another method to consider when CT scanning is nondiagnostic is a scintigraphic study with radio-labeled cholesterol. The combination of CT scanning and iodomethyl-cholesterol scanning has been found to be most accurate.(50) Finally, it should be emphasized that it is perfectly acceptable to move to surgical exploration (without any further testing) if an adrenal or ovarian mass is not identified by CT scanning.

Treatment of Hirsutism

Almost all patients presenting with hirsutism represent excess androgen production in association with the steady state of persistent anovulation. Treatment is directed toward interruption of the steady state. In those patients who wish to become pregnant, ovulation can be induced as discussed in Chapter 20. In patients in whom pregnancy is not desired, the steady state can be interrupted by suppression of ovarian steroidogenesis, by utilizing the potent negative feedback action on LH of progestational agents in birth control pills.

Androgen production in hirsute women is usually an LH-dependent process.(1) Suppression of ovarian steroidogenesis depends upon adequate LH suppression. In addition to the inhibitory action of the progestational component, further benefit is achieved by an increase in SHBG levels induced by the estrogen component in birth control pills. The increase in SHBG results in a greater testosterone binding capacity with a decrease in free testosterone levels. Testosterone levels decrease by 6 months of treatment. This reduction is associated with a gratifying clinical improvement in the progression of hirsutism.

Plasma testosterone levels can be effectively decreased with any combination type birth control pill, including the new low dose pills.(51) The new multiphasic pills appear equally effective. Although monophasic combination pills increase SHBG levels to a

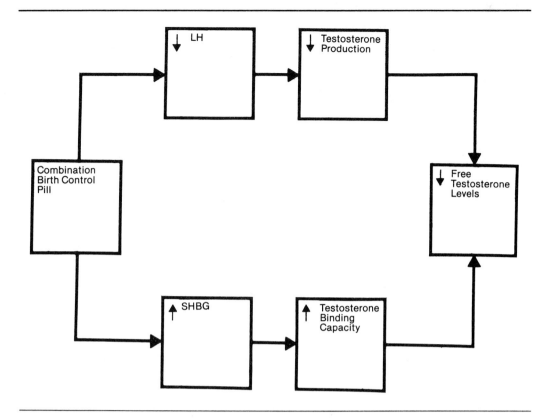

greater level, this very high SHBG concentration does not result in a further reduction in free testosterone.(52) Thus a similar decrease in total and free testosterone is achieved with all of the new low dose birth control pills, monophasics and multiphasics.

In the patient in whom oral contraceptive pills are contraindicated or unwanted, good results can be achieved with the use of depo-medroxyprogesterone acetate, 150 mg intramuscularly every 3 months, or the use of oral medroxyprogesterone acetate, 30 mg daily. The mechanism of action of medroxyprogesterone acetate is slightly different from that of the birth control pill. Suppression of gonadotropins is less intense, hence ovarian follicular activity continues. Even though LH suppression is not as great, some reduction in LH results in a decreased testosterone production rate. In addition, testosterone clearance from the circulation is increased.(53) This latter effect is due to an induction of liver enzyme activity. Medroxyprogesterone acetate also decreases SHBG (to the point where the percent free testosterone increases), but the suppression of total testosterone is so great that the actual amount of free testosterone decreases.(54) The overall effect yields a clinical result comparable to that achieved with the birth control pill.

A noteworthy feature of hirsutism is the slow response to treatment. Because of the hair growth cycle, change takes time. The patient should be cautioned that treatment with hormonal suppression will be necessary for at least 6 months before an observable diminution in hair growth occurs. Combined treatment with electrolysis is not recommended, therefore, until hormonal suppression has been used at least 6 months (except with extreme hirsutism).

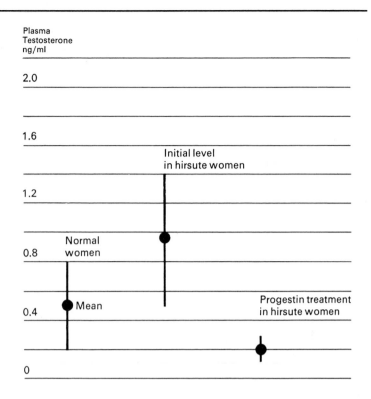

Plasma
Testosterone
ng/ml

2.0

1.6

Initial level
in hirsute women

1.2

Normal
0.8   women

Mean

0.4

Progestin treatment
in hirsute women

0

New hair follicles will no longer be stimulated to grow but hair growth which has been previously established will not disappear with hormone treatment alone. This may be affected temporarily by shaving, tweezing, waxing, or the use of depilatories. None of these tactics alters the inherent growth of the hair; therefore, they must be reapplied at frequent intervals. Permanent removal of hair can be accomplished only by electrocoagulation of dermal papillae. Some patients return after a period of treatment expressing disappointment because hair is still present. The effect of the treatment (prevention of new hair growth) may not be apparent unless the previously established hair is removed. The combination of ovarian suppression preventing new hair growth, and electrolysis removing the old hair, yields the most complete and effective treatment of hirsutism.

How long should treatment be continued? After 1-2 years it is worthwhile to stop the medication and observe the patient for a return of ovulatory cycles. Even in those patients who continue to be anovulatory, testosterone suppression may continue for 6 months to 2 years after discontinuing treatment.

The really resistant patient deserves further consideration. Combination therapy with one of the alternative approaches discussed below is worthwhile.

In most patients DHAS levels are suppressed by progestational treatment.(55-57) The mechanism is not definitely known, but there are several possible explanations. If the original stimulus for the increased DHAS secretion is the steady estrogen state of anovulation, then the change in the endocrine milieu of the adrenal gland brought about by the suppression of ovarian steroidogenesis will restore a normal adrenal secretory pattern. With the combination pill, an effect on the adrenal by the estrogen may be blocked by the progestin component. A combination birth control pill may be associated with subtle but significant alterations in ACTH stimulation or response in the adrenal gland.

The effectiveness of adrenal suppression in inducing ovulatory cycles in some anovulatory patients can be attributed to a lowering of circulating androgen levels due to a decrease in the adrenal contribution. The intraovarian androgen level is decreased, therefore lowering the inhibitory action of androgens on follicular growth and development. In terms of ovulation, the frequency of successful response with this type of treatment does not match that of the first drug of choice, clomiphene. In terms of treatment of hirsutism, progestin suppression of ovarian steroidogenesis is more effective and should remain the first therapeutic approach. Adrenal suppression should be reserved for patients with a clearly established diagnosis of an adrenal enzyme deficiency.

In an older woman who has no further desire for fertility, and in the woman in whom continued use of steroid medication is disturbing because of increasing risks with increasing age, serious consideration should be given to a surgical solution. A persistent problem of hirsutism, especially if it is progressive in severity, is a reasonable indication for hysterectomy and bilateral salpingo-oophorectomy. Patients with hyperthecosis respond poorly to suppression and are usually older. Surgical treatment for these patients is often very appropriate. Of course, these patients should accept an estrogen replacement program.

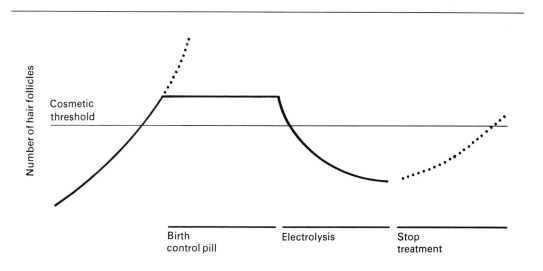

255

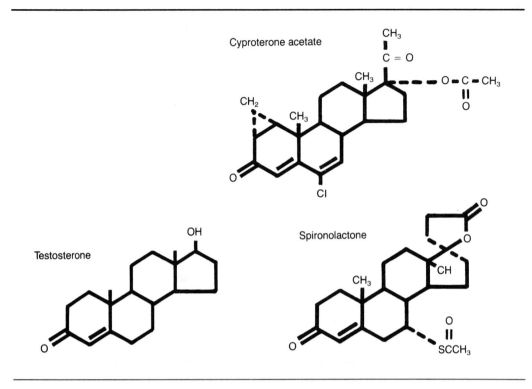

Cyproterone acetate

Testosterone

Spironolactone

Spironolactone. Spironolactone has multiple actions, inhibiting the ovarian and adrenal biosynthesis of androgens, competing for the androgen receptor in the hair follicle, and directly inhibiting 5α-reductase activity. The inhibition of steroidogenesis is achieved through an effect on the cytochrome p450 system, but the steroid suppressive effects are so variable that it is more likely that the receptor-blocking action is more important.(58) It is probably for this reason that cortisol, DHA, and DHAS levels are not significantly changed, even though androstenedione levels are decreased. (59) The impact on hirsutism is related to dosage, and a better effect is seen with a dose of 200 mg daily.(60,61) After a period of time, one can attempt lowering spironolactone to a maintenance dose of 25-50 mg daily. As with progestational agents, the response is relatively slow, and a maximal effect can be demonstrated only after 6 months of treatment. Side effects are minimal, including diuresis in the first few days of use, occasional complaints of fatigue, and dysfunctional uterine bleeding.

We use spironolactone when patients find birth control pills unacceptable or the response is disappointing. Indeed it makes sense to combine the peripheral tissue action of spironolactone with birth control pills to achieve a more dramatic result.(62) Acne has been effectively treated with the local application of a cream containing 2-5% spironolactone.(63) One word of caution: with inhibition of androgen secretion, ovulation can occur. In view of the unknown impact of spironolactone on a fetus, effective contraception is important. Theoretically, spironolactone interference with testosterone action could result in the feminization of a male fetus.

Cyproterone Acetate. Cyproterone acetate is a potent progestational agent. In many parts of the world, it is used in an oral contraceptive agent called "Diane" (2 mg cyproterone acetate and 50 μg ethinyl estradiol). A method popular in Europe for the treatment of hirsutism utilizes a so-called "reversed sequential regimen." (64) Cyproterone acetate, 100 mg daily, is given on days 5-15, with ethinyl estradiol, 50 μg daily, on days 5-26. The Canadians compared the use of Diane with high dose (100 mg) cyproterone acetate treatment in an excellent double blinded, randomized study.(65) The therapeutic effect was greater with the higher dose, and there was a similar incidence of side effects at both doses. The most common reactions included fatigue, edema, loss of libido, weight gain, and mastalgia. Significant improvement in facial hirsutism was seen by the third month of treatment. Others have noted a high relapse rate unless the 100 mg dose was maintained, as well as a relatively high rate of side effects (migraine, depression, nausea, and mastalgia).(66) The effect of this potent progestational agent on carbohydrate metabolism and the lipoprotein profile is similar to the adverse impact of the older high dose birth control pills. There is at least one study which concludes that a monophasic birth control pill combined with spironolactone 100 mg daily is as effective as cyproterone acetate.(67)

Dexamethasone. Dexamethasone suppression of endogenous ACTH secretion is used in women who have an adrenal enzyme deficiency. Dexamethasone is given nightly (to achieve maximal suppression of the CNS-adrenal axis which peaks during sleep) in a dose of 0.5 mg. An equivalent dose of prednisone is 5-7.5 mg. If this treatment suppresses the morning blood cortisol level below 2.0 μg/dl, the dose should be reduced to avoid an inability to react to stress. Fortunately, adrenal androgen secretion is more sensitive to suppression by dexamethasone than is cortisol secretion.(68) Patients with adrenal hyperplasia may require higher doses to normalize the steroid blood levels. With higher doses, alternate day therapy can still accomplish significant adrenal androgen suppression without affecting cortisol secretion.(69)

Other Agents. Cimetidine has also been used to treat hirsutism, but it is the least potent of the androgen receptor blockers.(70) The use of a skin cream containing progesterone is effective, but it must be applied frequently (because of rapid metabolic clearance) and its action is very concentrated at the point of application.(71) It is not surprising that turning off the pituitary-ovarian axis with a GnRH agonist is therapeutic.(72) The problem is to balance the response against the unwanted consequences of an hypoestrogenic state.

End Organ Hypersensitivity (Idiopathic Hirsutism)

There are some patients who present with hirsutism, but ovulate regularly. This category of patients has in the past been labeled idiopathic or familial hirsutism, and is more pronounced in certain geographic areas and among certain ethnic groups. The only satisfactory explanation for this distressing problem is hypersensitivity of the skin's hair apparatus to normal levels of androgens, probably due to increased 5α-reductase activity.(2) Because of this excessive sensitivity, normal levels of androgen stimulate hair growth. Even in these cases, hirsutism responds to ovarian suppression with a combination birth control pill. Suppression of normal female androgen levels to subnormal concentrations diminishes the stimulus to the hair follicles, yielding the same stabilizing results seen in other hirsute women. Spironolactone is also effective for this group of patients. Clinical response to pharmacologic treatment correlates with the circulating levels of 3α-AG, supporting the target tissue (hair follicle) locus of the problem.(73) While hirsutism due to an endocrine disorder requires control, end organ hypersensitivity is treated only for the purpose of cosmetic improvement. Electrolysis is a useful adjunct in this group of patients.

Limitations and Pitfalls

We have outlined a simple, straightforward approach for the evaluation of the hirsute woman, however as in all of medicine, exceptions occur.

1. Occasionally testosterone levels may be extremely elevated with anovulation, leading to very heavy hair growth and even masculinization. A level over 200 ng/dl does not absolutely indicate the presence of a tumor.

2. Enlarged ovaries are not necessary for the clinical syndrome of anovulation and excessive androgen production. On the other hand the presence of enlarged, polycystic ovaries does not assure the diagnosis of anovulation and excess ovarian production of androgen. They may be associated with adrenal disease or exogenous androgen ingestion.

3. Laparoscopy and ovarian biopsy are not indicated procedures in the evaluation of hirsutism.

4. The association of elevated testosterone production and hirsutism with normal ovulatory cycles should make the clinician suspicious of an adrenal problem.

5. Suppression of elevated androgens by progestin treatment does not rule out the presence of an ovarian tumor, since functional ovarian tumors are usually gonadotropin-dependent and responsive.

6. Failure of progestin treatment to suppress hair growth and testosterone levels after 6-12 months raises the suspicion of adrenal disease or a very small ovarian tumor.

References

1. **Chang RJ,** Ovarian steroid secretion in polycystic ovarian disease, Seminars Reprod Endocrinol 2:244, 1984.

2. **Serafini P, Lobo R,** Increased 5α-reductase activity in idiopathic hirsutism, Fertil Steril 43:74, 1985.

3. **Serafini P, Ablan F, Lobo RA,** 5α-Reductase activity in the genital skin of hirsute women, J Clin Endocrinol Metab 60:349, 1985.

4. **Greep N, Hoopes M, Horton R,** Androstanediol glucuronide plasma clearance and production rates in normal and hirsute women, J Clin Endocrinol Metab 62:22, 1986.

5. **Bardin CW, Lipsett M,** Testosterone and androstenedione blood production rates in normal women and women with idiopathic hirsutism and polycystic ovaries, J Clin Invest 46:891, 1967.

6. **Barcia-Bunuel R, Berek JS, Woodruff JD,** Luteomas of pregnancy, Obstet Gynecol 45:407, 1975.

7. **Crapo L,** Cushing's syndrome: a review of diagnostic tests, Metabolism 28:955, 1979.

8. **White FE, White MC, Drury PL, Fry IK, Besser GM,** Value of computed tomography of the abdomen and chest in investigation of Cushing's syndrome, Brit Med J 284:771, 1982.

9. **Chetkowski RJ, Judd HL, Jagger PI, Nieberg RK, Chang RJ,** Autonomous cortisol secretion by a lipoid cell tumor of the ovary, JAMA 254:2628, 1985.

10. **Lobo RA, Paul WL, Goebelsmann U,** Dehydroepiandrosterone sulfate as an indicator of adrenal androgen function, Obstet Gynecol 57:69, 1981.

11. **Cumming DC, Rebar RW, Hopper BR, Yen SSC,** Evidence for an influence of the ovary on circulating dehydroepiandrosterone sulfate levels, J Clin Endocrinol Metab 54:1069, 1982.

12. **Lobo RA, Kletsky OA, Kaptein EM, Goebelsmann U,** Prolactin modulation of dehydroepiandrosterone sulfate secretion, Am J Obstet Gynecol 138:632, 1980.

13. **Schiebinger RJ, Chrousos GP, Cutler GB Jr, Loriaux DL,** The effect of serum prolactin on plasma adrenal androgens and the production and metabolic clearance rate of dehydroepiandrosterone sulfate in normal and hyperprolactinemic subjects, J Clin Endocrinol Metab 62:202, 1986.

14. **Vermeulen A, Ando S, Verdonck L,** Prolactinomas, testosterone-binding globulin and androgen metabolism, J Clin Endocrinol Metab 54:409, 1982.

15. **Glickman SP, Rosenfield RL, Bergenstal RM, Helke J,** Multiple androgenic abnormalities, including elevated free testosterone, in hyperprolactinemic women, J Clin Endocrinol Metab 55:251, 1982.

16. **Kamilaris TC, DeBold CR, Manolas KJ, Hoursanidis A, Panageas S, Yiannatos J,** Testosterone-secreting adrenal adenoma in a peripubertal girl, JAMA 258:2558, 1987.

17. **Abraham GE,** Ovarian and adrenal contribution to peripheral androgens during the menstrual cycle, J Clin Endocrinol Metab 39:340, 1974.

18. **Brodie BL, Wentz AC,** Late onset congenital adrenal hyperplasia: a gynecologist's perspective, Fertil Steril 48:175, 1987.

19. **White PC, New MI, Dupont B,** Congenital adrenal hyperplasia, New Eng J Med 316:1519, 1580, 1987.

20. **New MI, Speiser PW,** Genetics of adrenal steroid 21-hydroxylase deficiency, Endocrin Rev 7:331, 1986.

21. **Kohn B, Levine LS, Pollack MS, Pang S, Lorenzen F, Levy DJ, Lerner AJ, Gian FR, Dupont B, New MI,** Late-onset steroid 21-hydroxylase deficiency: a variant of classical congenital adrenal hyperplasia, J Clin Endocrinol Metab 55:817, 1982.

22. **Speiser PW, Dupont B, Rubenstein P, Piazza A, Kastelan A, New MI,** High frequency of non-classical steroid 21-hydroxylase deficiency, Am J Hum Genet 37:650, 1985.

259

23. **Cobin RH, Futterweit, W, Fiedler RP, Thornton JC,** Adrenocortico-tropic hormone testing in idiopathic hirsutism and polycystic ovarian disease: A test of limited usefulness, Fertil Steril 44:224, 1985.

24. **Kuttenn F, Couillin P, Girard F, Billaud L, Vincens M, Boucekkine C, Thalabarad J-C, Maudelonde T, Spritzer P, Mowszowicz I, Boue A, Mauvais-Jarvis P,** Late-onset adrenal hyperplasia in hirsutism, New Eng J Med 313:224, 1985.

25. **Benjamin F, Deutsch S, Saperstein H, Seltzer VL,** Prevalence of and markers for the attenuated form of congenital adrenal hyperplasia and hyperprolactinemia masquarading as polycystic ovarian disease, Fertil Steril 46:215, 1986.

26. **Lobo RA,** The role of the adrenal in polycystic ovary syndrome, Seminars Reprod Endocrinol 2:251, 1984.

27. **New MI, Lorenzen F, Lerner AJ, Kohn B, Oberfield SE, Pollack MS, Dupont B, Stoner E, Levy DJ, Pang S, Levine LS,** Genotyping steroid 21-hydroxylase deficiency: hormonal reference data, J Clin Endocrinol Metab 57:320, 1983.

28. **Rosenfield RL, Helke J, Lucky AW,** Dexamethasone preparation does not alter corticoid and androgen responses to adrenocorticotropin, J Clin Endocrinol Metab 60:585, 1985.

29. **Pang S, Lerner AJ, Stoner E, Levine LS, Oberfield SE, Engel I, New MI,** Late-onset adrenal steroid 3β-hydroxysteroid dehydrogenase deficiency. I. A cause of hirsutism in pubertal and postpubertal women, J Clin Endocrinol Metab 60:428, 1985.

30. **Sobrino L, Kase N, Grunt J,** Changes in adrenocortical function in patients with gonadal dysgenesis after treatment with estrogen, J Clin Endocrinol Metab 33:110, 1971.

31. **Abraham G, Maroulis G,** Effect of exogenous estrogen on serum pregnenolone, cortisol and androgens in postmenopausal women, Obstet Gynecol 45:271, 1975.

32. **Lucky AW, Marynick SP, Rebar RW, Cutler GB, Glen M, Johnson-baugh E, Loriaux DL,** Replacement oral ethinyloestradiol therapy for gonadal dysgenesis: growth and adrenal androgen studies, Acta Endocrinol 91:519, 1979.

33. **Lobo RA, March CM, Goebelsmann U, Mishell DR Jr,** The modulating role of obesity and of 17β-estradiol (E_2) on bound and unbound E_2 and adrenal androgens in oophorectomized women, J Clin Endocrinol Metab 54:320, 1982.

34. **Lobo RA, Goebelsmann U, Brenner PF, Mishell DR Jr,** The effects of estrogen on adrenal androgens in oophorectomized women, Am J Obstet Gynecol 142:471, 1982.

35. **Rosenfield RL, Fang IS,** The effects of prolonged physiologic estradiol therapy on the maturation of hypogonadal teenagers, J Pediatr 85:830, 1974.

36. **Anderson D, Yen SSC,** Effects of estrogens on adrenal 3β-hydroxysteroid dehydrogenase in ovariectomized women, J Clin Endocrinol Metab 43:561, 1976.

37. **Rose DP, Fern M, Liskowski L, Milbrath JR,** Effect of treatment with estrogen conjugates on endogenous plasma steroids, Obstet Gynecol 49:80, 1977.

38. **Steingold K, De Ziegler D, Cedars M, Meldrum DR, Lu JKH, Judd HL, Chang RJ,** Clinical and hormonal effects of chronic gonadotropin-releasing hormone agonist treatment in polycystic ovarian disease, J Clin Endocrinol Metab 65:773, 1987.

39. **Fujieda K, Faiman C, Reyes FI, Winter JSD,** The control of steroidogenesis by human fetal adrenal cells in tissue culture: IV. The effects of exposure to placental steroids, J Clin Endocrinol Metab 54:89, 1982.

40. **Chang RJ, Mandel FP, Wolfren AR, Judd HL,** Circulating levels of plasma adrenocorticotropin in polycystic ovary disease, J Clin Endocrinol Metab 54:1265, 1982.

41. **Byrne GC, Perry YS, Winter JSD,** Steroid inhibitory effects upon human adrenal 3β-hydroxysteroid dehydrogenase activity, J Clin Endocrinol Metab 62:413, 1986.

42. **Vermesh M, Silva PD, Rosen GF, Vijod AG, Lobo RA,** Effect of androgen on adrenal steroidogenesis in normal women, J Clin Endocrinol Metab 66:128, 1988.

43. **Easterling WE Jr, Talbert LM, Potter HD,** Serum testosterone levels in the polycystic ovary syndrome, Am J Obstet Gynecol 120:385, 1974.

44. **Meldrum DR, Abraham GE,** Peripheral and ovarian venous concentrations of various steroid hormones in virilizing ovarian tumors, Obstet Gynecol 53:36, 1979.

45. **Gabrilove JL, Seman AT, Sabet R, Mitty HA, Nicolis GL,** Virilizing adrenal adenoma with studies on the steroid content of the adrenal venous effluent and a review of the literature, Endocrin Rev 2:462, 1981.

46. **Friedman CI, Schmidt GE, Kim MH, Powell J,** Serum testosterone concentrations in the evaluation of androgen-producing tumors, Am J Obstet Gynecol 153:44, 1985.

47. **Moltz L, Schwartz U,** Gonadal and adrenal androgen secretion in hirsute females, Clinics Endocrinol Metab 15:229, 1986.

48. **Brumsted JR, Chapitis J, Riddick D, Gibson M,** Norethindrone inhibition of testosterone secretion by an ovarian Sertoli-Leydig cell tumor, J Clin Endocrinol Metab 65:194, 1987.

49. **Copeland PM,** The incidentally discovered adrenal mass, Ann Surg 199:116, 1984.

50. **Taylor L, Ayers JWT, Gross MD, Peterson EP, Menon KMJ,** Diagnostic considerations in virilization: iodomethyl-norcholesterol scanning in the localization of androgen secreting tumors, Fertil Steril 46:1005, 1986.

51. **Raj SG, Raj MH, Talbert LM, Sloan CS, Hicks B,** Normalization of testosterone levels using a low estrogen-containing oral contraceptive in women with polycystic ovary syndrome, Obstet Gynecol 60:15, 1982.

52. **Jung-Hoffman C, Kuhl H,** Divergent effects of two low-dose oral contraceptives on sex hormone-binding globulin and free testosterone, Am J Obstet Gynecol 156:199, 1987.

53. **Gordon GG, Southren AL, Tochimoto S, Olivo J, Altman K, Rand J, Lemberger L,** Effect of medroxyprogesterone acetate (Provera) on the metabolism and biological activity of testosterone, J Clin Endocrinol Metab 30:449, 1970.

54. **Wortsman J, Khan MS, Rosner W,** Suppression of testosterone-estradiol binding globulin by medroxyprogesterone acetate in polycystic ovary syndrome, Obstet Gynecol 67:705, 1986.

55. **Madden JD, Milewich L, Parker CR Jr, Carr BR, Boyar RM, MacDonald PC,** The effect of an oral contraceptive treatment on the serum concentration of dehydroisoandrosterone sulfate, Am J Obstet Gynecol 132:380, 1978.

56. **Carr BR, Parker CR Jr, Madden JD, MacDonald PC, Porter JC,** Plasma levels of adrenocorticotropin and cortisol in women receiving oral contraceptive steroid treatment, J Clin Endocrinol Metab 49:346, 1979.

57. **Wild RA, Umstot ES, Andersen RN, Givens JR,** Adrenal function in hirsutism: II. Effect of an oral contraceptive, J Clin Endocrinol Metab 54:676, 1982.

58. **Young RL, Goldzieher JW, Elkind-Hirsch K,** The endocrine effects of spironolactone used as an antiandrogen, Fertil Steril 48:223, 1987.

59. **Serafini P, Lobo RA,** The effects of spironolactone on adrenal steroidogenesis in hirsute women, Fertil Steril 44:595, 1985.

60. **Lobo RA, Shoupe D, Serafini P, Brinton D, Horton R,** The effects of two doses of spironolactone on serum androgens and anagen hair in hirsute women, Fertil Steril 43:200, 1985.

61. **Evans DJ, Burke CW,** Spironolactone in the treatment of idiopathic hirsutism and the polycystic ovary syndrome, J Roy Soc Med 79:453, 1986.

62. **Pittaway DE, Maxson WS, Wentz AC,** Spironolactone in combination drug therapy for unresponsive hirsutism, Fertil Steril 43:878, 1985.

63. **Messina M, Manieri C, Rizzi G, Gentile L, Milani P,** Treating acne with antiandrogens: the confirmation of the validity of a percutaneous treatment with spironolactone, Curr Ther Res 38:269, 1985.

64. **Miller JA, Jacobs HS,** Treatment of hirsutism and acne with cyproterone acetate, Clinics Endocrinol Metab 15:373, 1986.

65. **Belisle S, Love EJ,** Clinical efficacy and safety of cyproterone acetate in severe hirsutism: results in a multicentered Canadian study, Fertil Steril 46:1015, 1986.

66. **Holdaway IM, Croxson MS, Ibbertson HK, Sheehan A, Knox B, France J,** Cyproterone acetate as initial treatment and maintenance therapy for hirsutism, Acta Endocrinol 109:522, 1985

67. **Chapman MG, Dowsett M, Dewhurst CJ, Jeffcoate SL,** Spironolactone in combination with an oral contraceptive: an alternative treatment for hirsutism, Brit J Obstet Gynaecol 92:983, 1985.

68. **Rittmaster RS, Loriaux DL, Cutler GB Jr,** Sensitivity of cortisol and adrenal androgens to dexamethasone suppression in hirsute women, J Clin Endocrinol Metab 61:462, 1985.

69. **Avgerinos PC, Cutler GB Jr, Tsokos GC, Gold PW, Feuillan P, Gallucci WT, Pillemer SR, Loriaux DL, Chraousos GP,** Dissociation between cortisol and adrenal androgen secretion in patients receiving alternate day prednisone therapy, J Clin Endocrinol Metab 65:24, 1987.

70. **Eil C, Edelson SK,** The use of human skin fibroblasts to obtain potency estimates of drug binding to androgen receptors, J Clin Endocrinol Metab 59:51, 1984.

71. **Rowe TC, Mezei M, Hilchie J,** Treatment of hirsutism with liposomal progesterone, Prostate 5:346, 1984.

72. **Andreyko JL, Monroe SL, Jaffe RB,** Treatment of hirsutism with a gonadotropin-releasing hormone agonist (Nafarelin), J Clin Endocrinol Metab 63:854, 1986.

73. **Kirschner MA, Samojlik E, Szmal E,** Clinical usefulness of plasma androstanediol glucuronide measurements in women with idiopathic hirsutism, J Clin Endocrinol Metab 65:597, 1987.

8   Dysfunctional Uterine Bleeding

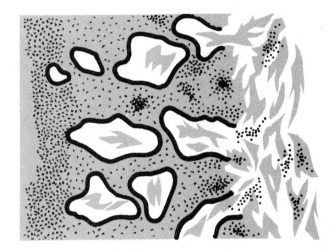

The thesis advanced in this chapter is that dysfunctional uterine bleeding, defined as a variety of bleeding manifestations of anovulatory cycles, can be confidently managed, without surgical intervention, by therapeutic regimens founded on sound physiologic principles. This formulation is based on knowledge of how the postovulatory menstrual function is naturally controlled, and utilizes pharmacologic application of sex steroids to reverse the abnormal tissue factors which lead to the excessive and prolonged flow typical of anovulatory cycles.

Three major categories of dysfunctional endometrial bleeding are dealt with:

1. Estrogen breakthrough bleeding,

2. Estrogen withdrawal bleeding, and

3. Progestin breakthrough bleeding.

In each instance, the manner in which the endometrium deviates from the norm is depicted and specific steroid therapy is recommended to counter the difficulties each situation presents.

This mode of clinical management has been in regular use for many years, and failure to control vaginal bleeding with this therapy, despite appropriate application and utilization, excludes the diagnosis of dysfunctional uterine bleeding. If this occurs, attention is directed to a pathologic entity within the reproductive tract as the cause of abnormal bleeding.

265

In the following pages we will substantiate our thesis in a more detailed fashion. First, a review of the endometrial changes associated with an ovulatory cycle will be offered. Second, endometrial-sex steroid interactions will be listed. Finally, typical clinical situations will be presented, and specific acute and long-term management programs will be described.

Histologic Changes in Endometrium during an Ovulatory Cycle

The sequence of endometrial changes associated with an ovulatory cycle has been carefully studied by Noyes in the human and Bartlemez and Markee in the subhuman primate.(1-3) From these data a theory of menstrual physiology has developed based upon specific anatomic and functional changes within glandular, vascular, and stromal components of the endometrium. These changes will be discussed in five phases: 1) menstrual endometrium, 2) the proliferative phase, 3) the secretory phase, 4) preparation for implantation, and finally 5) the phase of endometrial breakdown. While these distinctions are not entirely arbitrary, it must be recalled that the entire process is an integrated evolutionary cycle of endometrial growth and regression, which is repeated some 300-400 times during the adult life of the human female.

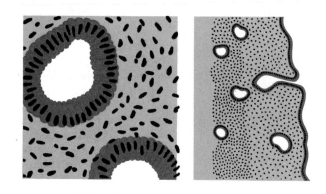

Menstrual Endometrium

The menstrual endometrium is a relatively thin but dense tissue. It is composed of the stable, nonfunctioning basalis component and a variable amount of residual stratum spongiosum. At menstruation, this latter tissue displays a variety of functional states including disarray and breakage of glands, fragmentation of vessels and stroma with persisting evidence of necrosis, white cell infiltration, and red cell interstitial diapedesis. Even as the remnants of menstrual shedding dominate the overall appearance of this tissue, evidence of repair in all tissue components can be detected. The menstrual endometrium is a transitional state bridging the more dramatic exfoliative and proliferative phases of the cycle. Its density implies that the shortness of height is not entirely due to desquamation. Collapse of the supporting matrix also contributes significantly to the shallowness. Reticular stains in rhesus endometrium confirm this "deflated" state. Nevertheless, as much as two-thirds of the functioning endometrium may be lost during menstruation. The more rapid the tissue loss, the shorter the duration of flow. Delayed or incomplete shedding is associated with heavier flow and greater blood loss.

Proliferative Phase

The proliferative phase is associated with ovarian follicle growth and increased estrogen secretion. Undoubtedly as a result of this steroidal action, reconstruction and growth of the endometrium are achieved. The glands are most notable in this response. At first they are narrow and tubular, lined by low columnar epithelium cells. Mitoses become prominent and pseudostratification is observed. As a result, the glandular epithelium extends peripherally and links one gland segment with its immediate neighbor. A continuous epithelial lining is formed facing the endometrial cavity. The stromal component evolves from its dense cellular menstrual condition through a brief period of edema to a final loose syncytial-like status. Coursing through the stroma, spiral vessels extend unbranched to a point immediately below the epithelial binding membrane. Here they form a loose capillary network.

During proliferation, the endometrium has grown from approximately 0.5 mm to 3.5-5.0 mm in height. Restoration of tissue constituents has been achieved by estrogen-induced new growth as well as incorporation of ions, water, and amino acids. The stromal ground substance has reexpanded from its menstrual collapse. While true tissue growth has occurred, a major element in achievement of endometrial height is "reinflation" of the stroma.

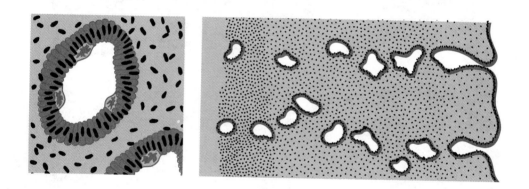

Secretory Phase

The endometrium now demonstrates a combined reaction to estrogen and progesterone activity. More impressive is that total endometrial height is fixed at roughly its preovulatory extent despite continued availability of estrogen. This restraint or inhibition is believed to be induced by progesterone. Individual components of the tissue continue to display growth, but confinement in a fixed structure leads to progressive tortuosity of glands and intensified coiling of the spiral vessels. The secretory events within the glandular cells, with progression of vacuoles from intracellular to intraluminal appearance, are well-known and take place approximately over a 7 day postovulatory interval. At the conclusion of these events the glands appear exhausted, the tortuous lumina variably distended, and individual cell surfaces fragmented and lost (sawtooth appearance). Stroma is increasingly edematous and spiral vessels are prominent and densely coiled.

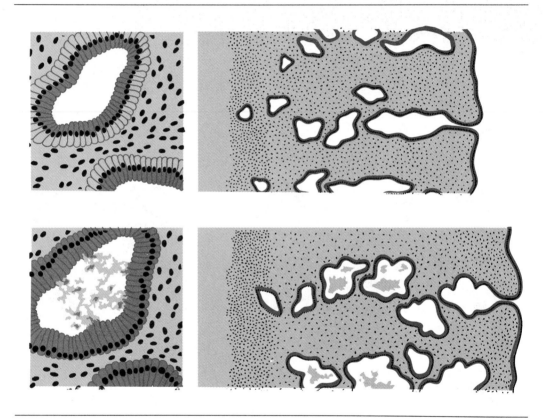

Implantation Phase

Significant changes occur within the endometrium from the 8th to the 13th day postovulation. At the onset of this period, the distended tortuous secretory glands have been most prominent with little intervening stroma. By 13 days postovulation, the endometrium has differentiated into three distinct zones. Something less than one-fourth of the tissue is the unchanged basalis fed by its straight vessels and surrounded by indifferent spindle-shaped stroma. The midportion of the endometrium (approximately 50% of the total) is the lace-like stratum spongiosum, composed of loose edematous stroma with tightly coiled but ubiquitous spiral vessels and exhausted dilated glandular ribbons. Overlying the spongiosum is the superficial layer of the endometrium (about 25% of the height) called the stratum compactum. Here the prominent histologic feature is the stromal cell which has become large and polyhedral. In its cytoplasmic expansion one cell abuts the other forming a compact, structurally sturdy layer. The necks of the glands traversing this segment are compressed and less prominent. The subepithelial capillaries and spiral vessels are engorged.

Phase of Endometrial Breakdown

In the absence of fertilization, implantation, and the consequent lack of sustaining quantities of human chorionic gonadotropin from the trophoblast, the otherwise fixed life-span of the corpus luteum is completed and estrogen and progesterone levels wane. The withdrawal of estrogen and progesterone initiates three endometrial events: vasomotor reactions, tissue loss, and menstruation. The most prominent immediate effect of this hormone withdrawal is a modest shrinking of the tissue height and remarkable spiral arteriole vasomotor responses. The following vascular sequence has been constructed from direct observations of rhesus endometrium. With shrinkage of height, blood flow within the spiral vessels diminishes, venous drainage is decreased, and vasodilatation ensues. Thereafter, the spiral arterioles undergo rhythmic vasoconstriction and relaxation. Each successive spasm is more prolonged and profound, leading eventually to endometrial blanching. Within the 24 hours immediately preceding menstruation, these reactions lead to endometrial ischemia and stasis. White cells migrate through capillary walls, at first remaining adjacent to vessels, but then extending throughout the stroma. During arteriolar vasomotor changes, red blood cells escape into the interstitial space. Thrombin-platelet plugs also appear in superficial vessels.

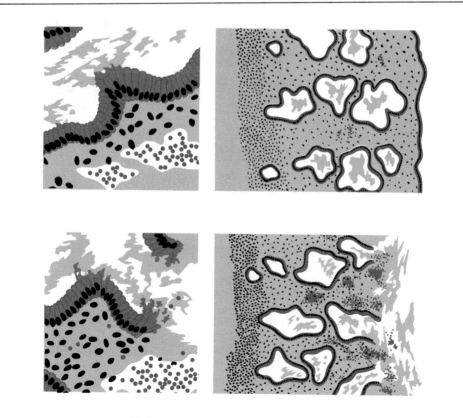

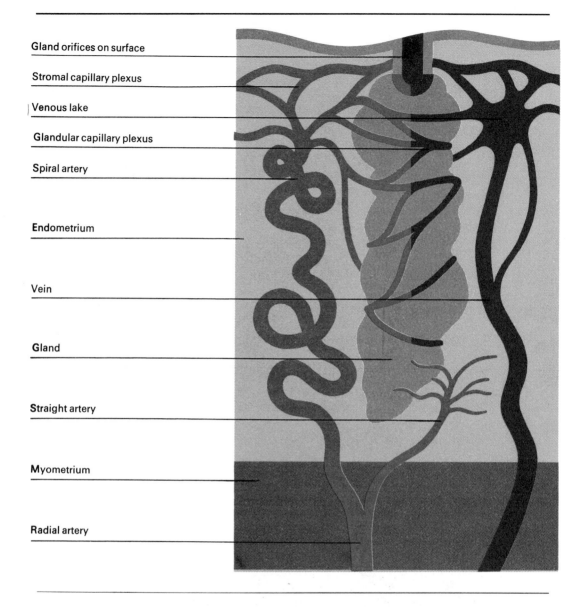

Gland orifices on surface

Stromal capillary plexus

Venous lake

Glandular capillary plexus

Spiral artery

Endometrium

Vein

Gland

Straight artery

Myometrium

Radial artery

Eventually considerable leakage occurs as a result of diapedesis, and finally, interstitial hemorrhage occurs due to breaks in superficial arterioles and capillaries. As ischemia and weakening progress, the continuous binding membrane is fragmented and intercellular blood is extruded into the endometrial cavity. New thrombin-platelet plugs form upstream at the shedding surface, limiting blood loss. With further tissue disorganization, the endometrium shrinks further and coiled arterioles are buckled. Additional ischemic breakdown ensues with necrosis of cells and defects in vessels adding to the menstrual effluvium. A natural cleavage point exists between basalis and spongiosum and, once breached, the loose, vascular, edematous stroma of the spongiosum desquamates and collapses. In the end, the typical deflated shallow dense menstrual endometrium results. Menstrual flow stops as a result of the combined effects of prolonged vasoconstriction, tissue collapse, vascular stasis and estrogen-induced ''healing.'' Resumption of estrogen secretion with its healing effects leads to clot formation over the decapitated stumps of endometrial vessels. Within 13 hours, the endometrial height shrinks from 4 mm to 1.25 mm.(4)

Most of the endometrium remains during menses, and repair takes place from the spongiosa. The remaining endometrium is protected from the lytic enzymes in the menstrual fluid by a mucinous layer of carbohydrate products which are discharged from the glandular and stromal cells.(5)

Teleologic Theory Endometrial- Menstrual Events

An unabashedly teleologic view of the events just described has been offered by Rock et al.(6) The basic premise of this thesis is that every endometrial cycle has, as its only goal, support of an early embryo. Failure to accomplish this objective is followed by orderly elimination of unutilized tissue and prompt renewal to achieve a more successful cycle.

The ovum must be fertilized within 12-24 hours of ovulation. Over the next 2 days, it remains unattached within the tubal lumen utilizing tubal fluids and residual cumulus cells to sustain nutrition and energy for early cellular cleavage. After this stay, the solid ball of cells (morula) which is the embryo leaves the tube and enters the uterine cavity. Here the embryo undergoes another 2-3 days of unattached, but active existence. Fortunately, by this time endometrial gland secretions have filled the cavity and they bathe the embryo in nutrients. This is the first of many neatly synchronized events that mark the egg-endometrial relationship. By 6 days after ovulation the embryo (now a blastocyst) is ready to attach and implant. At this time it finds an endometrial lining of sufficient depth, vascularity, and nutritional richness to sustain the important events of early placentation to follow. Just below the epithelial lining, a rich capillary plexus has been formed and is available for creation of the trophoblast-maternal blood interface. Later, the surrounding zona compactum, occupying more and more of the endometrium, will provide a sturdy splint to retain endometrial architecture despite the invasive inroads of the burgeoning trophoblast.

Failure of the appearance of human chorionic gonadotropin, despite otherwise appropriate tissue reactions, leads to the vasomotor changes associated with estrogen-progesterone withdrawal and menstrual desquamation. However, not all the tissue is lost, and, in any event, a residual basalis is always available, making resumption of growth with estrogen a relatively rapid process. Indeed, even as menses persists, early regeneration can be seen. As soon as follicle maturation occurs (in as short a time as 10 days), the endometrium is ready to perform its reproductive function.

Endometrial Responses to Steroid Hormones: Physiologic and Pharmacologic

Obviously estrogen and progesterone withdrawal is not the only type of endometrial bleeding provoked by the presence of sex steroids and their effects on the endometrium. There are clinical examples for estrogen withdrawal bleeding and estrogen breakthrough bleeding, as well as for progesterone withdrawal and breakthrough bleeding. These events can be summarized.

Estrogen Withdrawal Bleeding

This category of uterine bleeding can occur after bilateral oophorectomy, radiation of mature follicles, or administration of estrogen to a castrate and then discontinuation of therapy. Similarly, the bleeding that occurs postcastration can be delayed by concomitant estrogen therapy. Flow will occur on discontinuation of exogenous estrogen.

Estrogen Breakthrough Bleeding

Here a semiquantitative relationship exists between the amount of estrogen stimulating the endometrium and the type of bleeding that can ensue. Relatively low doses of estrogen yield intermittent spotting which may be prolonged, but is generally light in quantity of flow. On the other hand, high levels of estrogen and sustained availability lead to prolonged periods of amenorrhea followed by acute, often profuse bleeds with excessive loss of blood.

Progesterone Withdrawal Bleeding

Removal of the corpus luteum will lead to endometrial desquamation. Pharmacologically, a similar event can be achieved by administration and discontinuation of progesterone or a nonestrogenic progestin derivative. Progesterone withdrawal bleeding occurs only if the endometrium is initially proliferated by endogenous or exogenous estrogen. If estrogen therapy is continued as progesterone is withdrawn, the progesterone withdrawal bleeding still occurs. Only if estrogen levels are increased 10-20-fold will progesterone withdrawal bleeding be delayed.

Progestin Breakthrough Bleeding

Progestin breakthrough bleeding occurs only in the presence of an unfavorably high ratio of progesterone to estrogen. In the absence of sufficient estrogen, continuous progestin therapy will yield intermittent bleeding of variable duration, similar to low dose estrogen breakthrough bleeding noted above.

Of all the types of hormonal-endometrial relationships, the most stable endometrium and the most reproducible menstrual function in terms of quantity and duration occurs with postovulatory estrogen-progesterone withdrawal bleeding. It is so controlling that many women over the years come to expect a certain characteristic flow pattern. Any slight deviations, such as plus or minus 1 day in duration or minor deviation from expected napkin or tampon utilization, are causes for major concern in the patient. So ingrained is the expected flow that considerable physician reassurance may be required in some instances of minor variability. The usual duration of flow is 4-6 days, but many women flow as little as 2 days, and as much as 8 days. While the postovulatory phase averages 14 days, greater variability in the proliferative phase produces a distribution in the duration of a menstrual cycle. The normal volume of menstrual blood loss is 30 ml.(7) Greater than 80 ml is abnormal. Most of the blood loss occurs during the first 3 days of a period, so that excessive flow may exist without prolongation of flow.(8,9).

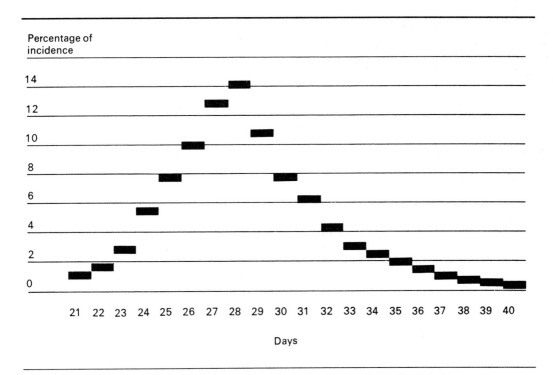

There are three reasons for the self-limited character of estrogen-progesterone withdrawal bleeding.

1. It is a universal endometrial event. Because the onset and conclusion of menses are related to a precise sequence of hormonal events, menstrual changes occur almost simultaneously in all segments of the endometrium.

2. The endometrial tissue which has responded to an appropriate sequence of estrogen and progesterone is structurally stable, and random breakdown of tissue due to fragility is avoided. Furthermore, the events leading to ischemic disintegration of the endometrium are orderly and progressive, being related to rhythmic waves of vasoconstriction of increasing duration.

3. Inherent in the events that start menstrual function following estrogen-progesterone are the factors involved in stopping menstrual flow. Just as waves of vasoconstriction initiate the ischemic events provoking menses, so will prolonged vasoconstriction abetted by the stasis associated with endometrial collapse enable clotting factors to seal off the exposed bleeding sites. Additional and significant effects are obtained by resumed estrogen activity.

Platelets and fibrin play a direct part in the hemostasis achieved in a bleeding menstrual endometrium. Deficiencies in these constituents cause the increased blood loss seen in von Willebrand's disease and in thrombocytopenia. The blood loss at menses in afibrinogenemia indicates the importance of fibrin generating and fibrinolytic factors in the menstrual process. Intravascular thrombi are observed in the functional layers and are localized to the shedding surface of the tissue. These are known as impeding "plugs" in that blood may flow past these only partially occlusive barriers. Therefore, thrombi continue to develop within the menstrual blood

273

accounting for the platelets and large amounts of fibrin found in this effluent. Fibrinolysis occurs in the endometrial tissue, limiting fibrin deposition in the proximal, still unshed layer. Despite large holes in vessel walls, with blood exposed to collagen surfaces, no occlusive surface binding thrombus is formed. After early dependence on thrombin plugs to restrain blood loss, later generalized vasoconstrictive hemostasis without thrombin plugs occur. The healing endometrium is pale, collapsed, and disorderly, but no thrombi and no fibrin deposits are seen.

The mechanisms of tissue breakdown, as well as clearance of debris and restructuring of the endometrium, are thought to proceed via sex steroid effects on the endometrial cell lysosomes.(10) With reduced steroids, lysosomal membrane destabilization and leakage of lysosomal prostaglandin synthetase enzymes, proteases, and collagenases occur. These cause breakdown of endometrial structures, dissolution of ground substance and cell walls, and vasoconstriction. Further "liquefaction" permits efficient absorption and possible recycling of protein components.

Hyperplasia vs. Neoplasia

The classical teaching that hyperplasia is the background from which endometrial neoplasia develops is being challenged. Ferenczy argues that there are two separate and biologically unrelated diseases: hyperplasia and neoplasia.(11) He suggests that all hyperplasia without atypia be referred to as *endometrial hyperplasia*, and this is not a precursor of carcinoma. He further proposes that lesions with cytologic atypia be referred to as *endometrial intraepithelial neoplasia (EIN)*. In these cases, persistence after multiple curettings or high-dose progestin therapy is approximately 75%. EIN would replace the following terms: atypical adenomatous hyperplasia and carcinoma in situ of the endometrium. This lesion is characterized by nuclear atypia of the cells lining the endometrial glands (enlargement, rounding, and pleomorphism of the nuclei with aneuploid DNA content). Invasive carcinoma is distinguished from EIN by stromal invasion.

EIN is best treated surgically! If future pregnancy is desired, daily progestin therapy (30 mg medroxyprogesterone acetate daily) should be followed by repeat endometrial aspiration curettage in 3-4 months. If EIN is still present, the choice is between surgery and high dose progestin (200 mg medroxyprogesterone acetate daily or 500 mg megestrol acetate biweekly, or depot medroxyprogesterone acetate 1000 mg weekly) with repeat biopsy surveillance.

Thus the benign lesions include all of the following traditional interpretations: anovulatory, proliferative, cystic glandular hyperplasia, simple hyperplasia, adenomatous hyperplasia without atypia. These lesions are basically the same (perhaps exaggerations at most) as preovulatory, proliferative endometrium. This hyperplasia regresses spontaneously, after curettage, or with hormonal treatment.(12) **This argument is an important one: benign lesions do not progress to cancer. Only the presence of cytonuclear atypia should raise concern for progression to cancer.**

274

Suggestions as to Why Anovulatory Bleeding is Excessive

Most instances of anovulatory bleeding are examples of estrogen withdrawal or estrogen breakthrough bleeding. Furthermore, the heaviest bleeding is secondary to high sustained levels of estrogen associated with the polycystic ovary syndrome, obesity, immaturity of the hypothalamic-pituitary-ovarian axis as in postpubertal teenagers, and late anovulation, usually involving women in their late 30s and early 40s. In the absence of growth limiting progesterone and periodic desquamation, the endometrium attains an abnormal height without concomitant structural support. The tissue increasingly displays intense vascularity, back to back glandularity, but without an intervening stromal support matrix. This tissue is fragile, and will suffer spontaneous superficial breakage and bleeding. As one site heals, another, and yet another new site of breakdown will appear. The typical clinical picture is that of a pale frightened teenager who has bled for weeks. Also frequently encountered is the older woman with prolonged bleeding who is deeply concerned over this experience as a manifestation of cancer.

In these instances the usual endometrial control mechanisms are missing. This bleeding is not a universal event, but rather it involves random portions of the endometrium at variable times and in asynchronous sequences. The fragility of the vascular adenomatous hyperplastic tissue is responsible for this experience, in part because of excessive growth, but mostly because of irregular stimulation in which the structural rigidity of a well-developed stroma or stratum compactum does not occur. Finally, the flow is prolonged and excessive not only because there is a large quantity of tissue available for bleeding, but more importantly because there is a disorderly, abrupt, random, accidental breakdown of tissue with consequent opening of multiple vascular channels. There is no vasoconstrictive rhythmicity, no tight coiling of spiral vessels, no orderly collapse to induce stasis. The anovulatory tissue can only rely on the "healing" effects of endogenous estrogen to stop local bleeds. However, this is a vicious cycle in that this healing is only temporary. As quickly as it rebuilds, tissue fragility and breakdown recur at other endometrial sites.

Alternate Hypothesis

Another explanation for the control of postovulatory endometrial bleeding and regeneration has been presented. (13) Based on light and scanning electron microscopy of hysterectomy specimens, this thesis favors nonhormone-related regeneration of surface epithelium from basal glands and cornual area residual tissue with restoration of the continuous binding membrane as the critical events in cessation of blood flow. By this account, estrogen withdrawal or breakthrough bleeding is uncontrolled because there is insufficient stimulus (loss of tissue) for binding surface restoration to occur. Furthermore, curettage is effective in this condition by reachieving sufficient basal glandular denudation (as is seen also in combined estrogen and progestin withdrawal) which stimulates regeneration of surface integrity, and thus controls blood flow.

Additional studies are needed to clarify the difference of opinion concerning the pathophysiology of dysfunctional uterine bleeding. The therapeutic approach favored in this book utilizes hormonal control of endometrial events and rarely finds it necessary to resort to surgery.

Treatment Program for Anovulatory Bleeding

The immediate objective of medical therapy in anovulatory bleeding is to retrieve the natural controlling influences missing in this tissue: universal, synchronous endometrial events, structural stability, and vasomotor rhythmicity.

Progestin Therapy

Most women will, at sometime, either fail to ovulate or not sustain adequate corpus luteum function or duration. This occurs with increased frequency in the decade prior to menopause. The usual clinical presentation is oligomenorrhea with terminal bouts of menorrhagia or polymenorrhea. Women correctly seek medical advice promptly because these menstrual aberrations suggest unplanned pregnancy or uterine pathology. Therefore, it is uncommon to find significant blood loss or excessive tissue proliferation in these women. Under most circumstances, progestin therapy will suffice to control the abnormality once uterine pathology is ruled out.

Progesterone and progestins are powerful antiestrogens when given in pharmacologic doses. Gurpide has shown that progestins induce enzymes in endometrial cells which convert estradiol to estrone sulfate.(14) Progestins also diminish estrogen effects on target cells by inhibiting the augmentation of estrogen receptors which ordinarily accompanies estrogen action (receptor replenishment inhibition).(15) These influences account for the antimitotic, antigrowth impact of progestins on the endometrium (prevention and reversal of hyperplasia, limitation of growth postovulation, and the marked atrophy during pregnancy or in response to combined birth control pills).

In the treatment of oligomenorrhea, orderly limited withdrawal bleeding can be accomplished by administration of a progestin such as medroxyprogesterone acetate, 10 mg daily for 10 days every month. Absence of induced bleeding requires workup. In the treatment of dysfunctional menometrorrhagia or polymenorrhea, progestins are prescribed for 10 days to 2 weeks (to induce stabilizing predecidual stromal changes) followed by a withdrawal flow—the so-called "medical curettage." Thereafter, repeat progestin is offered cyclically the first 10 days of each month to ensure therapeutic effect. Failure of progestin to correct irregular bleeding requires diagnostic reevaluation.

Combined Birth Control Therapy

In young women, anovulatory bleeding may be associated with prolonged endometrial buildup, delayed diagnosis, and heavy blood loss. In these cases, combined progestin-estrogen therapy is used in the form of birth control pills. Any of the oral combination tablets are useful. Whatever dose is available or chosen, therapy is administered as one pill 4 times a day for 5-7 days. This therapy is maintained despite cessation of flow within 12-24 hours. If flow does not abate, other diagnostic possibilities (polyps, incomplete abortion, and neoplasia) should be reevaluated by examination under anesthesia, and dilatation and curettage (D and C).

If flow does diminish rapidly, the remainder of the week of treatment can be given over to the evaluation of causes of anovulation, investigation of hemorrhagic tendencies, and blood replacement or initiation of iron therapy. In addition, the week provides time to prepare the patient for the progestin-estrogen withdrawal flow that will soon be induced. For the moment, therapy has produced the

276

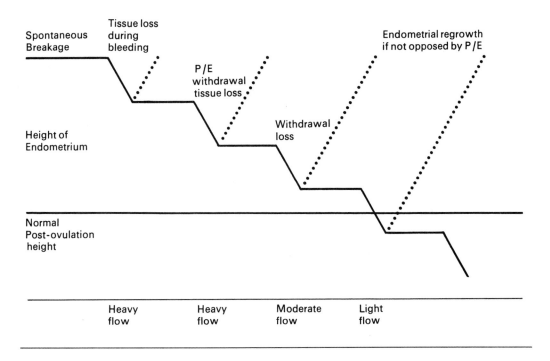

Therapy   P/E × 7 days   P/E × 21 days   P/E × 21 days   P/E × 21 days

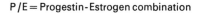

P/E = Progestin-Estrogen combination

Spontaneous Breakage

Tissue loss during bleeding

Endometrial regrowth if not opposed by P/E

P/E withdrawal tissue loss

Withdrawal loss

Height of Endometrium

Normal Post-ovulation height

Heavy flow   Heavy flow   Moderate flow   Light flow

structural rigidity intrinsic to the compact pseudodecidual reaction. Continued random breakdown of formerly fragile tissue is avoided and blood loss stopped. However, a large amount of tissue remains to react to progestin-estrogen withdrawal. The patient must be warned to anticipate a heavy and severely cramping flow 2-4 days after stopping therapy. If not prepared in this way, it is certain that the patient will view the problem as recurrent disease or failure of hormonal therapy.

In successful therapy, on the 5th day of flow, a low dose cyclic combination birth control medication (one pill a day) is started. This will be repeated for several (usually three) 3-week treatments, punctuated by 1-week withdrawal flow intervals. A decrease in volume and pain with each successive cycle is reassuring. Birth control pills reduce menstrual flow by at least 60% in normal uteri.(16) Early application of the progestin-estrogen combination limits growth and allows orderly regression of excessive endometrial height to normal controllable levels. If the progestin-estrogen combination is not applied, abnormal endometrial height and persistent excessive flow will recur.

In the patient not exposed to potential pregnancy, in whom cyclic progestin-estrogen for 3 months has reduced endometrial tissue to normal height, the pill may be discontinued and unopposed endogenous estrogen permitted to reactivate the endometrium. In the absence of spontaneous menses, the recurrence of the anovulatory state is suspected, and a brief preemptive course of an orally active progestin is administered to counter endometrial proliferation. Once

277

pregnancy is ruled out, medroxyprogesterone acetate, 10 mg orally daily for 10 days, is given monthly. Reasonable flow (progestin withdrawal flow) will occur 2-7 days after the last pill. With this therapy, excessive endometrial buildup is avoided, and an increased risk of endometrial and breast cancer is avoided. If contraception is desired, routine use of birth control pills is warranted and will also be of prophylactic value.

Estrogen Therapy

Intermittent vaginal spotting is frequently associated with minimal (low) estrogen stimulation (estrogen breakthrough bleeding). In this circumstance, where minimal endometrium exists, the beneficial effect of progestin treatment is not achieved, because there is insufficient tissue on which the progestin can exert action. A similar circumstance also exists in the younger anovulatory patient in whom prolonged hemorrhagic desquamation leaves little residual tissue.

In these circumstances, high dose estrogen therapy is applied using as much as Premarin 25 mg intravenously every 4 hours until bleeding abates (up to three doses can be given).(17) This is the sign that the ''healing'' events are initiated to a sufficient degree. Progestin treatment must be started at that time. Where bleeding is less, lower oral doses of estrogen (1.25 mg of conjugated estrogens daily for 7-10 days) can be prescribed initially. All estrogen therapy must be followed by progestin coverage.

Estrogen therapy is also useful in two examples of problems associated with progestin breakthrough bleeding. These are the breakthrough bleeding episodes occurring with use of birth control pills or with depot forms of progestational derivatives. In the absence of sufficient endogenous and exogenous estrogen, the endometrium shrinks by pharmacologically induced pseudoatrophy. Furthermore, it is composed almost exclusively of pseudodecidual stroma and blood vessels with minimal glands. Peculiarly, experience has shown that this type of endometrium also leads to the fragility bleeding more typical of pure estrogen stimulation. The usual clinical story is a patient on long-standing oral contraception who, after experiencing marked diminution or absence of withdrawal flow in the pill free interval, begins to see breakthrough bleeding while on medication.

Another frequently encountered problem is the progestin breakthrough bleeding experienced with chronic depot administration of progestin. This therapy is used not only for contraception, but also in the treatment of endometriosis and the prevention of menses during chemotherapy. In 75% of recipients, continuous therapy is not associated with abnormal menstrual bleeding. In the remainder, breakthrough progestin bleeding occurs. Judicious use of estrogen is the appropriate and effective therapy in these instances.

Estrogen therapy (ethinyl estradiol 20 μg or conjugated estrogens 2.5 mg daily for 7 days) during, and in addition to, the usual birth control pill administration is useful. This rejuvenates the endometrium and intermenstrual flow stops.

The Use of Antiprostaglandins

There seems little doubt that prostaglandins (PG) have important actions on the endometrial vasculature and presumably on endometrial hemostasis. The concentrations of PGE_2 and $PGF_{2\alpha}$ increase progressively in human endometrium during the menstrual cycle, and PG synthetase inhibitors decrease menstrual blood loss (18) perhaps by altering the balances between the platelet proaggregating vasoconstrictor thromboxane A_2 (TXA_2) and the antiaggregating vasodilator prostacyclin (PGI_2). Excessive bleeding in women with menorrhagia can be reduced by approximately 50%.(19)

Whatever the exact mechanism, PG synthetase inhibitors diminish menstrual bleeding in normal women as well as in the bleeding secondary to intrauterine device (IUD) use.

Summary of Key Points in Therapy of Anovulatory Dysfunctional) Bleeding

Teenager	Adult
Preliminary:	*Preliminary:*
Pelvic or rectal examination	Pelvic examination
	PAP smear
	Endometrial biopsy

1. Intense progestin-estrogen therapy for 7 days

2. Cyclic low dose oral contraceptive for 3 months

3. If exposed to pregnancy, continue oral contraception

4. If not exposed to pregnancy, medroxyprogesterone acetate, 10 mg daily for 10 days every month.

If bleeding has been prolonged:
If biopsy yields minimal tissue:
If patient is on progestin medication:
If follow-up is uncertain:

Premarin, 25 mg intravenously every 4 hours until bleeding stops, or significantly slows, then proceed to Step 1 above. If no response in 12-24 hours, proceed to D and C.

279

The clinical problem of dysfunctional bleeding is associated with either anovulation and estrogen withdrawal or breakthrough bleeding, or with anovulation due to exogenous progestin medication and bleeding due to progestational endometrial breakthrough. Both categories of bleeding lack the three important characteristics of normal estrogen-progesterone withdrawal bleeding:

1. Universal, simultaneous change in all segments of the endometrium;

2. An orderly progression of events involving a rigid, compact structure; and

3. Vasomotor rhythmicity with vasoconstriction, structural collapse, and clotting.

Evaluation and examination include biopsies where appropriate. One should keep in mind that as many as 20% of adolescents with dysfunctional uterine bleeding will have a coagulation defect.(20) An increase in menstrual problems has been noted in women with a history of previous abnormal periods who underwent tubal sterilization in the early 70s.(21) The increase appeared 2 or more years after the operation. It is likely that the newer techniques utilizing clips, bands, or bipolar coagulation have less risk. Few women who have normal menstrual periods before sterilization have abnormal function afterwards.

Therapy involves an initial choice between intensive progestin-estrogen combination medication or high doses of estrogen. The progestin-estrogen combination will be ineffective unless endometrium of sufficient quantity and responsiveness to allow the formation of pseudodecidual tissue is present. Therefore, the initial choice of therapy should be high doses of estrogen (Premarin, 25 mg intravenously every 4 hours until bleeding stops or for 24 hours) in the following situations:

1. When bleeding has been heavy for many days and it is likely that the uterine cavity is now lined only by a raw basalis layer;

2. When the endometrial curet yields minimal tissue;

3. When the patient has been on progestin medication (oral contraceptives, intramuscular progestins) and the endometrium is shallow and atrophic; and

4. When follow-up is uncertain, because estrogen therapy will temporarily stop all categories of dysfunctional bleeding.

If high dose estrogen therapy does not significantly abate flow within 12-24 hours, reevaluation is mandatory, and the need for curettage is likely.

Once the acute bleeding episode in an anovulatory patient is under control, the patient should not be forgotten. With persistent anovulation, recurrent hemorrhage is a common pattern and, more importantly, chronic unopposed estrogen stimulation to the endometrium can eventually lead to atypical tissue changes. It is absolutely necessary that the patient undergo periodic progestational withdrawal, either with a routine oral contraceptive regimen, or if exposure to pregnancy is not a consideration, a progestational agent (medroxyprogesterone acetate, 10 mg daily for 10 days) should be administered every month.

Curettage is *not* the first line of defense, but rather the last. The utilization of appropriate steroids for the clinical management of dysfunctional bleeding is based upon a physiologic understanding of the endometrium and its responses to hormones. Adherence to this program will avoid D and C except in a rare case of dysfunctional bleeding, and except in those cases where bleeding is due to a pathologic entity within the reproductive tract where D and C is truly indicated and necessary.

If a patient has recurrent bleeding despite repeated medical therapy, submucous myomas or endometrial polyps must be suspected. Thorough curettage can miss such pathology and further diagnostic study can be helpful. Either hysterosalpingography with slow instillation of dye and careful fluoroscopic examination or hysteroscopy may reveal a myoma or polyp. A pathologic problem such as this should especially be suspected in the puzzling case of the patient who has abnormal bleeding and ovulatory cycles.

References

1. **Noyes RW, Hertig AW, Rock J,** Dating the endometrial biopsy, Fertil Steril 1:3, 1950.

2. **Bartlemez GW,** The phases of the menstrual cycle and their interpretation in terms of the pregnancy cyle, Am J Obstet Gynecol 74:931, 1957.

3. **Markee JE,** Morphological basis for menstrual bleeding, Bull NY Acad Med 24:253, 1948.

4. **Sixma JJ, Cristiens GCML, Haspels AS,** The sequence of hemostatic events in the endometrium during normal menstruation, in *WHO Symposium on Steroid Contraception and Endometrial Bleeding,* Diczfalusy E, Fraser IS, Webb FTG, editors, 1980, p 86.

5. **Wilborn WH, Flowers CE Jr,** Cellular mechanisms for endometrial conservation during menstrual bleeding, Seminars Reprod Endocrinol 2:307, 1984.

6. **Rock J, Garcia CR, Menkin M,** A theory of menstruation, Ann NY Acad Sci 75:830, 1959.

7. **Hallberg L, Hogdahl A, Nilsson L, Rybo G,** Menstrual blood loss—a population study, Acta Obstet Gynecol Scand 45:320, 1966.

8. **Rybo G,** Menstrual blood loss in relation to parity and menstrual pattern, Acta Obstet Gynecol Scand 7:119, 1966.

9. **Haynes PJ, Hodgson H, Anderson ABM, Turnbull AC,** Measurement of menstrual blood loss in patients complaining of menorrhagia. Brit J Obstet Gynecol 84:763, 1977.

10. **Wilson EW,** Lysosome function in normal endometrium and endometrium exposed to contraceptive steroids, in *WHO Symposium on Steroid Contraception and Endometrial Bleeding,* Diczfalusy E, Fraser IS, Webb FTG, editors, 1980, p 201.

11. **Ferenczy A, Gelfand MM, Tzipris F,** The cytodynamics of endometrial hyperplasia and carcinoma, a review, Ann Path 3:189, 1983.

12. **Kurman RJ, Kaminski PT, Norris HJ,** The behavior of endometrial hyperplasia. A long-term study of "untreated" hyperplasia in 170 patients, Cancer 56:403, 1985.

13. **Ferenczy A,** Studies on the cytodynamics of human endometrial regeneration: I. Scanning electron microscopy. Am J Obstet Gynecol 124:64, 1976.

14. **Gurpide E, Gusberg S, Tseng L,** Estradiol binding and metabolism in human endometrial hyperplasia and adenocarcinoma, J Steroid Biochem 7:891, 1976.

15. **Hsueh AJW, Peck EJ, Clark JH,** Progesterone antagonism of the estrogen receptor and estrogen-induced uterine growth. Nature 254:337, 1975.

16. **Nelson L, Rybo G,** Treatment of menorrhagia. Am J Obstet Gynecol 110:713, 1971.

17. **DeVore GR, Owens O, Kase N,** Use of intravenous premarin in the treatment of dysfunctional uterine bleeding—a double-blind randomized control study, Obstet Gynecol 59:285, 1982.

18. **Anderson ABM, Haynes PJ, Guilleband J, Turnbull AC,** Reduction of menstrual blood loss by prostaglandin synthetase inhibitors, Lancet 1:774, 1976.

19. **Hall P, Maclachlan N, Thorn N, Nudd MWE, Taylor CG, Garrioch DB,** Control of menorrhagia by the cyclo-oxygenase inhibitors naproxen sodium and mefenamic acid, Brit J Obstet Gynaecol 94:554, 1987.

20. **Claessens EA, Colwell CA,** Acute adolescent menorrhagia, Am J Obstet Gynecol 139:277, 1981.

21. **DeStefano IF, Perlman JA, Peterson HB, Diamond EL,** Long-term risk of menstrual disturbances after tubal sterilization, Am J Obstet Gynecol 152:835, 1985.

9   The Breast

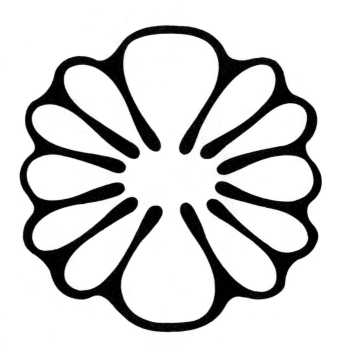

The form, function, and pathology of the human female breast are major concerns of medicine and society. As mammals, we define our biologic class by the function of the breast in nourishing our young. Breast contours occupy our attention. As obstetricians, we seek to enhance or diminish function, and as gynecologists, the appearance of inappropriate lactation (galactorrhea) may signify serious disease. Finally, an issue of growing magnitude, cancer of the breast is the most frequent cancer in women.

In this chapter, the factors involved in normal growth and development of the breast will be reviewed, including the physiology of normal lactation. A description of the numerous factors leading to inappropriate lactation will follow, and finally, the endocrine aspects of breast cancer will be considered.

Growth and Development

The basic component of the breast lobule is the hollow alveolus or milk gland lined by a single layer of milk-secreting epithelial cells, derived from an ingrowth of epidermis into the underlying mesenchyme at 10-12 weeks of gestation. Each alveolus is encased in a crisscrossing mantle of contractile myoepithelial strands. Also surrounding the milk gland is a rich capillary network.

The lumen of the alveolus connects to a collecting intralobular duct by means of a thin nonmuscular duct. Contractile muscle cells line the intralobular ducts that eventually reach the exterior via 15-25 apertures in the areola.

Growth of this milk-producing system is dependent on numerous hormonal factors which occur in two sequences, first at puberty and then in pregnancy. Although there is considerable overlapping of hormonal influences, the differences in quantities of the stimuli in each circumstance and the availability of entirely unique inciting factors (human placental lactogen (HPL) and prolactin) during pregnancy permit this chronologic distinction.

The major influence on breast growth at puberty is estrogen. In most girls, the first response to the increasing levels of estrogen is an increase in size and pigmentation of the areola and the formation of a mass of breast tissue just underneath the areola. Breast tissue binds estrogen in a manner similar to the uterus and vagina. The development of estrogen receptors in the breast does not occur in the absence of prolactin. The primary effect of estrogen in subprimate mammals is to stimulate growth of the ductal portion of the gland system. Progesterone in these animals influences growth of the alveolar components of the lobule. However, neither hormone alone, or in combination, is capable of yielding optimal breast growth and development. Full differentiation of the gland requires insulin, cortisol, thyroxine, prolactin, and growth hormone.(1) Changes occur routinely in response to the estrogen-progesterone sequence of a normal menstrual cycle. *Consequently, breast examination is most effective during the follicular phase of the cycle.*

The pubertal response is a manifestation of closely synchronized central (hypothalamus-pituitary) and peripheral (ovary-breast) events. For example, gonadotropin releasing hormone (GnRH) is known to stimulate prolactin release, and this action is potentiated by estrogen.(2) This suggests a paracrine interaction between gonadotrophs and lactotrophs, linked by estrogen, ultimately with an impact on the breast.

The estrogen-induced impetus to mammary epithelial stem cell division requires the presence of insulin. Final differentiation of the alveolar epithelial cell into a mature milk cell is accomplished in the presence of prolactin, but only after prior exposure to cortisol and insulin. The complete reaction depends on the availability of minimal quantities of thyroid hormone. Thus, the endocrinologically intact individual in whom estrogen, progesterone, thyroxine, cortisol, insulin, prolactin, and growth hormone are available can have appropriate breast growth. Mild deficiencies in any of the hormones, short of severe restrictions or total absence, can be compensated for by excess prolactin. Furthermore, the growth of the breast and breast function can be incited by an excess of prolactin.

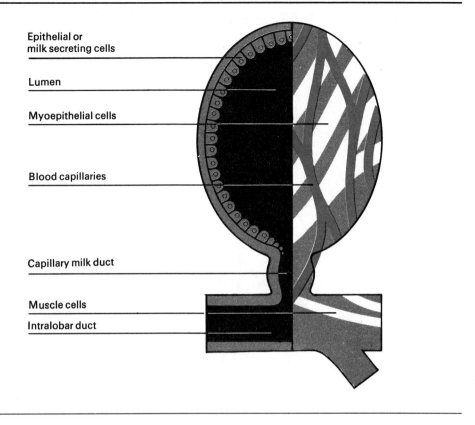

Epithelial or
milk secreting cells

Lumen

Myoepithelial cells

Blood capillaries

Capillary milk duct

Muscle cells

Intralobar duct

Abnormal Shapes and
Sizes

Early differentiation of the mammary gland anlage is under fetal hormonal control. Abnormalities in adult size or shape may reflect the impact of hormones (especially the presence or absence of testosterone) during this early period of development. Occasionally, the breast bud will begin to develop on one side first. Similarly, one breast may grow faster than the other. These inequalities usually disappear by the time development is complete. However, exact equivalence in size usually is never attained. Significant asymmetry is correctable only by the plastic surgeon. Likewise hypoplasia and hypertrophy can be treated only by corrective surgery. With one exception, hormone therapy is totally ineffective in producing a permanent change in breast shape or size. Of course in patients with primary amenorrhea secondary to deficient ovarian function, estrogen replacement will induce significant and gratifying breast growth.

Accessory nipples can be found anywhere from the knees to the neck. They occur in approximately 1% of women and require no therapy.

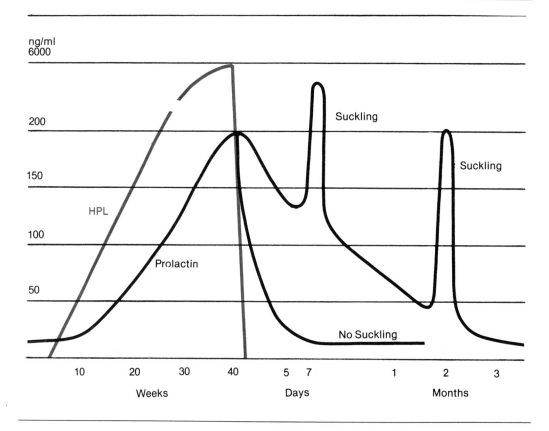

ng/ml
6000

200

150

100

50

HPL

Prolactin

Suckling

Suckling

No Suckling

| 10 | 20 | 30 | 40 | 5 | 7 | 1 | 2 | 3 |

Weeks

Days

Months

Pregnancy and Milk Secretion

The differentiation of terminal alveolar cells into active milk-secreting units requires the availability of insulin, prolactin, and cortisol, as well as estrogen and progesterone. (1) During pregnancy, prolactin levels rise from the normal level of 10-25 ng/ml to high concentrations, beginning about 8 weeks and reaching a peak of 200-400 ng/ml at term.(3) Made by the placenta and actively secreted into the maternal circulation from the 6th week of pregnancy, HPL rises progressively reaching a level of approximately 6000 ng/ml at term. HPL, though displaying less activity than prolactin, is produced in such large amounts that it may exert a lactogenic effect.

Although prolactin stimulates significant breast growth, and is available for lactation, only colostrum (composed of desquamated epithelial cells and transudate) is produced during gestation. Full lactation is inhibited by progesterone which interferes with prolactin action at the alveolar cell prolactin receptor level. Both estrogen and progesterone are necessary for the expression of the lactogenic receptor, but progesterone antagonizes the positive action of prolactin on its own receptor while progesterone and pharmacologic amounts of androgens reduce prolactin binding.(4,5)

Amniotic fluid concentrations of prolactin parallel maternal serum concentration until the 10th week of pregnancy, rise markedly until the 20th week, and then decrease. Maternal prolactin does not pass to the fetus in significant amounts. Indeed the source of amniotic fluid prolactin is neither the maternal pituitary nor the fetal pituitary. The failure of bromocriptine to suppress amniotic fluid prolactin levels, and studies with in vitro culture systems, indicate a primary decidual source with transfer via amnion receptors to the amniotic fluid, requiring the intactness of amnion, chorion, and adherent decidua. This decidual synthesis of prolactin is initiated by progesterone, but once decidualization is established, prolactin secretion continues in the absence of both progesterone and estradiol.(6) It is hypothesized that amniotic fluid prolactin plays a role similar to its regulation of sodium transport and water movement across the gills in fish (allowing the ocean dwelling salmon and steelhead to return to fresh water streams for reproduction). Thus prolactin would protect the human fetus from dehydration by control of salt and water transport across the amnion. Prolactin reduces the permeability of the human amnion in the fetal to maternal direction by a receptor-mediated action on the epithelium lining the fetal surface.(7)

There is marked variability in maternal prolactin levels in pregnancy, with a diurnal variation similar to that found in nonpregnant persons. The peak level occurs 4-5 hours after the onset of sleep.(8) The initial rise at 7-8 weeks of gestation correlates with the rising levels of estradiol which appear to act at the hypothalamic level to increase prolactin secretion.(9,10)

The principal hormone involved in milk biosynthesis is prolactin. Without prolactin, synthesis of the primary protein, casein, will not occur, and true milk secretion will be impossible. The hormonal trigger for initiation of milk production within the alveolar cell and its secretion into the lumen of the gland is the rapid disappearance of estrogen and progesterone from the circulation after delivery. The clearance of prolactin is much slower, requiring 7 days to reach nonpregnant levels in a nonbreast-feeding woman. These discordant hormonal events result in removal of the progesterone inhibition of prolactin action on the breast. Breast engorgement and milk secretion begin 3-4 days postpartum when steroids have been sufficiently cleared. Maintenance of steroidal inhibition (progestin or androgen) or rapid reduction of prolactin secretion (bromocriptine, 2.5 mg b.i.d. for 2 weeks) are effective in preventing postpartum milk synthesis and secretion. Augmentation of prolactin (by TRH or sulpiride, a dopamine receptor blocker) results in increased milk yield.

In the first postpartum week, prolactin levels in breast-feeding women decline approximately 50% (to about 100 ng/ml). Suckling elicits increases in prolactin, which are important in initiating milk production. Until 2-3 months postpartum, basal levels are approximately 40-50 ng/ml, and there are large (about 10-20-fold) increases after suckling. At least through 6 months (and probably throughout breast-feeding) baseline prolactin levels remain elevated, and suckling produces a twofold increase that is essential for continuing milk production.(11) The failure to lactate within the first 7 days postpartum may be the first sign of Sheehan's syndrome (hypopituitarism following intrapartum infarction of the pituitary gland).

Maintenance of milk production at high levels is dependent on the joint action of both anterior and posterior pituitary factors. By mechanisms to be described in detail shortly, suckling causes the release of both prolactin and oxytocin as well as thyroid stimulating hormone (TSH).(12) Prolactin sustains the secretion of casein, fatty acids, lactose and the volume of secretion, while oxytocin contracts myoepithelial cells and empties the alveolar lumen, thus enhancing further milk secretion and alveolar refilling. The increase in TSH with suckling response suggests that TRH may play a role in the prolactin response to suckling (see below, "Prolactin Releasing Factor"). The optimal quantity and quality of milk are dependent upon the availability of thyroid, insulin, cortisol, and the dietary intake of nutrients and fluids.

Frequent emptying of the lumen is important for maintaining an adequate level of secretion. Indeed, after the 4th postpartum month, suckling appears to be the only stimulant required; however environmental and emotional states also are important for continued alveolar activity.

The ejection of milk from the breast does not occur as the result of a mechanically induced negative pressure produced by suckling. Tactile sensors concentrated in the areola activate, via thoracic sensory nerve roots 4, 5, and 6, an afferent sensory neural arc which stimulates the paraventricular and supraoptic nuclei of the hypothalamus to synthesize and transport oxytocin to the posterior pituitary. The efferent arc (oxytocin) is blood-borne to the breast alveolus-ductal systems to contract myoepithelial cells and empty the alveolar lumen. Milk contained in major ductal repositories is ejected from openings in the nipple. This rapid release of milk is called "letdown". In many instances, the activation of oxytocin release leading to letdown does not require initiation by tactile stimuli. The central nervous system can be conditioned to respond to the presence of the infant, or to the sound of the infant's cry, by inducing activation of the efferent arc.

The oxytocin effect is a release phenomenon acting on secreted and stored milk. Prolactin must be available in sufficient quantities for continued secretory replacement of ejected milk. This requires the transient increase in prolactin associated with suckling. The amount of milk produced correlates with the amount removed by suckling. The breast can store milk for a maximum of 48 hours before production diminishes.

Vitamin A, vitamin B_{12}, and folic acid are significantly reduced in the breast milk of women with poor dietary intake. As a general rule approximately 1% of any drug ingested by the mother appears in breast milk.

Breast Feeding by Adoptive Mothers

Adopting mothers occasionally request assistance in initiating lactation.(13) Successful breast-feeding can be achieved by approximately half of the women by ingestion of 25 mg chlorpromazine t.i.d. together with vigorous nipple stimulation every 1-3 hours. Milk production will not appear for several weeks. This preparation ideally should be practiced for several months.

Prolactin Inhibiting Factor (PIF)

Suckling suppresses the formation of a hypothalamic substance, prolactin inhibiting factor (PIF). This intrahypothalamic effect is either mediated by dopamine, or, in contrast to the peptide nature of other hypothalamic hormones, PIF is dopamine itself.(14) Dopamine is secreted by the basal hypothalamus into the portal system and conducted to the anterior pituitary. Dopamine binds specifically to lactotroph cells and suppresses the secretion of prolactin into the general circulation; in its absence, prolactin is secreted. Suckling, therefore, acts to refill the breast by activating both portions of the pituitary (anterior and posterior) causing the breast to produce new milk and to eject milk.

Prolactin Releasing Factor (PRF)

Prolactin may also be influenced by a positive hypothalamic factor (prolactin releasing factor, PRF). PRF does exist in various fowl (e.g. pigeon, chicken, duck, turkey, and the tricolored blackbird). While the identity of this material has not been elucidated, or its function substantiated in normal human physiology, it is possible that TRH is a potent stimulant of prolactin secretion in man. The smallest doses of TRH which are capable of producing an increase in TSH, also increase prolactin levels, a finding which supports a physiologic role for TRH in the control of prolactin secretion. However, except in hypothyroidism, normal physiologic changes as well as abnormal prolactin secretion are best explained and understood in terms of variations in the inhibiting factor, PIF. A large collection of peptides has been reported to stimulate the release of prolactin in vitro. These include growth factors, angiotensin II, GnRH, vasopressin, and others. But it is unknown whether these peptides participate in the normal physiologic regulation of prolactin secretion.

Cessation of Lactation

Lactation can be terminated by discontinuing suckling. The primary effect of this cessation is loss of milk letdown via the neural evocation of oxytocin. With passage of a few days, the swollen alveoli depress milk formation probably via a local pressure effect. With resorption of fluid and solute, the swollen engorged breast diminishes in size in a few days. In addition to the loss of milk letdown the absence of suckling reactivates dopamine (PIF) production so that there is less prolactin stimulation of milk secretion. Routine use of bromocriptine for postpartum suppression of lactation is not recommended because of reports of hypertension, seizure, myocardial infarctons, and strokes associated with the postpartum use of bromocriptine.

Contraceptive Effect of Lactation

A moderate contraceptive effect accompanies lactation. (15) It is well known that this is temporary and at best an effect of low reliability. The contraceptive effectiveness of lactation, i.e. the length of the interval between births, depends on the level of nutrition of the mother (if low, the longer the contraceptive interval), the intensity of suckling, and the extent to which supplemental food is added to the infant diet. If suckling intensity and/or frequency is diminished, contraceptive effect is reduced. Approximately 40-75% of breast-feeding women resume menstrual function while still nursing and most will ovulate shortly thereafter. When breast-feeding is used exclusively and menstrual bleeding has not appeared, ovulation usually does not occur before the end of the 10th postpartum week. The mechanism of the contraceptive effect is of interest because a similar interference with normal pituitary-gonadal function is seen with elevated prolactin levels in nonpregnant women, the syndrome of galactorrhea and amenorrhea. Women who wish to breast-feed and also avoid pregnancy should use some method of contraception beginning at 4-5 weeks postpartum.

Prolactin concentrations are increased in response to the repeated suckling stimulus of breast-feeding. Given sufficient intensity and frequency, prolactin levels will remain elevated. Under these conditions, follicle-stimulating hormone (FSH) concentrations are in the normal range (having risen from extremely low concentrations at delivery to follicular range in the 3 weeks postpartum) and luteinizing hormone (LH) values are in the low normal range. Despite the presence of gonadotropin, the ovary during lactational hyperprolactinemia does not display follicular development and does not secrete estrogen.

Earlier experimental evidence suggested that the ovaries might be refractory to gonadotropin stimulation during lactation, and in addition, the anterior pituitary might be less responsive to GnRH stimulation. Other studies, done later in the course of lactation, indicated, however, that the ovaries as well as the pituitary were responsive to adequate tropic hormone stimulation.[16]

These observations suggest that high concentrations of prolactin work at both central and ovarian sites to produce lactational amenorrhea and anovulation. Prolactin appears to affect granulosa cell function in vitro by inhibiting synthesis of progesterone. It also may change the testosterone:dihydrotestosterone ratio, thereby reducing aromatizable substrate and increasing local antiestrogen concentrations. Nevertheless, a direct effect of prolactin on ovarian follicular development does not appear to be a major factor. The central action predominates.

Elevated levels of prolactin inhibit the pulsatile secretion of GnRH.[17] Prolactin excess has short loop positive feedback effects on dopamine. Increased dopamine reduces GnRH by suppressing arcuate nucleus function, perhaps in a mechanism mediated by endogenous opioid activity.[18]

At weaning, as prolactin concentrations fall to normal, gonadotropin concentrations increase and estradiol secretion rises. This prompt resumption of ovarian function is also indicated by the occurrence of ovulation within 14-30 days of weaning.

In nonbreast-feeding women, gonadotropin levels remain low during the early puerperium and return to normal concentrations during the 3rd to 5th week when prolactin levels have returned to normal. In an assessment of this important physiologic event (in terms of the need for contraception), the mean delay before first ovulation was found to be approximately 45 days, while no woman ovulated before 25 days after delivery.[19] Of the 22 women, 11 ovulated before the 6th postpartum week, underscoring the need to move the traditional postpartum medical visit to 3 weeks after delivery.

Inappropriate Lactation-Galactorrheic Syndromes

Galactorrhea refers to the mammary secretion of a milky fluid which is nonphysiologic in that it is inappropriate (not immediately related to pregnancy or the needs of a child), persistent, and sometimes excessive. Although usually white or clear, the color may be yellow or even green. In the latter circumstance, local breast disease also should be considered. To elicit breast secretion, pressure should be applied to all sections of the breast beginning at the base of the breast and working up toward the nipple. The quantity of secretion is not an important criterion. Any galactorrhea demands evaluation in a nulliparous woman, and, if at least 12 months have elapsed since the last pregnancy or weaning in a parous woman. Galactorrhea can involve both breasts, or just one breast. Amenorrhea does not necessarily accompany galactorrhea, even in the most serious provocative disorders.

Differential Diagnosis

The differential diagnosis of galactorrhea syndromes is a difficult and complex clinical challenge. The difficulty arises from the multiple factors involved in the control of prolactin release. Before proceeding, it would be useful to reemphasize the mechanisms controlling prolactin secretion. In most pathophysiologic systems the final common pathway leading to galactorrhea is an inappropriate augmentation of prolactin release. Prolactin is under a chronic tonic inhibition due to the hypothalamic secretion into the pituitary portal system of PIF. The following considerations are important:

1. Excessive estrogen (e.g. birth control pills) can lead to milk secretion via hypothalamic suppression, causing reduction of PIF and release of pituitary prolactin. Galactorrhea developing during birth control pill administration may be most noticeable during the days free of medication (when the steroids are cleared from the body and the prolactin interfering action of the estrogen and progestin on the breast wanes). Galactorrhea caused by excessive estrogen disappears within 3-6 months after discontinuing medication. This is now a rare occurrence with the lower dose pills. A longitudinal study of 126 women did demonstrate a 22% increase in prolactin values over mean control levels, but the response to low dose oral contraceptives was not out of the normal range.(20)

2. Prolonged intensive suckling can also release prolactin, via hypothalamic reduction of PIF. Similarly, thoracotomy scars, cervical spinal lesions, and herpes zoster can induce prolactin release by activating the afferent sensory neural arc, thereby simulating suckling.

3. A variety of drugs can also inhibit hypothalamic PIF. (21) There are nearly 100 phenothiazine derivatives with indirect mammotropic activity of this type. In addition, there are many phenothiazine-like compounds, reserpine derivatives, amphetamines, and an unknown variety of other drugs (opiates, diazepams, butyrophenones, α-methyldopa, and tricyclic antidepressants) which can initiate galactorrhea via hypothalamic suppression. The final action of these compounds is either to deplete dopamine levels or to block dopamine receptors. Chemical features common to many of these drugs are an aromatic ring with a polar substituent as in estrogen and at least two additional rings or structural attributes making spatial arrangements similar to estrogen. Thus, these compounds may

291

act in a manner similar to estrogens to decrease PIF. In support of this conclusion, it has been demonstrated that estrogen and phenothiazine derivatives compete for the same receptors in the median eminence. Prolactin is uniformly elevated in patients on therapeutic amounts of phenothiazines. Approximately 30-50% will exhibit galactorrhea which should not persist beyond 3-6 months after drug treatment is discontinued.

4. Stresses can inhibit hypothalamic PIF, thereby inducing prolactin secretion and galactorrhea. Trauma, surgical procedures, and anesthesia can be seen in temporal relation to the onset of galactorrhea.

5. Hypothalamic lesions, stalk lesions, or stalk compression (events that physically reduce production or delivery of PIF to the pituitary) allow release of excess prolactin leading to galactorrhea.

6. Hypothyroidism (juvenile or adult) can be associated with galactorrhea. With diminished circulating levels of thyroid hormone, hypothalamic TRH is produced in excess and acts as a PRF to release prolactin from the pituitary. Reversal with thyroid hormone is strong circumstantial evidence to support the conclusion that TRH stimulates prolactin.

7. Increased prolactin release may be a consequence of prolactin elaboration and secretion from pituitary tumors which function independently of the otherwise appropriate restraints exerted by PIF from a normally functioning hypothalamus. This infrequent, but potentially dangerous tumor, which has endocrine, neurologic, and ophthalmologic liabilities that can be disabling, makes the differential diagnosis of persistent galactorrhea a major clinical challenge. Beyond producing prolactin, the tumor may also suppress pituitary parenchyma by expansion and compression, interfering with the secretion of other tropic hormones. Other pituitary tumors may be associated with lactotroph hyperplasia and present with the characteristic syndrome of hyperprolactinemia and amenorrhea.

8. Increased prolactin concentrations may result from nonpituitary sources such as lung and renal tumors, and even a uterine leiomyoma. Severe renal disease requiring hemodialysis is associated with elevated prolactin levels due to the decreased glomerular filtration rate.

Clinical Problem of Galactorrhea

A variety of eponymic designations have been applied to variants of the lactation syndromes. These are based on the association of galactorrhea with intrasellar tumor (Forbes, Henneman, Griswold, and Albright, 1951), antecedent pregnancy with inappropriate persistence of galactorrhea (independently reported by Chiari and Frommel in 1852), and in the absence of previous pregnancy (Argonz and del Castillo, 1953). In all, the association of galactorrhea with eventual amenorrhea was noted.

On the basis of currently available information, categorization of individual cases according to these eponymic guidelines is neither helpful nor does it permit discrimination of patients who have serious intrasellar or suprasellar pathology.

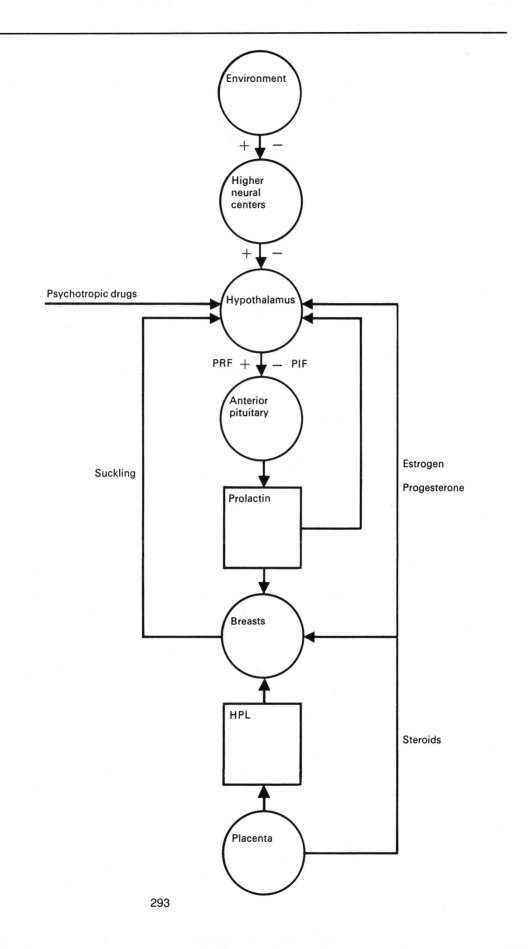

Hyperprolactinemia may be associated with a variety of menstrual cycle disturbances, oligoovulation, corpus luteum insufficiency, as well as amenorrhea. About one-third of women with secondary amenorrhea will have elevated prolactin concentrations. Pathologic hyperprolactinemia inhibits the pulsatile secretion of GnRH, and the reduction of circulating prolactin levels restores menstrual function.

Mild hirsutism may accompany ovulatory dysfunction due to hyperprolactinemia. Whether excess androgen is stimulated by a prolactin effect on adrenal cortex synthesis of DHA (dehydroepiandrosterone) and its sulfate (DHAS) or is primarily related to the chronic anovulation of these patients (and hence ovarian androgen secretion) is not settled.

Not all patients with hyperprolactinemia display galactorrhea. The reported incidence is about 33%. (Chapter 5) The disparity may not be due entirely to the variable zeal with which the presence of nipple milk secretion is sought for during physical examination. The absence of galactorrhea may be due to the usual accompanying hypoestrogenic state. A more attractive explanation focuses on the concept of heterogeneity of tropic hormones (Chapter 1). The radioimmunoassay for prolactin may not discriminate between heterogeneous molecules of prolactin. A high circulating level of prolactin may not represent material capable of interacting with breast prolactin receptors. On the other hand, galactorrhea can be seen in women with normal prolactin serum concentrations. Episodic fluctuations and sleep increments may account for this clinical discordance, or, in this case, bioactive prolactin may be present which is immunoactively not detectable. In the pathophysiology of male hypogonadism, hyperprolactinemia is much less common and the incidence of actual galactorrhea quite rare. Hyperprolactinemia in men usually presents as decreased libido and potency.

If galactorrhea has been present for 6 months to 1 year, or hyperprolactinemia is noted in the process of working up menstrual disturbances, infertility, or hirsutism, the probability of a pituitary tumor must be recognized. The workup of hyperprolactinemia is presented in detail in Chapter 5, "Amenorrhea." Nevertheless, it is worth reemphasizing the salient clinical issues here.

With the current diagnostic techniques there is no difficulty in discovering and monitoring the size and function of a pituitary prolactin secreting "tumor." With few exceptions the combination of elevation in basal levels of prolactin and radiographic imaging offers complete confidence in diagnosing sellar pathology. The major concern remains in determining management—medical, surgical, or expectant? The considerations that influence management include:

1. Microadenomas, if exclusively prolactin producing, rarely progress to macroadenoma size. Most are exceedingly slow growing or stable.

2. The histology of many so-called tumors is not one of neoplasia. Most contain nodular or diffuse hyperplasia of basically normal lactotrophs.

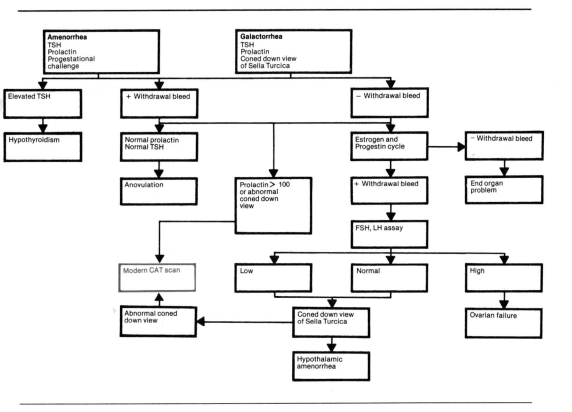

3. It is possible that a primary hypothalamic dysfunction which drives the lactotroph to hyperfunction and hyperplasia is the fundamental factor in the genesis of these "tumors." Thus, uncertain long-term cures, recurrence, and new tumor formation remain possibilities.

4. Some tumors regress spontaneously. Medical therapy (the dopamine agonist, bromocriptine) shrinks tumors and can prevent growth, although complete elimination of a tumor by bromocriptine does not occur, and rapid regrowth can follow discontinuation of bromocriptine treatment.

5. Transsphenoidal microsurgery is a very safe procedure, but there is a high recurrence rate.

As a result of these considerations, many patients can be observed, others treated medically, and rarely some treated with surgery, with or without prior medically induced tumor reduction (see Chapter 5).

Treatment of
Galactorrhea

Galactorrhea as an isolated symptom of hypothalamic dysfunction existing in an otherwise healthy woman does not require treatment. Periodic prolactin levels will, if within normal range, confirm the stability of the underlying process. However, some patients find the presence or amount of galactorrhea sexually, cosmetically, and emotionally burdensome. Treatment with combined birth control pills, androgens, danazol and progestins has met with minimal success. Bromocriptine, therefore, is clearly the drug of choice. Even with normal prolactin concentrations and a normal skull x-ray, treatment with bromocriptine can eliminate galactorrhea.

We have adopted a conservative approach of close surveillance for pituitary prolactin-secreting adenomas, recommending surgery only for those tumors that display rapid growth or those tumors that are already large and do not shrink in response to bromocriptine. If the prolactin level is greater than 100 ng/ml, or if the coned-down view of the sella turcica is abnormal, we recommend CT scan evaluation. If the CT scan rules out an empty sella syndrome or a suprasellar problem, surgical intervention after preoperative bromocriptine treatment is then dictated by the patient's desires, the size of the tumor, and the response of the tumor to bromocriptine. Patients with prolactin levels less than 100 ng/ml and with normal coned-down views of the sella turcica are offered a choice between bromocriptine therapy and surveillance. An annual prolactin level and periodic coned-down views are indicated for continued observation to detect a growing tumor. Bromocriptine therapy is recommended for patients wishing to achieve pregnancy, and for those patients who have galactorrhea to the point of discomfort.

The Management of Mastalgia

The cyclic occurrence of breast discomfort is a common problem and is usually associated with dysplastic, benign histologic changes in the breast. Medical treatment of mastalgia has historically included a bewildering array of options. Several are of questionable value. Diuretics have little impact, and thyroid hormone replacement is indicated only when hypothyroidism is documented. Steroid hormone treatment has been tried in many combinations, mostly unsupported by controlled studies. An old favorite, with many years of clinical experience testifying to its effectiveness, is testosterone. One must be careful, however, to avoid virilizing doses. A good practice is to start with small doses, such as 5 mg methyltestosterone every other day during the time of discomfort. In recent years, however, these methods have been supplanted by several new approaches.

Danazol in a dose of 200 mg/day is effective in relieving discomfort as well as decreasing nodularity of the breast.(22) A daily dose is recommended for a period of 6 months. This treatment may achieve long-term resolution of the histologic changes in addition to the clinical improvement. Doses below 400 mg daily do not assure inhibition of ovulation, and a method of effective contraception is necessary because of possible teratologic effects of the drug. Significant improvement has been noted with vitamin E, 600 units/day of the synthetic tocopheral acetate. No side effects have been noted, and the mechanism of action is unknown. Bromocriptine 2.5-5.0 mg/day) and antiestrogens such as tamoxifen (20 mg daily) are also effective for treating mammary discomfort and benign disease.(22,23)

Clinical observations had suggested that abstinence from methylxanthines leads to resolution of symptoms. Methylxanthines are present in coffee, tea, chocolate, and cola drinks. In controlled studies, however, a significant placebo response rate (30-40%) has been observed. Careful assessments of this relationship have failed to demonstrate a link between methylxanthine use and mastalgia, mammographic changes, or atypia (premalignant tissue changes).(24-26)

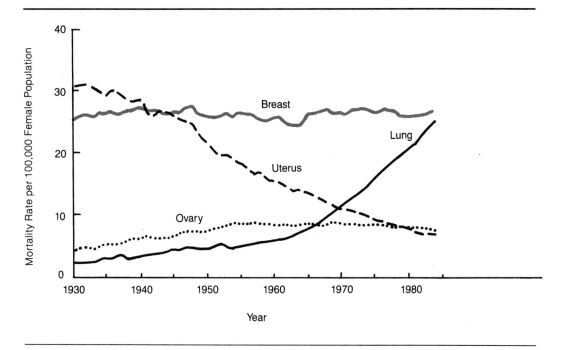

Cancer of the Breast

Scope of the Problem

One of every 10 American women will develop breast cancer during her lifetime. The incidence has been increasing over the past 2 decades and mortality rates have remained disappointingly constant. The breast is the leading site of cancer in women (28% of all cancers), and is now unfortunately (because smoking is obviously the reason) exceeded by lung cancer as the the leading cause of death from cancer in women.(27)

Cancer Site Incidence in U.S. Women:		
	Breast	**- 28%**
	Rectum	**- 16%**
	Lung	**- 11%**
	Uterus	**- 10%**
	Ovary	**- 4%**

Cancer Deaths in U.S. Women:		
	Lung	**- 20%**
	Breast	**- 18%**
	Rectum	**- 14%**
	Ovary	**- 5%**
	Uterus	**- 4%**

Breast cancer has an increasing frequency with age—a woman at age 70 has almost 10 times the risk as a 40-year-old woman. Over the years breast cancer has continued this deadly impact despite advances in surgical and diagnostic techniques. No more than 25% of breast cancer patients are "cured."

Classically, the single most useful prognostic information in women with operable breast cancer has been the histologic status of the axillary lymph nodes.(28) At 10 years only 25% of patients with positive nodes are free of disease compared to 75% of patients with negative nodes. If more than 3 nodes are involved, the 10 year

297

survival rate drops from about 38% to 13%. Because of this recognition for the importance of the axillary nodes, the traditional approach to breast cancer (the Halsted surgical approach) was based on the concept that breast cancer is a disease of stepwise progression. *There is an important change in concept. Breast cancer is now viewed as a systemic disease, with spread to local and distant sites at the same time. Breast cancer is best viewed as occultly metastatic at the time of presentation.* Therefore, dissemination of tumor cells has occurred by the time of surgery in many patients, and it is not surprising that radical mastectomy and local irradiation do not prevent metastatic disease.

Because we have been dealing with a disease which has already reached the point of dissemination in most patients, we must move the diagnosis forward several years in order to have an impact on breast cancer mortality. Earlier diagnosis requires that we be aware of what it is that makes a high risk patient.

Risk Factors

A constellation of factors influences the risk for breast cancer.(29) These include: reproductive experience, ovarian activity, benign breast disease, familial tendency, genetic differences, dietary considerations, and specific endocrine factors.

Reproductive Experience. The risk of breast cancer increases with the increase in age at which a woman bears her first full-term child. A woman pregnant before the age of 18 has about one-third the risk of one who first delivers after the age of 35. To be protective, pregnancy must occur before the age of 30. In fact, women over the age of 30 years at the time of their first birth have a greater risk than women who never become pregnant. There is, however, a significant protective effect with increasing parity, present even when adjusted for age at first birth and other risk factors.(30)

The fact that pregnancy early in life is associated with reduced breast cancer implies that etiologic factors are operating during that period of life. The protection afforded by the first pregnancy suggests that the first full-term pregnancy has a trigger effect which either produces a permanent change in the factors responsible for breast cancer, or changes the breast tissue and makes it less susceptible to malignant transformation. There is evidence for a lasting impact of a first pregnancy on a woman's hormonal milieu. A small but significant elevation of estriol, a decrease in DHA and DHAS, and lower prolactin levels all persist for many years after delivery.(31,32) These changes take on great significance when viewed in terms of the endocrine factors considered below.

Lactation offers a weak to moderate protective effect (20% reduced risk) only for premenopausal breast cancer. (33) There is a unique and helpful study of the Chinese Tanka, who are boat people living on the coast of southern China.(34) The women of the Chinese Tanka wear clothing with an opening only on the right side, and they breast-feed only with the right breast. All breast cancers were in postmenopausal women, and the cancers were equally distributed between the two sides.

Ovarian Activity. Women who have an oophorectomy have a lower risk and the lowered risk is greater the younger a woman is when ovariectomized. There is a 70% risk reduction in women who have surgery before age 35. There is a small increase in risk with early menarche and with late natural menopause, indicating that ovarian activity plays a continuing role throughout reproductive life. Obese women have earlier menarche and later menopause, higher estrone production rates and free estradiol levels (lower sex hormone binding globulin (SHBG)), and greater risk for breast cancer.(35)

Benign Breast Disease. With obstruction of ducts (probably by stromal fibrosis), ductule-alveolar secretion persists, the secretory material is retained, and cysts form from the dilatation of terminal ducts (duct ectasia) and alveoli. Women with cystic mastitis have about 4 times the breast cancer rate of comparable normal women. Despite their risk, women with prior benign breast disease form only a small proportion of breast cancer patients—approximately 5%.

There is strong support to eliminate the phrase: fibrocystic disease of the breast. In a review of over 10,000 breast biopsies in Nashville, Tennessee, 70% of the women were found to not have a lesion associated with an increased risk for cancer.(36) The most important variable on biopsies is the degree and character of the epithelial proliferation. Women with atypical hyperplasia had a relative risk of 5.3, while women with atypia and a family history of breast cancer had a relative risk of 11. The point is that we needlessly frighten patients with the use of the phrase fibrocystic disease. For most women, this is not a disease, but a physiologic change brought about by cyclic hormonal activity. *Let's call this problem FIBROCYSTIC CHANGE OR CONDITION.*

The College of American Pathologists supports this position and has offered this classification:(37)

Classification of Breast Biopsy Tissue According to Risk for Breast Cancer:

No increased risk: **Adenosis**
                                    Duct ectasia
                                    Fibroadenoma
                                    Fibrosis
                                    Mild hyperplasia (3-4 cells deep)
                                    Mastitis
                                    Periductal mastitis
                                    Squamous metaplasia

Slightly increased risk (1.5-2.0 times):
                                    Moderate or florid hyperplasia
                                    Papilloma

Risk increased 5 times:
                                    Atypical hyperplasia

Familial Tendency. Female relatives of women with breast cancer have 2-3 times the rate of the general population. There is an excess of bilateral disease among patients with a family history of breast cancer. Relatives of women with bilateral disease have about a 45% lifetime chance of developing breast cancer. In data from the CDC, these relative risks were observed:(38)

Affected aunt or grandmother — 1.5 relative risk.
Affected mother or sister — 2.3 relative risk.
Affected mother and sister —14.0 relative risk.

Fat in the Diet. The geographical variation in incidence rates of breast cancer is considerable (The United States has the highest rates and Japan the lowest), and it has been correlated with the amount of animal fat in the diet. Lean women, however, have been found to have an increased incidence of breast cancer, although this increase is limited to small, localized, and well-differentiated tumors.(39) Furthermore, studies have failed to find evidence for a positive relationship between breast cancer and dietary total or saturated fat or cholesterol intake.(40) Thus the epidemiologic literature provides little support for the hypothesis that dietary fat intake is related to the risk of breast cancer. This hypothesis was derived from international correlations between per capita fat intake and mortality rates for breast cancer, and has not withstood epidemiologic testing.

Alcohol in the Diet. There is a 60% increase in the risk for breast cancer with the consumption of one or more alcoholic drinks per day.(41) Almost all of many studies conclude that even moderate drinking increases the risk by 40-60%.

Specific Endocrine Factors.

1. *Adrenal Steroids.* Subnormal levels of etiocholanolone (a urinary excretion product of androstenedione) have been found from 5 months to 9 years before the diagnosis of breast cancer in women living on the island of Guernsey, off the English coast.(42) A subnormal excretion of this 17-ketosteroid was also found in sisters of patients with breast cancer. A 6-fold increase in the incidence of breast cancer was found between women excreting less than 0.4 mg of etiocholanolone and those excreting over 1 mg/24 hours. Measurement of this 17-ketosteroid might be a useful screening procedure to detect a high risk group of patients because approximately 25% of the population excretes less than 1 mg/24 hours.

2. *Endogenous Estrogen.* Estriol generally has failed to produce breast cancer in rodents, and in fact, estriol protects the rat against breast tumors induced by various chemical carcinogens. The hypothesis is that a higher estriol level protects against the more potent effects of estrone and estradiol. This might explain the protective effect of early pregnancies. Women having had an early pregnancy continue to excrete more estriol than nulliparous women. Premenopausal healthy Asiatic women have a lower breast cancer risk than Caucasians, and also have a higher rate of urinary estriol excretion.(43) When Asiatic women migrate to the United States, however, the risk of breast cancer increases, and their urinary excretion of estriol decreases.

300

The notion that normal estrogen stimulation unopposed by adequate progesterone secretion is a factor in the pathogenesis of breast cancer was first stated by Sherman and Korenman.(44) Although theoretically appealing on the basis of presumed correlation with epidemiologic risks (infertility, late menopause) clinical research has not always confirmed the thesis.(45) Young women at high genetic risk for breast cancer had normal luteal phases, and a group of premenopausal women with breast cancer also had normal luteal phases. On the other hand, a long-term follow-up study of infertile women with a history of progesterone deficiency indicated a 5.4 times increase in risk of premenopausal breast cancer, while a survey of anovulatory women detected a 3-4 times increase in the risk of cancer which appeared after the age of 50. (46,47)

The logic and epidemiologic support for an estrogen link are impressive arguments. Whether the important factor is the total amount of estrogen, the amount of estrogen unopposed by progesterone, or some other combination is not known. More modern studies implicate biologically available estrogen as a factor. Women who develop breast cancer have higher levels of nonbound estradiol and lower levels of sex hormone binding globulin (SHBG). (48) Perhaps SHBG measurements should be added to our screening efforts.

3. *Exogenous Estrogen.* Epidemiologic and other information continue to suggest some estrogen-related promoter function. These include: a) the condition is 100 times more common in women than in men, b) breast cancer invariably occurs after puberty, c) untreated gonadal dysgenesis and breast cancer are mutually exclusive, d) a 65% excess rate of breast cancer has been observed among women who have had an endometrial cancer, and e) breast tumors contain estrogen receptors which are biologically active as indicated by the presence of progesterone receptors in tumor tissue. Taken together, these data suggest an element of estrogen dependence, if not provocation, in many breast cancers. What is the evidence that exogenous estrogen therapy can provide the same stimulus in vulnerable recipients?

Early studies had in general found little overall effect, but higher risks were suggested for special sub-categories—high parity, nulliparous women, and women with benign breast disease. In several studies, the risk was higher with natural menopause; in one study the risk was highest for menopause due to oophorectomy.

The divergent results are probably due to study size, with positive results based on small numbers. We now have available 2 large studies with comforting results. Data from both the Boston Drug Surveillance Program and the CDC Cancer and Sex Hormone Study indicate that postmenopausal use of estrogens does not increase the risk for breast cancer.(49,50) Even better, the studies were large enough to provide data in the various sub-categories. The absence of an effect was evident among all of the groups of women for which we have concern. Specifically, there was no evidence for an effect regardless of age at menarche, age at menopause, age of first pregnancy, menopause by surgery, family history of breast cancer, use of estrogen for many years, or use of high doses. The answer is rather definitive. Exogenous estrogen in appropriate doses does not increase the risk of breast cancer.

4. *Thyroid, Prolactin, Various Nonestrogen Drugs.* Despite isolated suggestions of increased risk, hypothyroidism, reserpine, or prolactin excess, whether spontaneous or drug induced, are not related to an enhanced risk of breast cancer.

5. *Birth Control Pills and Breast Cancer.* The large number of women taking or having taken oral contraceptive steroids, combined with the belief that steroids provoke or promote abnormal breast growth and possibly cancer, has provided a source of major concern for years. The Royal College of General Practitioners, Oxford Family Planning Association, and Walnut Creek studies have indicated no significant differences in breast cancer rates between users and non-users. However patients were enrolled in these studies at a time when oral contraceptives were used primarily by married couples spacing out their children. Because this population may not reflect use by younger women delaying their first pregnancy, several case-control studies focused on the use of oral contraceptives before the age of 25.(51-53) All reported an increased risk of breast cancer in early users of oral contraceptives. Another case-control study suggested that the risk of premenopausal breast cancer is increased by long-term use (12 or more years) in young women.(54)

These reports prompted the Centers for Disease Control in Atlanta to review information from its on-going case-control study on steroid use and cancer. No increased risk of breast cancer was found in women using oral contraceptives before the age of 20 with a duration of use greater than 4 years, or before the age of 25 with a duration of use greater than 6 years, or with greater than 4 years use before a first pregnancy.(55) In addition, no increased risk of breast cancer was found among any subgroups of users including women with benign breast disease or a family history of breast cancer.

In a further analysis of the CDC study, the largest on the subject, there was no increased risk associated with any specific type of oral contraceptive, progestin only pills, or the use of 2 or more types.(56) In addition, there was no increased risk associated with any specific progestin or estrogen component, and most importantly, it was demonstrated that long-term use (15 or more years) was not associated with an increased risk of breast cancer. The reliability of the CDC study is reinforced by the fact that the data confirmed the already well-known risk factors, such as nulliparity, late age at first birth, history of benign breast disease, and a family history of breast cancer. Finally, the CDC conclusions are supported by a significant national study from New Zealand.(57)

The results of the CDC study, because of its large size, are very reassuring. However, because the population at risk for breast cancer is the age group over 45 years old, and because of the long latent phase for breast cancer, data in the 1990's and 2000's will be required to answer one last very important question: the possibility of very late effects of use. Thus far, the CDC Cancer and Steroid Hormone Study has found no evidence for a latent effect on breast cancer risk through age 54.

Worth emphasizing is a protective effect on benign disease of the breast associated with the progestin component of the pill, an effect which becomes apparent after 2 years of continuous usage. After this time there is a progressive reduction in the incidence of fibrocystic changes in the breast with increasing duration of use. Women who take the pill are one-fourth as likely to develop benign breast disease as nonusers.

6. *Breast Cancer in Diethylstilbestrol (DES)-exposed Women.* Exposure to DES occurred in association with 2 million live births; therefore, the risk for induction of breast cancer during a period of breast differentiation could be significant if DES were a true breast carcinogen. The major study on this subject reported on the follow-up of women who participated in a controlled trial of DES in pregnancy between 1950 and 1952 at the University of Chicago. In this study, no significant association between breast cancer and DES exposure was found.(58) Reinterpretation post hoc in the public press led to a review of the original data and additional information from the national DESAD (DES plus adenosis) Project at the Mayo Clinic.(59) In this new study, among 408 women given DES, there were 8 confirmed cases of breast cancer, in comparison with an expected number of 8.1 based upon breast cancer incidence rates among parous women in the local population. The original Chicago report of no association was confirmed. However, a large collaborative study, involving approximately 6000 women, concluded that there is a small but significant increase in the risk of breast cancer many years later in life in women exposed to DES during pregnancy.(60) Certainly it would be wise to recommend to DES-exposed women that they adhere religiously to screening for breast cancer, including mammography as discussed below.

The Estrogen Window Hypothesis for the Etiology of Breast Cancer

Stanley G. Korenman has promulgated a most interesting thesis concerning the endocrinology of breast cancer. (61,62) Recognizing that the endocrine changes thought to be related to the promotion or provocation of breast cancer were small, inconsistent, did not persist in crossculture or single culture studies, and could hardly account for the 5-fold differential risk of breast cancer among populations, Korenman concluded that *endocrine status is related to breast cancer by influencing the patient's susceptibility to environmental carcinogens.* Recall the dimethylbenzanthracene inducer-promoter model of rodents in which a favorable endocrine environment both increased susceptibility to a single exposure to a known carcinogen and thereafter provided favorable conditions for maintenance and growth of the tumor. Similarly the estrogen window hypothesis in humans has the following components:

1. Human breast cancer is induced by environmental carcinogens in a susceptible mammary gland.

2. Unopposed estrogen stimulation is the most favorable state for tumor induction (the ''open'' window).

3. The duration of exposure to estrogens determines risk (how long the window is ''open'').

303

4. There is a long latent period between tumor induction and clinical expression.

5. Susceptibility to induction ("inducibility") declines with the establishment of normal luteal phase progesterone secretion and becomes very low during pregnancy. (The "open" window is closed, but if tumor has been induced during a previous "open" window period, the hormones which reduce susceptibility nevertheless may promote maintenance and growth.)

The two main induction "open window" periods are the pubertal years prior to the establishment of regular ovulatory menstrual cycles and the perimenopausal period of waning follicle maturation and ovulation. The prolongation of these open windows by obesity, infertility, delayed pregnancy, earlier menarche, and later menopause would be associated with increased susceptibility to an environmental carcinogen. Opposed estrogen (as in birth control pill users and DES exposure during pregnancy) would not increase susceptibility.

Korenman has cited independent support for the estrogen window hypothesis—breast cancer incidence studies of populations exposed to a single carcinogen superimposed on the normal environmental risks. Such data are reported in the extended life-span study of atomic bomb survivors from Hiroshima and Nagasaki, and women with tuberculosis receiving repeated fluoroscopies. Inducibility, the presence of windows, and a latency period between induction and clinical expression were demonstrated in each. In the A-bomb survivors, no breast cancer was seen in children irradiated under the age of 10; increased differences in risk occurred if exposure occurred between age 10 and 29 with an especially marked risk exposure period between 10 and 14 years—the period just before menarche.(63) Excess risk due to irradiation decreased rapidly so that, if exposure occurred between 30 and 49 years of age, there was no significant breast cancer increase over nonradiated controls. After age 50, increased inducibility seemed to reappear.

In the repeatedly fluoroscoped women with tuberculosis, the greatest incremental risk of breast cancer over un-x-rayed controls occurred in those exposed in the 15-20 year age group with no increase after age 30.(64) The greatest risk appeared 15 years after exposure and persisted at least 40 years.

While the estrogen window hypothesis is not proven it has appealing clarity as well as partial supportive data. It explains many, but not all the elements of risk in breast cancer. It reminds us of duration as well as the intensity of inducer and promoter substances. It explains the lack of consistent hormonal findings in patients with established breast cancer even though a hormonal factor appears obvious in the pathogenesis of the disorder. It suggests that growth factors regulated by the endocrine environment may be determinants of breast cancer growth.

Progestational
Protection

There is a growing story that exposure to progestational agents is prophylactic against breast cancer. This is consistent with the open window hypothesis. It is progesterone which closes the window, and for that reason, the risk of breast cancer is increased with those factors associated with long-term exposure to unopposed estrogen. On the other hand, progestational agents have been implicated as causal factors for breast cancer. The situation is a very special one, being limited only to experiments with beagle dogs. Mammary tumors in the beagle dog are increased as a result of prolonged stimulation with large doses (up to 25 times human luteal phase levels) of progesterone or 17-hydroxyprogesterone derivatives (such as medroxyprogesterone acetate). This has not been reported in any other species, and there is no clinical evidence for a relationship between progestin use and breast cancer in women. Indeed, World Health Organization follow-up of women using Depo-Provera for contraception indicates that exposure to Depo-Provera protects women against breast cancer.(65)

One would expect the same mechanism of estrogen receptor depletion to operate in both the endometrium and the breast, and that protection against abnormal mitotic activity should exist in both target tissues. In one long-term follow-up study and one prospective, controlled study, there is an indication that the addition of monthly progestational exposure to an estrogen replacement program lowers the incidence of breast cancer in postmenopausal women.(66,67) There are legitimate criticisms of these studies, and by no means should the conclusions be accepted as definitive. Nevertheless, there is logic to this contention. For example, progestational agents inhibit the in vitro multiplication of human breast cancer cells.(68)

Receptors and Clinical
Prognosis

There is an excellent correlation between the presence of estrogen receptors and certain clinical characteristics of breast cancer. Premenopausal and younger patients are more frequently receptor negative. Patients with receptor positive tumors survive longer and have longer disease-free intervals after mastectomy than those with receptor negative tumors. The presence of an estrogen receptor correlates with increased disease-free interval regardless of the presence of axillary nodes, or the size and location of the tumors. Similarly, patients without axillary lymph node metastases, but with an estradiol receptor negative tumor, have the same high rate of recurrence as do patients with axillary lymph node metastases.

It appears that patients with estrogen receptors are those with the more slowly growing tumors. Several reports indicate that estrogen receptor status correlates with the degree of differentiation of the primary tumor. A large proportion of highly differentiated Grade I carcinomas are receptor positive while the reverse is true of Grade III tumors.

Remember that it takes estrogen to make progesterone receptors. Therefore the presence of progesterone receptors proves that the estrogen receptor in the tumor is biologically active. Thus, it is not surprising that the presence of progesterone receptors has a correlation with disease free survival of patients only second to the number of positive nodes.(69) The best prognosis is seen in patients with positive progesterone receptors, even with subsequent disease, if the recurrent disease is still progesterone receptor positive. The loss of progesterone receptors is an ominous sign.

Treatment Selection

The receptor assay is a valuable prognostic indicator, which combined with lymph node status and tumor histologic grade, can be used in management of patients with breast cancer.

The correlation between the presence of estrogen and progesterone receptors and the clinical response to all types of endocrine therapy has been established. Between 50 and 60% of receptor positive postmenopausal patients responded to ablation of hormones which is almost double the response rate in unselected patients with breast cancer. Less than 10% of receptor negative tumors showed a response (scored as tumor size regression of 50% for a period exceeding a month). Receptor negative patients can be spared unnecessary surgery and months of fruitless trials of hormone therapy by the prompt initiation of chemotherapy.

Current guidelines from the U. S. National Cancer Institute are as follows:

Premenopausal Women:

Positive Nodes—treatment with chemotherapy regardless of receptor status.

Negative Nodes—adjuvant therapy considered only in high risk situations.

Postmenopausal Women:

Positive Nodes—positive receptor status: treat with tamoxifen. negative receptor status: consider chemotherapy.

Negative Nodes—adjuvant therapy considered only in high risk situations.

Some disagree with these recommendations (which they label as conservative), arguing that it makes sense to use aggressive adjuvant therapy for node-negative patients. The problem remains that at the time of diagnosis we are usually dealing with a disease which has reached the point of dissemination. Effective treatment requires earlier diagnosis.

Aspiration

Needle aspiration of breast lumps should be part of the practice of everyone who cares for women. The technique is easy. A small infiltrate of xylocaine is placed in the skin. Holding the lesion between thumb and index fingers with one hand, the other hand passes a 21 gauge needle attached to a 10 ml syringe several times through the lesion with continuous suction on the syringe. Air is forcibly ejected through the needle on to a cytology slide for smearing and fixing. The usual Pap smear fixative can be used.

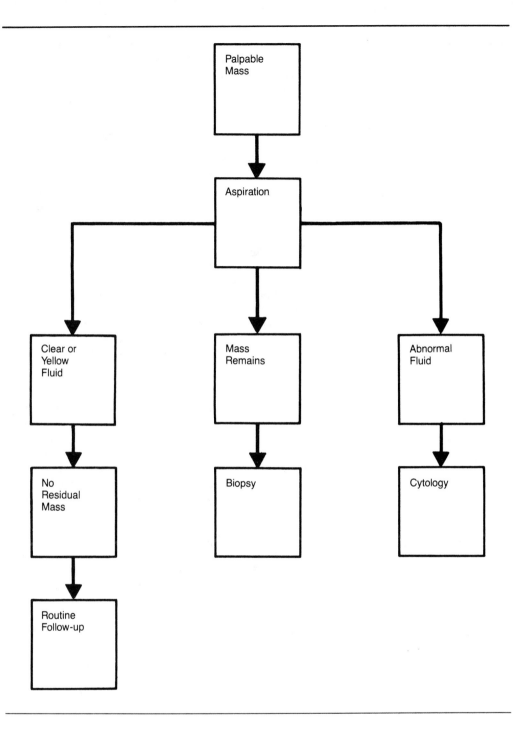

The procedure is very cost effective. When aspiration yields clear or yellow fluid and the mass disappears, the procedure is both diagnostic and therapeutic. Fluid of any other nature requires cytologic assessment. Failure to obtain material for histologic evaluation or the persistence of a mass requires biopsy. Locally recurrent cysts should be surgically removed.

Mammography

Mammography is a means of detecting the nonpalpable cancer. In the past few years technical advancements have significantly improved the mammographic image.(70) The doubling time of breast cancer is very variable, but in general, a tumor doubles in size every 100 days. Thus it takes a single malignant cell approximately 10 years to grow to a clinically detectable 1 cm mass, but by this time a tumor of 1 cm has already progressed through 30 of the 40 doublings in size which is estimated to be fatal. (71) Furthermore, the average size at which a tumor is detected (70-75% of tumors are found by patients themselves) is 2.5 cm, a size which has a 50% incidence of lymph node involvement. To decrease the mortality from breast cancer, we must utilize a technique to find the tumors when they are smaller. Mammography is the answer.

In the 1970s, xeromammography significantly reduced the amount of radiation delivered with x-ray mammography. In the 1980s, the film screen system (using special film against a fluorescent screen) now delivers approximately 0.1 rad per examination. With this amount of irradiation, there is no longer a concern for the radiation dose. From a diagnostic point of view, there is no difference between the film screen technique and xeromammography, however xeromammography delivers more radiation (although the slight increase with the very latest xeromammographic technique is probably insignificant).

Mammography is the technique of choice. Thermography has a high rate of false positive findings, and at best, should be considered experimental. Ultrasound can rarely reveal malignant lesions under 1 cm in size. It is useful, however, to guide the aspiration of lesions. CT scanning has 2 serious limitations. The x-ray dose is large, and the slices are too thick to detect early lesions. Finally, magnetic resonance imaging is not practical because of the long scan times that are necessary.

Mammography is the only method that detects clustered microcalcifications. These calcifications are less than 1 mm in diameter and are frequently associated with malignant lesions. More than 5 calcifications in a cluster are associated with cancer 25% of the time and require biopsy.

Mammography has a false negative rate of 8 to 10%. This means that masses are palpable but not visible. Mammography cannot and should not replace examination by patient and physician. Cancer commonly presents as a solitary, solid, painless, hard, unilateral, irregular nonmobile mass. A mass requires biopsy regardless of the mammographic picture.

A pattern of dysplasia on the mammogram carries with it an increased risk (2.0-3.5 times normal) of breast cancer. The risk is similar to that seen with the other known risk factors.(72)

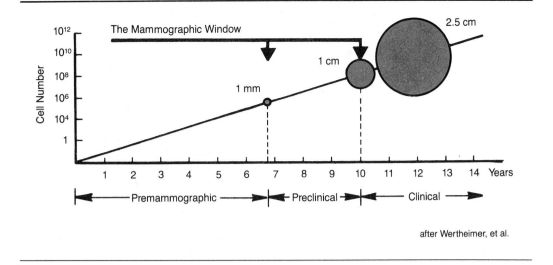

after Wertheimer, et al.

The Effectiveness of Mammography. It is now apparent that mammography is effective in reducing the mortality of breast cancer. The Health Insurance Plan of New York screening program demonstrated a 30% decrease in mortality in the screened group over 50 years old.(73) There are currently large scale trials ongoing, but preliminary results are very impressive. In Nijmegan, the breast cancer mortality rate in women of 35 and over was reduced by 50% by annual mammographic screening.(74) In Utrecht, the relative risk of dying from breast cancer among screened women was reduced by 70%.(75)

The first randomized, controlled trial of mammography was begun in Sweden in 1977. Results to the end of 1984 demonstrated a 31% reduction in mortality and a 25% reduction in more advanced breast disease, with a further acceleration of this reduction by the end of 1985.(76,77) Most impressively, these results were obtained with a screening only every 2-3 years and with only a single medio-lateral oblique view.

Until recently, it was questioned whether mammography screening was effective for women under 50. The American Breast Cancer Detection Demonstration Project has now demonstrated that screening is just as effective for women in their 40s as in women over 50.(78) This program whch was organized by the American Cancer Society and the National Cancer Institute began operating in 1973 in 27 locations throughout the United States, enrolling more than 280,000 women. Despite the fact that this is not an organized research study with a control group, the massive database permits many valuable conclusions. From 1977 to 1982, similar high survival rates (87%) for women in their 40s compared with women in their 50s verify that screening was just as effectve in the younger women. An important point made by this Project is the very significant role played by the women participating in the study. For an effective breast screening progam, women must be very active in their interaction with the process (including both the medical profession and the detection technology). Cooperation and alertness of the women are key ingredients for achieving success.

309

There are problems to be anticipated with extensive mammography screening. Small nonpalpable lesions have less than a 5% chance of being malignant, and overall, only about 20-30% of biopsy specimens contain carcinoma. That means there will be a large number of biopsies and mammograms performed (including the treatment of clinically irrelevant lesions), which involves costs to the health care system and cost to the individual in terms of stress and anxiety. Indeed, one analysis of risks and benefits concludes that because breast cancer is relatively infrequent under the age of 50, it is not cost effective to screen all asymptomatic women aged 40-49.(79) Nevertheless mammography is the most potent weapon we possess in the battle against breast cancer. Mammography not only lowers mortality, but it also decreases morbidity because less radical surgery is necessary for smaller lesions.

Every woman should be regarded as at risk. Health care professionals who interact with women have the opportunity to initiate an aggressive program of preventive health care. The major deterrent to patient use of mammography is the absence of physician recommendations. We urge you to follow these suggested guidelines:

SCREENING FOR BREAST CANCER

All women should be taught self-breast examination by age 20. Because of the changes which occur routinely in response to the hormonal sequence of a normal menstrual cycle, breast examination is most effective during the follicular phase of the cycle.

All women over the age of 35 should have an annual breast examination.

A baseline mammogram should be obtained by age 40, or earlier if high risk factors are present.

From ages 40 to 50, mammography should be performed every 2 years in low risk women and every year in women with significant risk factors.

Annual breast examination and annual mammography should be performed in all women over age 50.

SIGNIFICANT HIGH RISK FACTORS

Family history of breast cancer in mother or sister.

Proliferative disease of the breast by biopsy.

First childbirth after age 30.

Dysplasia on mammography.

Relatively low SHBG levels.

References

1. **Topper YL,** Multiple hormone interactions in the development of the mammary gland in vitro, Recent Prog Horm Res 26:287, 1970.

2. **Christiansen E, Veldhuis JD, Rogol AD, Stumpf P, Evan WS,** Modulating actions of estradiol on gonadotropin-releasing hormone-stimulated prolactin secretion in postmenopausal individuals, Am J Obstet Gynecol 157:320, 1987.

3. **Tyson JE, Hwang P, Guyda H, Friesen HG,** Studies of prolactin secretion in human pregnancy, Am J Obstet Gynecol 113:14, 1972.

4. **Murphy LJ, Murphy LC, Stead B, Sutherland RL, Lazarus L,** Modulation of lactogenic receptors by progestins in cultured human breast cancer cells, J Clin Endocrinol Metab 62:280, 1986.

5. **Simon WE, Pahnke VG, Holzel F,** In vitro modulation of prolactin binding to human mammary carcinoma cells by steroid hormones and prolactin, J Clin Endocrinol Metab 60:1243, 1985.

6. **Daly DC, Kuslis S, Riddick DH,** Evidence of short-loop inhibition of decidual prolactin synthesis by decidual proteins, Part I, Am J Obstet Gynecol 155:358, 1986.

7. **Raabe MA, McCoshen JA,** Epithelial regulation of prolactin effect on amnionic permeability, Am J Obstet Gynecol 154:130, 1986.

8. **Tyson JE, Friesen HG,** Factors influencing the secretion of human prolactin and growth hormone in menstrual and gestational women, Am J Obstet Gynecol 116:377, 1973.

9. **Barberia JM, Abu-Fadil S, Kletzky OA, Nakamura RM, Mishell DR Jr,** Serum prolactin patterns in early human gestation, Am J Obstet Gynecol 121:1107, 1975.

10. **Ehara Y, Siler TM, Yen SSC,** Effects of large doses of estrogen on prolactin and growth hormone release, Am J Obstet Gynecol 125:455, 1976.

11. **Battin DA, Marrs RP, Fleiss PM, Mishell DR Jr,** Effect of suckling on serum prolactin, luteinizing hormone, follicle-stimulating hormone, and estradiol during prolonged lactation, Obstet Gynecol 65:785, 1985.

12. **Dawood MY, Khan-Dawood FS, Wahl RS, Fuchs F,** Oxytocin release and plasma anterior pituitary and gonadal hormones in women during lactation, J Clin Endocrinol Metab 52:678, 1981.

13. **Auerbach KG, Avery JL,** Induced lactation, Am J Dis Child 135:340, 1981.

14. **Ben-Jonathan N,** Dopamine: A prolactin-inhibiting hormone, Endocrin Rev 6:564, 1985.

15. **McNeilly AS,** Effects of lactation on fertility, Brit Med Bull 35:151, 1979.

16. **Tyson JE, Carter JN, Andreassen B, Huth J, Smith B,** Nursing mediated prolactin and luteinizing hormone secretion during puerperal lactation, Fertil Steril 30:154, 1978.

17. **Sauder SE, Frager M, Case GD, Kelch RP, Marshall JC,** Abnormal patterns of pulsatile luteinizing hormone secretion in women with hyperprolactinemia and amenorrhea: Responses to bromocriptine, J Clin Endocrinol Metab 59:941, 1984.

18. **Petraglia F, De Leo V, Nappi C, Facchinetti F, Montemagno U, Brambilla F, Genazzani AR,** Differences in the opioid control of luteinizing hormone secretion between pathological and iatrogenic hyperprolactinemic states, J Clin Endocrinol Metab 64:508, 1987.

19. **Gray RH, Campbell OM, Zacur HA, Labbok MH, MacRae SL,** Postpartum return of ovarian activity in nonbreastfeeding women monitored by urinary assays, J Clin Endocrinol Metab 64:645, 1987.

20. **Hwang PLH, Ng CSA, Cheong ST,** Effect of oral contraceptives on serum prolactin: A longitudinal study in 126 normal premenopausal women, Clin Endocrinol 24:127, 1986.

21. **Sherman L, Fisher A, Klass E, Markowitz S,** Pharmacologic causes of hyperprolactinemia, Seminars Reprod Endocrinol 2:31, 1984.

22. **Pye JK, Mansel RE, Hughes LE,** Clinical experience of drug treatments for mastalgia, Lancet ii:373, 1985.

23. **Fentiman IS, Brame K, Caleffi M, Chaudary MA, Hayward JL,** Double-blind controlled trial of tamoxifen therapy for mastalgia, Lancet i:287, 1986.

24. **Ernster VL, Mason L, Goodson WH III, Sickles EA, Sacks ST, Selvin S, Dupuy ME, Hawkinson J, Hunt TK,** Effects of caffeine-free diet on benign breast disease: A randomized trial, Surgery 91:263, 1982.

25. **Lubin F, Ron E, Wax Y, Black M, Funaro M, Shitrit A,** A case-control study of caffeine and methylxanthines in benign breast disease, JAMA 253:2388, 1985.

26. **Schairer C, Brinton LA, Hoover RN,** Methylxanthines and benign breast disease, Am J Epidemiol 124:603, 1986.

27. **Silverberg E, Lubera J,** Cancer Statistics, 1988, CA 38:5, 1988.

28. **Henderson IC, Cannellos GP,** Cancer of the breast, New Eng J Med 302:17,78, 1980.

29. **Bland KI,** Risk factors as an indicator for breast cancer screening in asymptomatic patients, Maturitas 9:135, 1987.

30. **Pathak DR, Speizer FE, Willett WC, Rosner B, Lipnick RJ,** Parity and breast cancer risk: Possible effect on age at diagnosis, Int J Cancer 37:21, 1986.

31. **Musey VC, Collins DC, Brogan DR, Santos VR, Musey PI, Martino-Saltzman D, Preedy JRK,** Long term effects of a first pregnancy on the hormonal environment: Estrogens and androgens, J Clin Endocrinol Metab 64:111, 1987.

32. **Musey VC, Collins DC, Musey PI, Martino-Saltzman D, Preedy JRK,** Long-term effects of a first pregnancy on the secretion of prolactin, New Eng J Med 316:229, 1987.

33. **Byers T, Graham S, Rzepka T, Marshall J,** Lactation and breast cancer: Evidence for a negative association in premenopausal women, Am J Epidemiol 121:664, 1985.

34. **Ing R, Ho JHC, Petrakis NL,** Unilateral breast-feeding and breast cancer, Lancet ii:124, 1977.

35. **Sherman B, Wallace R, Beam J, Schlabaugh L,** Relationship of body weight to menarchial and menopausal age: Implication for breast cancer risk, J Clin Endocrinol Metab 52:488, 1981.

36. **Dupont WD, Page DL,** Risk factors for breast cancer in women with proliferative breast disease, New Eng J Med 312:146, 1985.

37. **Cancer Committee, College of American Pathologists,** Is 'fibrocystic disease' of the breast precancerous? Arch Path Lab Med 110:171, 1986.

38. **Sattin RW, Rubin GL, Webster LA, Huezo CM, Wingo PA, Ory HW, Layde PM,** Family history and the risk of breast cancer, JAMA 253:1908, 1985.

39. **Willett WC, Browne ML, Bain C, Lipnick RJ, Stampfer MJ, Rosner B, Colditz GA, Hennekens CH, Speizer FE,** Relative weight and risk of breast cancer among premenopausal women, Am J Epidemiol 122:731, 1985.

40. **Willett WC, Stampfer MJ, Colditz GA, Rosner BA, Hennekens CH, Speizer FE,** Dietary fat and the risk of breast cancer, New Eng J Med 316:22, 1987.

41. **Willett WC, Stampfer MJ, Colditz GA, Rosner BA, Hennekens CH, Speizer FE,** Moderate alcohol consumption and the risk of breast cancer, New Eng J Med 316:1174, 1987.

42. **Bulbrook RD,** Urinary androgen excretion and the etiology of breast cancer, JNCI 48:1039, 1972.

43. **Dickinson LE, MacMahon B, Cole P, Brown JB,** Estrogen profiles of Oriental and Caucasian women in Hawaii, New Engl J Med 291:1211, 1974.

44. **Sherman BM, Korenman SG,** Inadequate corpus luteum function: a pathophysiologic interpretation of human breast cancer epidemiology, Cancer 33:1306, 1974.

45. **McFayden IJ, Forrest APM, Prescott RJ, Golder MP, Groom GV, Fahmy DR,** Circulating hormone concentrations in women with breast cancer, Lancet i:1000, 1976.

46. **Cowan LD, Gordis L, Tonascia JA, Jones GS,** Breast cancer incidence in women with a history of progesterone deficiency, Am J Epidemiol, 114:209, 1981.

47. **Coulam CB, Annegars JF,** Chronic anovulation may increase postmenopausal breast cancer risk, JAMA 249:445, 1983.

48. **Cuzick J, Wang DY, Bulbrook RD,** The prevention of breast cancer, Lancet i:83, 1986.

49. **Kaufman DW, Miller DR, Rosenberg L, Helmrich SP, Stolley P, Schottenfeld D, Shapiro S,** Noncontraceptive estrogen use and the risk of breast cancer, JAMA 252:63, 1984.

50. **Wingo PA Layde PM, Lee NC, Rubin G, Ory HW,** The risk of breast cancer in postmenopausal women who have used estrogen replacment therapy, JAMA 257:209, 1987.

51. **Pike MC, Krailo MD, Henderson BE, Duke A, Roy S,** Breast cancer in young women and use of oral contraceptives: possible modifying effect of formulation and age at use, Lancet ii:926, 1983.

52. **McPherson K, Neil A, Vessey MP,** Oral contraceptives and breast cancer, Lancet ii:414, 1983.

53. **Olsson H, Landin-Olsson M, Moller TR, Ranstam J, Holm P,** Oral contraceptive use and breast cancer in young women in Sweden, Lancet i:748, 1985.

54. **Meirik O, Dami H, Christoffersen T, Lund E, Bergstrom R, Bergsjo P,** Oral contraceptive use and breast cancer in young women, Lancet ii:650, 1986.

55. **Stadel BV, Rubin GL, Webster LA, Schlesselman JJ, Wingo PA,** Oral contraceptives and breast cancer in young women, Lancet ii:970, 1985.

56. **Cancer and Steroid Hormone Study, CDC and NICHD,** Oral contraceptive use and the risk of breast cancer, New Eng J Med 315:405, 1986.

57. **Paul C, Skegg DCG, Spears GFS, Kaldor JM,** Oral contraceptives and breast cancer: a national study, Brit Med J 2923:723, 1986.

58. **Bibbo M, Haenszel W, Wied GL, Hubby M, Herbst AL,** A twenty-five year follow-up study of women exposed to DES during pregnancy, New Eng J Med 298:763, 1978.

59. **Brian OD, Tilley BC, LaBarthe DR, O'Fallon WM, Noller KL, Kurland LT,** Breast cancer in DES exposed mothers: Absence of association, Mayo Clin Proc 55:89, 1980.

60. **Greenburg ER, Barnes AB, Resseguie L, Barrett JA, Burnside S, Lanza LL, Neff RK, Stevens M, Young RH, Colton T,** Breast cancer in mothers given diethylstilbestrol in pregnancy, New Eng J Med 311:1393, 1984.

61. **Korenman SG,** The endocrinology of breast cancer, Cancer 46:874, 1980.

62. **Korenman SG,** Estrogen window hypothesis of the etiology of breast cancer, Lancet i:700, 1980.

63. **Tokunaga M, Norman JE, Asano M, Tokuoka S, Ezaki H, Nishimori I, Tsuji Y,** Malignant breast tumors among atomic bomb survivors, JNCI 62:1347, 1979.

64. **Boice JD, Monson RR,** Breast cancer in women after repeated fluoroscopic examinations of the chest, JNCI 59:823, 1977.

65. **W.H.O. Collaborative Study of Neoplasia and Steroid Contraceptives,** Breast cancer, cervical cancer, and depot medroxyprogesterone acetate, Lancet ii:1207, 1984.

66. **Gambrell RD Jr, Maier RC, Sanders BI,** Decreased incidence of breast cancer in postmenopausal estrogen-progestogen users, Obstet Gynecol 62:435, 1983.

67. **Nachtigall LE, Nachtigall RH, Nachtigall RB, Beckman M,** Estrogen replacement: II. A prospective study in the relationship to carcinoma and cardiovascular and metabolic problems, Obstet Gynecol 54:74, 1979.

68. **Vignon F, Bardon S, Chalbos D, Rochefort H,** Antiestrogenic effect of R5020, a synthetic progestin in human breast cancer cells in culture, J Clin Endocrinol Metab 56:1124, 1983

69. **McGuire WL, Clark LGM,** Role of progesterone receptors in breast cancer, CA 36:302, 1986.

70. **Kopans LDB, Meyer JE, Sadowsky N,** Breast imaging, New Eng J Med 310:960, 1984.

71. **Wertheimer MD, Costanza ME, Dodson TF, D'Orsi C, Pastides H, Zapka JG,** Increasing the effort toward breast cancer detection, JAMA 255:1311, 1986.

72. **Carlile T, Kopecky KJ, Thompson DJ, Whitehead JR, Gilbert FI Jr, Present AJ, Threatt BA, Krook P, Hadaway E,** Breast cancer prediction and the Wolfe classification on mammograms, JAMA 254:1050, 1985.

73. **Shapiro S, Venet W, Strax P, Venet L, Roeser R,** Ten to fourteen year effect of screening on breast cancer mortality, JNCI 69:329, 1982.

74. **Verbeek ALM, Holland R, Sturmans F, Hendriks JHCL, Miravunac M, Day NE,** Reduction of breast cancer mortality through mass screening with modern mammography, Lancet i:1222, 1984.

75. **Collette HJA, Rombach JJ, Day NE, De Waard F,** Evaluation of screening for breast cancer in non-randomized study (the DOM project by means of a case-control study), Lancet i:124, 1984.

76. **Tabar L, Gad A, Holmberg LH, Ljungquist U, Fagerberg CJG, Baldetorp L, Grontoft O, Lundstrom B, Manson JC, Eklund G, Dan NE, Petterson F,** Reduction in mortality from breast cancer after mass screening with mammography, Lancet i:829, 1985.

77. **Tabar L, Faberberg G, Day NE, Holmberg L,** What is the optimum interval between mammographic screening examinations?-An analysis based on the latest results of the Swedish two-county breast cancer screening trial, Brit J Cancer 55:547, 1987.

78. **Seidman H, Gelb SK, Silverberg E, LaVerda N, Lubera JA,** Survival experience in the breast cancer detection demonstration project, CA 37:258, 1987.

79. **Eddy DM, Hasselblad V, McGivney W, Hendee W,** The value of mammography screening in women under age 50 years, JAMA 259:1512, 1988.

10 The Endocrinology of Pregnancy

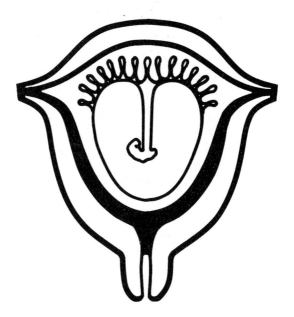

For the fetus, one of the crucial aspects of intrauterine life is its dependency on the effective exchange of nutritive and metabolic products with the mother. It is not surprising that mechanisms exist by which a growing fetus can influence or control the exchange process, and hence its environment. The methods by which a fetus can influence its own growth and development involve a variety of messages transmitted, in many cases, by hormones. Hormonal messengers from the conceptus can affect metabolic processes, uteroplacental blood flow, and cellular differentiation. Furthermore, a fetus may signal its desire and readiness to leave the uterus by hormonal initiation of parturition. *This chapter will review steroid and protein hormones of pregnancy, as well as perinatal thyroid physiology, and fetal lung maturation.*

Steroid Hormones in Pregnancy

Steroidogenesis in the fetal-placental unit does not follow the conventional mechanisms of hormone production within a single organ. Rather, the final products result from critical interactions and interdependence of separate organ systems which individually do not possess the necessary enzymatic capabilities. It is helpful to view the process as consisting of a fetal compartment, a placental compartment, and a maternal compartment. Separately the fetal and placental compartments lack certain steroidogenic activities. Together, however, they are complementary and form a complete unit, which utilizes the maternal compartment as a source of basic building materials and as a resource for clearance of steroids.

Progesterone

In its key location as a way station between mother and fetus, the placenta can utilize precursors from either mother or fetus to circumvent its own deficiencies in enzyme activity. The placenta converts little, if any, acetate to cholesterol or its precursors. Cholesterol as well as pregnenolone are obtained from the maternal blood stream for progesterone synthesis. The fetal contribution is negligible since progesterone levels remain high after fetal demise. Thus, the massive amount of progesterone produced in pregnancy depends upon placental-maternal cooperation.

Progesterone is largely produced by the corpus luteum until about 10 weeks of gestation. Indeed, until approximately the 7th week, the pregnancy is dependent upon the presence of the corpus luteum.(1) Exogenous support for an early pregnancy requires 200 mg progesterone daily. After a transition period of shared function between the 7th week to the 10th week, the placenta emerges as the major source of progesterone. At term, progesterone levels range from 100 to 200 ng/ml, and the placenta produces about 250 mg per day.

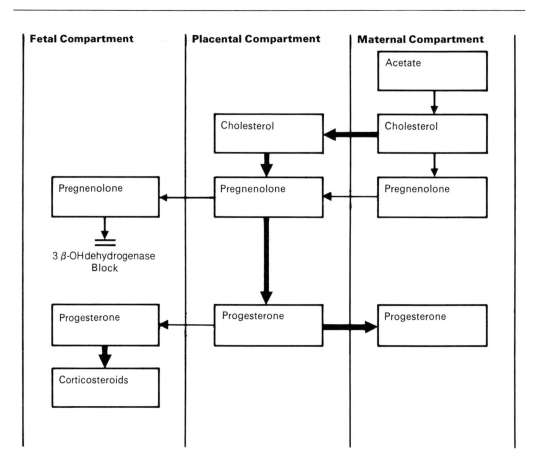

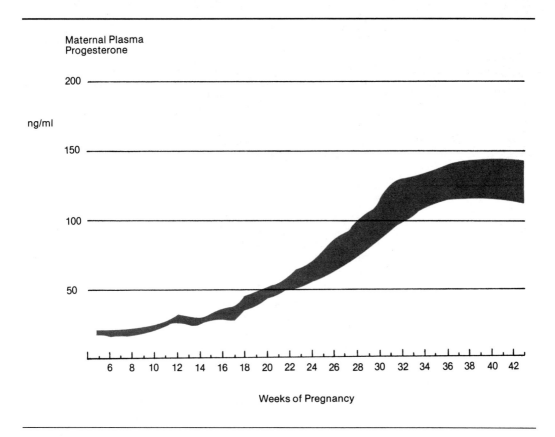

Maternal Plasma Progesterone

ng/ml

Weeks of Pregnancy

In contrast to estrogen, progesterone production by the placenta is largely independent of the quantity of precursor available, the uteroplacental perfusion, fetal well-being, or even the presence of a live fetus. This is because the fetus contributes essentially no precursor. The majority of placental progesterone is derived from maternal cholesterol which is readily available. At term a small portion (3%) is derived from maternal pregnenolone. The cholesterol utilized for progesterone synthesis enters the trophoblast from the bloodstream as low-density lipoprotein (LDL)-cholesterol, by means of the process of endocytosis (internalization) involving the LDL cell membrane receptors.(2,3) Hydrolysis of the protein component of LDL may yield amino acids for the fetus, and essential fatty acids may be derived from hydrolysis of the cholesterol esters.

The human decidua and fetal membranes also synthesize and metabolize progesterone.(4) In this case, neither cholesterol nor LDL-cholesterol are significant substrates; pregnenolone sulfate may be the most important precursor. This local steroidogenesis may play a role in regulating parturition.

Amniotic fluid progesterone concentration is maximal between 10 and 20 weeks, then decreases gradually. Myometrial levels are about 3 times higher than maternal plasma levels in early pregnancy, remain high, and are about equal to the maternal plasma concentration at term.

319

In early pregnancy the levels of 17-hydroxyprogesterone rise, marking the activity of the corpus luteum. By the 10th week of gestation this compound has returned to baseline levels, indicating that the placenta has little 17-hydroxylase activity. However, beginning about the 32nd week there is a second, more gradual rise in 17-hydroxyprogesterone, due to placental utilization of fetal precursors.

There are two active metabolites of progesterone which increase significantly during pregnancy. There is about a 10-fold increase of the 5α-reduced metabolite. 5α-pregnane-3,20-dione.(5) This compound contributes to the refractory state in pregnancy against the pressor action of angiotensin-II. The circulating level, however, is the same in normal and hypertensive pregnancies. The concentration of deoxycorticosterone (DOC) at term is 1200 times the nonpregnant levels. Some of this is due to the 3-4 fold increase in cortisol binding globulin during pregnancy, but a significant amount is due to 21-hydroxylation of circulating progesterone in the kidney.(6) This activity is significant during pregnancy because the rate is proportional to the plasma concentration of progesterone. The fetal kidney is also active in 21-hydroxylation of the progesterone secreted by the placenta into the fetal circulation. At the present time there is no physiologic role known for DOC during pregnancy.

Little is known about specific functions for the various steroids produced throughout pregnancy. Progesterone appears to have a role in parturition as will be discussed in Chapter 11. It also has been suggested that progesterone may be important in suppressing the maternal immunological response to fetal antigens, preventing maternal rejection of the trophoblast. Progesterone has an important role in allowing implantation. Whereas the human corpus luteum makes significant amounts of estradiol, it is progesterone and not estrogen that is required for successful implantation.(7) Since implantation normally occurs about 6-7 days after ovulation, and human chorionic gonadotropin (HCG) must appear by the 10th day after ovulation to rescue the corpus luteum, the blastocyst must successfully implant and secrete HCG within a narrow window of time. In the first 5-6 weeks of pregnancy, HCG stimulation of the corpus luteum results in the daily secretion of about 25 mg of progesterone and 0.5 mg of estradiol. Whereas estrogen levels begin to increase at 4-5 weeks due to placental secretion, progesterone production by the placenta does not increase significantly until about 10-11 weeks after ovulation.

Perhaps the most important role for progesterone is to serve as the principal substrate pool for fetal adrenal gland production of gluco- and mineralocorticoids. The fetal adrenal gland is extremely active, but produces steroids with a 3β-hydroxy-Δ^5 configuration like pregnenolone and dehydroepiandrosterone, rather than 3-keto-Δ^4 products such as progesterone. The fetus therefore lacks significant activity of the 3β-hydroxysteroid dehydrogenase, Δ^{4-5} isomerase system. Thus the fetus must borrow progesterone from the placenta to circumvent this lack, in order to synthesize the biologically important corticosteroids. In return the fetus supplies what the placenta lacks, 19 carbon compounds to serve as precursors for estrogens.

Estrogens

The basic precursors of estrogens are 19 carbon androgens. However, there is a virtual absence of 17-hydroxylation and 17-20 desmolase activity in the human placenta. As a result, 21 carbon products (progesterone and pregnenolone) cannot be converted to 19 carbon steroids (androstenedione and dehydroepiandrosterone). Like progesterone, estrogen produced by the placenta must derive its precursors from outside the placenta.

The androgen compounds utilized for estrogen synthesis in human pregnancy are, in the early months of gestation, derived from the maternal blood stream. By the 20th week of pregnancy, the vast majority of estrogen excreted in the maternal urine is derived from fetal androgens. In particular, approximately 90% of estriol excretion can be accounted for by dehydroepiandrosterone sulfate (DHAS) production by the fetal adrenal gland.(8)

The fetal endocrine compartment also is characterized by rapid and extensive conjugation of steroids with sulfate. Perhaps this is a protective mechanism, blocking the biologic effects of potent steroids present in such great quantities. In order to utilize fetal precursors, the placenta must be extremely efficient in cleaving the sulfate con-

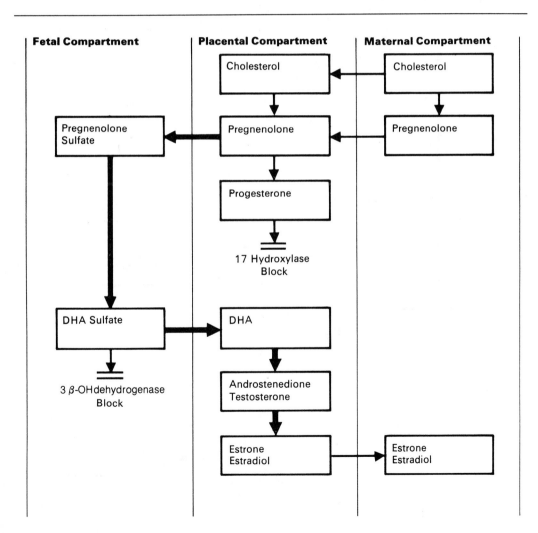

321

jugates brought to it via the fetal bloodstream. Indeed the sulfatase activity in the placenta is rapid and quantitatively very significant. It is recognized that a deficiency in placental sulfatase is associated with low estrogen excretion, giving clinical importance to this metabolic step. This syndrome will be discussed in greater detail later in this chapter.

The fetal adrenal provides DHAS as precursor for placental production of estrone and estradiol. The placenta lacks a 16α-hydroxylation ability, and estriol with its 16α-hydroxyl group must be derived from an immediate fetal precursor. The fetal adrenal, with the aid of 16α-hydroxylation in the fetal liver, provides the 16α-hydroxydehydroepiandrosterone sulfate for placental estriol forma-

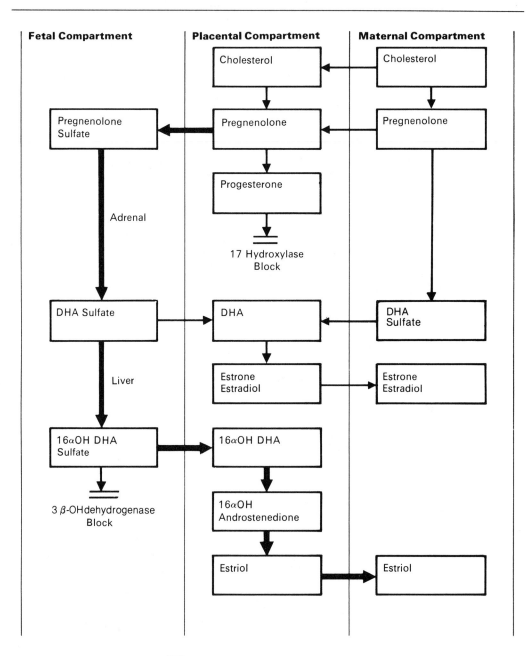

tion. After birth, neonatal 16-hydroxylation activity rapidly disappears. The maternal contribution of DHAS to total estrogen synthesis must be negligible because in the absence of normal fetal adrenal glands (as in an anencephalic infant) maternal estrogen levels and excretion are extremely low. The fetal adrenals secrete more than 200 mg of DHAS daily, about 10 times more than the mother.(9)

The profiles of the unconjugated compounds in the maternal compartment for the three major estrogens in pregnancy are:

1. A rise in estrone begins at 6-10 weeks and individual values range from 2 to 30 ng/ml at term.(10) This wide range in normal values precludes the use of estrone measurements in clinical applications.

2. Individual estradiol values vary between 6 and 40 ng/ml at 36 weeks of gestation, and then undergo an accelerated rate of increase.(11) At term, an equal amount of estradiol arises from maternal DHAS and fetal DHAS and its importance in fetal monitoring is negligible.

3. Estriol is first detectable at 9 weeks when the fetal adrenal gland secretion of precursor begins. Estriol concentrations plateau at 31-35 weeks, then increase again at 35-36 weeks.(11)

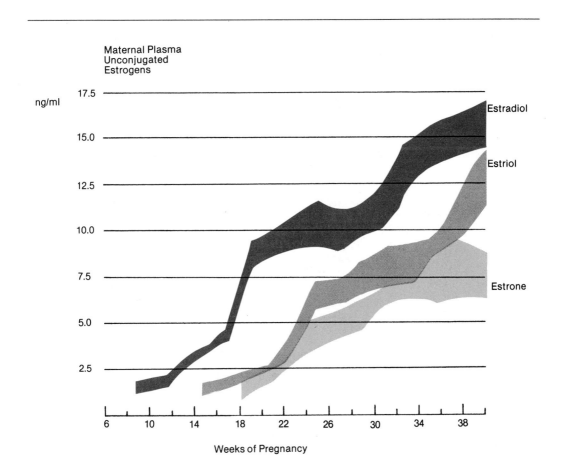

During pregnancy, estrone and estradiol excretion is increased about 100 times over nonpregnant levels. However, the increase in maternal estriol excretion is about a thousand-fold.

The estrogens presented to the maternal bloodstream are rapidly metabolized by the maternal liver prior to excretion into the maternal urine as a variety of more than 20 products. The bulk of these maternal urinary estrogens are composed of glucosiduronates conjugated at the 16-position. Significant amounts of the 3-glucosiduronate and the 3-sulfate-16-glucosiduronate are also excreted. Only approximately 8-10% of the maternal blood estriol is unconjugated.

The Fetal Adrenal Cortex

The fetal adrenal cortex is differentiated by 7 weeks into a thick inner fetal zone and thin outer definitive zone. Early in pregnancy, adrenal growth and development are remarkable, and the gland achieves a size equal to or larger than that of the kidney by the end of the first trimester. After the first trimester the adrenal glands slowly decrease in size until a second spurt in growth begins at about 34-35 weeks. The gland remains proportionately larger than the adult adrenal glands. After delivery, the fetal zone (about 85% of the bulk of the gland) rapidly involutes to be replaced by the adult definitive zone of the adrenal cortex. Thus, the specific steroidogenic characteristics of the fetus are associated with a specific morphologic change of the adrenal gland.

Fetal DHAS production rises steadily concomitant with the increase in fetal adrenal weight.(12) The well-known increase in maternal estrogen levels is significantly influenced by the increased availability of fetal DHAS as a precursor. Indeed, the accelerated rise in maternal estrogen levels near term can be explained in part by an increase in fetal DHAS. The stimulus for the substantial adrenal growth and steroid production has been a puzzle.

Early in pregnancy, the adrenal gland can function without ACTH, perhaps in response to HCG. After 20 weeks, fetal ACTH is required. However, during the last 12-14 weeks of pregnancy when fetal ACTH levels are declining, the adrenal quadruples in size.(13) Because pituitary prolactin is the only fetal pituitary hormone to increase throughout pregnancy, paralleling fetal adrenal gland size changes, it has been proposed that fetal prolactin is the critical tropic substance. In experimental preparations, however, only ACTH exerts a steroidogenic effect. There is no fetal adrenal response to prolactin, HCG, growth hormone, or melanocyte-stimulating hormone (MSH).(14,15) Furthermore, in patients treated with bromocriptine, fetal blood prolactin levels are suppressed, but DHAS levels are unchanged.(16) Nevertheless, interest in prolactin persists as both ACTH and prolactin can stimulate steroidogenesis in vivo in the fetal baboon.(17)

There is no question that ACTH is essential for the steroidogenic mechanism of the fetal adrenal gland.(18) ACTH activates adenylate cyclase, leading to steroidogenesis. Soon the supply of cholesterol becomes rate-limiting. Further ACTH action results in an increase in LDL receptors leading to an increased uptake of circulating LDL-cholesterol. With internalization of LDL-cholesterol, hydrolysis by lysosomal enzymes of the cholesterol ester makes choles-

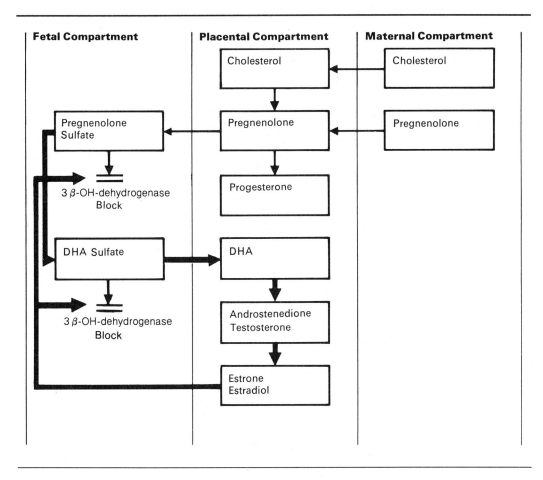

Fetal Compartment	Placental Compartment	Maternal Compartment
	Cholesterol	Cholesterol
Pregnenolone Sulfate	Pregnenolone	Pregnenolone
3 β-OH-dehydrogenase Block	Progesterone	
DHA Sulfate	DHA	
3 β-OH-dehydrogenase Block	Androstenedione Testosterone	
	Estrone Estradiol	

terol available for steroidogenesis. For this reason, fetal plasma levels of LDL are low, and after birth newborn levels of LDL rise as the fetal adrenal involutes. In the presence of low levels of LDL-cholesterol, the fetal adrenal is capable of synthesizing cholesterol de novo.(19) Thus near term, both de novo synthesis and utilization of LDL-cholesterol are necessary to sustain the high rates of DHAS and estrogen formation.

The unique features of the fetal adrenal gland can be ascribed to its high estrogen environment. A series of tissue culture studies has demonstrated that hormonal peptides of pituitary or placental origin are not the factors which are responsible for the behavior of the fetal adrenal gland.(20-22) Estrogens at high concentration inhibit 3β-hydroxysteroid dehydrogenase-isomerase activity in the fetal adrenal gland, and in the presence of ACTH enhance the secretion of dehydroepiandrosterone (DHA). Estradiol concentrations of 10-100 ng/ml are required to inhibit cortisol secretion.(23) The total estrogen concentrations in the fetus are easily in this range. A study of the kinetics of 3β-hydroxysteroid dehydrogenase activity in human adrenal microsomes reveals that all steroids are inhibitory, and most notably, estrone and estradiol at levels found in fetal life cause almost total inhibition. (24) The hyperplasia of the fetal adrenal cortex is the result of the high ACTH levels due to the relatively low cortisol levels, a consequence of the enzyme inhibition. With birth and loss of exposure to estrogen, the fetal adrenal gland quickly changes to the adult type of gland.

The principal mission of the fetal adrenal may be to provide DHAS as the basic precursor for placental estrogen production. Estrogen, in turn, feeds back to the adrenal to direct steroidogenesis along the Δ^5 pathway to provide even more of its precursor, DHAS. Thus far this is the only known function for DHAS.

Measurement of Estrogen in Pregnancy

Because pregnancy is characterized by a great increase in maternal estrogen levels, and estrogen production is dependent upon fetal and placental steroidogenic cooperation, the amount of estrogen present in the maternal blood or urine reflects both fetal and placental enzymatic capability and hence, well-being. Attention has been focused on estriol because 90% of maternal estriol is derived from fetal precursors. The end product to be assayed in the maternal blood or urine is influenced by a multitude of factors. Availability of precursor from the fetal adrenal gland is a prime requisite as well as the ability of the placenta to carry out its conversion steps. Maternal metabolism of the product as well as the efficiency of maternal renal excretion of the product can modify the daily amount of estrogen in the urine. Blood flow to any of the key organs in the fetus, placenta, and mother becomes important.(25,26) In addition, drugs or diseases can affect any level in the cascade of events leading up to assay of estrogen.

For years, measurement of estrogen in a 24-hour urine collection was the standard hormonal method of assessing fetal well-being. This was replaced by radioimmunoassay of unconjugated estriol in the plasma. Assays which measure the total plasma estriol show the same large variations from day to day as seen with the old urinary assays. It is important that the clinical use of the estrogen assay in pregnancy be limited to the measurement of unconjugated estriol.(27) Because of its short half-life (5-10 minutes) in the maternal circulation, unconjugated estriol shows less variation than urinary or total blood estriol.

Normal Values and Interpretation. There are two essential aspects to the clinical use of estriol assays. First, a single specimen is meaningless. Daily assays must be performed to provide a serial assessment of sequential changes. Second, to be significant, there must be a decrease of approximately 40% from the mean of the three highest consecutive values.(27,28) While estrogen levels in the mother are related to the size of the fetal adrenal gland and its production of precursor, there is a poor correlation between birth weight and plasma estriol levels. Macrosomia is not always associated with high estriol levels. On the other hand, excessive adrenal activity as in congenital adrenal hyperplasia can be associated with unusually high levels.

Problems. Drugs which affect the maternal estrogen level include corticosteroids and antibiotics. Corticosteroids administered to the mother cross the placenta poorly, and large amounts (the equivalent of 75 mg of cortisol daily) are required to suppress fetal adrenal production of estriol precursor. The synthetic steroids, dexamethasone and betamethasone, however, cross the placenta more easily, and maternal estriol assessment is not reliable for at least 1 week, and sometimes 2 weeks, after the last dose. Antibiotics which affect the flora of the maternal gastrointestinal tract depress maternal

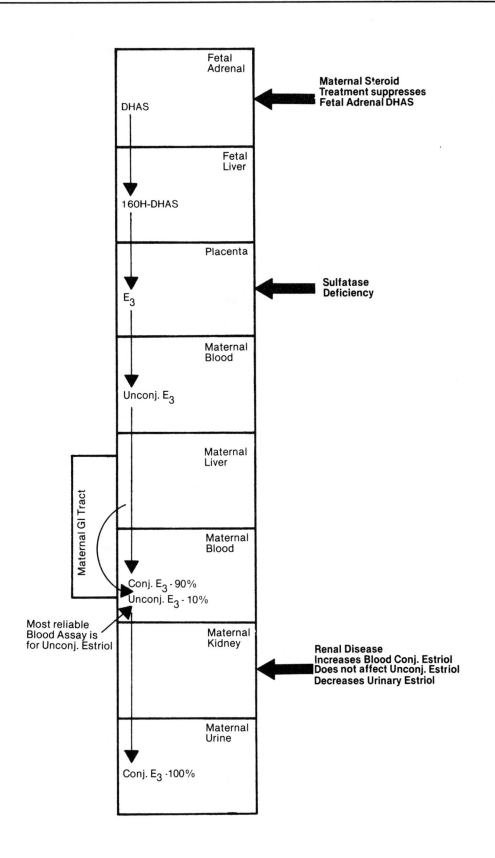

Fetal
Adrenal

Maternal Steroid
Treatment suppresses
Fetal Adrenal DHAS

DHAS

Fetal
Liver

16OH-DHAS

Placenta

Sulfatase
Deficiency

E_3

Maternal
Blood

Unconj. E_3

Maternal
Liver

Maternal GI Tract

Maternal
Blood

Conj. E_3 - 90%
Unconj. E_3 - 10%

Most reliable
Blood Assay is
for Unconj. Estriol

Maternal
Kidney

Renal Disease
Increases Blood Conj. Estriol
Does not affect Unconj. Estriol
Decreases Urinary Estriol

Maternal
Urine

Conj. E_3 ·100%

total estriol levels by interfering with the enterohepatic circulation. Such antibiotics inhibit the hydrolysis of the biliary estriol conjugates in the gut, preventing their reabsorption and reconjugation, leading to loss of estriol in the feces. Total blood and urinary estriol decline, but unconjugated estriol is unaffected. Falsely elevated blood total estriols will be encountered in the presence of renal disease or when a patient is receiving oxytocin for the induction of labor because of the antidiuretic action of oxytocin, but once again unconjugated estriol by a specific radioimmunoassay is the method of choice.

Clinical Uses of Estriol Assays

Assessment of maternal estriol levels has been superseded by various biophysical fetal monitoring techniques such as nonstress testing, stress testing, and measurement of fetal breathing and activity. Nevertheless, in certain clinical situations the addition of estriol assays is useful. The combination of a low estriol and a positive stress test is ominous. Certainly patients should not be managed by estriols alone. While a low estriol and a positive stress test indicate a fetus in jeopardy, a low estriol with a negative stress test allows postponement of intervention.

Amniotic Fluid Estrogen Measurements

Amniotic fluid estriol is correlated with the fetal estrogen pattern rather than the maternal. Most of the estriol in the amniotic fluid is present as 16-glucosiduronate or as 3-sulfate-16-glucosiduronate. A small amount exists as 3-sulfate. Very little unconjugated estriol is present in the amniotic fluid because free estriol is rapidly transferred across the placenta and membranes. Estriol sulfate is low in concentration because the placenta and fetal membranes hydrolyze the sulfated conjugates, and the free estriol is then passed out of the fluid.

Because the membranes and the placenta have no glucuronidase activity, the glucosiduronate conjugates are removed slowly from the fetus. The glucosiduronates therefore predominate in the fetal urine and the amniotic fluid. Because of the slow changes in glucosiduronates, measurements of amniotic fluid estriol have wide variations in both normal and abnormal pregnancies. An important clinical use for amniotic fluid estrogen measurements has not emerged.

Estetrol

Estetrol (15α-hydroxyestriol) is formed from fetal precursors, and is very dependent upon 15-hydroxylation activity in the fetal liver. The capacity for 15-hydroxylation of estrogens increases during fetal life, reaching a maximum at term. This activity then declines during infancy and is low, absent, or undetectable in adults. The clinical use of maternal blood and urine estetrol measurements is of no advantage over the usual estriol assessment.

Placental Sulfatase Deficiency

There is an X-linked metabolic disease expressed by a placental sulfatase deficiency, and postnatally, ichthyosis, occurring in about 1 in 2-6,000 newborns.(29) Patients with the placental sulfatase disorder are unable to hydrolyze DHAS or 16α-hydroxy-DHAS, and, therefore, the placenta cannot form normal amounts of estrogen. A deficiency in placental sulfatase is usually discovered when patients go beyond term and are found to have extremely low estriol levels and no evidence of fetal distress. The patients usually fail to go into labor and require delivery by cesarean section. Most striking is the failure of cervical softening and dilatation, thus a cervical dystocia occurs which is resistant to oxytocin stimulation. There are now over 100 case reports of this deficiency, almost all detected by finding low estriol levels. All newborn children, with a few exceptions, have been male. The steroid sulfatase X-linked recessive ichthyosis locus has been mapped on the distal short arm portion of the X-chromosome. There are no known geographic or racial factors which affect the gene frequency.

The characteristic steroid findings are as follows: extremely low estriol and estetrol in the mother with extremely high amniotic fluid DHAS and normal amniotic fluid DHA and androstenedione. The normal DHA and androstenedione with a high DHAS rule out the adrenogenital syndrome. The small amount of estriol which is present in these patients probably arises from 16-hydroxylation of DHAS in the maternal liver, thus providing 16-hydroxylated DHA to the placenta for aromatization to estriol. Measurement in maternal urine of steroids derived from fetal sulfated compounds is a simple and reliable means of prenatal diagnosis. Demonstration of a high level of DHAS in the amniotic fluid is reliable. To establish the diagnosis with certainty, a decrease in sulfatase activity should be demonstrated in an in vitro incubation of placental tissue. The clinician should keep in mind that fresh tissue is needed for this procedure as freezing lowers enzyme activity. Alternatively, steroid sulfatase activity can be assayed in leukocytes.

It is now recognized that steroid sulfatase deficiency is present in other tissues and can persist after birth. These children develop ichthyosis, characterized by hyperkaratosis (producing scales on the neck, trunk, and palms), and associated with corneal opacities, pyloric stenosis, and cryptorchidism. The skin fibroblasts have a low activity of steroid sulfatase, and scale formation which occurs early in the first year of life is thought to be due to an alteration in the cholesterol:cholesterol ester ratio (due to the accumulation of cholesterol sulfate). This inherited disorder thus represents a single entity: placental sulfatase deficiency and X-linked ichthyosis, both reflecting a deficiency of microsomal sulfatase. A family history of scaling in males (as well as repeated postdate pregnancies and cesarean sections) should prompt an effort to establish a diagnosis prenatally.

Protein Hormones of the Placenta

Human Chorionic Gonadotropin (HCG)

Human chorionic gonadotropin is a glycoprotein, a peptide framework to which carbohydrate sidechains are attached. Alterations in the carbohydrate components (about one-third of the molecular weight) change the biologic properties. For example, the long half-life of HCG is approximately 24 hours as compared to 2 hours for luteinizing hormone (LH), a 10-fold difference which is due mainly to the greater sialic acid content of HCG. As with the other glycoproteins, follicle-stimulating hormone (FSH), LH, and thyroid stimulating hormone (TSH), HCG consists of two noncovalently linked subunits, called alpha (α) and beta (β). The α subunits in these glycoprotein hormones are virtually identical, consisting of

92 amino acids. Unique biological activity as well as specificity in radioimmunoassays must be attributed to the molecular differences in the β subunits.

The 30 terminal amino acids of the β-HCG subunit are unique and different from the sequence on LH. Despite this difference (which allows specific antisera to discriminate between HCG and LH in assays), HCG is biologically similar to LH. To this day, the only definitely known function for HCG is support of the corpus luteum, taking over for LH on about the 8th day after ovulation when β-HCG first can be detected in maternal blood.

Continued survival of the corpus luteum is totally dependent upon HCG, and, in turn, the survival of the pregnancy is dependent upon steroids from the corpus luteum until the 7th week of pregnancy.(1) From the 7th week to the 10th week, the corpus luteum is gradually replaced by the placenta, and by the 10th week, removal of the corpus luteum will not be followed by steroid withdrawal abortion.

It is very probable, but not conclusively proven, that HCG stimulates steroidogenesis in the early fetal testes, so that androgen production will ensue and masculine differentiation can be accomplished.(30) It also appears that the function of the inner fetal zone of the adrenal cortex may depend upon HCG for steroidogenesis early in pregnancy. The mechanism for control of placental steroidogenesis is unknown and it is not certain whether the presence of HCG is necessary.

HCG is secreted by the syncytiotrophoblast, reaching a maximal level of 50,000-100,000 mIU/ml at 10 weeks of gestation. Why does the corpus luteum involute at the time that HCG is reaching its highest levels? One possibility is that a specific inhibitory agent becomes active at this time. Another is down-regulation of receptors by the high levels of HCG. In early pregnancy, down-regulation may be avoided because HCG is secreted in an episodic fashion.(31) For unknown reasons, the fetal testes escape desensitization; no receptor down regulation takes place.(30)

The maternal circulating HCG concentration is approximately 100 mIU/ml at the time of the expected but missed menses. HCG levels decrease to about 10,000-20,000 mIU/ml by 20 weeks and remain at that level to term. HCG levels close to term are higher in women bearing female fetuses. This is true of serum levels, placental content, urinary levels, and amniotic fluid concentrations. The mechanism and purpose of this difference are not known.

The old bioassay tests for pregnancy have been replaced by sensitive monoclonal antibody immunological tests for the presence of HCG in maternal urine and blood. There are two clinical conditions in which blood HCG titers are very helpful, trophoblastic disease and ectopic pregnancies. Early pregnancy is characterized by the sequential appearance of HCG, followed by β-HCG, and then α-HCG.(32) The ratio of beta to whole HCG remains constant after early pregnancy. Trophoblastic disease is distinguished by very high β-HCG levels (3-100 times higher than normal pregnancy). Ectopic production of α and β HCG by nontrophoblastic tumors is rare.

Previous studies with polyclonal antisera suggesting ectopic production were not accurate. The production of whole HCG in such tumors may not occur.

Following molar pregnancies the HCG titer should fall to a non-detectable level by 16 weeks in patients without persistent disease. Patients with trophoblastic disease show an abnormal curve (a titer greater than 500 mlU/ml) frequently by 3 weeks and usually by 6 weeks.(33) A diagnosis of gestational trophoblastic disease is made when the β-HCG plateaus or rises over a 2 week period, or a continued elevation is present 16 weeks after evacuation. In the United States, the rare occurrence of this disease mandates consultation with a certified subspecialist in gynecologic oncology. Following treatment, HCG should be measured monthly for at least a year, then twice yearly for 5 years.

In order to avoid unnecessary treatment (prophylactic chemotherapy) of the 80-85% of patients who undergo spontaneous remission, there is a need to identify those at high risk for persistent disease. A radioimmunoassay for the free beta subunit of HCG may serve this need in that persistent trophoblastic disease is associated with excessive production of the free β subunit.(34)

Virtually 100% of patients suspected of an ectopic pregnancy, but not having the condition, will have a negative blood HCG assay.(35) A positive test also can be utilized in diagnosis. The HCG level increases at different rates in normal and ectopic pregnancies. In the first 6 weeks of normal pregnancy, the concentration of HCG in the maternal blood follows a well-recognized pattern. When the HCG titer is below 6000 mlU/ml and abdominal ultrasound examination fails to identify an intrauterine pregnancy, a patient may be managed expectantly if the HCG titer approximately doubles in 2 days.(36,37) If the titer does not double, laparoscopy may be indicated. Laparoscopy is also indicated when the titer is above 6000 mlU/ml and ultrasound shows no evidence of an intrauterine pregnancy, or of course, in the presence of signs and symptoms of rupture and bleeding.

The doubling time is not sacrosanct; the rate of increase is nonlinear, changing with advancing gestational age and increasing HCG concentrations.(38) While the HCG level approximately doubles every 2 days below a level of 1200 mlU/ml, from 1200-6000 mlU/ml, it takes nearly 3 days to double, and above 6000 mlU/ml, about 4 days.(39) Furthermore, the zone at which a gestational sac is seen by ultrasound varies for different assays and different reference preparations. One should be sure that the discriminatory zone of 6000 mlU/ml applies to your local assay. In addition, vaginal ultrasonography is more sensitive; the discriminatory zone is considerably lower as gestational sacs can be identified with HCG concentrations less than 1000 mlU/ml.

With the use of modern sensitive assays, it is now appreciated that virtually all normal human tissues produce the intact HCG molecule. HCG can be detected in the blood of normal men and women, where it is secreted in a pulsatile fashion in parallel with LH, and apparently, the source of this circulating HCG is the pituitary gland.(40) The concentration of HCG normally reaches the sensitivity of the usual modern assay only in a rare postmenopausal woman with high LH levels.

Human Placental
Lactogen (HPL)

Human placental lactogen (HPL), also secreted by the syncytiotrophoblast, is a single chain polypeptide held together by two disulfide bonds. It is about 85% similar to human growth hormone (HGH), but has only 3% of HGH somatotropin activity. Although HPL has about 50% of the lactogenic activity of sheep prolactin in certain bioassays, its lactogenic contribution in human pregnancy is uncertain. Its half-life is short, about 15 minutes; hence its appeal as an index of placental problems. The level of HPL in the maternal circulation is correlated with fetal and placental weight, plateauing in the last 4 weeks of pregnancy. There is no circadian variation, and only minute amounts of HPL enter the fetal circulation. Very high maternal levels are found in association with multiple gestations; levels up to 40 μg/ml have been found with quadruplets and quintuplets. An abnormally low level is anything less than 4 μg/ml in the last trimester.

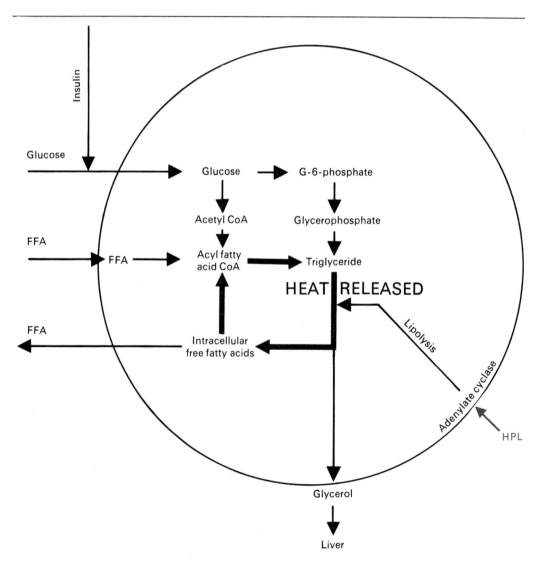

Fed State

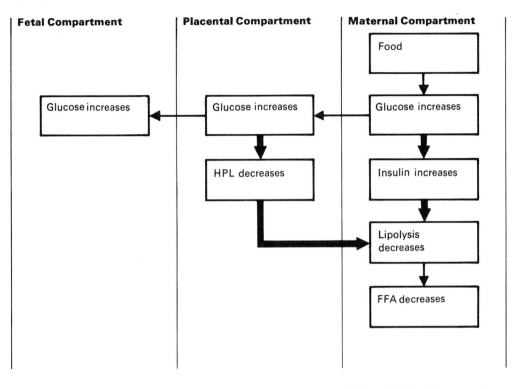

Physiologic Function. Experimentally, the maternal level of HPL can be altered by changing the circulating level of glucose. HPL is elevated with hypoglycemia and depressed with hyperglycemia. This information and studies in fasted pregnant women have led to the following formulation for the physiologic function of HPL.(41-46)

The metabolic role of HPL is to mobilize lipids as free fatty acids. In the fed state, there is abundant glucose available, leading to increased insulin levels, lipogenesis, and glucose utilization. This is associated with decreased gluconeogenesis, and a decrease in the circulating free fatty acid levels, as the free fatty acids are utilized in the process of lipogenesis to deposit storage packets of triglycerides (see Chapter 14, "Obesity").

Pregnancy has been likened to a state of "accelerated starvation," (43) characterized by a relative hypoglycemia in the fasting state. This state is due to two major influences:

1. Glucose provides the major, although not the entire, fuel requirement for the fetus. A difference in gradient causes a constant transfer of glucose from the mother to the fetus.

2. Placental hormones, specifically estrogen and progesterone, and especially HPL, interfere with the action of maternal insulin. In the second half of pregnancy when HPL levels rise approximately 10-fold, HPL is a major force in the diabetogenic effects of pregnancy. The latter is characterized by increased levels of insulin associated with decreased cellular response.

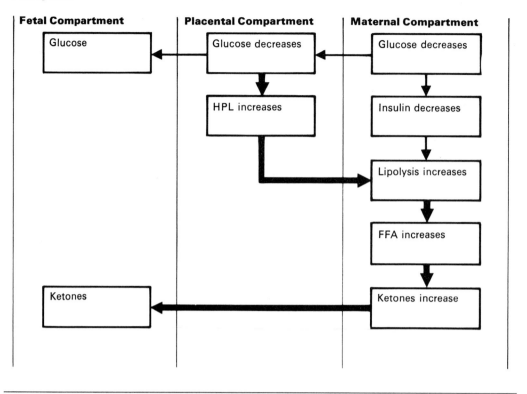

As glucose decreases in the fasting state, HPL levels rise. This stimulates lipolysis leading to an increase in circulating free fatty acids. Thus, a different fuel is provided for the mother so that glucose and amino acids can be conserved for the fetus. With sustained fasting, maternal fat is utilized for fuel to such an extent that maternal ketone levels rise. There is limited transport of free fatty acids across the placenta. Therefore, when glucose becomes scarce for the fetus, fetal tissues utilize the ketones which do cross the placenta. Thus, decreased glucose levels lead to decreased insulin and increased HPL, increasing lipolysis and ketone levels. HPL also may enhance the fetal uptake of ketones and amino acids. The mechanism for the insulin antagonism by HPL may be the HPL-stimulated increase in free fatty acid levels, which in turn directly interferes with insulin-directed entry of glucose into cells.

This mechanism can be viewed as an important means to provide fuel for the fetus between maternal meals. However, with a sustained state of inadequate glucose intake the subsequent ketosis may impair fetal brain development and function. Pregnancy is not the time to severely restrict caloric intake.

The lipid, lipoprotein, and apolipoprotein changes during pregnancy are positively correlated with changes in estradiol, progesterone, and HPL.(47) The lipolytic activity of HPL is an important factor as HPL also is linked to the maternal blood levels of cholesterol, triglycerides, and phospholipids.

The increases of insulin-like growth factors (IGF) which occur in pregnancy are probably due to the growth hormone activity of HPL. In addition, there is an IGF binding protein in the blood and amniotic fluid which is growth hormone dependent. This protein in amniotic fluid appears to be derived from the decidualized endometrium. (48,49)

HPL Clinical Uses. Blood levels of HPL are related to placental function. While some studies indicated that HPL was valuable in screening patients for potential fetal complications, others did not support the use of HPL measurements. Even though utilization of the HPL assay can have an impact on perinatal care, (50) fetal heart rate monitoring techniques are more reliably predictive and sensitive for assessing fetal well-being. Furthermore, a totally uneventful pregnancy has been reported despite undetectable HPL.(51)

Previous suggestions that a low or declining level of HPL and a high level of HCG are characteristic of trophoblastic disease were not accurate. Because of the rapid clearance of HPL, aborting molar pregnancies are likely to have low levels of HPL, while the level of HCG is still high. However, intact molar pregnancies may have elevated levels of both HPL and HCG.(52)

Human Chorionic Thyrotropin (HCT)

The human placenta contains two thyrotropic substances. One is called human chorionic thyrotropin (HCT), similar in size and action to pituitary TSH. The content in the normal placenta is very small. HCT differs from the other glycoproteins in that it does not appear to share the common α subunit. Antiserum generated to α-HCG does not neutralize the biologic activities of HCT, but it does that of HCG and pituitary TSH.

Rarely, patients with trophoblastic disease have hyperthyroidism. Studies have indicated that HCG has intrinsic thyrotropic activity, suggesting that HCG is the second placental thyrotropic substance.(53) On a molecular basis it has been calculated that HCG contains approximately 1/4000th of the thyrotropic activity of human TSH, although this is debated, and it has not been definitively demonstrated that HCG is thyrotropic in women.(54,55) In conditions with very elevated HCG levels, the thyrotropic activity can be sufficient to produce hyperthyroidism, but this may not be a simple HCG mechanism.

Human Chorionic Adrenocorticotropin Hormone

The rise in free cortisol that takes place throughout pregnancy may be due to ACTH production by the placenta.(56) The placental content of ACTH is higher than can be accounted for by the contribution of sequestered blood. In addition, cortisol levels in pregnant women are resistant to dexamethasone suppression, suggesting that there is a component of maternal ACTH that does not originate in the maternal pituitary gland. One can speculate that placental ACTH raises maternal adrenal activity in order to provide the basic building blocks (cholesterol and pregnenolone) for placental steroidogenesis.

335

Other Placental Peptides	The human placenta contains a number of releasing and inhibiting hormones, including gonadotropin releasing hormone (GnRH), thyroid releasing hormone (TRH) and somatostatin.(57) Immunoreactive GnRH can be localized in the cytotrophoblast. Evidence indicates that placental GnRH regulates placental steroidogenesis, and release of prostaglandin as well as HCG.(58-60)

The placental binding site for GnRH has a lower affinity than that of GnRH receptors in the pituitary, ovary, and testis.(61) This reflects the situation in which the binding site is in close proximity to the site of secretion for the regulatory hormone. A higher affinity is not necessary because of the large amount of GnRH available in the placenta, and the low affinity receptors avoid response to the low levels of circulating GnRH.

The trophoblast secretes a pregnancy-specific β_1-globulin into the maternal circulation. It appears shortly after implantation and increases steadily until term. The placenta pours a flood of other proteins into the maternal circulation, and it remains to be seen whether their identity and function can be sorted out.

Alpha-Fetoprotein

Alpha-fetoprotein (AFP) is a relatively unique glycoprotein derived largely from fetal liver, and partially from the yolk sac until it degenerates at about 12 weeks. Its function is unknown but it may serve as a protein carrier of steroid hormones in fetal blood. Peak levels are reached early in the second trimester (16-18 weeks), then levels decrease gradually until term. Maternal blood levels of AFP reflect the amniotic fluid level. Because AFP is highly concentrated in the fetal CNS, abnormal direct contact of CNS with the amniotic fluid (as with neural tube defects) results in elevated amniotic fluid and maternal blood levels. Other fetal abnormalities, such as intestinal obstruction, omphalocele, and congenital nephrosis, are also associated with high levels of AFP in the amniotic fluid. Because of a high incidence of false positive results in maternal serum AFP screening programs, each patient with a high blood level requires ultrasound evaluation to detect anencephaly, oligohydramnios, fetal kidney abnormalities, multiple gestation, erroneous dating or intrauterine demise, and then, if necessary, amniocentesis to measure the amniotic fluid AFP. An elevated amniotic fluid AFP deserves further meticulous ultrasound examination, because not all of these cases are associated with an abnormal fetus.

Not all fetal abnormalities are manifested by inappropriately high levels of AFP. Indeed, the risk of Down's syndrome is inversely correlated with maternal AFP levels, and this is probably also true for other trisomies.(62) When the level of AFP according to established standards indicates a trisomy risk of 1 in 250 or greater (the risk in a 35 year old woman at 15-20 weeks gestation), amniocentesis is recommended. There is a high false positive rate which is a costly and stressful problem. Other factors that cause a low AFP include: incorrect dates, fetal demise, trophoblastic disease, and diabetes mellitus.

Relaxin

Relaxin is a peptide hormone produced by the corpus luteum of pregnancy, and not detected in men or nonpregnant women. While it has been argued that the human corpus luteum is the sole source of relaxin in pregnancy, it has also been identified in human placenta, decidua, and chorion.(63-65) The maternal serum concentration rises during the first trimester and declines in the second trimester.(66) This suggests a role in maintaining early pregnancy, but its function is not really known. In animals, relaxin softens the cervix, inhibits uterine contractions, and relaxes the pubic symphysis. The cervical changes are comparable to those seen with human labor. (67)

Prolactin

Following ovulation, the endometrium becomes a secretory organ and remains so throughout pregnancy. As time passes we will probably discover more and more important endometrial products. For example, decidualized endometrium secretes renin which may play a role in the regulation of water and electrolytes in the amniotic fluid, and relaxin which may influence prostaglandin production in the membranes. One of the best studied special endocrine functions of the decidual endometrium is the secretion of prolactin. Prolactin is synthesized by endometrium during a normal menstrual cycle, but this synthesis is not initiated until histologic decidualization begins about day 23.(68,69) The control of prolactin secretion by decidual tissue has not been definitively established. Some argue that once decidualization is established, prolactin secretion continues in the absence of either progesterone or estradiol, although there is evidence for an inhibitory feedback by decidual proteins (perhaps prolactin itself). (69,70) Others indicate that endometrial prolactin production requires the combined effects of progestin and estrogen hormones plus the presence of relaxin.(71)

During pregnancy, prolactin secretion is limited to the fetal pituitary, the maternal pituitary, and the uterus. Neither trophoblast nor fetal membranes synthesize prolactin, but both the myometrium and endometrium can produce prolactin. The endometrium requires the presence of progesterone to initiate prolactin, while progesterone suppresses prolactin synthesis in the myometrium. Prolactin derived from the decidua is the source of prolactin found in the amniotic fluid.(72)

Amniotic fluid concentrations of prolactin parallel maternal serum concentration until the 10th week of pregnancy, rise markedly until the 20th week, and then decrease. The maternal and fetal blood levels of prolactin are derived from the respective pituitary glands. Bromocriptine suppression of pituitary secretion of prolactin throughout pregnancy produces minimal maternal and fetal blood levels, yet there is normal fetal growth and development, and amniotic fluid levels are unchanged.(73) Fortunately decidual secretion of prolactin is unaffected by bromocriptine because decidual prolactin may be important for fluid and electrolyte regulation of the amniotic fluid. This decidual prolactin is transported across the membranes in a process which requires the intact state of amnion and chorion with adherent decidua.

No clinical significance can be attached to maternal and fetal blood levels of prolactin in abnormal pregnancies. Decidual and amniotic fluid prolactin levels are lower, however, in hypertensive pregnancies and in patients with polyhydramnios.(74,75) Prolactin receptors are present in the chorion laeve, and their concentration is lower in patients with polyhydramnios.(76) Prolactin reduces the permeability of the human amnion in the fetal to maternal direction. This receptor-mediated action takes place on the epithelium lining the fetal surface.(77)

Endogenous Opiates and Pregnancy

The endogenous opiates probably originate from the pituitary glands, and are secreted in parallel with ACTH, in response to corticotropin releasing hormone.(78) There is reason to believe that in pregnancy the intermediate lobe of the maternal pituitary gland is a major source of elevated circulating endorphin levels. The placenta is also a source of opiates, especially β-endorphin and enkephalins. The maternal blood levels of endogenous opiates increase progressively with advancing gestation. Maximal values are reached during labor, coinciding with full cervical dilatation. The maternal levels also correlate with the degree of pain perception and use of analgesia. On the fetal side, hypoxia is a potent stimulus for endorphin release.

There are many hypotheses surrounding the function of endogenous opiates in pregnancy. These include: roles related to stress, inhibition of oxytocin, vasopressin and gonadotropins, the promotion of prolactin secretion, and of course, a natural analgesic agent during labor and delivery.

Other Pregnancy Peptides (Nonplacental)

The circulating levels of prorenin, the inactive precursor of renin, increase (10-fold) during the early stages of pregnancy, the result of ovarian stimulation by HCG.(79,80) This increase in prorenin from the ovary is not associated with any significant change in the blood levels of the active form, renin. Possible roles for this ovarian prorenin-renin-angiotensin system include the following: stimulation of steroidogenesis to provide androgen substrate for estrogen production, regulation of calcium and prostaglandin metabolism, and stimulation of angiogenesis. This system may affect vascular and tissue functions both in and outside the ovary. Prorenin also originates in chorionic tissues and is highly concentrated in the amniotic fluid.

Atrial natriuretic peptide (ANP) is derived from human atrial tissue. It is a potent natriuretic, diuretic, and smooth muscle relaxant peptide which circulates as a hormone. Maternal ANP increases during labor, and cord levels higher on the arterial side suggest that ANP is a circulating hormone in the fetus.(81)

338

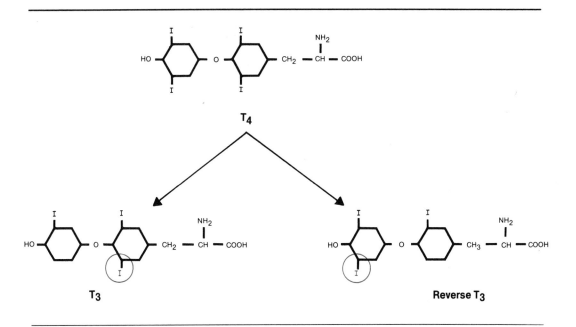

T_4

T_3

Reverse T_3

The human fetal thyroid gland develops the capacity to concentrate iodine and synthesize hormone between 10 and 13 weeks of gestation, the same time that the pituitary begins to synthesize TSH.(82) Some thyroid development and hormone synthesis are possible in the absence of the pituitary gland, but optimal function requires TSH. By 12-14 weeks, development of the pituitary-thyroid system is complete. Function is minimal, however, until an abrupt increase in fetal TSH occurs at 20 weeks. As with gonadotropin and other pituitary hormone secretion, this thyroid function correlates with the maturation of the hypothalamus and the development of the pituitary portal vascular system, which makes releasing hormones available to the pituitary gland.

Fetal TSH reaches a plateau at 28 weeks, and remains at relatively high levels to term. The free thyroxine (T_4) concentration increases progressively. At term, fetal T_4 levels exceed maternal levels. Thus a state of fetal thyroidal hyperactivity exists near term.

Placental transfer of TSH, T_4, and 3,5,3'-triiodothyronine (T_3) is severely limited in both directions. Indeed, the placenta is essentially impermeable to these substances no matter whether the fetus is euthyroid or hypothyroid. Slight transfer may occur, however, at pharmacologic concentrations.

Removal of one iodine from the phenolic ring of T_4 yields T_3, while removal of an iodine from the nonphenolic ring yields reverse T_3 (RT_3) which is biologically inactive. In a normal adult, about one-third of the T_4 secreted daily is deiodinated to T_3, while about 45% is converted to RT_3. About 83% of T_3 is produced from T_4 in peripheral tissues, while 17% is secreted by the thyroid. T_3 is 3-5 times more potent than T_4, and virtually all the biologic activity of T_4 can be attributed to the T_3 generated from it. While T_4 may have some intrinsic activity of its own, it serves mainly as a prohormone of T_3. Carbohydrate calories appear to be the primary determinant

339

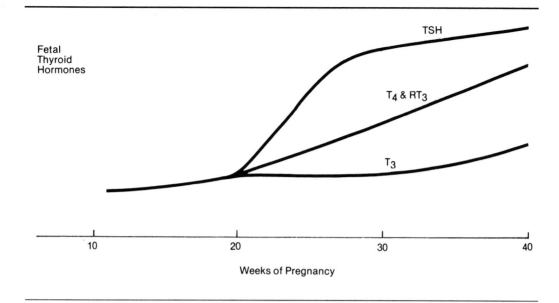

Fetal
Thyroid
Hormones

TSH

T_4 & RT_3

T_3

10	20	30	40

Weeks of Pregnancy

of T_3 levels in adults. A reciprocal relationship exists between T_3 and RT_3. Low T_3 and elevated RT_3 are seen in a variety of illnesses such as febrile diseases, burn injuries, malnutrition, and anorexia nervosa.

The major thyroid hormone secreted by the fetus is T_4. Total T_3 and free T_3 levels are low throughout gestation; however, levels of RT_3 are elevated, paralleling the rise in T_4. Like T_3, this compound is derived predominantly from conversion of T_4 in peripheral tissues. The increased production of T_4 in fetal life is compensated by rapid conversion to the inactive RT_3, allowing the fetus to conserve its fuel resources.

Treatment of maternal hyperthyroidism with propylthiouricil, even with moderate doses of 100-200 mg daily, suppresses T_4 and increases TSH levels in the newborns. (83) The infants are clinically euthyroid, however, and their laboratory measurements are normal by the 4th to 5th day of life. In addition, follow-up assessment has indicated unimpaired intellectual development in children whose mothers received propylthiouricil during pregnancy.(84)

With delivery, the newborn moves from a state of relative T_3 deficiency to a state of T_3 thyrotoxicosis. Shortly after birth serum TSH concentrations increase rapidly to a peak at 30 minutes of age. They fall to baseline values by 48-72 hours. In response to this increase in TSH, total T_4 and free T_4 increase to peak values by 24-48 hours of age. T_3 levels increase even more, peaking by 24 hours of age. By 3-4 weeks, the thyroidal hyperactivity has disappeared.

340

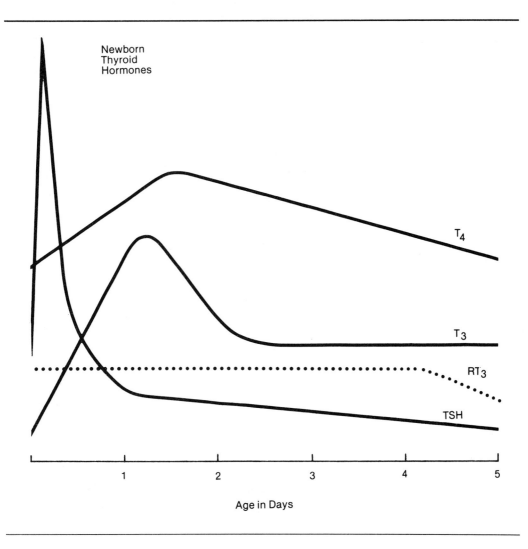

Newborn Thyroid Hormones

T_4

T_3

RT_3

TSH

Age in Days

The postnatal surge in TSH is accompanied by a prolactin surge, suggesting that both are increased in response to TRH. The TRH surge is thought to be a response to rapid neonatal cooling. A puzzle is the fact that the early increase in T_3 is independent of TSH and is tied in some way to cutting of the umbilical cord. Delaying cord cutting delays the increase in T_3, but TSH levels still reach their peak at 30 minutes. In some way cord cutting augments peripheral (largely liver) conversion of T_4 to T_3. The later increases in T_3 and T_4 (after 2 hours) are due to increased thyroid gland activity. These thyroid changes after birth probably represent defense mechanisms against the sudden entry into the cold world. The high RT_3 levels during pregnancy continue during the first 3-5 days of life, then fall gradually to normal adult levels by 2 weeks.

Summary of Fetal and Newborn Thyroid Changes:

1. TSH and T_4 appear in the fetus at 10-13 weeks. Levels are low until an abrupt rise at 20 weeks.

2. T_4 rises rapidly and exceeds maternal values at term.

341

3. T_3 levels rise, but concentrations are relatively low, similar to hypothyroid adults.

4. RT_3 levels exceed normal adult levels.

5. The fetal pattern of low T_3 and high RT_3 is similar to that seen with calorie malnutrition.

6. After delivery, TSH peaks at 30 minutes of age, followed by a T_3 peak at 24 hours and a T_4 peak at 24-48 hours. The T_3 increase is independent of the TSH change.

7. High RT_3 levels persist for 3-5 days, after delivery, then reach adult values by 2 weeks.

Newborn Screening for Hypothyroidism

The incidence of neonatal hypothyroidism is about 1/4000 live births. The problem is that congenital hypothyroidism is not apparent clinically at birth. Fortunately, infants with congenital hypothyroidism have low T_4 and high TSH concentrations easily detected in blood, and early treatment before 3 months of age is associated with normal mental development.(85,86) There is a familial tendency for hypothyroidism, and if the diagnosis is made in the antepartum period, weekly intraamniotic injections of thyroxine can raise fetal levels of thyroid hormone. Amniotic fluid iodothyronines reflect fetal plasma levels, and normal values have been established which allow prenatal diagnosis of fetal hypothyroidism by amniocentesis.(87) This is important because there is a concern that prenatal hypothyroidism can affect some aspects of development, for example the full function of physical skills.

Fetal Lung Maturation

The pulmonary alveoli are lined with a surface-active phospholipid-protein complex called pulmonary surfactant that is synthesized in the type II pneumocyte of mature lungs. It is this surfactant which decreases surface tension, thereby facilitating lung expansion and preventing atelectasis. In full-term fetuses, surfactant is present at birth in sufficient amounts to permit adequate lung expansion and normal breathing. In premature fetuses, however, surfactant is present in lesser amounts, and when insufficient, postnatal lung expansion and ventilation are frequently impaired, resulting in progressive atelectasis, the clinical syndrome of respiratory distress.

Phosphatidylcholine (lecithin) has been identified as the most active and most abundant lipid of the surfactant complex. The second most active and abundant material is phosphatidylglycerol (PG), which significantly enhances surfactant function. Both are present in only small concentrations until the last 5 weeks of pregnancy. Beginning at 20-22 weeks of pregnancy, a less stable and less active lecithin, palmitoylmyristoyl lecithin, is formed. Hence, a premature infant does not always develop respiratory distress syndrome; however, in addition to being less active, synthesis of this lecithin is decreased by stress and acidosis, making the premature infant more susceptible to respiratory distress. At about the 35th week of gestation, there is a sudden surge of dipalmitoyl lecithin, the major surfactant lecithin, which is stable and very active. Since secretion by the fetal lungs contributes to the formation of amniotic fluid and the sphingomyelin concentration of amniotic fluid changes relatively little throughout pregnancy, assessment of the lecithin/sphingomyelin (L/S) ratio in amniotic fluid at approximately 34-36 weeks of pregnancy can determine the amount of dipalmitoyl lecithin available and thus the degree to which the lungs will adapt to newborn life.

Gluck et al were the first to demonstrate that the L/S ratio correlates with pulmonary maturity of the fetal lung.(88) In normal development, sphingomyelin concentrations are greater than those of lecithin until about gestational week 26. Prior to 34 weeks, the L/S ratio is approximately 1:1. At 34-36 weeks, with the sudden increase in lecithin, the ratio rises acutely. In general, a ratio of 2.0 or greater indicates pulmonary maturity and that respiratory distress syndrome will not develop in the newborn. Respiratory distress syndrome associated with a ratio greater than 2.0 usually follows a difficult delivery with a low 5-minute Apgar score, suggesting that severe acidosis can inhibit surfactant production. A ratio in the transitional range (1.0 to 1.9) indicates that respiratory distress syndrome may develop, but that the fetal lung has entered the period of lecithin production, and a repeat amniocentesis in 1 or 2 weeks usually reveals a mature L/S ratio. The rise from low to high ratios may actually occur within 3-4 days.

An increase in the surfactant content of phosphatidylglycerol at 34-36 weeks marks the final maturation of the fetal lung. When the L/S ratio is greater than 2.0 and PG is present, the incidence of RDS is virtually zero. The assessment of PG is especially helpful when the amniotic fluid is contaminated in that the analysis is not affected by meconium, blood, or vaginal secretions.

Abnormalities of pregnancy may affect the rate of maturation of the fetal lung, resulting either in an early mature L/S ratio or a delayed rise in the ratio. Accelerated maturation of the ratio is associated with hypertension, advanced diabetes, hemoglobinopathies, heroin addiction, and poor maternal nutrition. Delayed maturation is seen with diabetes without hypertension, and Rh-sensitization. In general, accelerated maturation is associated with reductions in utero-placental blood flow (and presumably increased fetal stress). With vigorous and effective control of maternal diabetes, the risk of RDS in the newborns is not significantly different from infants born to nondiabetics.

Previously it was believed that delivery by cesarean section was associated with a greater incidence of respiratory distress syndrome when groups were corrected for gestational age. Since respiratory distress syndrome is related to the maturity of the fetal lung, and the L/S ratio is an index of pulmonary maturity, comparison of mode of delivery with the L/S ratio has allowed a more accurate appraisal of this problem. Gabert et al (89) and Donald et al (90) demonstrated that the maturity of the lungs indicated by the L/S ratio determines the potential for the respiratory distress syndrome regardless of the mode of delivery.

Since Liggins observed survival of premature lambs following the administration of cortisol to the fetus, it has become recognized that fetal cortisol is the principal requisite for surfactant biosynthesis. This is true despite the fact that no increase in fetal cortisol can be demonstrated to correlate with the increases in fetal lung maturation. For that reason, fetal lung maturation can be best viewed as the result of not only cortisol, but the synergistic action of cortisol, prolactin, T_4, estrogens, prostaglandins, growth factors, and perhaps other yet unidentified agents. Insulin partially antagonizes this stimulatory effect, which explains the delay in L/S ratio maturation associated with hyperglycemia in pregnancy (although this effect can be overcome by the stress associated with advanced diabetes).

In general, maximal benefit in terms of enhanced fetal pulmonic maturity has been demonstrated with glucocorticoid administration under 32 weeks of gestational age, with some benefit between 32-34 weeks, and no benefit beyond 34 weeks. The optimal effect requires that 48 hours elapse after initation of therapy, and this benefit is lost after 7 days. Most clinicians restrict antenatal steroid treatment for premature labor to pregnancies between 28-32 weeks with intact membranes.

References

1. **Csapo AL, Pulkkinen MO, Wiest WG,** Effects of luteectomy and progesterone replacement in early pregnant patients, Am J Obstet Gynecol 115:759, 1973.

2. **Simpson ER, Bilheimer DW, MacDonald PC,** Uptake and degradation of plasma lipoproteins by human choriocarcinoma cells in culture, Endocrinology 104:8, 1979.

3. **Parker CR, Illingworth DR, Bissonnette J, Carr BR,** Endocrine changes during pregnancy in a patient with homozygous familial hypobetalipoproteinemia, New Eng J Med 314:557, 1986.

4. **Mitchell BF, Challis JRG, Lukash L,** Progesterone synthesis by human amnion, chorion, and decidua at term, Am J Obstet Gynecol 157:349, 1987.

5. **Parker CR, Everett RB, Quirk JG, Whalley PJ, Gant NF,** Hormone production during pregnancy in the primigravid patient: I. Plasma levels of progesterone and 5α-pregnane-3,20-dione throughout pregnancy of normal women and women who developed pregnancy-induced hypertension. Am J Obstet Gynecol 135:778, 1979.

6. **Parker CR, Everett RB, Whalley PJ, Quirk JG, Gant NF, MacDonald PC,** Hormone production during pregnancy in the primigravid patient: II. Plasma levels of deoxycorticosterone throughout pregnancy of normal women and women who developed pregnancy-induced hypertension. Am J Obstet Gynecol 138:626, 1980.

7. **Rothchild I,** Role of progesterone in initiating and maintaining pregnancy, in Bardin CW, Milgrom E, Mauvais-Jarvis P, editors, *Progesterone and Progestins*, Raven Press, New York, 1983, pp 219-229.

8. **Siiteri PK, MacDonald PC,** Placental estrogen biosynthesis during human pregnancy, J Clin Endocrinol Metab 26:751, 1966.

9. **Madden JD, Gant NF, MacDonald PC,** Study of the kinetics of conversion of maternal plasma dehydroisoandrosterone sulfate to 16α-hydroxydehydroisoandrosterone sulfate, estradiol, and estriol, Am J Obstet Gynecol 132:392, 1978.

10. **Buster JE, Abraham GE,** The applications of steroid hormone radioimmunoassays to clinical obstetrics, Obstet Gynecol 46:489, 1975.

11. **Buster JE, Sakakini J Jr, Killam AP, Scragg WH,** Serum unconjugated estriol levels in the third trimester and their relationship to gestational age, Am J Obstet Gynecol 125:672, 1975.

12. **Parker CR Jr, Leveno K, Carr BR, Hauth J, MacDonald PC,** Umbilical cord plasma levels of dehydroepiandrosterone sulfate during human gestation, J Clin Endocrinol Metab 54:1216, 1982.

13. **Winters AJ, Oliver C, Colston C, MacDonald PC, Porter JC,** Plasma ACTH levels in the human fetus and neonate as related to age and parturition, J Clin Endocrinol Metab 39:269, 1974.

14. **Walsh SW, Norman RL, Novy MJ,** In utero regulation of rhesus monkey fetal adrenals: effects of dexamethasone, adrenocorticotropin, thyrotropin-releasing hormone, prolactin, human chorionic gonadotropin, and α-melanocyte-stimulating hormone on fetal and maternal plasma steroids, Endocrinology 104:1805, 1979.

15. **Abu-Hakima M, Branchaud CL, Goodyer CG, Murphy BEP,** The effects of human chorionic gonadotropin on growth and steroidogenesis of the human fetal adrenal gland in vitro, Am J Obstet Gynecol 156:681, 1987.

16. **del Pozo E, Bigazzi M, Calaf J,** Induced human gestational hypoprolactinemia: lack of action on fetal adrenal androgen synthesis, J Clin Endocrinol Metab 51:936, 1980.

17. **Walker ML, Pepe GJ, Albrecht ED,** Regulation of baboon fetal adrenal androgen formation by pituitary peptides at mid- and late gestation, Endocrinology 122:546, 1988.

18. **Carr BR, Simpson ER,** Lipoprotein utilization and cholesterol synthesis by the human fetal adrenal gland, Endocrin Rev 2:306, 1981.

19. **Mason JI, Rainey WE,** Steroidogenesis in the human fetal adrenal: A role for cholesterol synthesized *de novo,* J Clin Endocrinol Metab 64:140, 1987.

20. **Fujieda K, Faiman C, Reyes FI, Winter JSD,** The control of steroidogenesis by human fetal adrenal cells in tissue culture: I. Responses to adrenocorticotropin, J Clin Endocrinol Metab 53:34, 1981.

21. **Fujieda K, Faiman C, Reyes FI, Thliveris J, Winter JSD,** The control of steroidogenesis by human fetal adrenal cells in tissue culture: II. Comparison of morphology and steroid production in cells of the fetal and definitive zones. J Clin Endocrinol Metab 53:401, 1981.

22. **Fujieda K, Faiman C, Reyes FI, Winter JSD,** The control of steroidogenesis by human fetal adrenal cells in tissue culture: III. The effects of various hormonal peptides. J Clin Endocrinol Metab, 53:690, 1981.

23. **Fujieda K, Faiman C, Reyes FI, and Winter JSD,** The control of steroidogenesis by human fetal adrenal cells in tissue culture: IV. The effects of exposure to placental steroids, J Clin Endocrinol Metab 54:89, 1982.

24. **Byrne GC, Perry YS, Winter JSD,** Steroid inhibitory effects upon human adrenal 3β-hydroxysteroid dehydrogenase activity, J Clin Endocrinol Metab 62:413, 1986.

345

25. **Fritz MA, Stanczyk FZ, Novy MJ,** Relationship of uteroplacental blood flow to the placental clearance of maternal dehydroepiandrosterone through estradiol formation in the pregnant baboon, J Clin Endocrinol Metab 61:1023, 1985.

26. **Fritz MA, Stanczyk FZ, Novy MJ,** Maternal estradiol response to alterations in uteroplacental blood flow, Am J Obstet Gynecol 155:1317, 1986.

27. **Distler W, Gabbe SG, Freeman RK, Mestman JH, Goebelsmann U,** Estriol in pregnancy: V. Unconjugated and total plasma estriol in the management of pregnant diabetic patients, Am J Obstet Gynecol 130:424, 1978.

28. **Whittle MJ, Anderson D, Lowensohn RI, Mestman JH, Paul RH, Goebelsmann U,** Estriol in pregnancy: VI. Experience with unconjugated plasma estriol assays, Am J Obstet Gynecol 135:764, 1979.

29. **Bradshaw KD, Carr BR,** Placental sulfatase deficiency: Maternal and fetal expression of steroid sulfatase deficiency and X-linked ichthyosis, Obstet Gynecol Survey 41:401, 1986.

30. **Leinonen PJ, Jaffee RB,** Leydig cell desensitization by human chorionic gonadotropin does not occur in the human fetal testis, J Clin Endocrinol Metab 61:234, 1985.

31. **Owens OM, Ryan KJ, Tulchinsky D,** Episodic secretion of human chorionic gonadotropin in early pregnancy, J Clin Endocrinol Metab 53:1307, 1981.

32. **Ozturk M, Bellet D, Manil L, Hennen G, Frydman R, Wands J,** Physiological studies of human chorionic gonadotropin (HCG), α-HCG, and β-HCG as measured by specific monoclonal immunoradiometric assays, Endocrinology 120:549, 1987.

33. **Schlaerth JB, Morrow CP, Kletzky OA, Nalick RH, D'Ablaing GA,** Prognostic characteristics of serum human chorionic gonadotropin titer regression following molar pregnancy. Obstet Gynecol 58:478, 1981.

34. **Khazaeli MB, Hedayat MM, Hatach KD, To ACW, Soong S-j, Shingleton HM, Boots LR, LoBuglio AF,** Radioimmunoassay of free β-subunit of human chorionic gonadotropin as a prognostic test for persistent trophoblastic disease in molar pregnancy, Am J Obstet Gynecol 155:320, 1986.

35. **Schwartz RO, DiPietro DL,** β-HCG as a diagnostic aid for suspected ectopic pregnancy, Obstet Gynecol 56:197, 1980.

36. **Romero R, Kadar N, Copel JA, Jeanty P, DeCherney AH, Hobbins JC,** The value of serial human chorionic gonadotropin testing as a diagnostic tool in ectopic pregnancy, Am J Obstet Gynecol 155:392, 1986.

37. **Kadar N, Romero R,** Observations on the log human chorionic gonadotropin-time relationship in early pregnancy and its practical implications, Am J Obstet Gynecol 157:73, 1987.

38. **Fritz MA, Guo S,** Doubling time of human chorionic gonadotropin (hCG) in early normal pregnancy: Relationship to hCG concentration and gestational age, Fertil Steril 47:584, 1987.

39. **Pittaway DE, Wentz AC,** Evaluation of early pregnancy by serial chorionic gonadotropin determinations: A comparison of methods by receiver operating characteristic curve analysis, Fertil Steril 43:529, 1985.

40. **Odell WD, Griffin J,** Pulsatile secretion of human chorionic gonadotropin in normal adults, New Eng J Med 317:1688, 1987.

41. **Grumbach MM, Kaplan SL, Vinik A,** Chapter 2, HCS, in *Peptide Hormones*, Vol 2B, Berson SA, Yalow RS, editors, North-Holland, Amsterdam, 1973, pp 797-819.

42. **Spellacy WN, Buhi WC, Schram JC, Birk SA, McCreary SA,** Control of human chorionic somatomammotropin levels during pregnancy, Obstet Gynecol 37:567, 1971.

43. **Felig P,** Maternal and fetal fluid homeostasis in human pregnancy, Am J Clin Nutr 26:998, 1973.

44. **Felig P, Lynch V,** Starvation in human pregnancy: hypoglycemia, hypoinsulinemia, and hyperketonemia, Science 170:990, 1970.

45. **Kim YJ, Felig P,** Plasma chorionic somatomammotropin levels during starvation in mid-pregnancy, J Clin Endocrinol Metab 32:864, 1971.

46. **Felig P, Kim YJ, Lynch V, Hendler R,** Amino acid metabolism during starvation in human pregnancy, J Clin Invest 51:1195, 1972.

47. **Desoye G, Schweditsch MO, Pfeiffer KP, Zechner R, Kostner GM,** Correlation of hormones with lipid and lipoprotein levels during normal pregnancy and postpartum, J Clin Endocrinol Metab 64:704, 1987.

48. **Koistinen R, Kalkkinen N, Huhtala M-L, Seppala M, Bohn H, Rutanen E-M,** Placental protein 12 is a decidual protein that binds somatomedin and has an identical N-terminal amino acid sequence with somatomedin-binding protein from human amniotic fluid, Endocrinology 118:1375, 1986.

49. **Baxter RC, Martin JL, Wood MH,** Two immunoreactive binding proteins for insulin-like growth factors in human amniotic fluid: Relationship to fetal maturity, J Clin Endocrinol Metab 65:423, 1987.

50. **Spellacy WN, Buhi WC, Birk SA,** The effectiveness of human placental lactogen measurements as an adjunct in decreasing perinatal deaths, Am J Obstet Gynecol 121:835, 1975.

51. **Nielsen PV, Pedersen H, Kampmann E,** Absence of human placental lactogen in an otherwise uneventful pregnancy, Am J Obstet Gynecol 135:322, 1979.

52. **Dawood MY, Teoh ES,** Serum human chorionic somatomammotropin in unaborted hydatidiform mole, Obstet Gynecol 47:183, 1976.

53. **Nisula BC, Morgan FJ, Canfield RE,** Evidence that chorionic gonadotropin has intrinsic thyrotropic activity, Biochem Biophys Res Commun 59:86, 1974.

54. **Norman RJ, Lowings C, Oliver T, Chard T,** Doubts about human chorionic gonadotropin as a thyroid stimulator, Lancet i:1096, 1985.

55. **Pekonen F, Alfthan H, Stenman U, Ylikorkala O,** Human chorionic gonadotropin (hCG) and thyroid function in early human pregnancy: Circadian variation and evidence for intrinsic thyrotropic activity of hCG, J Clin Endocrinol Metab 66:853, 1988.

56. **Rees LH, Buarke CW, Chard T, Evans SW, Letchorth AT,** Possible placental origin of ACTH in normal human pregnancy, Nature 254:620, 1975.

57. **Siler-Khodr TM, Khodr GS,** Production and activity of placental releasing hormones, in *Fetal Endocrinology,* Novy MJ, Resko JA, eds, Academic Press, New York, 1981, pp 183-210.

58. **Siler-Khodr TM, Kuehl TJ, Vickery BH,** Effects of a gonadotropin-releasing antagonist on hormone levels in the pregnant baboon and on fetal outcome, Fertil Steril 41:448, 1984.

59. **Siler-Khodr TM, Khodr GS, Harper MJK, Rhode J, Vickery BH, Nestor JJ Jr,** Differential inhibition of human placental prostaglandin release in vitro by a GnRH antagonist, Prostaglandins 31:1003, 1986.

60. **Belisle S, Guevin J-F, Bellabarba D, Lehoux J-G,** Luteinizing hormone-releasing hormone binds to enriched placental membranes and stimulates in vitro the synthesis of bioactive human chorionic gonadotropin, J Clin Endocrinol Metab 59:119, 1984.

61. **Iwashita M, Evans MI, Catt KJ,** Characterization of a gonadotropin-releasing hormone receptor site in term placenta and chorionic villi, J Clin Endocrinol Metab 62:127, 1986.

62. **DiMaio MS, Baumgarten A, Greenstein RM, Saal HM, Mahoney MJ,** Screening for fetal Down's syndrome in pregnancy by measuring maternal serum alpha-fetoprotein levels, New Eng J Med 317:342, 1987.

63. **Weiss G, O'Byrne EM, Hochman J, Steinetz BG, Goldsmith L, Flitcraft JG,** Distribution of relaxin in women during pregnancy, Obstet Gynecol 52:569, 1978.

64. **Fields PA, Larkin LH,** Purification and immunohistochemical localization of relaxin in the human term placenta, J Clin Endocrinol Metab 52:79, 1981.

65. **Lopez Bernal A, Bryant-Greenwood GD, Hansell DJ, Hicks BR, Greenwood FC, Turnbull AC,** Effect of relaxin on prostaglandin E production by human amnion: Changes in relation to the onset of labour, Brit J Obstet Gynaecol 94:1045, 1987.

66. **Quagliarello J, Steinetz BG, Weiss G,** Relaxin secretion in early pregnancy, Obstet Gynecol 53:62, 1979.

67. **MacLennan AH, Katz M, Creasy R,** The morphologic characteristics of cervical ripening induced by the hormones relaxin and prostaglandin $F_{2\alpha}$ in a rabbit model, Am J Obstet Gynecol 152:691, 1985.

68. **Maslar IA, Ansbacher R,** Effects of progesterone on decidual prolactin production by organ cultures of human endometrium, Endocrinology 118:2102, 1986.

69. **Daly DC, Kuslis S, Riddick DH,** Evidence of short-loop inhibition of decidual prolactin synthesis by decidual proteins, Part I, Am J Obstet Gynecol 155:358, 1986.

70. **Daly DC, Kuslis S, Riddick DH,** Evidence of short-loop inhibiton of decidual prolactin synthesis by decidual proteins, Part II, Am J Obstet Gynecol 155:363, 1986.

71. **Huang JR, Tseng L, Bischof P, Janne OA,** Regulation of prolactin production by progestin, estrogen, and relaxin in human endometrial stromal cells, Endocrinology 121:2011, 1987.

72. **McCoshen JA, Barc J,** Prolactin bioactivity following decidual synthesis and transport by amniochorion, Am J Obstet Gynecol 153:217, 1985.

73. **Ho Yuen B, Cannon W, Lewis J, Sy L, Woolley S,** A possible role for prolactin in the control of human chorionic gonadotropin and estrogen secretion by the fetoplacental unit, Am J Obstet Gynecol 136:286, 1980.

74. **Luciano AA, Varner MW,** Decidual, amniotic fluid, maternal, and fetal prolactin in normal and abnormal pregnancies, Obstet Gynecol 63:384, 1984.

75. **Golander A, Kopel R, Lasebik N, Frenkel Y, Spirer Z,** Decreased prolactin secretion by decidual tissue of pre-eclampsia in vitro, Acta Endocrinol 108:111, 1985.

76. **Healy DL, Herington AC, O'Herlihy C,** Chronic polyhydramnios is a syndrome with a lactogen receptor defect in the chorion laeva, Brit J Obstet Gynaecol 92:461, 1985.

77. **Raabe MA, McCoshen JA,** Epithelial regulation of prolactin effect on amnionic permeability, Am J Obstet Gynecol 154:130, 1986.

78. **Hung TT,** The role of endogenous opioids in pregnancy and anesthesia, Seminars Reprod Endocrinol 5:161, 1987.

79. **Derkx FHM, Stuenkel C, Schalekamp MPA, Visser W, Huisveld IH, Schalekamp MADH,** Immunoreactive renin, prorenin, and enzymatically active renin in plasma during pregnancy and in women taking contraceptives, J Clin Endocrinol Metab 63:1008, 1986.

80. **Derkx, FHM, Alberda AT, De Jong FH, Zeilmaker FH, Makovitz JW, Schalekamp MADH,** Source of plasma prorenin in early and late pregnancy: Observations in a patient with primary ovarian failure, J Clin Endocrinol Metab 65:349, 1987.

81. **Yamaji T, Hirai N, Ishibashi M, Takaku F, Yanaihara T, Nakayama T,** Atrial natriuretic peptide in umbilical cord blood: Evidence for a circulating hormone in human fetus, J Clin Endocrinol Metab 63:1414, 1986.

82. **Fisher DA, Dussault JH, Sack J, Chopra IJ,** Ontogenesis of hypothalamic-pituitary-thyroid function and metabolism in man, sheep, and rat, Recent Prog Horm Res, 33:59, 1977.

83. **Cheron RG, Kaplan MM, Larsen PR, Selenkow HA, Crigler JF Jr,** Neonatal thyroid function after propylthiouracil therapy for maternal Graves' disease, New Eng J Med 304:525, 1981.

84. **Burrow GN, Klatskin EH, Genel M,** Intellectual development in children whose mothers received proplythiouracil during pregnancy, Yale J Biol Med 51:151, 1978.

85. **New England Congenital Hypothyroidism Collaborative,** Neonatal hypothyroidism screening: Status of patients at 6 years of age, J Pediatrics 107:915, 1985.

86. **Illig R, Largo RH,** European collaborative study on mental development in children with congenital hypothyroidism diagnosed by neonatal screening, Pediatric Res 19:73A, 1985.

87. **Klein AH, Murphy BEP, Artal R, Oddie TH, Fisher DA,** Amniotic fluid thyroid hormone concentrations during human gestation, Am J Obstet Gynecol 136:626, 1980.

88. **Gluck L, Kulovich MV, Borer RC, Brenner PH, Anderson GG, Spellacy WN,** Diagnosis of respiratory distress syndrome by amniocentesis, Am J Obstet Gynecol 109:440, 1971.

89. **Gabert HA, Bryson MJ, Stenchever MA,** The effect of cesarean section on respiratory distress in the presence of a mature lecithin/sphingomyelin ratio, Am J Obstet Gynecol 116:366, 1973.

90. **Donald IR, Freeman RK, Goebelsmann U, Chan WH, Nakamura RM,** Clinical experience with the amniotic fluid lecithin/sphingomyelin ratio, Am J Obstet Gynecol 115:547, 1973.

11   Prostaglandins

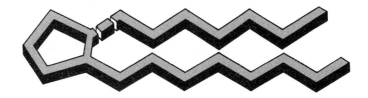

Prostaglandins play a fundamental role in the regulation of reproductive events. It is remarkable that most of the roles for prostaglandins predicted many years ago have come true. But what was once a relatively simple story has become exceedingly complex, especially from the biochemical point of view, as more and more members of the prostaglandin family are recognized.

This chapter will review the fundamental biochemistry of prostaglandins and focus on the roles prostaglandins play in pregnancy, specifically physiologic control mechanisms in luteal regression, the fetal circulation, parturition, uteroplacental blood flow, and maternal blood pressure.

Prostaglandin History

The historical evolution of the prostaglandin story is by now a familiar one. America can claim the first clue to the existence of prostaglandins because two New York gynecologists at Columbia, Kurzrok and Lieb, reported, in 1930, the effects of fresh human seminal fluid on strips of human uterus. This clue was overlooked, however, and the field was left for the pioneer work to come from Sweden and England, especially from the Karolinska Institute in Stockholm.

Goldblatt in England, in 1933, and von Euler in Sweden, in 1934, independently discovered that extracts of seminal vesicles stimulated smooth muscle preparations and also had vasodepressor activity. A year later, in 1935, von Euler reported that this biologic activity was due to an acidic lipid which he named prostaglandin. Nothing further was done until the late 1950s. World War II was certainly one reason for this hiatus, but also techniques were not sufficiently sensitive to measure and study prostaglandins which were available only in small amounts.

The supply problem was initially overcome by collecting large batches of sheep seminal vesicles and utilizing biosynthesis. This was an expensive and major logistic effort. The reward was the characterization and synthesis of prostaglandins in the early 1960s in the laboratory of Professor Sune Bergstrom, a student of von Euler's.

The discovery in 1970 that a coral (*Plexaura homomala*) off the coast of Florida contained large amounts of prostaglandin materials which could be used for the production of pure prostaglandins was a big boost for laboratory and clinical research. Shortly after, total synthesis of prostaglandins was achieved, and supply was no longer a problem.

During the 1970s the reproductive world was startled by the work of Sultan Karim. He was the first to use prostaglandins for the successful induction of labor and abortions, and this clinical application was responsible for a great surge of interest both clinically and in the laboratory. Recent history has centered on the new members of the prostaglandin family: thromboxane, prostacyclin, and the leukotrienes. The 1982 Nobel Prize in medicine was awarded jointly to Sune Bergstrom for his work with prostaglandins, Bengt Samuelsson for the leukotrienes, and John R. Vane for prostacyclin.

An appreciation for the make-up of this remarkable family is essential in order to understand the current prostaglandin world.

Prostaglandin Biochemistry

Biosynthesis

The family of prostaglandins with the greatest biologic activity is that having two double bonds, derived from arachidonic acid.[1] Arachidonic acid can be obtained from two sources, directly from the diet (from meats) or by formation from its precursor linoleic acid which is found in vegetables. In the plasma, 1-2% of the total free fatty acid content is free arachidonic acid. The majority of arachidonic acid is covalently bound in esterified form as a significant proportion of the fatty acids in phospholipids and in esterified cholesterol. Arachidonic acid is only a minor fatty acid in the triglycerides packaged in adipose tissue.

The rate-limiting step in the formation of the prostaglandin family is the release of free arachidonic acid. A variety of hydrolases may be involved in arachidonic acid release, but phospholipase A_2 activation is an important initiator of prostaglandin synthesis because of the abundance of arachidonate in the 2 position of phospholipids. Types of stimuli that activate such lipases include: burns, infusions of hyper and hypotonic solutions, thrombi and small particles, endotoxin, snake venom, mechanical stretching, catecholamines, bradykinin, angiotensin, and the sex steroids.

"Eicosanoids" refer to all the 20-carbon derivatives, while "prostanoids" indicate only those containing a structural ring. After the release of arachidonic acid the synthetic path can go in two different directions: the lipoxygenase pathway or the cyclooxygenase pathway. The leukotrienes are formed by 5-lipoxygenase oxygenation of arachidonic acid at C-5, forming an unstable intermediate, LTA_4. [2] LTB_4 is formed by hydration and LTC_4 by the addition of gluathione. The remaining leukotrienes are metabolites of LTC_4.

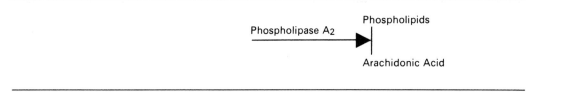

Phospholipase A$_2$

Phospholipids

Arachidonic Acid

The previously known slow reacting substance of anaphylaxis consists of a mixture of LTC$_4$, LTD$_4$, and LTE$_4$. The leukotrienes are involved in the defense reactions of white cells, and participate in hypersensitivity and inflammatory responses. LTB$_4$ acts primarily on leukocytes (stimulation of leukocyte emigration from the bloodstream), while LTC$_4$, LTD$_4$, and LTE$_4$ affect smooth muscle cells (bronchoconstriction in the lungs and reduced contractility in the heart). All leukotrienes increase microvascular permeability. Thus the leukotrienes are major agonists, synthesized in response to antigens and provoking asthma and airway obstruction. Leukotrienes are 100-1000 times more potent than histamine in the pulmonic airway. The future development of specific inhibitors has great potential for the treatment of immune and inflammatory responses.

The 12-lipoxygenase pathway leads to 12-HETE. Little is known about 12-HETE other than its function as a leukostatic agent. Finally, a new group of arachidonic acid products recently has been discovered, the lipoxins. (2) The lipoxins (LXA and LXB) inhibit natural killer cell cytotoxicity.

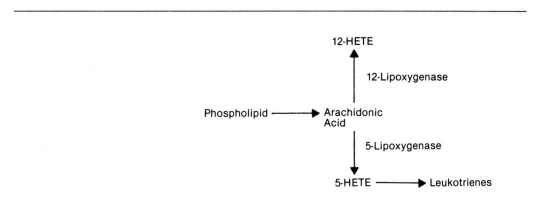

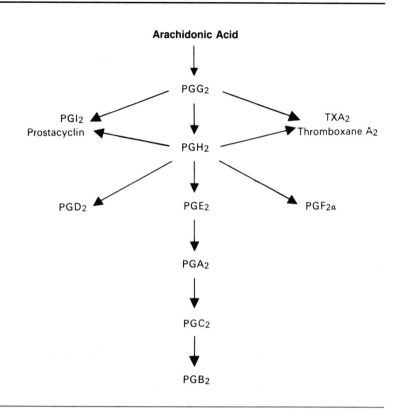

Arachidonic Acid

The cyclooxygenase pathway leads to the prostaglandins. The first true prostaglandin (PG) compounds formed are PGG_2 and PGH_2 (half-life of about 5 minutes), the mothers of all other prostaglandins. The numerical subscript refers to the number of double bonds. This number depends on which of the three precursor fatty acids has been utilized. Besides arachidonic acid, the other two precursor fatty acids are linoleic acid, which gives rise to the PG_1 series, and pentanoic acid, the PG_3 series. The latter two series are of less importance in physiology, hence the significance of the arachidonic acid family. The prostaglandins of original and continuing relevance to reproduction are PGE_2 and $PGF_{2\alpha}$ and possibly PGD_2. The A, B, and C prostaglandins either have little biologic activity, or do not exist in significant concentrations in biologic tissues. In the original work, the prostaglandin more soluble in ether was named PGE, while the one more soluble in phosphate (spelled with an F in Swedish) buffer was named PGF. Later, naming became alphabetical.

Thromboxane and
Prostacyclin

Thromboxanes are not true prostaglandins due to the absence of the pentane ring, but prostacyclin (PGI_2) is a legitimate prostaglandin. Thromboxane (TX) (half-life about 30 seconds) and PGI_2 (half-life about 2-3 minutes) can be viewed as opponents, each having powerful biologic activity which counters or balances the other. TXA_2 is the most powerful vasoconstrictor known, while PGI_2 is a potent vasodilator. These two agents also have opposing effects on platelet function. Platelets, lungs, and the spleen predominately synthesize TXA_2, while the heart, stomach, and blood vessels throughout the body synthesize PGI_2. The lungs are a major source of prostacyclin. Normal pulmonary endothelium makes prostacyclin while TXA_2

354

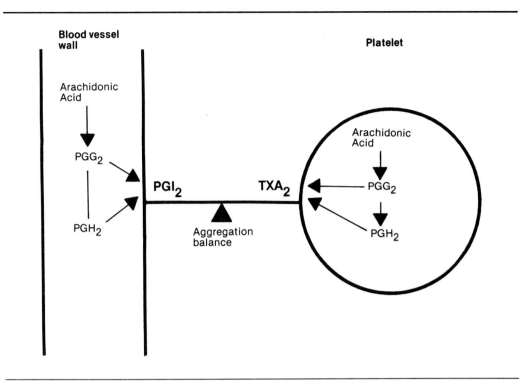

appears in response to pathological stimuli.(3) The pulmonary release of prostacyclin may contribute to the body's defense against platelet aggregation.

Let's take a closer look at platelets. The primary function of platelets is the preservation of the vascular system. Blood platelets stick to foreign surfaces or other tissues, a process called adhesion. They also stick to each other and form clumps; this process is called aggregation. Because platelets synthesize TXA_2, a potent stimulator of platelet aggregation, the natural tendency of platelets is to clump and plug defects and damaged spots. The endothelium, on the other hand, produces PGI_2 and its constant presence inhibits platelet aggregation and adherence, keeping blood vessels free of platelets and ultimately clots. Thus, prostacyclin has a defensive role in the body. It is 4-8 times more potent a vasodilator than the E prostaglandins, and it prevents the adherence of platelets to healthy vascular endothelium. However, when the endothelium is damaged, platelets gather, beginning the process of thrombus formation. Even in this abnormal situation, prostacyclin strives to fulfill its protective role as increased PGI_2 can be measured in injured endothelium, thrombosed vessels, and in the vascular tissues of hypertensive animals.

Conditions associated with vascular disease can be understood through the prostacyclin-thromboxane mechanism.(4) For example, atheromatous plaques and nicotine inhibit prostacyclin synthesis. Increasing the cholesterol content of human platelets increases the sensitivity to stimuli which cause platelet aggregation due to increased thromboxane production. The well-known association between low-density and high-density lipoproteins (LDL and HDL) and cardiovascular disease may also be explained in terms of PGI_2. LDL from men and postmenopausal women inhibits and HDL stimulates prostacyclin production.(5) Platelets from diabetics and from Class A

355

diabetic pregnant women make more TXA_2 than platelets from normal pregnant women. Platelets from women using oral contraceptives make more TXA_2 than controls. The same is true of smokers and people with strong family histories of cardiovascular disease. Incidentally, onion and garlic inhibit platelet aggregation and TXA_2 synthesis.(6) Perhaps the perfect contraceptive pill is a combination of progestin, estrogen, and some onion or garlic.

In some areas of the world there is a low incidence of cardiovascular disease. This can be directly attributed to diet and the protective action of prostacyclin.(7) The diet of Eskimos and Japanese has a high content of pentanoic acid and low levels of linoleic and arachidonic acids. Pentanoic acid is the precursor of prostaglandin products with 3 double bonds, and as it happens, PGI_3 is an active agent while TXA_3 is either not formed, or it is inactive. The fat content of most common fish is 8-12% pentanoic acid, and more than 20% in the more exotic (and expensive) seafoods such as scallops, oysters, and caviar.

Metabolism

The metabolism of prostaglandins occurs primarily in the lungs, kidney, and liver. The lungs are important in the metabolism of E and F prostaglandins. Indeed, there is an active transport mechanism which specifically carries E and F prostaglandins from the circulation into the lungs. Therefore, members of the prostaglandin family have a short half-life, and in most instances, exert their action at the site of their synthesis. Because of the rapid half-lives, studies are often carried out by measuring the inactive end products, for example 6-keto-$PGF_{1\alpha}$, the metabolite of prostacyclin, and TXB_2, the metabolite of thromboxane A_2.

Prostaglandin Inhibition

A review of prostaglandin biochemistry is not complete without a look at the inhibition of the biosynthetic cascade of products. Corticosteroids were previously thought to inhibit the prostaglandin family by stabilizing membranes and preventing the release of phospholipase. It is now believed that corticosteroids induce the synthesis of a substance which blocks the action of phospholipase.(8) Thus far, steroids and some local anesthetic agents are the only substances known to work at this step.

Aspirin is an irreversible inhibitor, selectively acetylating the fatty acid dioxygenase involved in prostaglandin synthesis. The other inhibiting agents, such as indomethacin, are reversible agents, forming a reversible bond with the active site of the enzyme. Acetaminophen inhibits cyclooxygenase only in the central nervous system. Thus, it is an analgesic and antipyretic agent, but has no anti-inflammatory properties nor does it affect platelets.

The analgesic, antipyretic, and anti-inflammatory actions of these agents are mediated by inhibition of the cyclooxygenase enzyme. Because of the irreversible nature of the inhibition by aspirin, aspirin exerts a long lasting effect on platelets, effectively maintaining inhibition in the platelet for its life-span (8-10 days). The sensitivity of the platelets to aspirin may explain the puzzling results in the early studies in which aspirin was given to prevent subsequent morbidity and mortality following thrombotic events. It takes only a little aspirin to effectively inhibit thromboxane synthesis in

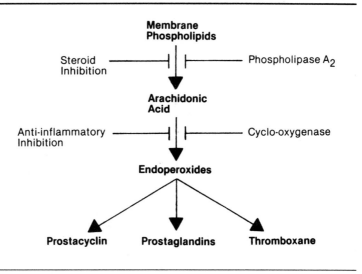

platelets. Going beyond this dose will not only inhibit thromboxane synthesis in platelets, but also the protective prostacyclin production in blood vessel walls. Controversy continues as to what dose of aspirin and what frequency of administration are best. Some suggest that a dose of 3.5 mg/kg (about half an aspirin tablet) given at 3-day intervals effectively induces maximal inhibition of platelet aggregation without affecting prostacyclin production by the vessel walls. (9) More recent evidence indicates that the dose which effectively and selectively inhibits platelet cyclooxygenase is 40 mg daily.(10) The major handicap with the use of inhibitors of PG synthesis is that they strike blindly and with variable effect from tissue to tissue. Obviously drugs which selectively inhibit TXA_2 synthesis will be superior to aspirin in terms of antithrombotic effects.

Prostaglandins and Luteal Regression

Prostaglandin $F_{2\alpha}$ causes luteal regression in many species. It is the agent responsible for terminating the life-span of the corpus luteum if fertilization fails to take place, so that a subsequent repeat ovulation can follow rapidly. The $PGF_{2\alpha}$ originates in the endometrium, and its synthesis is stimulated by the estrogen produced in growing follicles. It is transported directly to the corpus luteum through the vasculature connecting the ovary and the uterus, thus achieving an effective concentration at the corpus luteum and avoiding a systemic level with widespread actions.

The mechanism of $PGF_{2\alpha}$-induced luteolysis is 2-fold: a rapid anti-LH action followed by a loss of luteinizing hormone (LH) receptors in the corpus luteum.(11) The rapid action is expressed only in intact cells and appears to be the result of some mediator that blocks LH receptor activation of adenylate cyclase. The slower response is an indirect action, interfering with prolactin maintenance of LH receptors.

Luteolysis has not been demonstrated in the primate, and it is well known that removal of the uterus does not interfere with normal ovulatory cycles. However, high doses of estrogen can induce luteolysis in the monkey and perhaps in the human. In the monkey, estrogen induces a drop in progesterone during the luteal phase, mirrored by a rise in F prostaglandin. Furthermore, indomethacin can block this effect of estrogen.(12) There is considerable evidence to support a role for estrogen in the decline of the human corpus luteum. The premature elevation of circulating estradiol levels in the early luteal phase results in a prompt fall in progesterone concentrations. Direct injections of estradiol into the ovary bearing the corpus luteum induce luteolysis while similar treatment of the contralateral ovary produces no effect. Auletta postulates that prostaglandin $F_{2\alpha}$ produced within the ovary bearing the corpus luteum or within the corpus luteum serves as the luteolytic agent and the production of the prostaglandin is initiated by the luteal estrogen. (13-15)

The human application of these findings can be found in the use of postcoital estrogen for contraception. High doses of estrogen can decrease progesterone levels in human cycles. (16) It is important to remember that the mechanism of estrogen is through $PGF_{2\alpha}$, and since the mechanism of $PGF_{2\alpha}$ is antagonism of LH action, human chorionic gonadotropin (HCG) can overcome this effect of estrogen. Hence, the effective action of estrogen when used for postcoital contraception is limited to the 7 days prior to implantation, before the corpus luteum is subject to rescue by HCG.

Prostaglandins and the Fetal Circulation

The predominant effect of prostaglandins on the fetal and maternal cardiovascular system is to maintain the ductus arteriosus, renal, mesenteric, uterine, placental, and probably the cerebral and coronary arteries in a relaxed or dilated state. The importance of the ductus arteriosus can be appreciated by considering that 59% of the cardiac output flows through this connection between the pulmonary artery and the descending aorta.

Control of ductal patency and closure is mediated through prostaglandins. The arterial concentration of oxygen is the key to the caliber of the ductus. With increasing gestational age, the ductus becomes increasingly responsive to increased oxygen. In this area, too, attention has turned to PGI_2 and TXA_2.

Fetal lamb ductus homogenates produce mainly PGI_2 when incubated with arachidonic acid. PGE_2 and $PGF_{2\alpha}$ are formed in small amounts and TXA_2 not at all. Although PGE_2 is less abundant than PGI_2 in the ductus, it is a more potent vasodilator of the ductus and is more responsive to oxygen (decreasing vasodilatation with increasing oxygen).(17) Thus, PGE_2 appears to be the most important prostaglandin in the ductus from a functional point of view, while PGI_2, the major product in the main pulmonary artery, appears to be the major factor in maintaining vasodilatation in the pulmonary bed. The ductus is dilated maximally in utero by production of prostaglandins, and a positive vasoconstrictor process is required to close it. The source of the vasoconstrictor is probably the lung. With increasing maturation, the lung shifts to TXA_2 formation. This fits with the association of ductal patency with prematurity. With the onset of pulmonary ventilation at birth leading to vascular changes which deliver blood to the duct directly from the lungs, TXA_2 can now serve as the vasoconstrictor stimulus. The major drawback to this hypothesis is the failure of inhibitors to affect the constriction response to oxygen.

Administration of vasodilating prostaglandins can maintain patency after birth, while preparing an infant for surgery to correct a congenital lesion causing pulmonary hypertension. Infants with persistent ductus patency may be spared thoracotomy by treatment with an inhibitor of prostaglandin synthesis. The use of indomethacin to close a persistent ductus in the premature infant is successful about 40% of the time. (17) The variable success cannot be attributed to any single factor, and further studies are necessary. At least one important factor, however, is early diagnosis and treatment because with increasing postnatal age the ductus becomes less sensitive to prostaglandin inhibitors, probably because of more efficient clearance of the drug.(18) The highest incidence of sucessful indomethacin ductus closure has been with infants less than 30 weeks gestation and less than 10 days old.

This aspect of the use of prostaglandin inhibitors is of concern in considering the use of agents to inhibit premature labor. The drug half-life in the fetus and newborn is prolonged because the metabolic pathways are limited, and there is reduced drug clearance because of immature renal function. In utero constriction of the ductus can cause congestive heart failure and fetal pulmonary hypertension.(19) Prolonged ductus constriction leads to subendocardial ischemia and fibrotic lesions in the tricuspid valve muscles. Infants with persistent pulmonary hypertension have hypoxemia, cardiomegaly and right to left shunting through the foramen ovale or the ductus. Infants of mothers given either indomethacin or salicylates chronically have been reported to have this syndrome. Duration of exposure and dosage are critical. It takes occlusion of the ductus for more than 2 weeks to produce fetal pulmonary hypertension and cardiac hypertrophy. Side effects appear to be minimized when administration is limited to mothers less than 34 weeks pregnant, and long-term use is avoided.

Prostaglandins and Parturition

Perhaps the best example of the interplay among fetus, placenta, and the mother is the initiation and maintenance of parturition. Endocrine changes in the uteroplacental environment are the principal governing factors accounting for the eventual development of uterine contractions. The sequence of events has been repeatedly reviewed in detail, where references to the original work are available.(20,21)

Extensive work in the sheep has implicated the fetal pituitary-adrenal axis in normal parturition. The sequence of events in the sheep begins about 10 days prior to labor with elevation of fetal cortisol, probably in response to fetal pituitary ACTH. Fetal adrenalectomy or hypophysectomy prolongs pregnancy, while infusion of ACTH or glucocorticoids into the sheep fetus stimulates premature labor. Maternal stimulation of the fetal adrenal is not a factor because in sheep (and in human beings) there is little or no placental transfer of maternal ACTH into the fetal circulation.

Increased glucocorticoid secretion by the fetal adrenal gland presumably starts a chain of events associated with labor. The sequence of events continues in the sheep with a decline in progesterone. This change is brought about by the induction of 17α-hydroxylase enzyme activity in the sheep placenta.

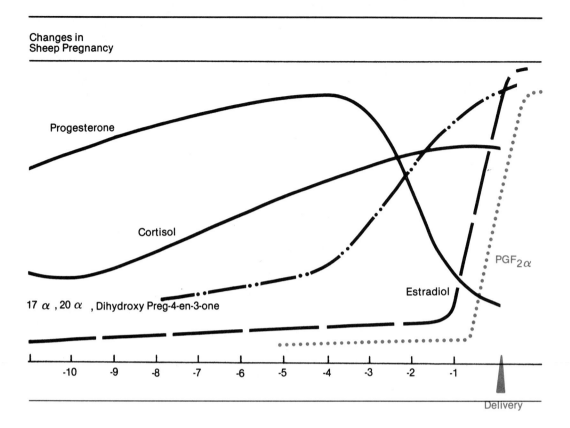

Glucocorticoid treatment of sheep placental tissue specifically increases the rate of production of $17\alpha,20\alpha$-dihydroxypregn-4-en-3-one. This dihydroxyprogesterone compound also has been identified in sheep placental tissue obtained after spontaneous labor. Thus, direct synthesis of progesterone does not decline, but increased metabolism to a 17-hydroxylated product results in less available progesterone. Progesterone withdrawal is associated with a decrease in the resting potential of myometrium, i.e., an increased response to electric and oxytocic stimuli. Conduction of action potential through the muscle is increased, and the myometrial excitability is increased.

Dihydroxyprogesterone also serves as a precursor for the rise in estrogen levels which occurs a few days prior to parturition. Estrogens enhance rhythmic contractions as well as increasing vascularity and permeability, and the oxytocin response. Thus, progesterone withdrawal and estrogen increase lead to an enhancement of conduction and excitation.

The final event is a rise in $PGF_{2\alpha}$ production hours before the onset of uterine activity. A cause-and-effect relationship between the rise in estrogen and the appearance of $PGF_{2\alpha}$ has been demonstrated in the sheep. These events indicate that the decline in progesterone, the rise in estrogen, and the increase in $PGF_{2\alpha}$ are all secondary to direct induction of a placental enzyme by a glucocorticoid.

The steroid events in human pregnancy are somewhat similar to events in the ewe, with a very important difference: a more extended time scale. Steroid changes in the sheep occur over the course of several days, while in human pregnancy the changes begin at approximately 34-36 weeks and occur over the last 5 weeks of pregnancy.

Cortisol rises dramatically in amniotic fluid, beginning at 34-36 weeks, and correlates with pulmonic maturation. Cord blood cortisol concentrations are high in infants born vaginally or by cesarean section following spontaneous onset of labor. In contrast, cord blood cortisol levels are lower in infants born without spontaneous labor, whether delivery is vaginal (induced labor) or by cesarean section (elective repeat section). In keeping with the extended time scale of events, administration of glucocorticoids is not followed acutely by the onset of labor in pregnant women (unless the pregnancy is past due).

It is unlikely that the cortisol increments in the fetus represent changes due to increased adrenal activity in the mother in response to stress. Although maternal cortisol crosses the placenta readily, it is largely (85%) metabolized to cortisone in the process. This, in fact, may be the mechanism by which suppression of the fetal adrenal gland by maternal steroids is avoided. In contrast to the maternal liver, the fetal liver has a limited capacity for transforming the biologically inactive cortisone to the active cortisol. On the other hand, the fetal lung does possess the capability of changing cortisone to cortisol, and this may be an important source of cortisol for the lung. Cortisol itself induces this conversion in lung tissue. Increased fetal adrenal activity is followed by changes in steroid levels as well as important developmental accomplishments (e.g., increased pulmonary surfactant production and the accumulation of liver glycogen.)

But the increased levels of fetal cortisol associated with labor appear to be secondary to the stress of the process, and at the present time there is no evidence that fetal cortisol production triggers human parturition. In human parturition the important contribution of the fetal adrenal, rather than cortisol, is probably its effect on placental estrogen production. The common theme in human pregnancies associated with failure to begin labor on time is decreased estrogen production, e.g. anencephaly and placental sulfatase deficiency. In contrast, mothers bearing fetuses who cannot form normal amounts of cortisol, such as those with congenital adrenogenital syndrome, deliver on time. (22)

An increase in estrogen levels in maternal blood begins at 34-35 weeks of gestation, but a late increase just prior to parturition (as in the sheep) has not been observed in human pregnancy. Perhaps a critical concentration is the signal in human pregnancy rather than a triggering increase; or the changes are taking place at a local level and are not reflected in the maternal circulation.(23) Although it has not been definitely demonstrated, increased or elevated estrogen levels are thought to play a key role in increasing prostaglandin production.

Progesterone maintenance of uterine quiescence and increased myometrial excitability associated with progesterone withdrawal ap-

361

pear to be firmly established as mechanisms of parturition in lower species. In primates, the role of progesterone is less clear, largely because of the inability to demonstrate a definite decline in peripheral blood levels of progesterone prior to parturition. Nevertheless, pharmacologic treatment with progesterone or synthetic progestational agents has proven effective in preventing premature labor.(24,25) There is reason to believe that progesterone concentration is regulated locally, and progesterone withdrawal can be accomplished by a combination of binding and metabolism.(26)

Evidence for a role of prostaglandin in parturition includes the following:

1. Prostaglandin levels in maternal blood and amniotic fluid increase in association with labor.

2. Arachidonic acid levels in the amniotic fluid also rise in labor, and arachidonate injected into the amniotic sac initiates parturition.

3. Patients taking high doses of aspirin have a highly significant increase in the average length of gestation, incidence of postmaturity, and duration of labor.

4. Indomethacin prevents the normal onset of labor in monkeys and stops premature labor in human pregnancies.

5. Stimuli known to cause the release of prostaglandins (cervical manipulation, stripping of membranes, and rupture of membranes) augment or induce uterine contractions.

6. Prostaglandins induce labor.

   Fetal respiratory movements are influenced by prostaglandins. The administration of indomethacin to fetal sheep increases, while infusion of PGE suppresses, fetal breathing movements. This may be the explanation for the decrease in fetal breathing movements observed during labor.

   The precursor fatty acid for prostaglandin production in part may be derived from storage pools in the fetal membranes, or the decidua, or both. Phospholipase A_2 has been demonstrated in both human chorioamnion and uterine decidua. Gustavii has suggested that progesterone withdrawal allows degeneration of decidual cells and release of lysosomal enzyme, leading to the activation of lipase enzyme.(27) Others believe the major source of arachidonic acid is the fetal membranes.(28,29) However, the precise mechanism for initiating prostaglandin synthesis, presumably by activation of the enzyme phospholipase A_2, remains unknown.

   The Texas thesis is that availability of arachidonic acid for prostaglandin production during parturition is due to stimulation of hydrolysis of phosphatidylethanolamine and phosphatidylinositol in decidual, amnion, and chorion laeve tissues.(30-32) Microsomes from amnion, chorion laeve, and decidua vera tissues contain lipases that hydrolyze fatty acids esterified in the 2 position. Specific phospholipase activity combined with a diacylglycerol lipase which also has a specificity for arachidonic acid, provides a mechanism

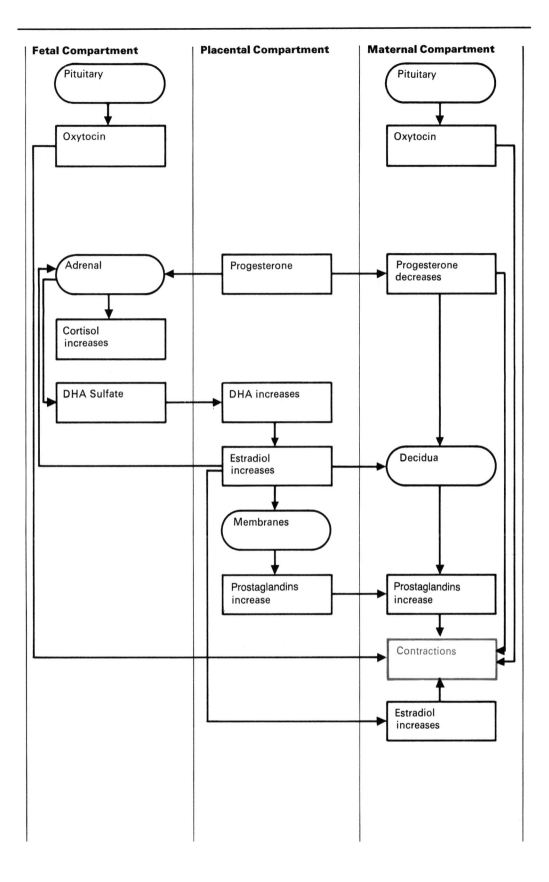

Fetal Compartment

Pituitary

Oxytocin

Adrenal

Cortisol increases

DHA Sulfate

Placental Compartment

Progesterone

DHA increases

Estradiol increases

Membranes

Prostaglandins increase

Maternal Compartment

Pituitary

Oxytocin

Progesterone decreases

Decidua

Prostaglandins increase

Contractions

Estradiol increases

for the release of arachidonic acid. The activity of these enzymes in fetal membranes and decidua vera tissue increases with increasing length of gestation.

The key may be the increasing formation of estrogen (both estradiol and estriol) in the maternal circulation as well as in the amniotic fluid, or more importantly, locally within the uterus. The marked rise in estrogen near term may affect the activity of the lipase enzymes, leading to the liberation of arachidonic acid.

The human fetal membranes and decidua are incredibly active. Human chorion and decidua produce estrogen utilizing a variety of substrates, especially estrone sulfate and dehydroepiandrosterone sulfate (DHAS), and this activity is increased around the time of parturition.(33,34) In addition, the human fetal membranes synthesize and metabolize progesterone.(35) The membranes contain a 17,20-hydroxysteroid dehydrogenase system. One active site converts 20α-dihydroxyprogesterone to progesterone, while another active site on this enzyme converts estrone to estradiol. Thus this enzyme can play an important role in altering the estrogen/progesterone ratio. The membranes and the decidua contain distinct cell populations with different biochemical activities (which change with labor).(36) Steroidogenic and prostaglandin interactions among these cells could produce the changes necessary for parturition without affecting the concentrations of circulating hormones. In addition, relaxin derived from decidua and/or chorion may exert a paracrine action on amnion prostaglandin production.(37) Finally, the fetus may take a very direct role in this scenario by secreting substances into the amniotic fluid, which interact with the fetal membranes to signal the initiation of parturition.

With labor, the arachidonic acid pathway in the fetal membranes shifts in the cyclooxygenase direction with a large increase in the production of PGE_2. A specific inhibitor of prostaglandin synthetase has been demonstrated in amniotic epithelium, and this inhibitor cannot be found in tissue from patients who have established labor.(38) The link between infection and the onset of labor may be due to the conversion by bacterial medium of arachidonic metabolism in the membranes to a condition associated with labor, marked by the production of PGE_2.(39,40)

During labor the circulating levels of PGE_2, $PGF_{2\alpha}$, and the $PGF_{2\alpha}$-metabolite are increased, a change which can be directly attributed to uterine production in that the gradient across the uterus for these substances is also increased. This increase in production of prostaglandins within the uterus must be the key factor, as the concentration and affinity of prostaglandin receptors do not change at parturition.(41) Meanwhile, prostacyclin and its metabolite are not increased. Prostacyclin is produced (at least in vitro) by a variety of tissues involved in pregnancy: endometrium, myometrium, placenta, amnion, chorion, decidua. As will be discussed later, this prostacyclin is probably more important in the vascular responses of mother and fetus, and in all likelihood does not play a role in initiating or maintaining uterine contractions.

The amnion appears to be a major source of prostaglandins leading to parturition. There is evidence for the transfer of prostaglandin E_2 across the membranes to the decidua and possibly the myometrium.(42) The paradox of PGE_2 production in the amnion being matched not by a PGE-metabolite in the maternal circulation, but by a $PGF_{2\alpha}$-metabolite, is explained by transfer across the membranes and conversion of PGE_2 to $PGF_{2\alpha}$ in the decidua.(43)

There is little evidence that increased maternal levels of oxytocin are responsible for initiating parturition, although a low fixed level may be an essential permissive factor. Once labor has begun, however, oxytocin levels do rise, especially during the second stage. Thus, oxytocin may be important for developing the more intense uterine contractions. Extremely high concentrations of oxytocin can be measured in the cord blood at delivery and, release of oxytocin from the fetal pituitary may also play a role during labor. Indeed, the magnitude of the fetal contribution to the maternal side is similar to the dose usually infused to induce labor.

It is likely that oxytocin action during the inital stages of labor may depend on myometrial sensitivity to oxytocin rather than on the levels of oxytocin in the blood. The concentration of oxytocin receptors in the myometrium is low in the nonpregnant state, and increases steadily throughout gestation (an 80-fold increase), and during labor the concentration doubles. This receptor concentration correlates with the uterine sensitivity to oxytocin. The mechanism for the increase is unknown, but it likely is due to a change in the hormonal milieu of the myometrium. Finally, oxytocin receptors in the decidua are thought to play a role in regulating prostaglandin production.

Animal studies have implicated the formation of low resistance pathways in the myometrium, called gap junctions, as an important action of steroids and prostaglandins during labor. In the gap junction, a pore forms which allows communication from cytoplasm to cytoplasm between two cells. Either substances or electrical current can follow this pathway. Thus, gap junctions provide a means of communication between myometrial cells allowing enhancement of electrical conductivity and synchronization of activity. Gap junction formation is related to the estrogen/progesterone ratio and to the presence of the stimulating prostaglandins, PGE_2 and $PGF_{2\alpha}$. Therefore it is not surprising that the number of gap junctions increases in the final weeks of pregnancy. But experimental evidence suggests that the number of gap junctions best correlates with the number of estrogen and progesterone receptors rather than the concentrations of the steroids themselves.

The final contraction of uterine muscle results from increased free calcium concentrations in the myofibril, the result of prostaglandin action, an action opposed to that of progesterone which promotes calcium binding in the sarcoplasmic reticulum.(44) Thus prostaglandins and oxytocin increase while progesterone decreases intracellular calcium levels. The intracellular calcium concentration is affected by cellular entry and exit of calcium as well as binding in the sarcoplasmic reticulum. It is the intracellular concentration of calcium which determines the rate of myosin light-chain phosphorylation and the contractile state of the myometrium. Tocolytic therapy (the use of β-adrenergic agents) stimulates adenylate cyclase activity which increases the levels of cellular cyclic AMP, which in turn decreases intracellular calcium concentration as well as inhibiting actin-myosin interaction by modulating kinase phosphorylation.

Treatment of Labor with Prostaglandin Inhibition

The key role for prostaglandins in parturition raises the potential for treatment of premature labor with inhibitors of prostaglandin synthesis. The concern has been that such treatment would result in intrauterine closure of the ductus arteriosus and pulmonary hypertension. Clinical studies, however, indicate that use of the nonsteroidal anti-inflammatory agents for short periods of time yields good results and does not result in this complicaiton.(45) Beyond 34 weeks, the fetus is more sensitive to this action, and treatment should be limited to pregnancies less than 34 weeks. Perhaps it is the treatment of choice for the inhibition of labor during a maternal transport. If the drug is failing, it should not be maintained because increased blood loss can occur at delivery. This treatment has also been used for polyhydramnios with good response and no effect on the newborn despite treatment for 2 to 11 weeks.(46)

Induction of Labor and Cervical Ripening

Pharmacologically and physiologically, prostaglandins have two direct actions associated with labor: ripening of the cervix and a direct oxytocic action. Successful parturition requires organized changes in both the upper uterus and in the cervix. The cervical changes are in response to the estrogen/progesterone ratio and the local release of prostaglandins. Whether relaxin plays a role in human parturition is not established.

Ripening of the cervix is the result of a change which includes an increase in hyaluronic acid and water, and a decrease in dermatan sulfate and chondroitin sulfate (these compounds hold the collagen fibers in a rigid structure). How prostaglandins are involved in this change is unknown, but enzyme activation must be involved. For ripening of the cervix, PGE_2 is very effective while $PGF_{2\alpha}$ has little effect. The purpose of achieving ripening of the cervix is to increase the success rate with induction of labor and lower the proportion of cesarean sections. Intravaginal prostaglandin E_2 gel has been compared with a synthetic cervical stent, and been found to be more effective.(47)

A major clinical application for the induction of labor in the United States is the use of intravaginal PGE_2 in cases of fetal demise and anencephalic fetuses. Based on our own experience, certain precautions have been developed. It is best to start slowly, using $\frac{1}{4}$-$\frac{1}{2}$ tablets every 2-4 hours. The patient should be well hydrated with an electrolyte solution to counteract the induced vasodilatation and decreased peripheral resistance. If satisfactory uterine activity is established, the next suppository should be withheld. And finally, because there is a synergistic effect when oxytocin is used shortly after prostaglandin administration, there should be a minimum of 12 hours between the last prostaglandin dose and beginning oxytocin augmentation.

Prostaglandins are used to induce term labor. Intravenous prostaglandins are not an acceptable method due to the side effects achieved by the high dosage necessary to reach the uterus. The intravaginal

366

and oral administration of PGE_2 is as effective as intravenous oxytocin, even including patients with previous cesarean sections. These methods, plus intracervical administration, are in routine use in many parts of the world.

Therapeutic Abortion

Prostaglandins are effective for postcoital contraception and first trimester abortion, but impractical due to the high incidence of side effects, including an unacceptable rate of incomplete abortions. For midtrimester abortions, intraamniotic prostaglandin, intramuscular methyl esters, and vaginal PGE suppositories are available. The major clinical problems have been the efficacy in accomplishing complete expulsion and the high level of systemic side effects. Overall, there is a higher risk of hemorrhage, fever, infection, antibiotic administration, readmission to the hospital, and more operative procedures when compared to saline abortions. These complications can be minimized if care is paid to two aspects of the clinician's technique. First, laminaria should be used to reduce the incidence of cervical injury and the need for retreatment. Second, aggressive management of the third stage is necessary. Removing the placenta with ring forceps, inspecting the cervix, and exploring the uterine cavity are necessasry immediately after expulsion of the fetus.

This aggressive management will minimize the most troublesome side effects, which are due to retained tissue. Prostaglandin E_2 and PGE analogues have proven to be most efficacious with the least side effects for the induction of labor, ripening of the cervix, and therapeutic abortion. The long-term instability of these compounds has been a major obstacle to commercial development. Attempts to solve this problem are focusing on improved gels as the physical base and on sustained release vaginal delivery systems.

Prostaglandins and Postpartum Hemorrhage

When routine methods of management for postpartum hemorrhage due to uterine atony have failed, an analogue of prostaglandin $F_{2\alpha}$ has been used with excellent results (80-90% successful).(48) Prostin 15 M is (15-S)-15-methyl prostaglandin $F_{2\alpha}$-tromethamine. The dose is 0.25-0.5 mg, repeated up to 4 times and given with equal efficiency either intramuscularly or directly into the myometrium. It can also be used after the replacement of an inverted uterus. Failures are usually associated with infections or magnesium sulfate therapy. It should not be used in patients with severe hypertension or symptomatic asthma. Diarrhea is a frequent side effect.

Prostaglandins, Uteroplacental Blood Flow, and Maternal Blood Pressure

A change must take place in the maternal vascular system to accommodate the volume and flow changes during pregnancy. The maternal plasma volume begins to increase about the 6th week of pregnancy. It rapidly expands during the second trimester, but increases only slightly in the last trimester until term. There is a greater increment in plasma volume as compared to the red cell volume in normal pregnancy (mean plasma volume increase of 1074 ml vs. 350 ml increase in red cell volume).(49) In order to accommodate the increase in volume (and cardiac output) without a significant increase in the maternal blood pressure, there must be a decrease in the peripheral vascular resistance. There are two mechanisms for the decrease in resistance. One is the increasing fraction of the cardiac output which passes through the uteroplacental circulation; the other is vasodilatation in the maternal vascular tree. Maintenance of normal maternal blood pressure and also maintenance of utero-placental blood flow (and therefore effective exchange functions across the placenta) depend upon vasodilatation, both in the systemic maternal circulation and locally with the uteroplacental unit. Prostacyclin may mediate this important function.

Toxemia of Pregnancy as a Chronic Disease

For the sake of nostalgia and for an economy of words, it continues to be useful to use "toxemia" of pregnancy interchangeably with pregnancy-induced hypertension. A more important change in our thinking has been the acceptance of the concept of toxemia as a chronic problem throughout pregnancy, not an acute disease arising at the time of hypertension. Measuring the metabolic clearance rate of dehydroepiandrosterone sulfate (DHAS), Gant et al demonstrated a decline in DHAS clearance prior to the development of clinically evident toxemia.(50) Subsequently, the same group showed that the pressor response to angiotensin II was different as early as 22 weeks in a group of primigravid women who went on to develop near term the typical clinical manifestations of toxemia.(51) Even the routine measurement of blood pressure, by a standardized technique that included a 5 minute rest period, was able to delineate a group of women who later became hypertensive, in that they had higher blood pressures throughout pregnancy.(52) Doppler blood flow studies confirm that in women destined to develop toxemia, changes occur early in pregnancy.(53)

The above studies indicate that toxemia of pregnancy is caused by or associated with a disturbance in a homeostatic mechanism responsible for maintenance of blood pressure and uteroplacental blood flow. The metabolic requirements of the fetus are best served by maintaining an adequate blood flow. In pregnancy, there is a need beyond the ordinary organ's concern with cellular function, there is the obligation of meeting the demands of the growing fetus. Toxemia is associated with a 40-60% reduction in blood flow through the uteroplacental unit in women, but it has been impossible to determine whether this is a primary or secondary event. If toxemia is due to the development of impaired blood flow over a period of time, it would seem that the clinical symptoms of the disease would be a late occurrence, and subclinical abnormalities should be detectable earlier in pregnancy (as in the above studies). Indeed, it has now been demonstrated that clearance of DHAS reflects a decrease in uteroplacental blood flow and therefore, reduced uteroplacental blood flow precedes the appearance of hypertension.(54)

Prostaglandins and Toxemia

Two properties of certain classes of prostaglandins are noteworthy in searching for the mechanism of vasodilatation and regulation of blood flow in pregnancy. First, E prostaglandins and prostacyclin are potent vasodilators, decreasing the peripheral resistance and systemic blood pressure by directly relaxing the smooth muscle of the arterial walls. Second, the majority of the activity of these prostaglandins appears to be limited to the immediate vicinity of the synthesizing tissue itself.

Initially, attention was focused on E and F prostaglandins. The important observations in the monkey (55-57), the sheep (58), the dog (59), and the rabbit (60), were as follows:

1. Angiotensin II increased uterine blood flow.

2. Angiotensin II increased PGE production by the pregnant uterus.

3. Inhibition of prostaglandin synthesis lowered basal blood flow, blocked the blood flow and PGE response to angiotensin II, and raised the systemic blood pressure.

These findings are consistent with a role for E prostaglandins in maintaining the resting uteroplacental and maternal vasomotor tone, and in moderating resistance to flow in response to vasoconstrictors. In the experiments in monkeys in the third trimester, angiotensin II-induced hypertension following treatment with indomethacin failed to increase uterine artery blood flow as had been noted after the initial infusion of angiotensin. A significant obstacle in the interpretation of these studies is the impact of surgical and anesthetic stress.

The entire renin-angiotensin-aldosterone system is increased in pregnancy, presumably due to a direct stimulation of substrate (angiotensinogen) synthesis by estrogen. It appears that this increase is the basic mechanism for producing the increased blood volume of pregnancy. The demonstration that blood vessels produce prostaglandins led to the speculation that vascular prostaglandins were responsible for the concomitant vasodilatation associated with the increased renin-angiotensin-aldosterone activity.(61) A pregnant woman's blood pressure at any point in time then reflected the balance of these various forces. A role for prostaglandins was supported by the demonstration that the administration of indomethacin or aspirin decreased the amount of angiotensin necessary to produce a pressor response in pregnant women.(62) This is consistent with the conclusion that pressor responsiveness to angiotensin II during pregnancy is determined by the degree of vascular resistance to the pressor agent. A hypothesis was then suggested linking estrogen, the renin-angiotensin system, and prostaglandins.(61)

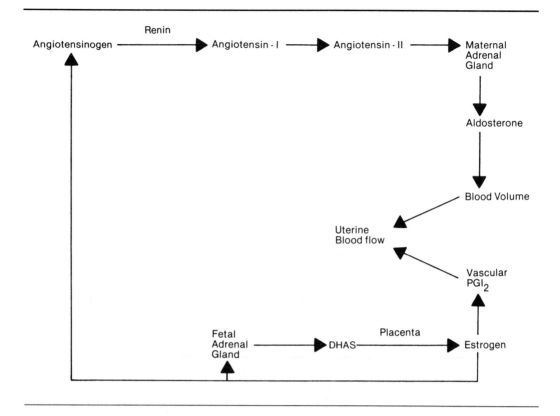

Estrogen can be viewed as a principal messenger for ensuring normal growth and development. Estrogen increases uterine blood flow, apparently via the mediation of a vasodilating prostaglandin. The major precursor for placental estrogen production is DHAS, secreted by the fetal adrenal gland. What regulates estrogen production has been an important question in placental physiology. This question appears to be answered, with the concept that the fetal adrenal-placental unit governs its own rate of estrogen production. (Chapter 10) The amount of precursor available for estrogen production may be the major rate-limiting factor. Estrogen itself circulates back to the fetus to increase the production of its precursor by suppressing the activity of the enzyme, 3β-hydroxysteroid dehydrogenase, thus diverting the steroidogenic pathway to DHAS. This mechanism allows ever increasing levels of estrogen production. The rising levels of estrogen increase the activity of the aldosterone system to expand blood volume, and at the same time may stimulate prostacyclin production within fetal and maternal blood vessels to maintain vasodilatation and blood flow. Toxemia of pregnancy may represent defective prostacyclin production, increased degradation of prostacyclin, a loss of response to prostacyclin, or a combination of these factors.

Prostacyclin and
Toxemia

The emergence of prostacyclin as a vasodilator even more potent than E prostaglandins directed attention to this new member of the prostaglandin family. In addition, it was appreciated that the prostacyclin metabolite migrates with E prostaglandins in separation systems. Therefore, previous studies implicating E prostaglandins may have been dealing with prostacyclin.

370

Many investigators have reported a general decrease in prostacyclin associated with pre-eclampsia.(63-65) Lower levels of this potent vasodilator and inhibitor of platelet activity could explain three of the most significant clinical consequences of toxemia: hypertension, platelet consumption, and reduced uteroplacental blood flow.

For years, investigators have implicated disseminated intravascular coagulation (DIC) as an important component of the symptom complex associated with toxemia. Pritchard has argued strongly that thrombocytopenia in toxemia is not an etiologic factor, but a consequence of the disease, most consistent with platelet adherence at sites of vascular endothelial damage.(66) A closer analysis reveals that the thrombocytopenia associated with toxemia is most similar to that seen with various microangiopathies, a consequence of abnormal platelet-endothelial interaction.(67) Such a mechanism for the thrombocytopenia of toxemia is consistent with a problem in prostacyclin production or function. Indeed modern assessments indicate that preeclampsia is associated with high fibronectin, low antithrombin III, and low alpha$_2$-antiplasmin, suggesting endothelial injury, clotting, and fibrinolysis, respectively.(68) The most marked resolution associated with delivery occurs with fibronectin the marker for endothelial injury.

	Disseminated Intravascular Coagulation	Microangiopathy
Etiology	Thromboplastins, thrombin, fibrin	Endothelial cell damage, platelet activation
Pathology	Intravascular fibrin	Intravascular platelet deposition
Fibrinogen levels	Low	Normal or high
Platelet count	Mild to moderately decreased	Moderate to markedly decreased
Red cells	Slight to moderate fragmentation	Moderate to marked fragmentation

As with blood pressure measurement, DHAS clearance, and angiotensin II pressor response, decreased platelet counts, when studied in a carefully controlled manner, also precede the development of hypertension. Early platelet consumption may be seen with preeclampsia before deterioration of urate clearance or elevation of blood pressure. The failure of heparin therapy to affect the clinical course of pre-eclampsia supports the fact that DIC is not the mechanism of the thrombocytopenia. Indeed, the reason that hypertension does not accompany coagulation disorders associated with intrauterine fetal demise and abruption placentae, may be that these classic problems are due to infusion of thromboplastin and DIC, and not due to an endothelial prostacyclin disorder.

The pathologic appearance of blood vessels in the placental bed in toxemic pregnancies bears significant resemblance to the blood vessels associated with microangiopathic syndromes.(69) Patients with the hemolytic uremic syndrome and thrombotic thrombocytopenic purpura share a common problem: defective prostacyclin activity.(70-72) Another similar syndrome has been reported, a problem

371

with a "lupus" anticoagulant. "Lupus" anticoagulant is a spontaneously acquired inhibitor of blood coagulation that interferes with activation of prothrombin. It is an immunoglobulin that is associated with an inhibition of prostacyclin synthesis in a variety of tissues. Although first recognized in patients with systemic lupus erythematosus, it has been detected in other clinical conditions as well. Lesions in the placenta and the placental vessels in this syndrome resembled those formerly believed to be only associated with hypertension in pregnancy. These lesions (fibrinoid necrosis, acute atherosis, and intraluminal thrombosis) have now been described in idiopathic intrauterine growth retardation, diabetic pregnancies, systemic lupus erythematosus, and toxemia. Are these examples of diseases of different mechanisms, but all having the same target: prostacyclin?

The precise problem may be more a reflection of the thromboxane/prostacyclin balance. Both thromboxane and prostacyclin production are increased during pregnancy, but the increase in prostacyclin far exceeds the increase in thromboxane.(10) The key may be the requirement for this excess of prostacyclin in normal pregnancy. A low dose of aspirin (40 mg daily) that selectively inhibits platelet cyclooxygenase results in a marked reduction in thromboxane levels in maternal blood (but not in fetal blood), with minimal but transient impact on prostacyclin metabolites and no impairment of prostacyclin synthesis in the umbilical artery.(73) Low doses of aspirin which inhibit thromboxane production (in platelets, and perhaps in trophoblastic tissue), unbalancing the ratio in favor of prostacyclin, do offer prophylaxis against toxemia of pregnancy.(74,75) This dose of aspirin appears to be safe for the fetus because it takes 100 mg daily to decrease levels of thromboxane in cord bloods (leaving prostacyclin unaffected) and 500 mg to inhibit both thromboxane and prostacyclin in the fetus.(76)

In a sheep model of toxemia, a specific inhibitor of thromboxane synthetase increased uterine blood flow and glomerular filtration rate, decreased proteinuria, and restored platelet counts to normal.(77) During the hypertension, both prostacyclin and thromboxane decreased (as measured by their metabolites), and after treatment with the inhibitor, prostacyclin increased even higher than baseline while thromboxane did not change. Finally, part of the beneficial impact of magnesium therapy for preeclampsia can be attributed to an effect on prostacyclin. Magnesium increases prostacyclin production in cultured human umbilical endothelial cells, and so does the plasma from preeclamptic patients undergoing magnesium sulfate treatment.(78)

In an in vitro model, inhibition of prostaglandin synthesis reduced placental transfer and a prostacyclin analogue reversed this effect.(79) The vasodilatation by prostacyclin may be at a very local level in the placental vascular bed. The use of a stable analogue offers pharmacologic promise over the use of the unstable parent prostacyclin. This study also raises caution regarding the use of prostaglandin inhibitors and probably the importance of dose.

Evidence is accumulating to link prostacyclin and thromboxane to the clinical and pathological manifestations of toxemia. Having recognized and accepted the concept that toxemia is a chronic disease, the current challenge is to discover a practical method for early diagnosis, long before the irreversible end stage represented by the classical triad of hypertension, proteinura and edema develops. Accurate early diagnosis would open the door for pharmacologic intervention.

References

1. **Ramwell PW, Foegh M, Loeb R, Leovey EMK,** Synthesis and metabolism of prostaglandins, prostacyclin, and thromboxanes: the arachidonic acid cascade, Seminars Perinatol 4:3, 1980.

2. **Samuelsson B, Dahlen S-E, Lindgren JA, Rouzer CA, Serhan CN,** Leukotrienes and lipoxins: Structures, biosynthesis, and biological effects, Science 237:1171, 1987.

3. **Gryglewski RJ, Korbut R, Oetkiewicz A, Splawinski J, Wojtaszek B, Swies J,** Lungs as a generator of prostacyclin-hypothesis on physiological significance, Arch Pharmacol 304:45, 1979.

4. **Moncada S, Vane JR,** Arachidonic acid metabolites and the interactions between platelets and blood vessel walls, New Eng J Med 300:1142, 1979.

5. **Beitz J, Muller G, Forster W,** Effect of HDL and LDL from pre and post menopausal women on prostacyclin synthesis, Prostaglandins 30:179, 1985.

6. **Makheja A, Vanderhoek JY, Bailey JM,** Inhibition of platelet aggregation and thromboxane synthesis by onion and garlic, Lancet i:781, 1979.

7. **Fischer S, Weber PC,** The prostacyclin/thromboxane balance is favourably shifted in Greenland Eskimos, Prostaglandins 32:235, 1986.

8. **Flower RJ, Blackwell GJ,** Anti-inflammatory steroids induce biosynthesis of the phospholipase A_2 inhibitor which prevents prostaglandin generation, Nature 278:456, 1979.

9. **Masotti G, Poggesi L, Galanti G, Abbate R, Neri Serneri GG,** Differential inhibition of prostacyclin production and platelet aggregation by aspirin, Lancet ii:1213, 1979.

10. **Fitzgerald DJ, Mayo G, Catella F, Entman SS, FitzGerald GA,** Increased thromboxane biosynthesis in normal pregnancy is mainly derived from platelets, Am J Obstet Gynecol 157:325, 1987.

11. **Behrman HR,** Prostaglandins in hypothalamo-pituitary and ovarian function, Ann Rev Physiol 41:685, 1979.

12. **Auletta FJ, Agins H, Scommegna A,** Prostaglandin $F_{2\alpha}$ mediation of the inhibitory effect of estrogen on the corpus luteum of the rhesus monkey, Endocrinology 103:1183, 1978.

13. **Auletta FJ, Caldwell BV, Speroff, L,** Estrogen-induced luteolysis in the rhesus monkey: Reversal with indomethacin, Prostaglandins 11:745, 1976.

14. **Auletta FJ, Kamps DL, Pories S, Bisset J, Gibson M,** An intra-ovarian site for the luteolytic action of prostaglandin $F_{2\alpha}$ in the rhesus monkey, Prostaglandins 27:285, 1984.

15. **Auletta FJ, Kamps DL, Wesley M, Gibson M,** Luteolysis in the rhesus monkey: Ovarian venous estrogen, progesterone, and prostaglandin $F_{2\alpha}$-metabolite, Prostaglandins 27:299, 1984.

16. **Gore BC, Caldwell BV, Speroff L,** Estrogen-induced human luteolysis, J Clin Endocrin Metab 36:615, 1973.

17. **Coceani F, Olley PM, Lock JE,** Prostaglandins, ductus arteriosus, pulmonary circulation: current concepts and clinical potential, Eur J Clin Pharmacol 18:75, 1980.

18. **Brash AR, Hickey DE, Graham TP, Stahlman MT, Oates JA, Cotton RB,** Pharmacokinetics of indomethacin in the neonate: relation of plasma indomethacin levels to response of the ductus arteriosus, New Eng J Med 305:67, 1981.

19. **Rudolph AM,** The effects of nonsteroidal antiinflammatory compounds on fetal circulation and pulmonary function, Obstet Gynecol 58:635, 1981.

20. **Challis JRG, Mitchell BF,** Hormonal control of pre-term and term parturition, Seminars Perinatol 5:192, 1981.

21. **Nelson GH, Fadel HE,** Prostaglandins and parturition, Seminars Reprod Endocrinol 3:231, 1985.

22. **Price HV, Cone BA, Keogh M,** Length of gestation in congenital adrenal hyperplasia, J Obstet Gynaecol Brit Common 78:430, 1971.

23. **Davidson BJ, Murray RD, Challis JRG, Valenzuela GJ,** Estrogen, progesterone, prolactin, prostaglandin E_2, prostaglandin $F_{2\alpha}$, 13,14-dihydro-15-keto-prostaglandin $F_{2\alpha}$, and 6-keto-prostaglandin $F_{1\alpha}$ gradients across the uterus in women in labor and not in labor, Am J Obstet Gynecol 157:54, 1987.

24. **Femini M, Borenstein R, Dreazen E, Apelman Z, Mogilner BM, Kessler I, Lancet M,** Pevention of premature labor by 17α-hydroxyprogesterone caproate, Am J Obstet Gynecol 151:574, 1985.

25. **Erny R, Pigne A, Prouvost C, Gamerre M, Malet C, Serment H, Barrat J,** The effects of oral administration of progesterone for premature labor, Am J Obstet Gynecol 154:525, 1986.

26. **Khan-Dawood FS,** In vitro converison of pregnenolone to progesterone in human term placenta and fetal membranes before and after onset of labor, Am J Obstet Gynecol 157:1333, 1987.

27. **Gustavii B,** Release of lysosomal acid phosphatase into the cytoplasm of decidual cells before the onset of labor in humans, Brit J Obstet Gynaecol 82:177, 1975.

28. **Schwarz BE, Schultz FM, MacDonald PC, Johnston JM,** Initiation of human parturition: III. Fetal membrane content of prostaglandin E_2 and $F_{2\alpha}$ precursor, Obstet Gynecol 46:564, 1975.

29. **Curbelo V, Bejar R, Benirschke K, Gluck L,** Premature labor: 1. Prostaglandin precursors in human placental membranes, Obstet Gynecol 57:473, 1981.

374

30. **Okazaki T, Sagawa N, Okita JR, Bleasdale JE, MacDonald PC, Johnston JM,** Diacylglycerol metabolism and arachidonic acid release in human fetal membranes and decidua vera, J Biol Chem 256:7316, 1981.

31. **Okazaki T, Sagawa N, Bleasdale JE, Okita JR, MacDonald PC, Johnston JM,** Initiation of human parturition: XIII. Phospholipase C, phospholipase A_2, and diacylglycerol lipase activities in fetal membranes and decidua vera tissues from early and late gestation, Biol Reprod 25:103, 1981.

32. **DiRenzo GC, Johnston JM, Okazaki T, Okita JR, MacDonald PC, Bleasdale JE,** Phosphatidylinositol specific phospholipase C in fetal membranes and uterine decidua, J Clin Invest 67:847, 1981.

33. **Romano WM, Lukash LA, Challis JRG, Mitchell BF,** Substrate utilization for estrogen synthesis by human fetal membranes and decidua, Am J Obstet Gynecol 155:1170, 1986.

34. **Chibbar R, Hobkirk R, Mitchell BF,** Sulfohydrolase activity for estrone sulfate and dehydroepiandrosterone sulfate in human fetal membranes and decidua around the time of parturition, J Clin Endocrinol Metab 62:90, 1986.

35. **Mitchell BF, Challis JRG, Lukash L,** Progesterone synthesis by human amnion, chorion, and decidua at term, Am J Obstet Gynecol 157:349, 1987.

36. **Challis JRG, Vaughan M,** Steroid synthetic and prostaglandin metabolizing activity is present in different cell populations from human fetal membranes and decidua, Am J Obstet Gynecol 157:1474, 1987.

37. **Lopez Bernal A, Bryant-Greenwood GD, Hansell DJ, Hicks BR, Greenwood FC, Turnbull AC,** Effect of relaxin on prostaglandin E production by human amnion: Changes in relation to the onset of labour, Brit J Obstet Gynaecol 94:1045, 1987.

38. **Mortimer G, Hunter IC, Stimson WH, Govan ADT,** A role for amniotic epithelium in control of human parturition, Lancet i:1074, 1985.

39. **Bennett PR, Rose MP, Myatt L, Elder MG,** Preterm labor: Stimulation of arachidonic acid metabolism in human amnion cells by bacterial productions, Am J Obstet Gynecol 156:649, 1987.

40. **Romero R, Emamian M, Wan M, Quintero R, Hobbins JC, Mitchell MD,** Prostaglandin concentrations in amniotic fluid of women with intra-amniotic infection and preterm labor, Am J Obstet Gynecol 157:1461, 1987.

41. **Giannopoulis G, Jackson K, Kredentser J, Tulchinsky D,** Prostaglandin E_2 and $F_{2\alpha}$ receptors in human myometrium during the menstrual cycle and in pregnancy and labor, Am J Obstet Gynecol 153:904, 1985.

42. **Nakla S, Skinner K, Mitchell BF, Challis JRG,** Changes in prostaglandin transfer across human fetal membranes obtained after spontaneous labor, Am J Obstet Gynecol 155:1337, 1986.

43. **Niesert S, Christopherson W, Korte K, Mitchell MD, MacDonald PC, Casey ML,** Prostaglandin E_2 9-ketoreductase activity in human decidua vera tissue, Am J Obstet Gynecol 155:1348, 1986.

44. **Carsten ME, Miller JD,** A new look at uterine muscle contraction, Am J Obstet Gynecol 157:1303, 1987.

375

45. **Niebyl JR, Witter FR,** Neonatal outcome after indomethacin treatment for preterm labor, Am J Obstet Gynecol 155:747, 1986.

46. **Cabrol D, Landesman R, Muller J, Uzan M, Sureau C, Saxena BB,** Treatment of polyhydramnios with prostaglandin synthetase inhibitor (indomethacin), Am J Obstet Gynecol 157:422, 1987.

47. **Johnson IR, Macpherson MBA, Welch CC, Filshie GM,** A comparison of Lamicel and prostaglandin E_2 vaginal gel for cervical ripening before induction of labor, Am J Obstet Gynecol 151:178, 1985.

48. **O'Leary JA,** Prostaglandins and postpartum hemorrhage, Seminars Reprod Endocrinol 3:247, 1985.

49. **Brinkman CR,** Physiology and pathophysiology of maternal adjustments to pregnancy, in *Clinical Perinatology,* Aladjem S, Brown AK, editors, C. V. Mosby, St. Louis, 1975.

50. **Gant NP, Hutchinson HT, Siiteri PK, MacDonald PC,** Study of the metabolic clearance of dehydroisoandrosterone sulfate in pregnancy, Am J Obstet Gynecol 111:555, 1971.

51. **Gant NF, Daley GL, Chand S, Whalley PJ, MacDonald PC,** A study of angiotensin II pressor response throughout primigravid pregnancy, J Clin Invest 52:2682, 1973.

52. **Gallery EDM, Ross M, Hunyor SN, Gyory AX,** Predicting the development of pregnancy-associated hypertension, the place of standardized blood pressure measurement, Lancet i:1273, 1977.

53. **Cohen-Overbeck T, Pearce JM, Campbell S,** The antenatal assessment of utero-placental and feto-placental blood flow using Doppler ultrasound, Ultrasound Med Biol 11:329, 1985.

54. **Fritz MA, Stanczyk FZ, Novy MJ,** Relationship of uteroplacental blood flow to the placental clearance of maternal dehydroepiandrosterone through estradiol formation in the pregnant baboon, J Clin Endocrinol Metab 61:1023, 1985.

55. **Franklin GO, Dowd AJ, Caldwell BV, Speroff L,** The effect of angiotensin II intravenous infusion on plasma renin activity and prostaglandins A, E, and F levels in the uterine vein of the pregnant monkey, Prostaglandins, 6:271, 1974.

56. **Speroff L, Haning RV Jr, Ewaschuk EJ, Alberino SL, Kieliszek FX,** Uterine artery blood flow studies in the pregnant monkey, in *Hypertension in Pregnancy*, Lindheimer MD, Katz AL, Zuspan FP, editors, John Wiley, New York, 1976, pp 315-327.

57. **Speroff L, Haning RV Jr, Levin RM,** The effect of angiotensin II and indomethacin on uterine artery blood flow in pregnant monkeys, Obstet Gynecol 50:611, 1977.

58. **McLaughlin MK, Brennan SC, Chez RA,** Effects of indomethacin on sheep uteroplacental circulations and sensitivity to angiotensin II, Am J Obstet Gynecol 132:430, 1978.

59. **Terragno NA, Terragno DA, Pacholxzyk D, McGiff JC,** Prostaglandins and the regulation of uterine blood flow in pregnancy, Nature 249:57, 1974.

60. **Venuto RC, O'Dorisio T, Stein JH, Ferris TF,** Uterine prostaglandin E secretion and uterine blood flow in the pregnant rabbit, J Clin Invest 55:193, 1975.

61. **Speroff L, Dorfman GS,** Prostaglandins and pregnancy hypertension, Clin Obstet Gynecol 4:635, 1977.

62. **Everett RB, Worley RJ, MacDonald PC, Gant NF,** Effect of prostaglandin synthetase inhibitors on pressor response to angiotensin II in human pregnancy, J Clin Endocrinol Metab 46:1007, 1978.

63. **Goodman RP, Killam AP, Brash AR, Branch RA,** Prostacyclin production during pregnancy: comparison of production during normal pregnancy and pregnancy complicated by hypertension, Am J Obstet Gynecol 142:817, 1982.

64. **Ylikorkala O, Pekonen F, Viinikka L,** Renal prostacyclin and thromboxane in normotensive and preeclamptic pregnant women and their infants, J Clin Endocrinol Metab 63:1307, 1986.

65. **Fitzgerald DJ, Entman SS, Mulloy K, FitzGerald GA,** Decreased prostacyclin biosynthesis preceding the clinical manifestations of pregnancy-induced hypertension, Circulation 75:956, 1987.

66. **Pritchard JA, Cunningham FG, Mason RA,** Coagulation changes in eclampsia: their frequency and pathogenesis, Am J Obstet Gynecol 124:855, 1976.

67. **Bern MM, Driscoll SG, Leavitt T Jr,** Thrombocytopenia complicating pre-eclampsia, Obstet Gynecol 57:28S, 1981.

68. **Saleh AA, Bottoms SF, Welch RA, Ali AM, Mariona FG, Mammen EF,** Preeclampsia, delivery, and the hemostatic system, Am J Obstet Gynecol 157:331, 1987.

69. **De Wolf F, Robertson WB, Brosens I,** The ultrastructure of acute atherosis in hypertensive pregnancy, Am J Obstet Gynecol 123:154, 1975.

70. **Jorgensen KA, Pedersen RS,** Familial deficiency of prostacyclin production stimulating factor in the hemolytic uremic syndrome of childhood, Thromb Res 21:311, 1981.

71. **Machin SJ, Defreyn G, Chamone DAF, Vermylen J,** Plasma 6-keto-$PGF_{1\alpha}$ levels after plasma exchange in thrombotic thrombocytopenic purpura, Lancet i:661, 1980.

72. **Remuzzi G, Imperti L, DeGaetano G,** Prostacyclin deficiency in thrombotic microangiopathy, Lancet ii:1422, 1981.

73. **Ritter JM, Farquhar C, Rodin A, Thom MH,** Low dose aspirin treatment in late pregnancy differentially inhibits cyclo-oxygenase in maternal platelets, Prostaglandins 34:717, 1987.

74. **Beaufils M, Donsimoni R, Uzan S, Colau JC,** Prevention of preeclampsia by early antiplatelet therapy, Lancet ii:240, 1985.

75. **Wallenburg HCS, Dekker GA, Makovitz JW, Rotmans P,** Low-dose aspirin prevents pregnancy-induced hypertension and preeclampsia in angiotensin-sensitive primigravidae, Lancet i:1, 1986.

76. **Ylidordala O, Makila U, Kaapa P, Viinikka L,** Maternal ingestion of acetylsalicylic acid inhibits fetal and neonatal prostacyclin and thromboxane in humans, Am J Obstet Gynecol 155:345, 1986.

77. **Keith JC, Thatcher CD, Schaub RG,** Beneficial effects of U-63,557A, a thromboxane synthetase inhibitor in an ovine model of pregnancy-induced hypertension, Am J Obstet Gynecol 157:199, 1987.

78. **Watson K, Moldow CG, Ogburn PL, Jacob HS,** Magnesium sulfate: Rationale for its use in preeclampsia, Proc Natl Acad Sci 83:1075, 1986.

79. **Kuhn DC, Stuart MJ,** Cyclooxygenase inhibition reduces placental transfer: Reversal by carbacyclin, Am J Obstet Gynecol 157:194, 1987.

12 Normal and Abnormal Sexual Development

Abnormalities of sexual differentiation are seen infrequently in an individual physician's practice. There are, however, few practitioners who have not been challenged at least once by a newborn with ambiguous genitalia or by a young woman with primary amenorrhea on a genetic basis. The categorization of the various syndromes in this area has been confusing, requiring constant reference to multiple textbooks, and dependence upon memory of eponym-laden, seemingly endless lists of syndromes. Happily, this "catalogue" state of affairs has changed; major advances in reproductive science have yielded clarification and consolidation. As a result, an informed basis for clinical practice has emerged and is readily applicable.

This chapter will present classification of the major problems and our clinical approach to diagnosis. Normal sexual differentiation will be considered in order to provide a basis of understanding for the various types of abnormal development. This is followed by a section on the diagnosis and management of ambiguous genitalia. Some subjects are discussed in other chapters, but brief descriptions will be repeated here in order to present a complete picture. The text by Jones and Rock (1) is recommended for greater detail, including descriptions of operative techniques used for the surgical repair of genital abnormalities. However, additional references to techniques for repair of hypospadias and reconstructive surgery should be noted.(2-4)

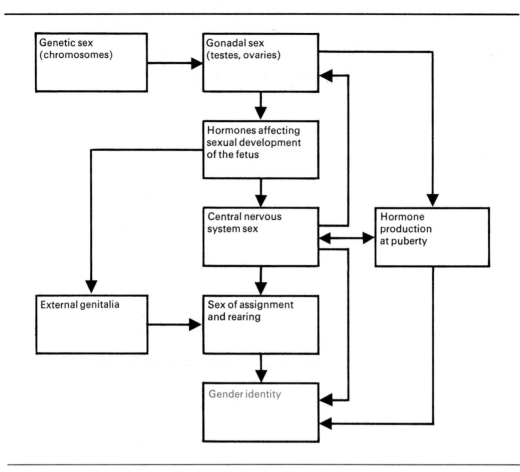

Genetic sex (chromosomes)		Gonadal sex (testes, ovaries)

Hormones affecting sexual development of the fetus

Central nervous system sex

Hormone production at puberty

External genitalia

Sex of assignment and rearing

Gender identity

Normal Sexual Differentiation

The gender identity of a person (whether an individual identifies as a male or a female) is the end result of genetic, hormonal and morphologic sex as influenced by the environment of the individual. It includes all behavior with any sexual connotation, such as body gestures and mannerisms, habits of speech, recreational preferences, and content of dreams. Sexual expression, both homosexual and heterosexual, can be regarded as the result of all influences on the individual, both prenatal and postnatal.

Prenatally, sexual differentiation follows a specific sequence of events. First is the establishment of the genetic sex. Second, under the control of the genetic sex the gonads differentiate, determining the hormonal environment of the embryo, the differentiation of internal duct systems, and the formation of the external genitalia. It has become apparent that the embryonic brain is also sexually differentiated, probably via a control mechanism very similar to that which determines the sexual development of the external genitalia. The inductive influences of hormones on the central nervous system may have an effect on the patterns of hormone secretion and sexual behavior in the adult.(5,6)

Gonadal Differentiation

In human embryos, the gonads begin development during the 5th and 6th weeks of gestation as protuberances overlying the mesonephric ducts. At 6 weeks, the migration of primordial germ cells into these gonadal ridges begins and is completed in a single week. Although germ cells do not induce gonadal development and simply take the form of the gonad in which they find themselves, if the germ cells fail to arrive, gonads do not develop and only the fibrous streak of gonadal agenesis will exist.(7) At 7 weeks of fetal life the gonads are indifferent but bipotential, possessing both cortical and medullary areas, and capable of differentiation into either testes or ovaries. They are composed of germ cells, special epithelia (potential granulosa/Sertoli cells), mesenchyme (potential theca/Leydig cells), and the mesonephric duct system. Wolffian and müllerian ducts exist side by side; external genitalia are undifferentiated.(8) Subsequent sexual differentiation requires direction by various genes, with a single gene determinant on the Y chromosome (testes-determining factor—TDF) necessary for testicular differentiation.(9,10)

The TDF gene, localized to the distal short arm (p) of the Y chromosome, has been identified in apes, monkeys, dogs, cattle, rabbits, goats, and there is a very similar gene in mice. Its gene product is a protein which reacts with other DNA as well as RNA, making this gene the primary "master switch" for male differentiation by its capacity to react with genes elsewhere on X, Y, and autosomes, as well as their diverse gene products. One such notable interaction is with the H-Y locus (or loci) with which TDF was originally thought to be identical. These H-Y genes induce a cell surface antigen, the H-Y antigen (Y-induced histocompatibility antigen). H-Y antigen is uniformly present in individuals with testes, and lacking in those without testes. However, it is not androgen induced and its derivation is uncertain, having been detected as early as the 8 cell stage embryo.

In the human, autosomal genes are also essential for gonadal development. These autosomal genes regulate migration of the germ cells, the processing or functioning of the H-Y antigen system, and coding of the steroidogenic enzymes. In the absence of a Y chromosome, the cortical zone develops and contains the germ cells, while the medullary portion regresses with its remnant being the rete ovarii, a compressed nest of tubules and Leydig cells in the hilus of the ovary. The formation of the testicle precedes any other sexual development in time, and a functionally active testis controls subsequent sexual development.

Testicular differentiation begins at 7 weeks; first with spermatogenic cords, then seminiferous tubules, followed by Leydig cell formation a week later. Human chorionic gonadotropin (HCG) stimulation produces Leydig cell hypertrophy, and peak fetal testosterone levels are seen at 12 weeks.(11)

In an XX individual, without the active influence of a Y chromosome, the bipotential gonad develops into an ovary about 2 weeks later than testicular development. The cortical zone differentiates and enlarges, and the germ cells proliferate by mitosis, reaching a peak of 5-7 million by 20 weeks. Medullary components regress to a hilar aggregation of rete tubules and residual nests of Leydig-like hilar cells. By 20 weeks, the fetal ovary achieves mature compartmentalization with primordial follicles containing oocytes, initial evidence of follicle maturation and atresia, and an incipient stroma. Degeneration (atresia) begins even earlier, and by birth, approximately 1-2 million germ cells remain. These have become surrounded by a layer of follicular cells, forming primordial follicles with oocytes which have entered the first meiotic division. Meiosis is arrested in the prophase of the first meiotic division until reactivation of follicular growth which may not occur until years later.

Excessively rapid atresia in gonadal dysgenesis (45,X) accounts for the streak gonad seen in these cases.(12) A complete 46,XX chromosomal complement is necessary for normal ovarian development.(13) Deletion of any portion of an X chromosome results in streak gonads. The short arm of the Y appears to contain loci similar to the short arm of the X chromosome. The absence of either results in short stature and gonadal dysgenesis.

Duct System Differentiation

The wolffian and müllerian ducts are discrete primordia which temporarily coexist in all embryos during the ambisexual period of development. One type of duct system persists normally and gives rise to special ducts and glands, whereas the other disappears during the 3rd fetal month, except for nonfunctional vestiges.

The elaboration of androgens by the medullary cells (forerunners of the Leydig cells) in the early testicle stimulates development of the wolffian duct system into epididymis, vas deferens, and seminal vesicles. Another substance (known as müllerian inhibiting factor, MIF) is responsible for regression of the müllerian duct system in the male. MIF is an incompletely characterized protein hormone which is the initial endocrine product of the testis. This influence from the fetal testis is unilateral. Duct system differentiation will proceed, therefore, according to the nature of the adjacent gonad.

The internal genitalia possess the intrinsic tendency to feminize. In the absence of a Y chromosome and a functional testis, the lack of MIF allows retention of the müllerian system and development of fallopian tubes, uterus, and upper vagina. In the absence of testosterone, the wolffian system regresses. In the presence of a normal ovary or the absence of any gonad, müllerian duct development takes place.

External Genitalia Differentiation

In the bipotential state (8th fetal week), the external genitalia consist of a urogenital sinus, two lateral labioscrotal swellings, and a genital tubercle. Unlike the internal genitalia where both duct systems initially coexist, the external genitalia are neutral primordia able to develop into either male or female structures depending on gonadal steroid hormone signals. Normally, this differentiation is under the active influence of androgen from the Leydig cells of the testis. The genital tubercle forms the penis, labioscrotal folds fuse to form a scrotum, and folds of the urogenital sinus form the penile urethra. The testis begins androgen secretion by 8-9 weeks; masculinization of the external genitalia is manifest 1 week later and is completed by 17 weeks. To achieve this morphologic change, external genitalia target tissue cells must convert testosterone to dihydrotestosterone (DHT) by the intracellular enzyme 5α-reductase. In the male, DHT mediates the following androgen events: temporal hairline recession, growth of facial and body hairs, development of acne, and development of the external genitalia and prostate.

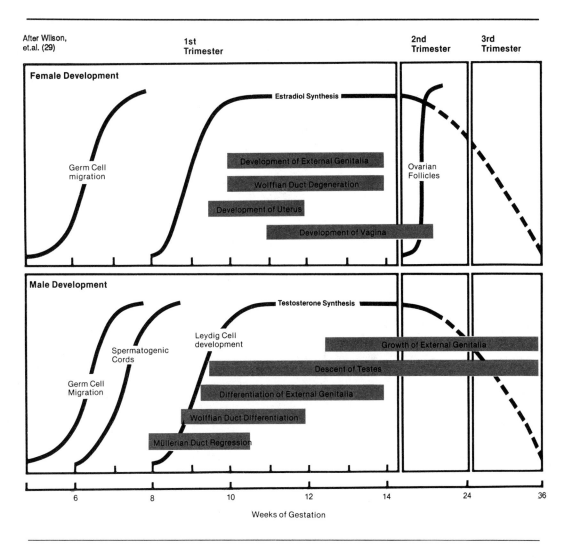

1st Trimester **2nd Trimester** **3rd Trimester**

Female Development

Estradiol Synthesis

Germ Cell migration

Development of External Genitalia

Wolffian Duct Degeneration

Development of Uterus

Development of Vagina

Ovarian Follicles

Male Development

Testosterone Synthesis

Spermatogenic Cords

Leydig Cell development

Germ Cell Migration

Growth of External Genitalia

Descent of Testes

Differentiation of External Genitalia

Wolffian Duct Differentiation

Müllerian Duct Regression

6   8   10   12   14   24   36

Weeks of Gestation

In the absence of this androgen effect (the absence of a Y chromosome, the presence of an ovary, the absence of a gonad, abnormalities in androgen receptor or postreceptor events, or defects of the 5α-reductase enzyme), the folds of the urogenital sinus remain open, forming the labia minora, the labioscrotal folds form the labia majora, the genital tubercle forms the clitoris, and the urogenital sinus differentiates into the vagina and the urethra. Thus, the lower vagina is formed as part of the external genitalia.

Exposure to androgens at critical time periods leads to variable masculinization. Androgen superimposes variable external ambiguity on the basic female phenotype (clitoral hypertrophy, hypospadias, scrotalization of nonfused labia). By the same token, if sufficient local androgen concentration or activity is not achieved by the 12th week in the male, incompletely masculinized genitalia will result. Because of shared common tissue origin, male-female external genital structural ambiguities reflect abnormal androgen impact—males too little, females too much.

383

Genital tubercle

Urogenital slit

Anal pit

Tail

Urethral folds

Labioscrotal swelling

Bipotential Stage

Glans

Genital tubercle

Urogenital slit

Urethral folds

Labioscrotal swelling

Anus

Glans

Genital tubercle

Urogenital slit

Urethral folds

Labioscrotal swelling

Anus

Meatus

Glans penis

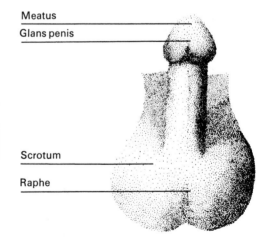

Clitoris

Urethral meatus

Labia minora

Vaginal orifice

Labia majora

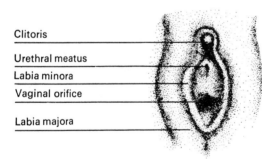

Scrotum

Raphe

Central Nervous System Differentiation	At the same time as the presence or absence of androgens is playing a critical role in genitalia development, the neuroendocrine mechanism of the central nervous system is also being influenced. Androgens present in sufficient amounts during the appropriate critical stage of development may program the CNS to induce the potential for male sexual behavior.(14) Experimental and analytical evidence suggests that a behavioral effect can be traced to this early androgen influence. Inappropriate fetal hormonal programming may contribute, therefore, to the spectrum of psychosexual behavior seen in humans.
Abnormal Sexual Differentiation	The standard classification of individuals with intersexuality (hermaphroditism) proceeds according to gonadal morphology. In this terminology, a *true hermaphrodite* possesses both ovarian and testicular tissue. A *male pseudohermaphrodite* has testes, but external and sometimes internal genitalia take on female phenotypic aspects. A *female pseudohermaphrodite* has ovaries, but genital development displays masculine characteristics. These classifications are modified to reflect gonadal abnormalities due to abnormal sex chromosome constitution or abnormalities of phenotype attributable to an inappropriate fetal hormone environment. Hypospadias in the absence of any other deformity is not included in this classification:

Disorders of Fetal Endocrinology

1. *Female pseudohermaphroditism (partial virilization)*
    a.   Congenital adrenal hyperplasia
        i.   21-Hydroxylase deficiency
        ii.   11β-Hydroxylase deficiency
        iii. 3β-Hydroxysteroid dehydrogenase deficiency
    b.   i.   Drug intake
        ii.   Maternal disease

2. *Male pseudohermaphroditism (inadequate virilization)*
    a.   Müllerian duct inhibitory factor defect
    b.   Impaired androgenization
        i.   Complete testicular feminization
        ii.   Incomplete testicular feminization
        iii. 5α-Reductase deficiency
    c.   Testosterone biosynthesis defects
        i.   20-22-Desmolase defect
        ii.   3β-Hydroxysteroid dehydrogenase deficiency
        iii. 17α-Hydroxylase deficiency
        iv.   17-20-Desmolase deficiency
        v.   17-Hydroxysteroid dehydrogenase deficiency

Disorders of Gonadal Development

1. *Male pseudohermaphroditism*
   a. Primary gonadal defect
   b. Y Chromosome defect

2. *True hermaphroditism*

3. *Gonadal dysgenesis*
   a. Turner's syndrome
   b. Mosaicism
   c. Structural abnormality—X chromosome
   d. Normal karyotype

Masculinized Females (Female Pseudohermaphrodites)

Masculinized females possess ovaries and are female by genetic sex (XX), but the external genitalia are not those of a normal female. Of all infants with ambiguous genitalia, 40-45% have adrenal hyperplasia. Rarer causes of female pseudohermaphroditism are excess maternal androgen caused by drug ingestion or tumor secretion.

The Adrenogenital Syndrome. The adrenogenital syndrome in females is characterized by masculinized external genitalia, and is diagnosed by demonstrating excessive androgen production by the adrenal cortex, due either to tumor or hyperplasia. The syndrome may appear in utero or develop postnatally.

The presence of excessive androgens is manifested by varying degrees of fusion of the labioscrotal folds, clitoral enlargement, and anatomical changes of the urethra and vagina. Generally, the urethra and vagina share a urogenital sinus formed by the fusion of labial folds. This sinus opens at the base of the clitoris which is usually enlarged. The degree of urogenital sinus deformity is related to the timing in prenatal development of the onset of masculinizing androgen effect. Only the external genitalia are affected because internal genitalia differentiation is completed by the 10th week of gestation while the adrenal cortex begins function by the 12th week. Since the female external genitalia phenotype is not completed until 140 days of fetal age, early androgen excess (7-12 weeks) may fully masculinize, whereas late (18-20 weeks) androgen may create limited ambiguity of the basically female appearance of the urogenital sinus and genital folds. The size of the clitoris depends on the quantity rather than timing of androgen excess. Cases of incorrect sex assignment in the female are due to the similarity between these external genitalia and hypospadias and bilateral cryptorchidism in a male infant.

If untreated, the female with adrenal hyperplasia will develop signs of progressive virilization. Pubic hair will appear by age 2-4, followed by axillary hair, then body hair and beard. Bone age is advanced by age 2, and because of early epiphyseal closure, height in childhood is achieved at the expense of shortened stature in adulthood. Progressive masculinization continues with the development of the male habitus, acne, deepened voice, and primary amenorrhea and infertility.

In addition to sexual changes, patients may present with metabolic disorders such as salt-wasting, hypertension, or rarely, hypoglycemia. An electrolyte imbalance of the salt-losing type is usually apparent within a few days of birth and occurs in approximately one-third of patients with virilizing adrenal hyperplasia. Beginning with a refusal to feed, failure to thrive, apathy, and vomiting, the infant goes on to an Addisonian-like crisis with hyponatremia, hyperkalemia, and acidosis. Rapid diagnosis and treatment are necessary to save these infants. Less frequent is hypertension, which occurs in approximately 5% of patients with virilizing adrenal hyperplasia.

Pathophysiology. Virilizing adrenal hyperplasia is the result of an inherited abnormality of steroid biosynthesis which results in an inability to synthesize glucocorticoids. The hypothalamic-pituitary axis reacts to the low level of cortisol by elevated ACTH secretion in a homeostatic response to achieve normal levels of cortisol production. This stimulation causes a hyperplastic adrenal cortex which produces androgens as well as corticoid precursors in abnormal quantities. Therefore, one can see a well-compensated infant who has achieved normal cortisol levels, but at the expense of extensive masculinization. In summary, the clinical picture resulting from a specific enzyme deficiency is due to the effects of both the inadequate production of cortisol and excess accumulation of precursors.

Although the most common defects are the 21-hydroxylase and 11β-hydroxylase types, each of the enzymatic steps from cholesterol to cortisol can be expressed in specific clinical disease.(15) Some affect the adrenal only, while others affect adrenal and ovarian steroid synthesis. It should be noted here that similar defects occur in males as well as females. Both excessive and insufficient androgenization can be seen in affected males.

Enzyme Defect in Adrenal Only: Deficient 21-Hydroxylase. The 21-hydroxylase block is the most common form of congenital adrenal hyperplasia (90% of cases), the most frequent cause of sexual ambiguity, and the most frequent endocrine cause of neonatal death. With severe uncompensated blocks of this type, salt-wasting and shock accompany significant virilization. In less severe variations, when sufficient cortisol can be produced, virilization due to excess androgen is present in utero, at birth, or later in life. Three different clinical forms are recognized: the salt-wasting, the simple virilizing, and the late-onset (also known as nonclassic, attenuated, or acquired adrenal hyperplasia). The first and second are associated with female pseudohermaphroditism at birth, while the third usually becomes apparent at adolescence or beyond, and causes hirsutism, menstrual irregularities, and infertility.

Recent developments in molecular biology and genetics have greatly expanded our understanding of this condition. As a result of the close genetic linkage between 21-hydroxylase deficiency and the HLA (human leukocyte antigen) complex located on the short arm of chromosome 6, we have learned the following:

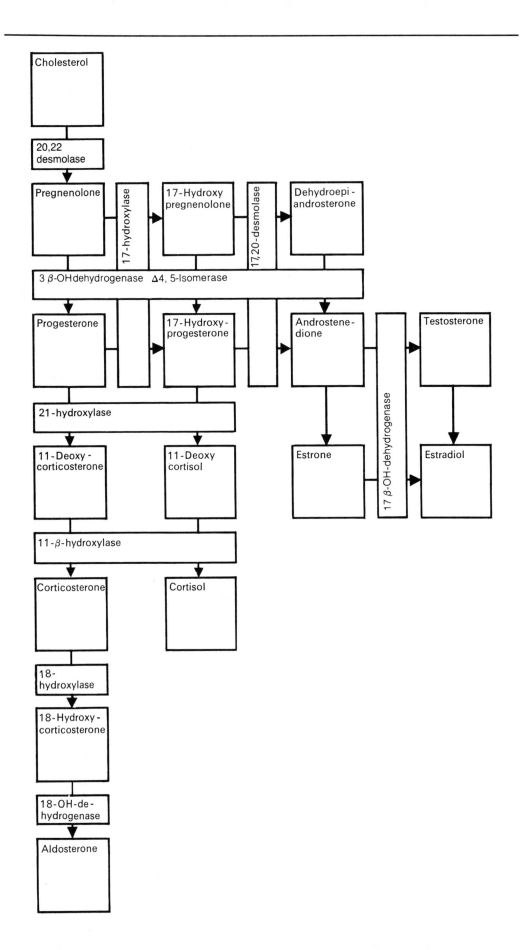

1. The disorder is inherited as a monogenic autosomal recessive trait.

2. HLA typing can be used to determine the carrier status of family members and for early prenatal diagnosis prior to virilization.

3. Two 21-hydroxylase genes exist (21-OHA and 21-OHB), located on chromosome 6 between HLA-B and DR, and are in tandem duplication with the Class III genes encoding the fourth component of complement. Only 21-OHB is active in adrenal steroidogenesis and 21-OHA is not involved.

4. A variety of mutations affecting 21-OHB (deletions, gene conversion, point mutations) lead to 21-hydroxylase deficiency.

5. 21-Hydroxylase deficiency is often found in association with specific HLA antigens or combinations of antigens (haplotypes). For example, salt-wasting 21-hydroxylase deficiency is associated with HLA-Bw60, classical deficiency with HLA-B47, and late-onset deficiency with a significantly increased frequency of HLA-B14, DR1.

By combined HLA genotyping and ACTH stimulation testing (see 17-OHP nomogram in Chapter 7) of families that contained patients with late-onset and classic disease, a concept of allelic variants at the 21-hydroxylase locus evolved.(16,17) Salt-wasting, simple virilizing, and late-onset alleles, respectively, caused the most, less, and least deficiency of 21-hydroxylase. Some family members exhibited abnormal responses to ACTH and, while some of these had clinical evidence of androgen excess, others were entirely normal and represented a "cryptic" form of 21-hydroxylase deficiency. Finally, heterozygotes for either the mild or severe deficiency allele exhibited the mildest enzyme deficiency and were clinically asymptomatic.

In summary, a useful classification has been proposed. (16) There are 3 alleles for 21-hydroxylase deficiency:

1. 21-hydroxylase deficiency^{normal}.

2. 21-hydroxylase deficiency^{mild}.

3. 21-hydroxylase deficiency^{severe}.

Classical disease results when an individual is homozygous for the severe allele. All of the recent terms (late-onset, attenuated, acquired, nonclassical, including the cryptic form) refer to individuals who are either homozygous for the mild allele or carry one mild and one severe allele. Simple virilizing denotes a reduction of cortisol production alone, while in salt-wasting, both cortisol and aldosterone production are impaired. Despite the absence of symptoms, individuals with cryptic 21-hydroxylase deficiency are biochemically indistinguishable from those with the late-onset form and carry the same genotypes. Heterozygotes for either the mild or severe deficiency allele also possess a normal allele.

Enzyme Defect in Adrenal Only: Deficient 11β-Hydroxylase. The final step in cortisol synthesis is blocked in this condition. In classic 11β-hydroxylase deficiency, 11-deoxycortisol is not converted to cortisol. Accumulated precursors are shunted into androgen biosynthesis with virilization similar to that seen with 21-hydroxylase deficiency. However, a parallel defect also exists so that desoxycorticosterone (DOC) is not converted to corticosterone. This pathway is used in the zona glomerulosa to synthesize aldosterone, and the degree to which aldosterone levels are affected lends clinical heterogeneity to the classic presentation of 11β-hydroxylase deficiency.

Usually as a result of 11β-hydroxylase deficiency, metabolically active precursors of corticosterone and cortisol add to excess androgen synthesis as further liabilities of ACTH-induced hyperplasia. Hypertension and hypokalemia are induced by elevated DOC with reduced renin and aldosterone. Virilization is caused by androgens of the "deoxy" type (dehydroepiandrosterone [DHA], dehydroepiandrosterone sulfate [DHAS], and androstenedione). The diagnosis is confirmed by high plasma DOC and compound S (11-deoxycortisol) levels, and increased urinary excretion of their tetrahydro derivatives.

About two-thirds of untreated patients with 11β-hydroxylase deficiency become hypertensive, usually of mild to moderate degree (150/90 mm Hg), and only after several years of life. A mild nonclassic form of 11β-hydroxylase deficiency, as in 21-hydroxylase defects, has also been documented; it is characterized by mild biochemical abnormalities, and the patients are only mildly virilized and rarely hypertensive.

Enzyme Defect in Adrenal and Ovary: Deficient 17α-Hydroxylase. With block of the 17α-hydroxylase enzyme, synthesis of cortisol, androgens, and estrogens is curtailed. Only the non-17-hydroxylated corticoids, DOC and corticosterone, are formed.(18) The resulting syndrome is composed of hypertension, hypokalemia, infantile female external genitalia, which do not mature at puberty, and primary amenorrhea with elevated follicle-stimulating hormone (FSH) and luteinizing hormone (LH). Genital ambiguity is a problem only in male infants.

Enzyme Defect in Adrenal and Ovary: Deficient 3β-Hydroxysteroid Dehydrogenase. Lack of this essential step in the formation of all biologically active steroids affects both the adrenal cortex and the ovary. Thus, there is decreased synthesis of corticoids, androgens, and estrogens. These infants are severely ill at birth and rarely survive. The external genitalia ambiguity presumably results from the massive increase in DHA which is androgenic when available in excess, and also can be utilized to form more potent androgens in peripheral tissues. Thus females may be slightly virilized and males incompletely masculinized with a variable degree of hypospadias. As in 21-hydroxylase deficiency, milder nonclassic cases may be common with mild hirsutism and elevated DHA (and DHAS) being the only distinguishing features.

390

Enzyme Defect in Adrenal and Ovary: Deficient 20-22-Desmolase.
A block in this step prevents conversion of cholesterol to pregnenolone, the necessary precursor to all biologically active steroids. The adrenals are enlarged and filled with cholesterol esters. Predictably, the internal and external genitalia are female, and death occurs.

Genetic Aspects. The genetic defect in virilizing adrenal hyperplasia is an autosomal recessive gene. Within families, the clinical picture is uniform, the type of syndrome (simple, salt-wasting, hypertensive) is always the same in affected siblings. The ratio in offspring of unaffected parents is one affected to three nonaffected individuals. Treated patients have a 1:100 to 1:200 chance of producing an affected infant. Males and females are at equal risk. The overall incidence of the 21-hydroxylase deficiency is between 1:5,000 and 1:15,000.

As Brodie and Wentz (19) have noted in an excellent review, the incidence of 21-hydroxylase deficiency is variable. One out of every 100 caucasians is likely to be a genetic carrier of the classic type. For the nonclassic types, frequency rates established by the usual methodology (neonatal screening, case surveys) are likely to markedly underestimate what may be one of the most common autosomal recessive disorders in humans. Extrapolations from ACTH testing suggest the following frequencies:

	Nonclassical Disease	Heterozygous Carrier
Eastern European Jews:	1 in 30	1 in 3
Hispanics	1 in 40	1 in 4
Yugoslavs	1 in 50	1 in 5
Italians	1 in 333	1 in 9
Others	1 in 1000	1 in 14

The diagnosis of congenital adrenal hyperplasia due to 21-hydroxylase deficiency may be obtained prenatally by demonstrating elevated levels of 17-OHP, 21-deoxycortisol, and androstenedione in the amniotic fluid. HLA genotyping of amniotic cells may yield confirmation by showing that the fetus is HLA identical to an affected sibling. The 11β-hydroxylase deficiency is associated with elevated levels of 11-deoxycortisol in amniotic fluid and tetrahydro-11-deoxycortisol in maternal urine, but this defect is not linked to HLA as the gene coding for this enzyme is found on the long arm of chromosome 8.(20)

More recently prenatal diagnosis of the 21-hydroxylase deficiency by chorion villus biopsy utilizing DNA probes offers the timely options of termination or in utero therapy.(21) The relative frequency of the 21-hydroxylase deficiency merits consideration for a neonatal screening program (utilizing an assay for 17-OHP).

Diagnosis. For years the demonstration of a metabolic defect and its location depended upon the study of urinary steroid excretion. The table shows the normal and abnormal values of 17-ketosteroids. Notice that, in the first few days of life, the excretion of 17-ketosteroids is normally slightly higher; however, pregnanetriol excretion is not elevated.

Urinary 17-Ketosteroid Excretion (mg per 24 hours)		
Age	Normal Values	Values in Virilizing Adrenal Hyperplasia
1–10 days	0.5–5.0	
2–3 weeks	0.5–1.0	2–6
1–6 months	0.5	1–10
7–12 months	0.5	3–10
1–5 years	1.0	4–30
6–9 years	2.0	11–40
10–15 years	4–10	16–50
Over 15 years	7–13	21–80

Further study of the urine will reveal abnormal levels of pregnanetriol with 21- and 11β-hydroxylase blocks, elevated levels of tetrahydro-S and DOC in the hypertensive type (11β-hydroxylase block), and elevated levels of DHA in the 3β-hydroxysteroid dehydrogenase defect. Total excretion of 17-ketosteroids may not be impressively elevated with the 3β-hydroxysteroid dehydrogenase block.

In recent years, the radioimmunoassay of blood 17-OHP has proved useful in the diagnosis and management of congenital adrenal hyperplasia. With the 21- and 11β-hydroxylase blocks, the 17-OHP level may be 50-400-fold above normal.

17-OHP must be measured first thing in the morning to avoid later elevations due to the diurnal pattern of ACTH secretion. The baseline 17-OHP level should be less than 300 ng/dl. Levels greater than 300 ng/dl, but less than 800 ng/dl, require ACTH testing (discussed in Chapter 7). Levels over 800 ng/dl are virtually diagnostic of the 21-hydroxylase deficiency. The DHAS level is usually normal. The hallmarks of late-onset adrenal hyperplasia are elevated levels of 17-OHP and a dramatic increase after ACTH stimulation. The elevated levels of 17-OHP are often not impressive (e.g. overlapping with those found in women with polycystic ovaries due to anovulation), and a simple ACTH stimulation test must be utilized.

During delivery of affected infants, the concentration of 17-OHP is elevated in cord blood (1000-3000 ng/dl), but it rapidly decreases to 100-200 ng/dl after 24 hours. A delay in measurement gains accuracy. In contrast to 17-ketosteroids where the delay must be several days, with 17-OHP the delay need be only a day or two. In affected patients, 17-OHP levels range from 3000 to 40,000 ng/dl. Of course, in patients with 3β-hydroxysteroid dehydrogenase or 17-hydroxylase blocks the 17-OHP level will not be elevated. With the

392

3β-hydroxysteroid dehydrogenase block, the blood levels of DHA and DHA sulfate (DHAS) will be markedly increased.

Treatment. Treatment of adrenal hyperplasia is to supply the deficient hormone, cortisol. This decreases ACTH secretion and lowers production of androgenic precursors. The addition of salt-retaining hormone to glucocorticoid therapy has improved the control of the disease. When the plasma renin activity is normalized, ACTH and androgen levels are further decreased, and a decrease in the glucocorticoid dose is also possible. Therefore, the modern management of hormonal control requires the measurement of the blood levels of 17-OHP, androstenedione, testosterone, and plasma renin activity. (15) The drugs of choice are hydrocortisone and 9-fluorohydrocortisone. This method of treatment and monitoring applies to all forms of adrenal hyperplasia. Minor stresses will cause brief elevations of adrenal androgens, but usually do not require readjustment of dosage. With major stress, such as surgery, additional hormonal support is necessary.

The surgical treatment of the anatomical abnormalities should be carried out in the first few years of life, when the patient is still too young to remember the procedure and too young to have developed psychological problems centered about the abnormal external genitalia. If clitoridectomy is necessary, it is important to know that women who undergo total clitoral amputations have no subsequent impairment of erotic responsiveness or capacity for orgasm. If significant vaginal reconstruction is necessary, this is best accomplished after puberty when mature compliance is possible.

Normal reproduction is possible with replacement therapy of the cortisol deficiency. Unfortunately poor compliance with therapy and less than satisfactory surgical reconstruction of the vagina result in decreased fertility and sexuality.(22) Greater attention to these factors is needed to improve the sexual experience and fertility of these women. Many cases come to cesarean section because normal anatomy of the perineum may be obscured by scar tissue from earlier plastic surgery; therefore, greater blood loss and the risk of a hematoma with a vaginal delivery are significant factors. A masculine pelvis is not expected since the adult form and size of the inlet of the pelvis are assumed largely during the growth spurt in puberty. However, a small pelvis might be anticipated if the bone age is up to age 13-14 when treatment is initiated.

The maintenance steroid dose usually does not need to be changed during pregnancy. Urinary 17-ketosteroids do not alter appreciably during pregnancy, and may be used for monitoring the patient. The dosage of steroids used in the treatment of this syndrome replaces the approximate amount normally produced, and, therefore, is a physiologic dose. At these low doses, teratogenic effects would be unlikely, and none have been noted.

The need for additional steroids during the stress of labor and delivery is obvious, and is usually met by the administration of cortisone acetate intramuscularly and cortisol intravenously. Infection and impaired wound healing have not been problems. Aside from the liability associated with genetic transmission of this syndrome,

393

the children born to patients with adrenal hyperplasia have been normal. The newborn should be closely observed for adrenal insufficiency due to steroid crossover and suppression of the fetal adrenal in utero.

Masculinization Due to Elevated Androgens in Maternal Circulation

Masculinization of the female fetus, while in most cases due to fetal virilizing adrenal hyperplasia, may be produced by an androgen-secreting maternal tumor, or may be due to the intake of exogenous androgenic substances, such as progestins and danazol. When not caused by an error in the metabolism of the fetal adrenal gland, virilization is not progressive, urinary 17-ketosteroids and blood steroids are not elevated, and no hormonal therapy is needed. Subsequent development will be normal. Therefore, surgical correction of abnormalities in the external genitalia is the only indicated treatment.

The occurrence of an androgen-secreting tumor in a mother during pregnancy is rarely seen. On the other hand, the iatrogenic cause of masculinization is a well-known story. The majority of these cases resulted from antenatal maternal treatment of threatened or recurrent abortion with various progestin compounds. In view of the lack of evidence for positive results with such therapy, the use of progestin compounds in pregnancy is contraindicated.

Incompletely Masculinized Males (Male Pseudohermaphrodites)

Incompletely masculinized males are male by genetic sex (XY) and possess testicles, but the external genitalia are not normally male. Male pseudohermaphrodites may arise in one of three ways:

1. Defective responses in androgen dependent tissues—Androgen Insensitivity.

2. Abnormal androgen synthesis.

3. Absent or defective müllerian inhibiting factor.

Syndromes of Androgen Insensitivity

Factors that influence the response to androgens in specific target cells include the following:

1. The intracellular concentration of androgen.

2. The relative binding affinity of these steroids to their nuclear androgen receptors.

3. The binding capacity of the receptor.

4. The nuclear content of androgen receptors.

5. The cellular concentrations of catabolic and/or synthetic enzymes (e.g. 5α-reductase, aromatase, 17β-hydroxysteroid dehydrogenase).

6. The adequacy of the nuclear (chromatin) acceptor site.

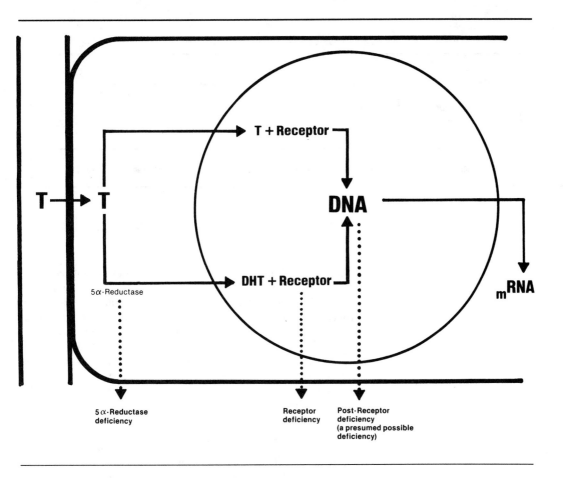

7. The adequacy of regulatory molecules controlling chromatin "read" of the androgen message.

8. RNA processing and translation.

9. The quality of the protein gene product.

Defects in androgenization of targets doubtless occur as a result of failure in any of these steps. Three major clinical conditions are worthy of detailed review.

Complete Androgen Insensitivity—Testicular Feminization. The phenotype of this condition (also discussed in Chapter 5) is female because there is a congenital insensitivity to androgens, transmitted by means of a maternal X-linked recessive gene responsible for the androgen intracellular receptor. Therefore, androgen induction of wolffian duct development does not occur. However, MIF activity is present, and the individual does not have müllerian development (a natural experiment which indicates the presence of an MIF). The vagina is short (derived from the urogenital sinus only) and ends blindly. The uterus and tubes are absent. There is no problem of sex assignment as there is no trace of androgen activity. This syndrome accounts for about 10% of all cases of primary amenorrhea. The hormone profile in these individuals is typical: high LH, normal to slightly elevated male testosterone levels, high estradiol (for men), and normal to elevated FSH.

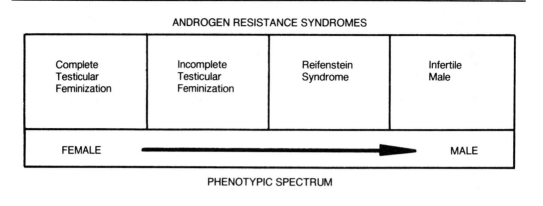

ANDROGEN RESISTANCE SYNDROMES

Complete Testicular Feminization	Incomplete Testicular Feminization	Reifenstein Syndrome	Infertile Male
FEMALE			MALE

PHENOTYPIC SPECTRUM

The "complete" form indicates that there is no androgen response; therefore, normal external female development occurs, and these infants should be reared as females. The testes (azoospermic with hyperplastic Leydig cells) may be present in the inguinal canals. Children with inguinal hernias and/or inguinal masses should be suspected of testicular feminization. There is no virilization at puberty because of the lack of androgen response. In contrast to dysgenetic gonads with a Y chromosome, the occurrence of gonadal tumors is relatively late.(23) Therefore, gonadectomy should be performed at approximately age 16-18, to allow endogenous hormonal changes and a smooth transition through puberty.

Because of the importance of prophylactic gonadectomy, detection of this syndrome demands careful investigation for other affected family members. Future apparent sisters of affected individuals have a 1 in 3 chance of being XY; female offspring of a normal sister of an affected individual have a 1 in 6 chance of being XY. About a third of the patients have negative family histories and presumably represent new mutations.

Incomplete Androgen Insensitivity. A spectrum of disorders, all due to an X-linked recessive trait, are known as incomplete forms of testicular feminization. (24) The clinical presentation ranges from almost complete failure of virilization to essentially complete phenotypic masculinization. Toward the feminine end of the spectrum is Lub's syndrome, while toward the masculine end is Reifenstein's syndrome. Recently, males have been described whose only indication of androgen insensitivity was azoospermic or severe oligospermic infertility. Indeed the incidence may approach 40% or more of men with infertility due to azoospermia or severe oligospermia. However, the defect in androgen receptor function may be so subtle that some affected men are fertile.(25) The diversity of presentation represents variable manifestations of the same mutant gene. The biochemical abnormality lies in the degree of function of the androgen receptor or postreceptor events.(26)

Sex assignment may be a problem when ambiguous genitalia exist because of a partial response of the receptor. If sex assignment is female, early gonadectomy is performed to avoid neoplasia. In the Reifenstein syndrome, the phallus may be large enough to allow a male sex assignment at birth, despite the perineal hypospadias. After puberty, however, the inadequate androgen receptor resource becomes evident and feminization with gynecomastia occurs. The receptor function is inadequate to respond to the surge of androgen at puberty; without androgen effect, estrogen activity prevails. These individuals are infertile and cannot react to exogenous androgen, the karyotype is male XY, distinguishing it from other feminizing syndromes of puberty in phenotypic males (e.g. Klinefelter's syndrome).

The endocrine profiles of both the complete and incomplete forms are similar: high blood levels of testosterone, LH, and estradiol.

5α-Reductase Deficiency. This form of familial incomplete male pseudohermaphroditism is due to an autosomal recessive trait characterized by severe perineal hypospadias and underdevelopment of the vagina. (27) In the past it was known as pseudovaginal perineoscrotal hypospadias (PPH). It differs from the incomplete forms of testicular feminization because, at puberty, masculinization occurs. Normal testicular function occurs, and there is no lack of response to endogenous or exogenous androgen. At birth, however, the external genitalia are similar to that of incomplete testicular feminization; i.e. hypospadias, varying failure of fusion of labioscrotal folds and a urogenital opening, or separate urethral and vaginal openings. The cleft in the scrotum appears to be a vagina (there are no müllerian ducts), and these patients have been reared as girls with an enlarged clitoris. At birth, steroid levels are normal, ruling out adrenal disorders. Diagnosis can be established by demonstrating an elevated T/DHT ratio based upon the blood levels of testosterone and dihydrotestosterone, especially after HCG stimulation. The karyotype is XY, and, as with other incompletely masculinized males, the sex assignment is female if the phallus is inadequate. Gonadectomy is necessary to avoid not only neoplasia but the virilization that is certain to appear at puberty. The deficiency is believed to be due to the homozygous state, manifest clinically only in males. Homozygous 46,XX females have normal fertility. At least 3 "types" of enzyme deficiency have been described in affected families: (1) abnormally low concentration of enzyme, (2) reduced enzyme activity due to enzyme instability, (3) normal enzyme concentration but defective affinity for testosterone and/or essential cofactors leading to reduced enzyme activity.

Study of this syndrome points out three important lessons in intersexuality.(28) In this condition, the wolffian duct virilizes in a normal male fashion, but the urogenital sinus and genital tubercle persist as female structures. The failure is due to inadequate DHT formation intracellularly in these external genitalia tissues at the time the normal male fetus virilizes. In the 5α-reductase deficiencies, the seminal vesicles, ejaculatory ducts, epididymis, and vas deferens which are all testosterone-dependent are present, whereas the DHT-dependent structures, external genitalia, urethra, and prostate, do not develop along male lines. Affected men have less facial and body hair, less temporal hairline recession and no problems with acne. However, spermatogenesis, muscle mass, male libido, deepening of the voice do occur in these men. DHT presence is a requirement only in the fetus, as indicated by the significant genital virilization these patients undergo at puberty and thereafter.(29) Whereas the conversion from male to female role is exceedingly traumatic psychologically, the reversal of sex identity (female to male) these patients undergo at puberty is apparently uncomplicated.(14) In one such case, a "double-life" was conducted. Although functioning in all public respects as a female, one 5α-reductase individual conducted numerous and prolonged heterosexual affairs, which were quite satisfactory, albeit clandestine. He had known of his male sexual identity since puberty, but delayed medical assistance for fear that exposure would bring shame and guilt to his religiously devoted elderly "old world" mother. He decided to keep his secret until his mother died. He finally sought diagnostic help at age 65, however, because his mother at age 93 continued to enjoy good health.

Abnormal Androgen Synthesis

Defective male development may stem from a secretory failure of the testes during the critical period of sex differentiation. In addition to the obvious specific and often familial defects in enzymatic steps leading to testosterone biosynthesis, a variety of other intrinsically testicular problems can lead to male pseudohermaphroditism. In all, the following conditions account for 4% of male pseudohermaphroditism:

1. Aberrations in testicular organogenesis (dysgenetic testes).

2. Defective synthesis, secretion, or response to müllerian inhibiting factor.

3. Testicular unresponsiveness to LH with Leydig cell hypoplasia

Defects in testosterone synthesis can be at any one of the five required enzymatic reactions which lead from cholesterol to testosterone; 20,22-desmolase; 3β-hydroxysteroid dehydrogenase; 17α-hydroxylase, 17,20-desmolase; and 17β-hydroxysteroid dehydrogenase. These defects are inherited as autosomal recessive traits, and the phenotypes range from partial to complete male pseudohermaphroditism.

Patients with male pseudohermaphroditism who are considered variants of testicular feminization upon partial virilization at puberty may actually have a defect in androgen synthesis. The diagnosis is made by demonstrating elevated 17-ketosteroids or elevated blood levels of androstenedione and estrogens, while the blood level of testosterone is low or low-normal.(30) When the enzyme involves a reaction which is active in the adrenal gland (all but the 17β-hydroxysteroid dehydrogenase), the adrenal blocks are usually severe with adrenal failure and death in the newborn period.

The male pseudohermaphrodite due to deficient testicular 17β-hydroxysteroid dehydrogenase activity has male internal genitalia and no müllerian structures. The characteristic clinical findings in these patients are external female genitalia at birth with testes usually located in the inguinal canal. Paradoxically, at puberty they may virilize (enlarged phallus, male body hair and muscle mass, voice changes) and/or feminize with gynecomastia depending on the extent of peripheral conversion of elevated androstenedione to either testosterone and/or estrogen. Early gonadectomy is required to avoid virilization at puberty and testicular neoplasia.

Gonadotropin Resistant Testes

Male pseudohermaphrodites due to agenesis or abnormal differentiation of Leydig cells include reduced responsiveness to LH/HCG, deficiency in the availability or function of receptors or post-receptor elements, such as regulatory guanyl nucleotides, cyclic AMP, crucial phosphokinases, cholesterol uptake, and esterase enzymes. All these cases could be termed "gonadotropin resistant testes." In general, the characteristics of the syndrome include basically female but ambiguous genitalia, male cryptorchid testes with degenerated Leydig cells, no müllerian ducts but present vas deferens and epididymis, elevated gonadotropins (FSH rises further after gonadectomy, indicating the presence of inhibin).(31) Although an absence or deficiency of LH receptors is postulated, an environmentally or autoimmune produced disappearance of the receptors on the Leydig cells is possible.

Abnormal Müllerian Inhibiting Factor

Hernia Uterine Inguinale (Uterine Hernia Syndrome). Individuals with this syndrome appear to be normal males, but relatively well-differentiated müllerian duct structures are found, usually a uterus and tubes in an inguinal hernia sac. This is due to a failure of MIF function either as a result of failure of Sertoli cell secretion of this polypeptide or an inability of the müllerian ducts to respond to MIF. It is inherited as a recessive trait, either X-linked or autosomal. Fertility is usually preserved. Other instances in which some müllerian duct retention is found include dysgenetic testes, ovotestes, mixed gonadal dysgenesis, müllerian duct and utricular cysts, and prenatal DES exposure.

Experimental evidence suggests that MIF may act as an anti tumor (ovarian and endometrial) agent, perhaps by causing tumor regression in a manner similar to its embryonic role.(32,33)

Abnormal
Gonadogenesis

The proper development and eventual function of the gonad depends on the presence of germ cells, the appropriate sex chromosome constitution, and appropriate gonadal ridge somatic cells. Errors in meiotic division can cause aneuploidy and abnormal sex chromosomes. These occur by nondisjunction, anaphase lag, translocation, breakage, rearrangements, or deletions. Mitosis can also be marred by nondisjunction and anaphase lag leading to mosaicism. Two or more different cell lines can persist and appear in different tissues. Finally, abnormal gonadogenesis may occur as a result of structural or disease related catastrophes leading to loss of fetal gonadal function.

A Clarification of Terminology (35)

Event	Time of Event (Days after Fertilization)	Nomenclature	Müllerian Duct	Wolffian Duct	External Genitalia
Early embryonic testicular regression	Before 43	Pure gonadal dysgenesis	Present	Absent	Female
Late embryonic testicular regression	43–59	Swyer syndrome	Present	Absent	Female
Early fetal testicular regression	60–69	Agonadism	Present	Absent	Ambiguous
	70–75	Testicular dysgenesis	Present	Present	Ambiguous
	75–84	Testicular regression	Absent	Present	Ambiguous
Midfetal testicular regression	90–120	Rudimentary testis	Absent	Present	Male infantile
Late fetal testicular regression	After 140	Vanishing testis, anorchia	Absent	Present	Male infantile

Bilateral Dysgenesis of the Testes (Swyer Syndrome). Affected individuals have an XY karyotype but normal (infantile) female external and internal genitalia.(34) There are fibrous bands in place of the gonads yielding primary amenorrhea and lack of secondary sexual development at puberty. It is a matter of prudent practice to avoid the possibility of virilization or neoplasm; therefore, laparotomy and removal of these band areas are advocated. Presumably, testes failed to develop or were eliminated (testicular regression) before internal or external genital differentiation in this syndrome.(35) Estrogen and progestin sequential therapy supports female secondary sex development. Menstruation occurs from endometrial cells with an XY chromosome.

True Agonadism. The pathogenesis of this condition, in view of a normal XY sex chromosome complement, must be complete testicular degeneration sometime between 6 and 12 weeks of pregnancy. If testicular loss is early, there is inadequate androgen stimulation (minimal wolffian development and female external genitalia), and müllerian ducts are preserved. The presence of a normal vagina, uterus, and tubes distinguishes this syndrome from testicular feminization variants. However, if testes loss occurs late, no gonads will be present, external genitalia will be ambiguous (but primarily female), and rudimentary components of both müllerian and wolffian internal ducts present.(35) Laparotomy (removal of bands) is required as a precaution against neoplasia.

Anorchia. Affected XY individuals have infantile unambiguous male external genitalia, male wolffian ducts, and lack müllerian ducts. There are, however, no detectable testes. Early testis function did occur (wolffian presence, MIF function), but was not sustained in sufficient amounts or duration to develop a normal size phallus. It

400

is frequently called "the disappearing testis syndrome." Sex of assignment depends on the extent of external genitalia development.

True Hermaphrodites

Abnormal sexual differentiation can occur as a result of a mixture of gonadal sex (true hermaphroditism) or complete uncertainty of gonadal sex (gonadal dysgenesis with some virilization).(36) A true hermaphrodite possesses both ovarian and testicular tissue. Both types may be contained in one gonad (ovotestis) or one side may be an ovary, the other a testis. The internal structures correspond to the adjacent gonad. In the majority, external genitalia are ambiguous with sufficient male character to allow male sex assignment. However, three-fourths develop gynecomastia and half menstruate post-puberty. Fifty percent are genetic females (XX), few are XY, the rest are mosaics with at least one cell line XX.

Gonadal Dysgenesis

Gonadal dysgenesis with bilateral rudimentary streak gonads due to the presence of only one X chromosome in all cell lines (X chromosome monosomy) is called Turner's syndrome. In the absence of gonadal development, the individuals are phenotypic females. The well-known characteristics are short stature (48-58 inches), sexual infantilism, and streak gonads. The streak gonad is composed of fibrous tissue, containing no ova or follicular derivatives. Other congenital problems in this syndrome are: a webbed neck, coarctation of the aorta, a high arched palate, cubitus valgus, a broad shield-like chest with widely spaced nipples, a low hairline on the neck, short fourth metacarpal bones, and renal abnormalities. Usually the diagnosis is not made until puberty when amenorrhea and lack of sexual development become apparent. At birth, however, lymphedema of the extremities may indicate the condition. About 98% of conceptuses with only one X chromosome abort. The remaining 2% account for an incidence of 45,X in about 1 in 10,000 liveborn girls.

A large variety of mosaic patterns is seen with gonadal dysgenesis. From analysis of the various combinations, it is apparent that short stature is related to loss of the short arm of one X chromosome. Thus X, XXp-, and XXqi are all short. Xqi designates an isochromosome for the long arms, and Xp-, deletion of the short arm. The loss of the long arm of one of the X chromosomes (XXq-) is associated with amenorrhea and streak gonads, but the patients are not always growth compromised, nor do they display other Turner somatic malformations. Thus, loss of material from the short arms of the X chromosome leads to short stature and the other stigmata of Turner's syndrome. Streak gonads result if any part of an X chromosome is missing. This suggests that normal ovarian development requires two loci, one on the long arm and one on the short arm; loss of either results in gonadal failure. Thyroid autoimmunity is common in Turner's syndrome, but Hashimoto's thyroiditis may be specific to the 46,XXqi cases.

The presence of menstrual function and reproduction in a patient with Turner's phenotype must be due to a mosaic complement, such as a 46,XX line in addition to 45,X. When pregnancy does occur in an X deficient subject, the incidence of aneuploidy in the conceptus is almost 50%.

401

Multiple X females (47,XXX) have normal development and reproductive function, although mental retardation may be more frequent. Secondary amenorrhea and/or eunuchoidism may be seen.

Just as X chromosome monosomy, with deletion of the second X chromosome, results in Turner's phenotype—female phenotype, sexual infantilism, and dysgenetic gonads—the same will apply to loss of the Y chromosome. The 45,X karyotype derived from leukocyte culture does not guarantee that a mosaic does not exist with a gonadal cell line containing XY. For this reason, annual pelvic examinations, β subunit HCG and α-fetoprotein levels are required to detect incipient signs of gonadal neoplasia as an adnexal mass. If a presumed 45,X (based on white cell culture karyotype) develops breasts or sexual hair *without* exogenous therapy, a gonadoblastoma or dysgerminoma should be considered and ruled out. Heterosexual signs require the same scrutiny in all 45,X individuals. The hope that clinical decisions could be eased by detection of the H-Y antigen has not been fulfilled. Newer Y-DNA probes may prove to be more useful.

Pure Gonadal
Dysgenesis

A normal XY karyotype can be found in a phenotypic female with sexual infantilism and streak gonads. The genetic content of the Y chromosome is abnormal despite its morphologic presence in these cases. Removal of streaks is required.

The problem of the 46,XX male and the 46,XY female is being scrutinized by sensitive molecular biology techniques.(37,38) Three-fourths of 46,XX males have been found to contain Y-DNA sequences. At the same time, 46,XY females have been shown to have precisely the same sequences deleted. These reciprocal findings are best understood by the presence of a specific testes determining gene on the Y chromosome.(10)

In gonadal dysgenesis, the gonadal structures are streak gonads, and the external genitalia are of infantile female type. In mixed gonadal dysgenesis, testicular tissue may be present on one side and a streak gonad on the other. Mosaicism is the likely underlying abnormality, though it may not be detected in the cell line studied. The external genitalia may be female, ambiguous, or almost normal male. Ambiguous genitalia are produced if testicular tissue is present, from clitoral hypertrophy to basically male with hypospadias. Internal genitalia are basically female with some müllerian regression (absent tube) expressed adjacent to the gonad with testicular components. Virilization and neoplasia dictate timely gonadectomy.

Noonan's Syndrome

Both affected males and females have apparently normal chromosome complements and normal gonadal function. The phenotypic appearance of the female is that of a patient with Turner's syndrome: short stature, webbed neck, shield chest, and cardiac malformations. The cardiac lesions, however, are different. Pulmonic stenosis is most frequent in Noonan's syndrome as opposed to aortic coarctation in Turner's. Apparently this syndrome results from a mutant gene or genes.(39) In the past these patients have been referred to as male Turner's or Turner's with normal chromosomes.

Both male and female Noonan's are fertile and transmit the trait as an autosomal dominant with variable expression.

Diagnosis of Ambiguous Genitalia

Ambiguous external genitalia in a newborn infant represent a major diagnostic challenge. The physician is involved in a pressure-filled situation because of the necessity for making such an influential decision as the sex of rearing. Diagnostic procedures may delay the decision, and it is well-recognized that a period of delay is far better than later reversal of the sex assignment. Parental education and guidance are essential in this anxiety-ridden situation.

The most important point to remember when confronted with a newborn infant with ambiguous genitalia, or an apparently male infant with bilateral cryptorchidism, is that the prime diagnosis until ruled out is congenital adrenal hyperplasia. The reason is clear: adrenal hyperplasia is the only condition which is life-threatening. Signs of adrenal failure such as vomiting, diarrhea, dehydration, and shock may develop rapidly.

The history of a previously affected relative may aid in the diagnosis of testicular feminization or any of its variants. Similarly, the history of a sibling with genital ambiguity or the history of a previous neonatal death in a sibling strongly suggest the possibility of adrenal hyperplasia. A history of maternal exposure to androgenic compounds may be difficult to elicit. The mother may be unaware of the nature of her medications, and the obstetrician should be consulted.

Careful examination of the phallus may differentiate between a clitoris and a penis. The penis has a midline ventral frenulum, while the clitoris has two folds which extend from the lateral aspects of the clitoris to the labia minora. The position of the urethral meatus may range from a mild hypospadias to an opening in the perineal area into a urogenital sinus.

Palpation of the genital and inguinal regions is the most important part of the physical examination. Ovaries are not found in scrotal folds or in the inguinal regions. Therefore, palpable masses in these locations represent testicles. The testicles, however, may be intraabdominal. If testicles are not palpable, the infant should be considered to have virilizing adrenal hyperplasia until demonstrated otherwise. A uterus may be palpable on rectal examination, especially shortly after birth when the uterus is a little enlarged in response to maternal estrogen.

Rapid testing of the karyotype along with serum electrolytes, serum 17-OHP, urinary 17-ketosteroids or serum androstenedione and DHAS should be ordered immediately in all newborns with ambiguous genitalia.

Because both masculinized females and incompletely masculinized males can result from enzyme blocks in the adrenal, urinary 17-ketosteroids or serum androgens, and 17-OHP are necessary regardless of the karyotype. In 3β-hydroxysteroid dehydrogenase and 17-hydroxylase enzyme blocks, the 17-OHP will not be elevated. 21-Hydroxylase and 11β-hydroxylase deficiencies will be associated

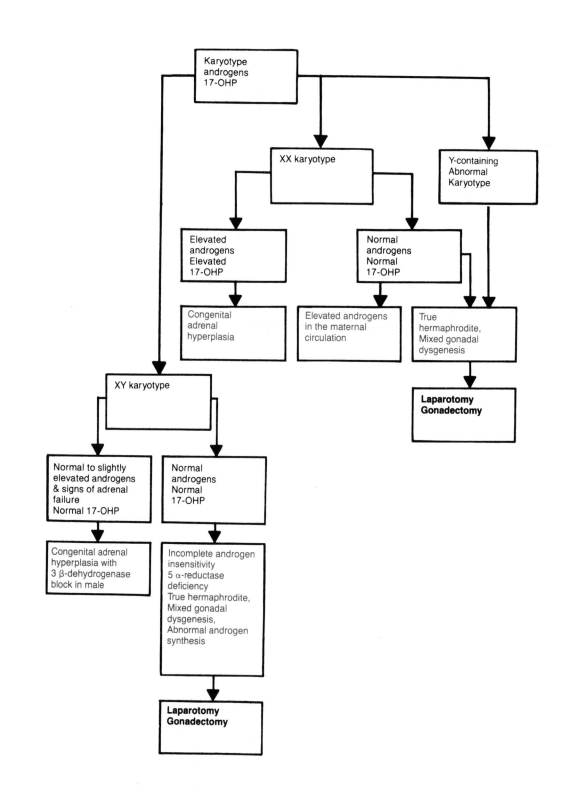

with massive elevations of 17-OHP in blood. The serum androgens and 17-ketosteroids may not be impressively increased with a 3β-hydroxysteroid dehydrogenase block, but serum levels of DHA and 17-hydroxypregnenolone should be elevated. *Clinical signs of adrenal failure indicate that the newborn has adrenal hyperplasia regardless of the steroid pattern.* The diagnosis is certain if such an infant is hyperkalemic and hyponatremic.

Endoscopy and special x-ray studies are not necessary for assigning sex; however, the information gained will be helpful in delineating the exact structures and abnormalities present.

Although laparotomy is not necessary for assignment of sex, it may be the only way to arrive at a definitive diagnosis. Laparotomy is indicated in the following situations (laparoscopic evaluation is inadequate because gonads may be small and hidden in the inguinal canal):

1. The XX infant with ambiguous genitalia, normal androgens, in apparent good health, and no history of maternal androgen exposure. This is either a true hermaphrodite or a variant of mixed gonadal dysgenesis, and gonadectomy is indicated.

2. The XY patient with ambiguous genitalia, without palpable gonads, and normal androgens. The possibilities are incompletely masculinized males (variants of testicular feminization), a true hermaphrodite, mixed gonadal dysgenesis, and 5α-reductase deficiency. Sex of rearing will be female, and gonadectomy is necessary to avoid virilization at puberty and the propensity to develop gonadal neoplasia.

Assignment of Sex Rearing

In a newborn who presents a problem of correct sex of assignment, it is better to delay than to reverse the sex assignment at a later date. Generally, the decision can be made within a few days, at most a few weeks. In dealing with the parents, terms with unfortunate connotations, such as hermaphrodite, should be avoided. An easy way to explain ambiguous genital development to parents is to indicate that the genitals are unfinished, rather than abnormal from a sexual point of view. Chromosome discrepancies are probably best left unmentioned.

The future fertility in all masculinized females is unaffected. With proper treatment, reproduction is possible, since the internal genitalia and gonads are those of a normal female. Therefore, all masculinized females should be reared as females.

The only other category of patients with ambiguous genitalia with reproductive capability consists of males with 1) isolated hypospadias, 2) the male with repaired isolated cryptorchidism, and 3) the male with the uterine hernia syndrome.

All other patients with ambiguous genitalia will be sterile. Except for salt-wasting adrenal hyperplasia, the physician's prime concern is not with physical survival, but to enable the patient to grow into a psychologically normal, healthy, and well-adjusted adult. The sex

405

of assignment depends upon only one judgment: can the phallus ultimately develop into a penis adequate for intercourse. The success of a penis is dependent upon erectile tissue, and the genitalia should not only be serviceable, but also erotically sensitive. Technically, the construction of female genitalia is easier, and therefore, the physician must be convinced that a functional penis is possible.

All decisions regarding sex of rearing and the overall treatment program should be made early in life. If a case has been neglected, sex reassignments must be made according to the gender identity in which a child has developed. Reassignment of sex can probably be made safely up to age 18 months.

It is recommended that older individuals requesting sexual changes be referred to research-oriented clinical programs established in university medical centers.

References

1. **Jones WH Jr, Rock JA,** *Reparative and Constructive Surgery of the Female Generative Tract,* Williams & Wilkins, Baltimore, 1983.

2. **Duckett JW Jr,** Transverse preputial island flap technique for repair of severe hypospadias, Urol Clin North Am 7:423, 1980.

3. **Donakoe PK, Hendren WH,** Perineal reconstruction and ambiguous genitalia of infants raised as females, Ann Surg 200:371, 1984.

4. **Jeffs RD, Gearhart JP,** Reconstructive surgery of male external genitalia, Seminars Reprod Endocrinol 5:315, 1987.

5. **Money J, Devore H, Norman BF,** Gender identity and gender transposition: Longitudinal outcome study of 32 male hermaphrodites assigned as girls, J Sex Marital Ther 12:165, 1986.

6. **Money J, Norman BF,** Gender identity and gender transposition: Longitudinal outcome study of 24 male hermaphrodites assigned as boys, J Sex Marital Ther 13:75, 1987.

7. **Magre S, Jost A,** Dissociation between testicular morphogenesis and endocrine cyto-differentiation of Sertoli cells, Proc Natl Acad Sci 81:7831, 1984.

8. **Van Wagenen G, Simpson ME,** *Embryology of the Ovary and Testis, Homo Sapiens and Mucaca Mulatta,* Yale University Press, 1965.

9. **Simpson E, Chandler P, Galoumy Y, Disteche CM, Ferguson-Smith MA, Page DC,** Separation of the genetic loci for the H-Y antigen and for testes determination on the human Y chromosome, Nature 326:876, 1987.

10. **Page DC, Mosher R, Simpson EM, Fisher EMG, Mardon G, Pollack J, McGillivray B, de la Chapelle A, Brown LG,** The sex determining region of the human Y chromosome encodes a finger protein, Cell 51:1091, 1987.

11. **Wilson JD, Griffin JE, George FW, Leshin M,** The role of gonadal steroids in sexual differentiation, Recent Prog Horm Res 37:1, 1981.

12. **Singh RP, Carr DH,** The anatomy and histology of XO human embryos and fetuses, Anat Rec 155:369, 1966.

13. **Krauss CM, Turksoy RN, Atkins L, McGlaughlin C, Brown LG, Page DC,** Familial premature ovarian failure due to an interstitial deletion of the long arm of the X chromosome, New Eng J Med 317:125, 1987.

14. **Imperato-McGinley J, Peterson RE, Gaultier T, Sturla E,** Androgens and the evolution of male gender identity among male pseudohermaphrodites with 5α-reductase deficiency. New Eng J Med 300:1233, 1979.

15. **White PC, New MI, DuPont B,** Congenital adrenal hyperplasia, New Eng J Med 316:1519,1580, 1987.

16. **Kohn B, Levine LS, Pollack MS, Pang S, Lorezen F, Levy DJ, Lerner AJ, Gian FR, DuPont B, New MI,** Late onset steroid 21-OH deficiency: A variant of classical congenital adrenal hyperplasia. J Clin Endocrinol Metab 55:817, 1982.

17. **Spenser PW, New MI,** Genotype and hormonal phenotype in nonclassical 21-OH deficiency, J Clin Endocrinol Metab 64:86, 1987.

18. **Biglieri EG, Herron MA, Brust N,** 17-Hydroxylation deficiency in man. J Clin Invest 45:1946, 1966.

19. **Brodie BL, Wentz AC,** Late onset congenital adrenal hyperplasia: A gynecologist's perspective, Fertil Steril 48:175, 1987.

20. **Rosler A, Weshler N, Leiberman E, Hochberg Z, Weidenfeld J, Sack J, Chemke J,** 11β-hydroxylase deficiency congenital adrenal hyperplasia: Update of prenatal diagnosis, J Clin Endocrinol Metab 66:830, 1988.

21. **Reindollar RH, Lewis JB, White PC, Fernhoff PM, McDonough PG, Whitney JB III,** Prenatal diagnosis of 21-hydroxylase deficiency by the complementary deoxyribonucleic acid probe for cytochrome P-450$_{C-21OH}$, Am J Obstet Gynecol 158:545, 1988.

22. **Mulaikal RM, Migeon CJ, Rock JA,** Fertility rates in female patients with congenital adrenal hyperplasia due to 21-hydroxylase deficiency, New Eng J Med 316:178, 1987.

23. **Manuel M, Katayama KP, Jones Jr HW,** The age of occurrence of gonadal tumors in intersex patients with a Y chromosome. Am J Obstet Gynecol 124:293, 1976.

24. **Wilson JD, Harrod MJ, Goldstein JL, Hemsell DL, MacDonald PC,** Familial incomplete male pseudohermaphroditism, type 1. New Eng J Med 290:1097, 1974.

25. **Grino PB, Griffin JE, Cushard WG Jr, Wilson JD,** A mutation of the androgen receptor associated with partial androgen resistance, familial gynecomastia, and fertility, J Clin Endocrinol Metab 66:754, 1988.

26. **Griffin JE, Wilson JD,** The syndromes of androgen resistance. New Eng J Med 302:198, 1980.

27. **Walsh PC, Madden JD, Harrod MJ, Goldstein JL, MacDonald PC, Wilson JD,** Familial incomplete male pseudohermaphroditism, type 2. New Eng J Med 291:949, 1974.

28. **Haseltine FP, Ohno S,** Mechanism of gonadal differentiation. Science 211:1272, 1981.

29. **Wilson JD, George FW, Griffin JE,** The hormonal control of sexual development. Science 211:1278, 1981.

30. **Goebelsmann U, Horton R, Mestman JH,** Male pseudohermaphroditism due to testicular 17β-hydroxysteroid dehydrogenase deficiency, J Clin Endocrinol Metab 30:867, 1973.

31. **Perez-Palacios G, Scaglia HE, Kofman-Alfaro S,** Inherited male pseudohermaphroditism due to gonadotropin unresponsiveness, Acta Endocrinol 98:148, 1981.

32. **Donahoe PK, Fuller AFJ, Scully RE,** Müllerian inhibiting substance inhibits growth of a human ovarian cancer in nude mice, Ann Surg 194:472, 1981.

33. **Liu H-C, Kreiner D, Rosenwaks Z,** Anti-müllerian hormone, Seminars Reprod Endocrinol 5:283, 1987.

34. **Swyer GIM,** Male pseudohermaphroditism: A hitherto undescribed form, Brit Med J II:709, 1955.

35. **Coulam CB,** Testicular regression syndrome. Obstet Gynecol 53:44, 1979.

36. **Simpson JL,** True hermaphroditism: etiology and phenotypic considerations. Birth Defects 14(6c):9, 1978.

37. **Page DC, de la Chapelle A,** The paternal origin of X chromosomes in XX males determined using restriction fragment length polymorphisms, Am J Hum Genet 36:565, 1984.

38. **Muller U, Latt SA, Donlon T,** Y-specific DNA sequences in male patients with 46,XX and 47,XXX karyotypes, Am J Med Genet 28:393, 1987.

39. **Allanson JE, Hall JG, Hughes HE, Preus M, Witt RD,** Noonan syndrome: The changing phenotype, Am J Med Genet 21:507, 1985.

13 Abnormal Puberty and Growth Problems

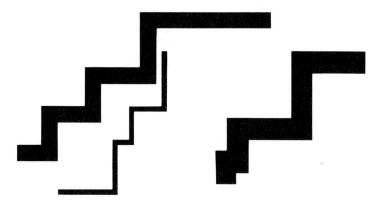

The ability to diagnose and manage disorders of female pubescence requires a thorough understanding of the physical and hormonal events which mark the evolution of the child into a sexually mature adult capable of reproduction. Abnormalities in this process of developmental endocrinology either lead to premature or retarded (delayed) puberty. *This chapter reviews the important landmarks and mechanisms of normal female maturation as well as the abnormalities which lead to precocious or delayed puberty.*

The Physiology of Puberty

The Period of Infancy and Childhood

There is good evidence that the hypothalamus, anterior pituitary gland, and gonads of the fetus, neonate, the prepubertal infant and child, are all capable of secreting hormones in adult concentrations. Even during fetal life, serum concentrations of follicle-stimulating hormone (FSH) and luteinizing hormone (LH) reach adult levels at midgestation but fall thereafter as the high level of pregnancy steroid hormones exerts inhibitory feedback.(1) Separation of the newborn from its sources of maternal and placental estrogen and progesterone at birth releases newborn FSH and LH from this negative feedback. A prompt rise in gonadotropin secretion follows which, in female neonates, may reach adult castrate levels by 3 months of life.(2) As a result, transient estradiol secretion equivalent to the level of mid-puberty is induced and is associated with waves of ovarian follicle maturation and atresia. Negative feedback is once more reasserted; ovarian steroids and gonadotropins decline and remain at very low levels until at least 8 years of age. During this period, the hypothalamic-pituitary system controlling gonadotropins (the "gonadostat") is highly sensitive to negative feedback of estrogen (estradiol concentration in these years remains low at 10 pg/ml). Studies on gonadal dysgenesis and other hypogonadal infants indicate that the "gonadostat" is 6-15 times more sensitive to negative feedback at this period than in the adult.(3) Therefore, gonadotropin secretion is in part restrained by extraordinarily low levels of estrogen.

This reduction in the infant's gonadotropins is not entirely due to exquisite sensitivity to negative feedback. Low levels of FSH and LH even exist in hypogonadal children (primarily gonadal dysgenesis) between the ages of 5 and 11 years and are the same as the low levels in normal infants of this age.(4) Because gonadotropin releasing hormone (GnRH) infusion stimulates moderate LH and FSH secretion in these agonadal subjects, a central nonsteroidal suppressor of endogenous GnRH and gonadotropin synthesis appears to be operative.(5)

Although peptide hormone concentrations are low throughout infancy and the prepubertal child, LH shows evidence of pulsatile control of secretion.(6) As noted, pituitary gonadotropins react with small but significant responses to exogenously administered GnRH which although quantitatively less than those achieved in puberty are nevertheless capable of inducing the immature gonad to respond with modest steroid secretion. Immaturity of the various endocrine components is not the rate-limiting step in the onset of puberty.

The Prepubertal Period

As puberty approaches, three critical changes in the low level endocrine homeostatic function of childhood emerge:

1. "Adrenarche."

2. Decreasing repression of the "gonadostat."

3. Gradual amplification of the peptide-peptide and peptide-steroid interactions leading to "gonadarche."

Adrenarche

The growth of pubic and axillary hair is due to an increased production of adrenal androgens at puberty. Thus, this phase of puberty is often referred to as adrenarche or pubarche. Premature pubarche by itself is occasionally seen, i.e., pubic and axillary hair without any other sign of sexual development. Premature thelarche (breast development) without other signs of puberty is very rare, but does occur. Increased adrenal cortical function, expressed by a rise in circulating dehydroepiandrosterone (DHA), dehydroepiandrosterone sulfate (DHAS), and androstenedione, occurs progressively in late childhood from about age 6 to adolescence (13-15 years of age).(7) This steroid secretion is associated with an increase in size and differentiation of the inner zone (zona reticularis) of the cortex. Generally, the beginning of adrenarche precedes by 2 years the linear growth spurt, the rise in estrogens and gonadotropins of early puberty, and menarche at midpuberty. Because of this temporal relationship, activation of adrenal androgen secretion has been suggested as a possible initiating event in the ontogeny of the pubertal transition.

Considerable evidence, however, supports a *dissociation* of the control mechanisms which initiate adrenarche and those governing GnRH-pituitary-ovarian maturation ("gonadarche"). Premature adrenarche (precocious appearance of pubic and axillary hair before age

8 years) is not associated with a parallel abnormal advancement of gonadarche.(8) In hypergonadotropic hypogonadism (gonadal dysgenesis) or in hypogonadotropic states such as Kallmann's syndrome, adrenarche occurs despite the absence of gonadarche. When adrenarche is absent, as in children with cortisol-treated Addison's disease (hypoadrenalism), gonadarche still occurs. Finally, in true precocious puberty occurring before 6 years of age, gonadarche precedes adrenarche.

Plasma levels of adrenal androgens change without corresponding changes in cortisol and ACTH during fetal life, puberty, and aging. Furthermore, in other circumstances such as chronic disease, surgical stress, recovery from secondary adrenal insufficiency, and anorexia nervosa, changes in ACTH-induced cortisol secretion are not accompanied by corresponding changes in plasma adrenal androgen levels.(9) Thus, adrenarche does not appear to be under direct control of gonadotropin, ACTH, or prolactin.

A pituitary adrenal androgen stimulating factor formed by cleavage of a high molecular weight precursor, proopiomelanocortin (POMC), which also contains ACTH and β-lipotropin, acting on an ACTH prepared and maintained adrenal, has been suggested as the agent stimulating adrenarche.(10) The name for this material is CASH, corticotropin androgen stimulating hormone. However, in a study confirming the dissociation between plasma adrenal androgens and cortisol in children and adolescents with Cushing's disease and ectopic ACTH producing tumors, all known proopiomelanocortin-related peptides, including ACTH, β-endorphin, and β-lipotropin did not have a determinative role in the initiation of adrenarche.(11) Thus, the control of adrenarche remains obscure. However, a study of the kinetics of the 3β-hydroxysteroid dehydrogenase enzyme in human adrenal microsomes suggests that the changes in adrenal secretion from fetal life to adulthood can be explained by local steroid inhibition of key enzymes within the adrenal, acting to a variable degree in different layers of the cortex and at different stages of development.(12)

Decreasing Repression of the "Gonadostat"

Regardless of its relation to adrenarche, factors which induce gonadarche in late prepuberty involve de-repression of the CNS-pituitary gonadostat, progressive responsiveness of the anterior pituitary to exogenous (and presumably endogenous) GnRH, and follicle reactivity to FSH and LH.

For approximately 8 years, from early infancy to the prepubertal period, LH and FSH are suppressed to very low levels. The mechanisms for this restraint on gonadotropin secretion are: a highly sensitive negative feedback of low level gonadal estrogen on hypothalamic and pituitary sites, and an intrinsic central inhibitory influence on GnRH which reduces basal gonadotropin concentrations even in agonadal children. Gonadal dysgenesis patients display marked elevations of gonadotropins for the first 2-3 years of life. Thereafter, a striking decline in concentrations of FSH and LH occurs, reaching a nadir at 6-8 years. By age 10-11 (at the time puberty would have occurred), however, gonadotropins are elevated once again to the castrate range. The overall pattern of basal gonadotropin secretion in agonadal children is qualitatively similar to that observed in normal females.

Whereas negative feedback inhibition may play the more important role in early childhood, the central intrinsic inhibitor becomes functionally dominant in midchildhood and persists up to prepuberty. Suppression of, or damage to, the neural source of this inhibition has been postulated in the pathogenesis of the precocious puberty secondary to hypothalamic lesions which compress or destroy posterior hypothalamic areas.(13) Thus normal pubertal timing of gonadarche, with the reactivation of gonadotropin synthesis and secretion, results from the combined reduction in intrinsic suppression of GnRH and decreased sensitivity to the negative feedback of estrogen.(14)

It has been suggested that the reversal of central intrinsic suppression is due to a reduction in melatonin secretion by the pineal gland. In lower animals affected by photoperiodicity, pineal melatonin appears to inhibit hypothalamic-pituitary gland secretion. While melatonin may play a role in the altered timing of puberty associated with pineal tumors, there is no evidence that it is important in the physiologic onset of normal puberty in humans. In a large study of circadian rhythms of serum melatonin from infancy to adulthood (1-18 years) the decline in the nocturnal surge of melatonin, thought to have been exclusively related to the pubertal conversion, was observed to begin in infancy and progressively decline through pubescence.(15) Pinealectomy in agonadal primates does not prevent the inhibition of FSH and LH seen during transition from infancy to childhood nor the return of gonadotropins with the advent of puberty.(16)

The fascinating search for the factor(s) involved in the de-repression of the "gonadostat" so crucial to the timing of puberty continues. POMC-related peptides do not appear to change during the transitional period.(17) Recently human growth hormone (GH) and other growth promoting peptides have been investigated in primate pubescence. In early data, it appears that both the nongonadal (central) control and estradiol feedback inhibition of basal LH begin and follow sustained elevation of serum growth hormone unrelated to a specific increment or threshold level of body growth or body weight.(18)

Alteration and Amplification of GnRH-Gonadotropin and Gonadotropin-Ovarian Steroid Interactions

Rhythmic pulses of GnRH given to immature rhesus monkeys will initiate activity of the pituitary-gonadal apparatus, supporting the primacy of endogenous GnRH in the establishment and maintenance of puberty. Similar effects have been demonstrated in prepubertal girls.(19) Normal pubertal maturation in girls is also accompanied by changes in the pattern of gonadotropin responses to the hypothalamic releasing hormone GnRH. FSH responses to GnRH are initially pronounced but decrease steadily throughout the onset of puberty. In contrast, LH responses are low in prepubertal girls and increase strikingly during puberty.(20) This is the basis of the observation that in general FSH rises initially and plateaus in midpuberty while LH tends to rise more slowly and reaches adult levels in late puberty. The increased amplitude and frequency of pulsatile GnRH are believed to provoke progressively enhanced responses of FSH and LH secretion. GnRH acts as a self-primer on the gonadotrope cells of the anterior pituitary by inducing cell surface receptors specific for GnRH and necessary for its action (up-regulation). Thus, gonadotrope cells increase their capacity to respond to

GnRH first by synthesis and later by secretion of gonadotropins. As gonadotropin secretion appears, ovarian follicle steroid synthesis is stimulated and estrogen secretion rises.

Elsewhere (see Chapter 2), the evidence for the dichotomous effects of estrogen feedback on the anterior pituitary has been reviewed. Suffice to say at this point, by midpuberty, estrogen enhances LH secretory responses to GnRH (positive feedback) while maintaining relative inhibition (negative feedback) of FSH response.

The amplification of peptide-steroid interactions during pubescence is not restricted to the GnRH impact on gonadotropin or steroid feedback on the pituitary and hypothalamus. As pubertal transition advances there is a disproportionate rise of biologically potent LH beyond the increase seen in immunologic LH. This marked increase in the bioactive to immunoactive ratio is due to molecular alterations in the glycosylation pattern of LH. (21)

The onset of significant GnRH pulses first occurs during sleep. There is sleep-associated release of LH in both sexes which correlates with the timing (early puberty) of LH responses to exogenous GnRH. Sleep-related LH pulses also are seen in children with idiopathic precocious puberty, in anorexia nervosa patients during intermediate stages of exacerbation and recovery, and also in agonadal patients during the pubertal age period when their gonadotropins are returning from midchildhood reductions. (22)

GnRH pulses appear and are maintained independent of steroid feedback. Positive estrogen feedback is established only in midpuberty just prior to menarche.

Puberty

The cascade of events initiated by the release of pulsatile GnRH from prepubertal feedback and central negative inhibition results in increased levels of gonadotropins and steroids with appearance of secondary sexual characteristics and eventual adult function (menarche, and later, ovulation). Between the ages of 10 and 16, the endocrine sequence observed includes first, pulsatile patterns of LH during sleep, followed by similar pulses of less amplitude occurring throughout the 24-hour day. Episodic peaks of estradiol result and menarche appears. By mid to late puberty, maturation of the positive feedback relationship between estradiol and LH is established leading to ovulatory cycles.

Timing of Puberty

Although the major determinant of the timing of puberty is genetic, other factors appear to influence the time of initiation and the rate of progression of puberty: geographic location, exposure to light, general health and nutrition, and psychologic factors. For example, children with a family history of early puberty do start early.(23) Children closer to the equator, at lower altitudes, those in urban areas, and mildly obese children start earlier than those in Northern latitudes, at higher elevations above sea level, in rural areas, and normal weight children, respectively. There is a fairly good correlation between the times of menarche of mothers and daughters and between sisters.(23)

The decline in the age of menarche displayed by children in developed countries undoubtedly reflects improved nutritional status. Frisch believes that a critical body weight (47.8 kg) must be reached by a girl to achieve menarche.(24) Possibly more important than total weight may be the shift in body composition to a greater percent fat (from 16.0 to 23.5%). Indeed, moderately obese girls (20-30% over normal weight) have earlier menarche than normal weight girls. Conversely, anorectics and intense exercisers (low weight or low percent fat component of weight) have delayed menarche or secondary amenorrhea. That other factors are involved is indicated by the delayed menarche experienced by morbidly obese girls (greater than 30% overweight), diabetics, and intense exercisers of normal weight. Intriguingly, blind girls experience earlier menarche. Furthermore, girls with idiopathic central precocious puberty may undergo menarche at a total body fat of 19%: children with hypothyroidism display sexual precocity despite a total body fat of 29%, while girls with no signs of puberty may have measured total body fat of 27%.(25) It is reasonable to hypothesize that central mechanisms bring about maturation of the hypothalamic-pituitary-ovarian axis which in turn stimulates growth to the critical weight as well as the increases in body fat composition. Evidence suggests that growth acceleration is due more to estrogen and concomitant increases in growth hormone production and secondary stimulation of somatomedin-C (insulin-like growth factor-I) levels.(26)

Stages of Pubertal
Development

On the average, the pubertal sequence of accelerated growth, breast development, pubarche, and menarche requires a period of 4.5 years (range 1.5 to 6 years). The largest body of data has been accumulated in healthy European girls; however, current North American Standards are approximately 6 months earlier for each stage.(27, 28)

In general, the first sign of puberty is an acceleration of growth followed by breast budding (thelarche) (median age 9.8 years). Although the sequence may be reversed, pubarche usually appears after the breast bud (median 10.5 years) with axillary hair growth 2 years later. In approximately 20% of children, pubic hair growth is the first sign of puberty. Menarche is a late event (median 12.8 years), occurring after the peak of growth has passed.

Growth

An adolescent girl's growth spurt occurs 2 years earlier than that of a boy, and in 1 year, her rate of growth doubles, yielding a height increment of between 6 to 11 cm (2 to 4 inches).(29) The average girl reaches this growth peak about 2 years after breast budding and 1 year prior to menarche. Hormonal requirements for this increased growth velocity include growth hormone and gonadal estrogen. Adrenal androgens are not involved because cortisol-repleted Addisonian patients display normal pubertal growth patterns.

In a remarkable study of African pygmies, it was discovered that the short stature of adult pygmies is due primarily to a failure of growth to accelerate during puberty, and that the principal factor responsible for normal pubertal growth is insulin-like growth factor-I (somatomedin-C), the mediator of sex steroid induction of growth.(30) Growth hormone exerts its action through circulating mediators, originally called somatomedins and now called insulin-

Height Gain in Centimeters

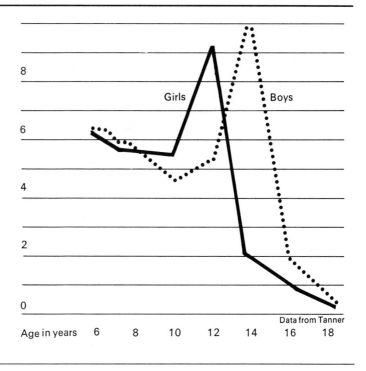

Data from Tanner

like growth factors. The current hypothesis states that growth hormone affects cartilage by means of insulin-like growth factor-I, which is thought to be synthesized in multiple distant sites. Normal growth at puberty requires the concerted action of growth hormone, insulin-like growth factor-I, and sex steroids. The increase in circulating insulin-like growth factor-I at puberty correlates with sexual development and results from the interaction between sex steroids and growth hormone. Specifically, the increase in sex steroids in turn increases the secretion of growth hormone, which stimulates the production of insulin-like growth factor-I.(31)

The amounts of estrogen required to stimulate long-bone cortical growth are incredibly small. Doses of 100 nanograms per kilogram body weight per day produce maximal growth in agonadal recipients. These doses are insufficient to cause breast budding, vaginal cornification, or an increase in sex hormone binding globulin.(32,33) These low dose effects are consistent with the observation that girls attain peak height velocity early in puberty at serum estradiol concentrations of 20 pg/ml which is one-sixth the mean level of adult women.

415

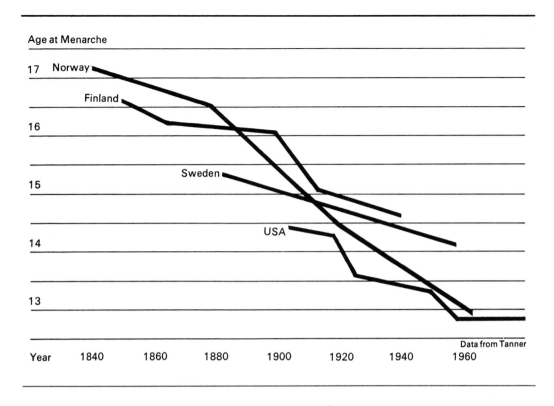

Age at Menarche

17 Norway

Finland

16

Sweden

15

USA

14

13

Year   1840   1860   1880   1900   1920   1940   1960

Data from Tanner

Menarche

As mentioned previously, environmental factors are important in the onset of puberty. Improved living standards and nutrition in the mother antenatally, and in children postnatally, have played a significant role in producing taller, heavier children with earlier maturation. Studies of identical twins and nonidentical twins show that the age at menarche is chiefly controlled by genetic factors when the environment is optimal. In affluent cultures, the trend toward lowering of the menarcheal age and puberty has now been halted.(28) In the 1700s, the mean age of voice change in the Boys' Bach Choir in Leipzig was 18, now it is 13.5 years.

The relationship between menarche and the growth spurt is relatively fixed: menarche occurs after the peak in growth velocity has passed. Hence slower growth (totaling no more than 6 cm (2.5 inches) is noted after initiation of menses.

The normal age range of menarche in American girls is 9.1-17.7 years with a median of 12.8.(28) The final endocrine hallmark of puberty is the development of positive estrogen feedback on the pituitary and hypothalamus. This feedback stimulates the midcycle surge of LH required for ovulation. Thus the menses following menarche are usually anovulatory, irregular, and occasionally heavy. Anovulation lasts as long as 12-18 months after menarche, but there are reports of pregnancy before menarche. Ovulation increases in frequency as menses occur and puberty progresses.

Summary of Pubertal Events	The onset of puberty is an evolving sequence of maturational steps. The hypothalamic-pituitary gonadotrope-gonadal system differentiates and functions during fetal life and early infancy. Thereafter, it is suppressed to low activity levels during childhood by a combination of hypersensitivity of the "gonadostat" to estrogen negative feedback and an intrinsic CNS inhibitor. All the components located below GnRH (below the CNS) are competent to respond at all ages (as will be seen in the pathogenesis of precocious puberty). After a decade of functional GnRH insufficiency (between late infancy and the onset of puberty), GnRH secretion is resumed and gonadarche (the reactivation of the CNS-pituitary-ovarian apparatus) appears. Prolongation of intrinsic CNS suppression or disability in any of the components of the gonadarche cascade leads to delayed or absent pubescence.

1. FSH and then LH levels rise moderately before the age of 10 and are followed by a rise in estradiol. Early gonadotropin LH pulses are seen only in sleep, but gradually extend throughout the day. In the adult, they occur at roughly 1.5-2 hourly intervals.

2. As gonadal estrogen increases (gonadarche), breast development, female fat distribution, and vaginal and uterine growth occur. Skeletal growth rapidly increases as a result of initial gonadal secretion of low levels of estrogen. Sex hormone binding globulin rises.

3. Adrenal androgen (adrenarche) and, to a lesser degree, gonadal androgen secretion cause pubic and axillary hair growth. Adrenarche plays little if any part in skeletal growth. While temporarily related to gonadarche, adrenarche is an independent, functionally unrelated biological event.

4. At midpuberty, sufficient gonadal estrogen secretion proliferates the endometrium, and the first menses (menarche) occurs. Estradiol positive feedback on LH secretion is demonstrable thereafter.

5. Postmenarchal cycles are initially anovulatory. Sustained, predictable positive gonadotropin responses to estradiol or clomiphene are late pubertal events.

Blood Hormone Concentrations During Female Puberty (34–40)				
Tanner Stage	*FSH mIU/ml*	*LH mIU/ml*	*Estradiol pg/ml*	*DHA ng/dl*
Stage 1	0.9–5.1	1.8–9.2	<1.0	19–302
Stage 2	1.4–7.0	2.0–16.6	7–37	45–1904
Stage 3	2.4–7.7	5.6–13.6	9–59	125–1730
Stage 4	1.5–11.2	7–14.4	10–156	153–1321
Adult: Follicular-	3–20	5–25	30–100	162–1620

417

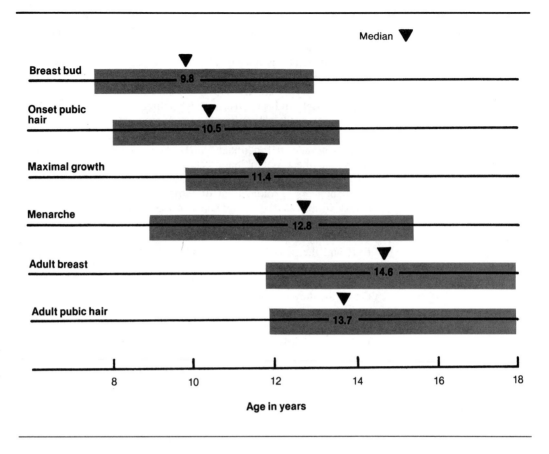

Median ▼

Breast bud — 9.8

Onset pubic hair — 10.5

Maximal growth — 11.4

Menarche — 12.8

Adult breast — 14.6

Adult pubic hair — 13.7

8   10   12   14   16   18

Age in years

Precocious Puberty

Puberty is the biologic transition between immature and adult reproductive function. Its timing, endocrine milieu, and physical expressions have been characterized sufficiently to set clinically reasonable time limits for the normal appearance of female maturity and to allow recognition of the pathogenesis and pathophysiology of most of the causes of premature or delayed pubescence.

If one accepts the mean ± 2.5 standard deviations as encompassing the normal range, then pubertal changes before the age of 8 are regarded as precocious. Increased growth is often the first change in precocious puberty. This is usually followed by breast development and growth of pubic hair. On occasion, pubarche, thelarche, and linear growth occur simultaneously. Menarche, however, may be the first sign.

Classically, precocious puberty has been divided into true sexual prococity in which the hormones are secreted by maturing gonads, and precocious pseudopuberty in which maturing normal gonads are not the source of the sex steroids. These classifications are of little practical use. Precocity occurs in girls 5 times more frequently than boys, and almost three-quarters of precocity in girls is idiopathic. In the face of any precocious development, the physician is obligated to rule out a serious disease process.

Sexual development does not require ovulatory capability. Evaluation of a patient's possible fertility, for example, with basal body temperatures or progesterone assays, is an unnecessary procedure.

More importantly, true sexual precocity with potential fertility and adult levels of gonadotropins does not rule out the possibility of a serious disease process (e.g. a CNS tumor). While it is true that the most common form of sexual precocity in females is constitutional precocity (true sexual precocity), this must be a diagnosis by exclusion with prolonged follow-up in an effort to detect slowly developing lesions of the brain, ovary, or adrenal gland.

Classification and Relative Occurrence of Precocious Puberty (41–45)

	Female	Male
Increased Gonadotropins (True Precocity)		
Idiopathic	74%	41%
Cerebral Problem	7%	26%
Ectopic Gonadotropin Production	0.5%	0.5%
Increased Sex Steroids (Precocious Pseudopuberty)		
Ovarian (cyst or tumor)	11%	—
Testicular	—	10%
McCune-Albright Syndrome	5%	1%
Adrenal Feminizing	1%	0
Adrenal Masculinizing	1%	22%

A classification of sexual precocity is presented above to provide a guide to the possible conditions and the relative incidences encountered. The cause of precocious development may be immediately suggested by the history and physical examination. A familial occurrence renders unlikely a variety of causes, mainly tumors.

Particular attention should be given to the following possibilities: drug ingestion, cerebral problems such as cranial trauma or encephalitis, retarded growth with symptoms of hypothyroidism, and a pelvic or abdominal mass. A left hand-wrist film (for use with atlases) should be obtained for bone age. Determination of thyroid function is indicated, and a blood level of DHAS should be measured. A CT scan and EEG are probably indicated in patients with precocious puberty, even in the face of a normal overall evaluation, including normal routine skull x-rays. Other procedures should be dictated by the clinical findings. Virilization, of course, demands a full adrenal evaluation.

Precocious
Development Due to
Stimulation of
Gonadotropin
Secretion: True
Precocious Puberty

The signs of *constitutional* sexual precocity are due to premature maturation of the hypothalamic-pituitary-ovarian axis, resulting in production of gonadotropins and sex steroids. Constitutional precocity runs in families and usually occurs very close to the "borderline" age of 8 years. On the other hand, *idiopathic* precocious puberty does not run in families and occurs much earlier in childhood. It must be reemphasized that these benign diagnoses should be made only by exclusion and deserve long-term follow-up, as cerebral abnormalities may not become apparent until adulthood.

Clinical presentation of true precocity may not follow the usual progression of breast and pubic hair growth, acceleration of growth rate and then menses. It is not unusual for pubarche or menarche to be the first sign with others following. This progression is variable, usually slower in idiopathic cases, but telescoped in precocity due to central disease.

Sexual precocity is consistent with normal reproductive life and it is not associated with premature menopause. The most serious effect of precocity is the resultant adult short stature. Because the skeleton is very sensitive to even the lowest levels of estrogen, these children are transiently tall for their age, but as a result of early epiphyseal fusion eventually short stature results. Fifty percent are less than 5 feet tall. Dental eruption correlates more with chronological rather than skeletal age.

Intellectual and psychosocial development are also commensurate with chronologic age rather than stage of puberty. Expectations of emotional, social, sexual and intellectual competence corresponding to their pubertal state leave these youngsters and their families with potentially serious difficulties on all levels of social and emotional function.

A number of *cerebral* problems, including abnormal skull development due to rickets, can cause true precocious development. Various tumors include: craniopharyngioma, optic glioma, astrocytoma, and suprasellar teratoma—all usually near the hypothalamus. Pineal tumors, for unknown reasons, have been seen only in male precocious puberty. Nontumorous causes include encephalitis, meningitis, hydrocephalus, and von Recklinghausen's disease. An injury to the skull may stimulate sexual development. The mechanism is unknown, and a latent period of 1-2 months is usually seen. A hamartoma is a hyperplastic malformation at the base of the hypothalamus which usually produces precocity in the first few years of life.

Ectopic gonadotropin production is a rare cause of sexual precocity accounting for less than 0.5% of cases. The most common tumors producing gonadotropins are chorioepithelioma and dysgerminoma of the ovary, and liver hepatoblastoma.(46,47) Tumor spread may be present at the time of pubertal development; pelvic and abdominal masses accompanied by ascites are usually detectable.

True sexual precocity occurs in a small number of children with long-standing hypothyroidism. In addition to short stature, galactorrhea may be present. The sella turcica is frequently enlarged, but with thyroid replacement pubertal development will stop and even regress. The sella films will return to normal. While reported cases have been severe and therefore clinically obvious, laboratory evaluation of thyroid function is indicated in all cases of sexual precocity.

Development Due to Availability of Sex Steroids: Precocious Pseudopuberty

Eleven percent of girls with precocious puberty have an ovarian tumor. The tumor is usually an estrogen-producing neoplasm or cyst. Five percent of granulosa cell tumors and 1% of theca cell tumors occur before puberty. However, gonadoblastomas, teratomas, lipoid cell tumors, cystadenomas and even ovarian cancers have been reported as causes of precocity. Bleeding is irregular and menorrhagic—clearly anovulatory. A pelvic mass is readily palpable in 80% of cases. The palpation of a pelvic or abdominal mass demands surgical exploration. Increasing use has been made of pelvic ultrasonography and whole body (abdominal) CT scan for the work-up of precocious puberty.

A feminizing adrenal tumor is very rare (1% of cases) and is associated with increased blood levels of DHAS.

Drug ingestion should be suspected when there is dark pigmentation of the nipples and breast areola, an effect of certain synthetic estrogens such as stilbestrol.

McCune-Albright syndrome (polyostotic fibrous dysplasia) accounts for 5% of female precocity and consists of multiple disseminated cystic bone lesions which easily fracture, cafe au lait skin areas of various sizes and shapes, and sexual precocity. Premature menarche may be the first sign of the syndrome. Skeletal abnormalities may become evident following the onset of puberty. The combination of multiple bone fractures, cafe au lait patches, and premature development should lead to the diagnosis. Sexual precocity in Albright syndrome is now demonstrated to be the result of autonomous early production of estrogen by the ovaries.(48) In addition, Cushing's disease, gigantism, and hyperthyroidism have been reported in this syndrome. The protean manifestations of this disorder suggest that the pathophysiology results from a basic defect in cellular regulation at the level of either cAMP generation or protein kinase function in affected tissues. Eventual fertility is unimpaired, and adult height appears to be normal. These positive factors must be considered in the choice of management of the syndrome.

Yet another example of precocity due to gonadotropin independent gonadal secretion of estrogen is by autonomous benign ovarian follicular or luteal cysts. (49) These children demonstrate an absence of gonadotropin pulsations, variable responses to GnRH, and a lack of suppression of puberty by a long-acting GnRH agonist. The cysts may enlarge and involute, and then recur so that signs of sexual precocity and vaginal bleeding remit and exacerbate. The cysts are unusually large and therefore palpable. GnRH testing is useful in differentiating the autonomous (nonreactive) cyst from those secondary to the FSH and LH stimulation of central true precocity (reactive).

Laboratory Findings in Disorders Producing Precocious Puberty

	Gonadal Size	Basal FSH/LH	Estradiol or Testosterone	DHAS	GnRH
Idiopathic:	Increased	Increased	Increased	Increased	Pubertal
Cerebral:	Increased	Increased	Increased	Increased	Pubertal
Gonadal:	Unilat. Incr.	Decreased	Increased	Increased	Flat
Albright:	Increased	Decreased	Increased	Increased	Flat
Adrenal:	Small	Decreased	Increased	Increased	Flat

Special Cases of Precocious Development	Special cases of precocious development include the isolated appearance of one sexual characteristic: premature adrenarche or pubarche (pubic hair), or premature thelarche (breast development). Sparse hair growth on the vulva does not represent precocious pubarche. Little is known about these conditions other than that they are associated with an increased incidence of central nervous system abnormalities, such as mental deficiency. The usual effort should be made to exclude a serious disease process. If the bone age is advanced, treatment is indicated. Isolated vaginal bleeding is rare. Careful local exam for foreign bodies, tumors or infections is required.
Diagnosis of Precocious Puberty	The cause of precocious development may be obvious by findings in the history or physical examination. Familial occurrence helps to exclude certain disease processes (tumors). Clinically, the nature of precocity dictates certain diagnostic priorities:

1. Rule out life-threatening disease. This includes neoplasms of the CNS, ovary, and adrenal.

2. Define the velocity of the process. Is it progressing or stabilized? Management decisions hinge on this determination. Isolated, non-endocrine causes of vaginal bleeding (trauma, foreign body, vaginitis, genital neoplasm) must be excluded.

The differential diagnosis of puberty is derived from the physical and laboratory findings as noted:

Differential Diagnostic Steps

Physical Diagnosis:

> Record of growth, Tanner stages.
> External genitalia changes.
> Abdominal, pelvic, neurologic examination.
> Signs of androgenization.
> Special findings: McCune-Albright, hypothyroidism.

Laboratory Diagnosis:

> Serial bone age.
> Skull film, CT scan, EEG.
> FSH, LH, HCG assay.
> Thyroid function tests (TSH and free T_4).
> Steroids (serum DHAS, testosterone, estradiol, progesterone, 17-OHP).

If the full signs of sexual precocity are present, and basal or GnRH-stimulated gonadotropins are in the pubertal range, a pituitary source of gonadotropins is suspected. Any abnormality on neurologic exam, skull x-rays or CT scan points toward cerebral precocious puberty. If these are all normal, idiopathic sexual precocity is the most likely diagnosis. It should be emphasized that basal serum gonadotropins may be in the prepubertal range in the early stages of idiopathic or cerebral precocious puberty; with time and progression of sexual development these will rise to the pubertal range. However, if serum gonadotropins are suppressed while estradiol is markedly elevated, an ectopic source of HCG should be considered; a situation easily confirmed by radioimmunoassay specific for the β-subunit of HCG. If the laboratory picture is more one of elevated adrenal androgens with only slightly elevated serum estradiol and suppressed serum gonadotropin, the rare feminizing adrenal tumor may be present.

If signs of sexual precocity are associated with accelerated growth and skeletal maturation, in the absence of virilization, the etiology may be an ovarian tumor or cyst. A pelvic mass is usually palpable. In this situation, serum FSH and LH are suppressed, while serum estradiol is usually elevated. An elevated serum progesterone suggests an ovarian luteoma. Pelvic ultrasound or CT scan can help to confirm the presence of an ovarian mass. Laparotomy is indicated to confirm the diagnosis and carry out surgical resection.

If signs of sexual precocity are accompanied by virilization, adrenal hyperplasia or a virilizing adrenal or ovarian tumor must be considered. With elevation of serum 17-hydroxyprogesterone (17-OHP) and adrenal androgens, the diagnosis of 21-hydroxylase deficient adrenal hyperplasia is established, whereas an elevation of serum 11-deoxycortisol (compound S) leads to the diagnosis of 11-hydroxylase deficient adrenal hyperplasia. If these two serum hormones are normal, while serum DHAS or androstenedione is elevated, an adrenal tumor or a virilizing ovarian tumor is suspect. Ultrasound examination and abdominal CT scan can be utilized to further localize the tumor.

If breast and genital development, pubic hair growth, and vaginal bleeding are seen in a short child with a *delayed* bone age, primary hypothyroidism is the most likely diagnosis. This can be confirmed by finding a low serum T_4 and elevated TSH concentration. Serum FSH and LH levels may be in the pubertal range, but these will decrease following thyroid treatment. Galactorrhea may be present along with elevated serum prolactin concentrations. These return to normal with thyroid treatment.

Treatment of Precocious Development

The drug with which there has been the greatest experience in the treatment of idiopathic central precocious puberty is medroxyprogesterone acetate (MPA). MPA is usually administered in a dose of 100-200 mg IM weekly, but it may be given orally at 20-40 mg per day. While MPA is successful in slowing breast and genital development and preventing menses, it is not usually successful in slowing the accelerated growth rate and skeletal maturation.(50) Further, it sometimes provokes signs of glucocorticoid excess.(51)

The current most effective treatment for central precocious puberty is a GnRH agonist. In the first week of treatment, increased gonadotropins and sex steroids are induced. This is followed by down regulation of gonadotropins and suppression of sex steroids back to the prepubertal range.(52) Long-term treatment results in a decrease in growth velocity and skeletal maturation leading to an increase in final adult height.(53) GnRH agonist, initially administered by daily subcutaneous injection, is now available in an intranasal preparation. Soon, long acting forms can be utilized. GnRH agonist treatment is not effective for non-central forms of precocious puberty such as McCune-Albright syndrome, gonadotropin-independent sexual precocity, or congenital adrenal hyperplasia. However, should patients with McCune-Albright syndrome or congenital adrenal hyperplasia mature their hypothalamic-pituitary-gonadal axis and develop sexual precocity, then GnRH agonist therapy is effective.(53,54)

If a specific etiology for precocious puberty is identified, treatment is aimed at curing the underlying disorder. Neurosurgical excision of hypothalamic, pituitary, optic nerve, or pineal tumors must be individualized in each patient. If these tumors are small and do not extend around or into vital brain structures, their removal may be successful. If complete surgical excision is not possible, radiation therapy should be considered. Although many tumors are said not to be radiosensitive, this may be the only treatment available, although new chemotherapy protocols are of benefit with some tumors. The tumors which secrete ectopic HCG, such as chorioepitheliomas, teratomas, hepatomas, should be managed in a manner consistent with current specific treatment protocols.

If an ovarian or adrenal tumor is identified, surgical excision is the treatment of choice. In the case of an ovarian cyst, it may be difficult to know whether the cyst is an autonomous source of estrogens or whether its growth is secondary to gonadotropin stimulation. If multiple bilateral cysts are discovered on ultrasound examination, these are usually secondary to central gonadotropin secretion. If the cyst is solitary and the contralateral ovary appears immature, then cyst resection is justified. With primary hypothyroidism, thyroid replacement will prevent further progression of sexual precocity. If adrenal hyperplasia is identified, treatment with appropriate doses of glucocorticoids (and mineralocorticoids if salt-wasting is present) will also prevent further progression of pubertal development. If these patients have a bone age of 11-12 years, glucocorticoid therapy may result in onset of sexual precocity.

Careful consideration must be given to the management of psychosocial problems in all children with precocious puberty. As mentioned previously, these children have intellectual, behavioral and psychosexual maturation in keeping with their chronological age, not their physical or pubertal age. They do not have early heterosexual activity or abnormal sexual libido. Unfortunately, parents, teachers, and peers may have unrealistic expectations of their intellectual and athletic abilities, and these children may even inappropriately be labeled as retarded. Careful explanation of these considerations must be given to parents. The children should be counseled that their secondary sexual characteristics are normal albeit early. If the child is bright, advancement in school may be possible with special tutoring and this may prove beneficial. Children with precocious puberty may place a stress on the marital or family relationship, and in these situations formal psychological counseling may be useful.

Prognosis

The prognosis for precocious puberty depends on the underlying cause. With primary hypothyroidism, the prognosis is excellent. Children with adrenal hyperplasia tend to be short as adults. Removal of benign ovarian tumors and adrenal tumors carries a good prognosis, while malignant carcinomas often have metastatic disease at the time of presentation, with consequent poor prognosis.

Approximately 20 percent of granulosa cell tumors are malignant, and the prognosis should be guarded for recurrences as late as 25 years after removal. Approximately 25 percent of ovarian Sertoli-Leydig cell tumors are malignant.

With cerebral causes of sexual precocity, the prognosis again depends on the exact etiology. If tumors of the CNS are completely resectable, the prognosis is good; however, this tends to be the exception rather than the rule. Some tumors, though, such as hamartomas, are slow growing and may only be discovered during a routine autopsy following death owing to other causes. Other tumors such as craniopharyngiomas, are developmental remnants rather than true neoplasms, and with partial resection and radiation therapy patients may go into remission for many years. With other conditions, such as congenital cysts, hydrocephalus, encephalitis, McCune-Albright syndrome, and neurofibromatosis, the prognosis is related to associated neurologic deficits.

Psychometric testing shows that girls with precocious puberty have higher verbal IQ scores. Behavioral testing shows that a majority of girls do not have problems; a minority may show a tendency toward social difficulties related to apparent age and physical maturation, such as depression, social withdrawal, moodiness, aggression and hyperactivity. However, with the exception of short stature as an adult, the prognosis for idiopathic sexual precocity remains good if the children enter adult life without psychosexual scars. The mean adult height in adult women is approximately 152 cm. Most women have normal menstrual cycles and fertility, and they do not have premature menopause.(55)

Tanner Staging

	Breast	Pubic Hair
Stage 1 (prepubertal)	Elevation of papilla only	No public hair
Stage 2	Elevation of breast and papilla as small mound, areola diameter enlarged. Median age: 9.8 years	Sparce, long, pigmented hair chiefly along labia majora. Median age: 10.5 years
Stage 3	Further enlargement without separation of breast and areola. Median age: 11.2 years	Dark, coarse, curled hair sparsely spread over mons. Median age: 11.4 years
Stage 4	Secondary mound of areola and papilla above the breast. Median age: 12.1 years	Adult-type hair, abundant but limited to the mons. Median age: 12.0 years
Stage 5	Recession of areola to contour of breast. Median age: 14.6 years	Adult type spread in quantity and distribution. Median age: 13.7 years

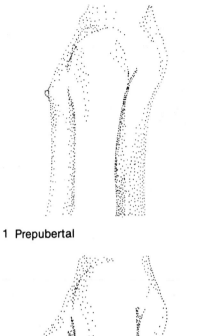

1 Prepubertal

2 Breast Bud

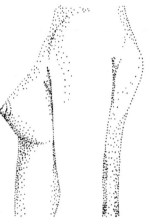

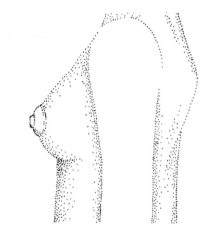

3 Breast Elevation

4 Areolar Mound

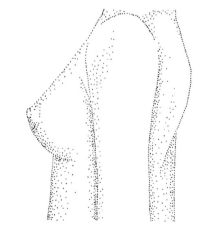

5 Adult Contour

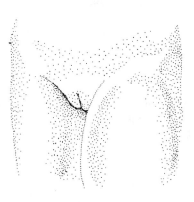

1 Prepubertal

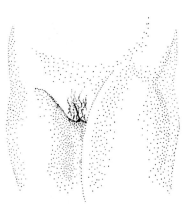

2 Presexual hair

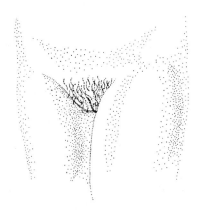

3 Sexual hair

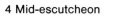

4 Mid-escutcheon

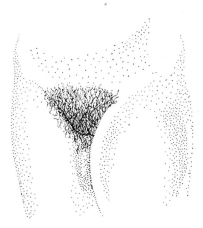

5 Female escutcheon

Delayed Puberty

Since there is such a wide variation in normal development, it is difficult to define the patient with abnormally delayed sexual maturation. Only 1% of all girls will not have had menarche by the age of 18, and complete absence of breast budding by the age of 13 is probably abnormal. However, some evaluation is needed whenever a patient or parents are concerned enough to seek a physician's advice.

Delayed puberty is a rare condition in girls, and a genetic problem or hypothalamic-pituitary disorder must be suspected. In addition, anatomic abnormalities of the target organ (uterus and endometrium) or outflow tract are unique but important elements to consider in amenorrheic but otherwise normal pubertal adolescents.

The history and physical examination are very useful in the diagnostic work-up of delayed puberty. In the history, special note should be taken of past general health, height and weight records, and the pubertal milestone experience of older siblings and parents. On physical examination, in addition to body measurements and Tanner staging of any secondary sexual characteristics present, a search for signs of hypothyroidism, gonadal dysgenesis, hypopituitarism or chronic illness should be made.

The failure of growth in stature suggests several possibilities. Isolated growth hormone deficiency is associated with somewhat delayed sexual maturity. Menarche may eventually occur, albeit delayed, but with bone age still discrepantly several years below chronologic age. More global pituitary hormone deficiency will result in total pubertal delay. Finally, gonadal dysgenesis (45,X) will be associated with decreased height and sexual infantilism with normal to slightly reduced bone age and hypergonadotropism.

Neurologic examination is important; evidence of intracranial disease, restricted visual fields, or absent sense of smell are key findings. Anatomic defects of the müllerian ducts must be sought, especially when a disparity between normal puberty and absent menses is encountered.

As will be seen in the discussion of the work-up, the diverse etiologic possibilities for delayed puberty are best classified by the level of gonadotropin encountered. The distribution of diagnostic frequencies in the three categories hyper-, hypo- and eugonadotropism are depicted below, representing the findings in 252 patients.(56)

Relative Frequency of Pubertal Abnormalities

Hypergonadotropic Hypogonadism	—	43%
Ovarian failure, abnormal karyotype	—	27%
Ovarian failure, normal karyotype	—	16%
(46,XX)	—	(14%)
(46,XY)	—	(2%)

Hypogonadotropic Hypogonadism	—	31%
Reversible:	—	20%
(Physiologic delay)	—	(14%)
(Weight loss/anorexia)	—	(2%)
(Primary hypothyroidism)	—	(1%)
(Congenital adrenal hyperplasia)	—	(1%)
(Cushing's syndrome)	—	(0.5%)
(Prolactinomas)	—	(1%)
Irreversible:	—	11%
(GnRH Deficiency)	—	(5%)
(Hypopituitarism)	—	(2%)
(Congenital CNS defects)	—	(1%)
(Other pituitary adenomas)	—	(1%)
(Craniopharyngioma)	—	(0.5%)
(Malignant pituitary tumor)	—	(0.5%)
(Postsurgical hypopituitarism)	—	(0.5%)
Eugonadism	—	26%
Müllerian agenesis	—	15%
Vaginal septum	—	3%
Imperforate hymen	—	1%
Androgen insensitivity syndrome	—	1%
Inappropriate positive feedback	—	6%

Laboratory Assessments of Delayed Puberty

Laboratory work-up of delayed puberty usually includes x-rays for bone age, skull films, and serum gonadotropin levels. If short stature (5 feet) exists, evaluation according to the program outlined in Chapter 5, "Amenorrhea," will lead to the proper diagnosis.

If gonadotropins are increased into the postmenopausal range (hypergonadotropin hypogonadism), then some type of gonadal deficiency usually is the basis of delayed maturation. In sickle cell disease, approximately 20% of patients have delayed puberty and hypergonadotropism. Also a 17 α-hydroxylase deficiency in steroid synthesis (affecting both adrenals and ovaries) will cause hypergonadotropic delayed puberty.

Hypergonadotropic Hypogonadism. The most common disorder of this type is gonadal dysgenesis. In the 45,X patient, the typical phenotypic stigmata of Turner's syndrome will be displayed. However, these may be minimal or absent in sex chromosome mosaicism or structural deletions of the X chromosome. A Y-bearing cell line requires laparotomy and gonadal excision as prophylaxis against the risk of gonadal malignancy.

A hypergonadotropic 45,XX individual presents interesting possibilities. If hypertension, sexual infantilism, and an elevated serum progesterone are found, 17α-hydroxylase deficiency in steroid synthesis is likely. Acquired ovarian damage from torsion or inflammation should be ruled out. Finally, the 46,XX patient may have pure gonadal dysgenesis (gonadal streaks) or the resistant ovary syndrome. See the discussion in Chapter 5 under Premature Ovarian Failure.

Hypogonadotropic Hypogonadism. Decreased secretion of LH (less than 6 mIU/ml), associated with depressed FSH, is seen in hypothalamic (amenorrhea and anosmia), pituitary (tumor) disorders, or nonpathologic constitutional delay in development. The typical patient with constitutional delay is short with appropriate bone maturation delay. As previously noted, constitutional delay is frequently seen in a familial pattern, with the expectation of a late but otherwise normal growth pattern and adult reproductive function.

Poor nutrition (anorexia nervosa, malabsorption, chronic illness, regional ileitis, renal disease) also may lead to hypogonadotropic delayed growth and development.

In the presence of normal olfaction, exclusion of pituitary or parapituitary tumor by specialized neuroradiologic procedures is necessary. If tumor or vascular malformation is not found, the possibility of pituitary insufficiency can be evaluated with GnRH stimulation.

Eugonadotropic Hypogonadism. Müllerian tube segmental discontinuities, müllerian agenesis, or androgen insensitivity syndrome will present as delayed menarche despite normal development of an adult female phenotype. Müllerian agenesis accounts for about one-fifth of cases of prolonged primary amenorrhea. Other obstructive anomalies of the müllerian ducts are less frequently seen (1%). Anovulation and the polycystic ovary, and androgen-producing adrenal disease, can present as primary amenorrhea.

Treatment of Sexual Infantilism (Delayed Puberty)

The first priority in therapy is removal or correction of the primary etiology when possible. In this regard, thyroid therapy for hypothyroidism, growth hormone for isolated GH deficiency, treatment of ileitis, are examples of specific therapy. In hypogonadism, cyclic estrogen and progestin therapy in the usual replacement doses will initiate and sustain maturation and function of secondary sexual characteristics. In XY individuals, properly timed gonadectomy followed by sex hormone replacement is required. In constitutional delay, reassurance that the anticipated development will occur is the only management step needed, although early hormonal treatment is worthwhile in order to minimize psychological stress.

Treatment with pulsatile GnRH is both a logical and effective means of inducing a physiologic puberty.(57) However this treatment regimen is not practical. While its expense is an important consideration, the technical aspects associated with the parenteral administration of GnRH pulses make this method too cumbersome and difficult.

Growth Problems in Normal Adolescents

Perhaps the worst thing about an adolescent growth problem is that it makes the individual "different." It is probably true that more than anyone else the adolescent does not like to be different. Therefore, excessive or insufficient growth is not a problem to be dismissed lightly, and psychologic support and reassurance are key features in the management of such problems. A willingness to listen to problems, together with an adult-to-adult attitude, will place the adolescent-physician relationship at the proper level of mutual respect.

The basic and essential laboratory procedure is a left hand-wrist x-ray for bone age. The Bayley-Pinneau tables predict future adult height, utilizing the bone age and present height.(58) To use the tables, one needs a measurement of height, the patient's age, and an x-ray of the left hand and wrist for bone age. All of the hand epiphyses and those of the distal end of the arm are used to determine the skeletal age. The Bayley-Pinneau tables begin on page 438.

To estimate a patient's adult height, use the tables as follows: Go down the left hand column to the patient's present height, follow this horizontal row to the column under the bone age which is given by 6 month intervals across the top. The number at the intersection represents the predicted adult height. If figures do not fall at the 1 inch or 6 month intervals used on the tables, the predicted height can be easily extrapolated.

It is important to use the table suitable for the rate of maturing. If the bone age is within 1 year of the chronologic age, use the table for average girls; if the bone age is accelerated 1 year or more, use the table for accelerated girls; if the bone age is retarded 1 year or more, use the table for retarded girls.

The tables are for use with bone age films of the hand and wrist only in conjunction with the Greulich-Pyle Atlas. Use with bone age determined by any other method is less accurate.

Short Stature. Thorough medical history and physical examination will eliminate the usual disorders associated with short stature: malnutrition, chronic urinary tract disease, chronic infectious disease, hypothyroidism, mental illness, panhypopituitarism, and gonadal dysgenesis. In the history, the heights and weights of parents, siblings, and relatives should be obtained along with timing of growth in the family, dietary history, daily activities, and sleep habits. Normal history and examination in an individual with a bone age only 1 year behind the chronologic age suggest a constitutional pattern which does not require treatment.

Generally, endocrine disease is an uncommon basis for impairment of growth. Congenital hypothyroidism is the most frequent problem of this type, followed by hypopituitarism, hypothyroidism with onset during childhood, and excess cortisol.

It is unlikely that a patient with congenital hypothyroidism will present undiagnosed and untreated as an adolescent. However, juvenile hypothyroidism must be suspected in an adolescent with obesity and short stature and normal early childhood development. Similarly, an adolescent with hypopituitarism due to a slow growing pituitary tumor may present with a failure to develop secondary sexual characteristics and a failure to grow. Cortisol excess may be due to Cushing's disease (rare in childhood) or to therapy with corticosteroids. Excess endogenous or exogenous corticosteroids suppress skeletal maturation and growth. Moderate overdosage of cortisol, for example when treating children with adrenal hyperplasia, may suppress growth.

431

Treatment of Short Stature. If the physician concludes that an adolescent suffers from a delay of normal growth and no disease process is present, support and observation are indicated. If the bone age is more than 1 year below the chronologic age, but the family history reveals a consistent pattern of retarded but eventual normal growth, reassurance is essential. It is helpful to point out the x-ray, indicating that the individual has 1 year or more of unused potential in which to catch up with her friends.

When continued failure to grow is evident in the absence of disease, hormone treatment can be considered. Presently the use of growth hormone is limited to use in growth hormone deficiency. Acceleration of growth has been attempted by administration of Human Growth Hormone Releasing Hormone, and by exogenous stimulators of HGH-RH (α-adrenergic agonists such as clonidine).(59) It is too early to assess effect and safety. Recently illicit sources of GH have been utilized by parents eager to "grow" big kids for athletic prowess. This dangerous practice all too often leads to growth but of fragile bones unsupported by the sought after muscular capacities. Fortunately, it is rare to see a female adolescent with this problem. More commonly it is an adolescent boy who is sensitive to reduced growth, and in whom the use of testosterone may be indicated. In cases of gonadal failure, estrogen may be used in a female to stimulate epiphyseal growth bringing the bone age to match the chronologic age. Ethinyl estradiol in a dose of 100 ng/kg/day has been shown to be effective in hypogonadal individuals (this is a much smaller dose than previously used). Patients should be observed at monthly intervals to document the pattern of growth and development. Hormone treatment may be discontinued when the bone age matches the chronologic age.

Tall Stature. This is rarely a problem in boys (basketball has provided a ready outlet, and fortunately participation in sports is now appealing to girls as well), but girls who are the daughters of very tall parents may come for help. The Bayley-Pinneau tables are accurate in predicting the height of tall girls. A predicted height greater than 6 feet probably deserves treatment.

A hand-wrist x-ray for bone age is necessary. The degree of development of secondary sexual characteristics is important, since the more mature a girl is, the less effective treatment is in influencing her eventual height.

Treatment of Tall Stature. It is difficult to make a decision for treatment, and parental participation in the decision is essential. In a case where some success can be achieved, the patient is relatively young and may find it hard to know what to think about the future problem.

Since the adolescent growth spurt precedes menarche, treatment must begin before menarche in order to be optimally successful. This would be as early as 8 or 9 years, and certainly before the age of 12. However, treatment begun after menarche may still achieve up to an inch of growth reduction.(60,61) Once begun, treatment must continue until epiphyses are fused. If treatment is stopped earlier, further growth will occur. The parents and patient must be informed of possible problems with menorrhagia, breast symptoms, water retention, etc.

Conjugated estrogen can be given in a dose of 10 mg daily from the 1st through the 25th of each month, and medroxyprogesterone acetate, 10 mg, is added on the 16th through the 25th to ensure consistent and predictable menstrual bleeding. Hand-wrist films should be taken every 6 months until epiphyseal closure is demonstrated. In view of the sensitivity of growth physiology to low levels of estrogen, it is not certain that these high doses are necessary. It would be reasonable to consider the usual replacement dose (0.625-1.25 mg conjugated estrogen), especially if the high doses elicit unpleasant symptoms.

References

1. **Kaplan SL, Grumbach MM, Aubert ML,** The ontogenesis of pituitary hormones and hypothalamic factors in the human fetus: Maturation of central nervous system regulation of anterior pituitary function, Rec Prog Hor Res 32:161, 1976.

2. **Winter JSD, Hughes IA, Reyes FI, Faiman C,** Pituitary-gonadal relations in infancy: 2. Patterns of serum gonadal steroid concentration in man from birth to two years of age. J Clin Endocrinol Metab 42:679, 1976.

3. **Winter JSD, Faiman C,** The development of cyclic pituitary-gonadal function in adolescent females. J Clin Endocrinol Metab 37:714, 1973.

4. **Conte FA, Grumbach MM, Kaplan SL, Reiter EO,** Correlation of LHRF induced LH and FSH release from infancy to 19 years with the changing pattern of gonadotropin secretion in agonadal patients: Relation to restraint of puberty, J Clin Endocrinol Metab 50:163, 1980.

5. **Roth JC, Kelch RP, Kaplan SL, Grumbach MM,** FSH and LH response to luteinizing hormone-releasing factor in prepubertal and pubertal children, adult males and patients with hypogonadotropic and hypergonadotropic hypogonadism. J Clin Endocrinol Metab 37:680, 1973.

6. **Jakacki RI, Kelch RP, Sander SE, Lloyd JS, Hopwood NJ, Marshall JC,** Pulsatile secretion of luteinizing hormone in children. J Clin Endocrinol Metab 55:453, 1982.

7. **Sizonenko PC, Paunier L, Carmignac D,** Hormonal changes during puberty: IV. Longitudinal study of adrenal androgen secretion. Hor Res 7:288, 1976.

8. **Sklar CA, Kaplan SL, Grumbach MM,** Evidence for dissociation between adrenarche and gonadarche: studies in patients with idiopathic precocious puberty, gonadal dysgenesis, isolated gonadotropin deficiency, and constitutionally delayed growth and adolescence. J Clin Endocrinol Metab 51:548, 1980.

9. **Zumoff B, Walsh BT, Katz JL,** Subnormal plasma dehydroiso androsterone to cortisol ratio in anorexia nervosa: a second hormonal parameter of ontogenetic regression. J Clin Endocrinol Metab 56:668, 1983.

10. **Pederson RC, Brownie AC, Ling N,** Pro-adrenocorticotropin/ endorphin derived peptides: coordinate action on adrenal steroidogenesis. Science 208:1044, 1980.

11. **Hauffa BP, Kaplan SL, Grumbach MM,** Dissociation between plasma adrenal androgens and cortisol in Cushing's disease and ectopic ACTH producing tumor: relation to adrenarche. Lancet i:1373, 1984.

433

12. **Byrne GC, Perry YS, Winter JSD,** Steroid inhibitory effects upon human adrenal 3β-hydroxysteroid dehydrogenase activity, J Clin Endocrinol Metab 62:413, 1986.

13. **Terasawa E, Noonan JJ, Nass TE, Loose MD,** Posterior hypothalamic lesions advance the onset of puberty in the female rhesus monkey. Endocrinology 115:224, 1984.

14. **Foster DL, Ryan KD,** Endocrine mechanisms governing transition into adulthood: a marked decrease in inhibitory feedback action of estradiol on tonic secretion of LH in the lamb during puberty. Endocrinology 105:896, 1979.

15. **Attanasio A, Borrelli P, Gupta D,** Circadian rhythms in serum melatonin from infancy to adolescence. J Clin Endocrinol Metab 61:388, 1985.

16. **Plant TM, Zorub DS,** Pinealectomy in agonadal infantile male rhesus monkeys does not interrupt initiation of the prepubertal hiatus in gonadotropin secretion. Endocrinology 118:227, 1986.

17. **Genazzani AR, Fachinetti F, Petraglia F, Pintor C, Corda R,** Hyperendorphinemia in obese children and adolescents. J Clin Endocrinol Metab 62:36, 1986.

18. **Wilson ME, Gordon TP, Collins DC,** Ontogeny of LH secretion and first ovulation in seasonal breeding rhesus monkeys. Endocrinology 118:293, 1986.

19. **Marshall JC, Kilch RP,** Low dose pulsatile GnRH in anorexia nervosa: a model of human pubertal development. J Clin Endocrinol Metab 49:712, 1979.

20. **Job JC, Garnier PE, Chaussain JL, Milhaud G,** Elevation of serum gonadotropins (LH and FSH) after releasing hormone (LH-RH) injection in normal children and in patients with disorders of puberty. J Clin Endocrinol Metab 35:473, 1972.

21. **Burstein S, Schaff-Blass E, Blass J, Rosenfield R,** Changing ratio of bioactive to immunoactive LH through puberty. J Clin Endocrinol Metab 61:508, 1985.

22. **Kapen S, Boyan RM, Hellman L, Weltzman ED,** 24-Hour patterns of LH secretion in humans: ontogenic and sexual consideration. Prog Brain Res 42:103, 1975.

23. **Tanner JM,** *Growth at Adolescence,* Ed 2, Blackwell Scientific Publications, Oxford, 1962.

24. **Frisch RE,** Body fat, menarche, and reproductive ability, Seminars Reprod Endocrinol 3:45, 1985.

25. **Crawford JD, Osler DC,** Body composition at menarche: The Frisch Revelle hypothesis revisited. Pediatrics 56:449, 1975.

26. **Harris DA, Van Vliet G, Egli LA, Grumbach MM, Kaplan SL, Styne DM, Vainsel M,** Somatomedin-C in normal puberty and in true precocious puberty before and after treatment with a potent luteinizing hormone-releasing hormone agonist. J Clin Endocrinol Metab 61:152, 1985.

27. **Marshall WA, Tanner JM,** Variations in the pattern of pubertal changes in girls. Arch Dis Child 44:291, 1969.

28. **Zacharias L, Rand WM, Wurtman RJ,** A prospective study of sexual development and growth in American girls: the statistics of menarche. Obstet Gynecol Surv 31:325, 1976.

29. **Fried RI, Smith EE,** Postmenarcheal growth patterns, J Pediat 61:562, 1962.

30. **Merimee TJ, Zapf J, Hewlett B, Cavalli-Sforza LL,** Insulin-like growth factors in Pygmies, New Eng J Med 316:906, 1987.

31. **Mansfield MJ, Rudlin CR, Crigler JF Jr, Karol KA, Crawford JD, Boepple PA, Crowley WF Jr,** Changes in growth and serum growth hormone and plasma somatomedin-C levels during suppression of gonadal sex steroid secretion in girls with central precocious puberty, J Clin Endocrinol Metab 66:3, 1988.

32. **Ross JL, Cassorla FG, Skerda MC, Valk IG, Loriaux L, Culter GB,** A preliminary study of the effect of estrogen dose on growth in Turner's syndrome. New Eng J Med 309:1104, 1983.

33. **Bohnet HG,** New aspects of oestrogen/gestagen-induced growth and endocrine changes in individuals with Turner syndrome, Eur J Pediatr 145:275, 1986.

34. **Sizonenko PC, Paunier L,** Hormonal changes in Puberty III: Correlation of plasma dehydroepiandrosterone, testosterone, FSH and LH with stage of puberty and bone age in normal boys and girls and in patients with Addison's disease or hypogonadism or premature or late adrenarche. J Clin Endocrinol Metab 41:894, 1975.

35. **Hung W, August GP, Glasgow AM,** *Pediatric Endocrinology,* Medical Examination Publishing Co., Garden City, Chap. 2, 1978.

36. **Jenner MR, Kelch RP, Kaplan SL, Grumbach MM,** Hormonal changes in puberty. IV. Plasma Estradiol, LH and FSH in prepubertal children, pubertal females, and in precocious puberty, premature thelarche, hypogonadism and in a child with a feminizing ovarian tumor. J Clin Endocrinol Metab 34:521, 1972.

37. **Raiti S, Johanson A, Light C, Migeon CJ, Blizzard RM,** Measurement of immunologically reactive follicle stimulating hormone in serum of normal male children and adults. Metabolism 18:234, 1969.

38. **Johanson J, Guyda H, Light C, Migeon CJ, Blizzard RM,** Serum luteinizing hormone by radioimmunoassay in normal children. J Pediatr 74:416, 1969.

39. **Frasier SD, Gafford F, Horton R,** Plasma androgens and adolescence. J Clin Endocrinol Metab 29:1404, 1969.

40. **Lee PA, Migeon CJ,** Puberty in boys: Correlation of plasma levels of gonadotropins (LH, FSH), androgens (testosterone, androstenedione, dehydroepiandrosterone and its sulfate), estrogens (estrone and estradiol) and progestins (progesterone and 17-hydroxyprogesterone). J Clin Endocrinol Metab 41:556, 1975.

41. **Thumdrup E,** *Precocious Sexual Development,* Charles C Thomas, Springfield, Illinois, 1961.

42. **Seckel HPG,** Precocious sexual development in children. Med Clin N Amer 30:183, 1946.

43. **Jolly H,** *Sexual precocity,* Charles C Thomas, Springfield, Illinois, 1955.

44. **Wilkins L,** *The Diagnosis and Treatment of Endocrine Disorders in Childhood and Adolescence,* Charles C Thomas, Springfield, Illinois, 3rd ed., 1965.

45. **Sigurjonsdottir TT, Hayles AB,** Precocious Puberty: A report of 96 cases. Am J Dis Child 115:309, 1968.

46. **Pomariede R, Finidori J. Czernichow P, Pfister A, Hirsch JF, Rappaport R,** Germinoma in a boy with precocious puberty: evidence of HCG secretion by the tumoral cells. Child Brain 11:298, 1984.

47. **Navarro C, Corretser JM, Sancho A, Rovira J, Morales L,** Paraneoplasic precocious puberty. Report of a new case with hepatoblastoma and review of the literature. Cancer 56:1725, 1985.

48. **Lee PA, Van Dop C, Migeon CJ,** McCune-Albright Syndrome: long-term follow-up. JAMA 256:290, 1986.

49. **Lightner ES, Kelch RP,** Treatment of precocious pseudopuberty associated with ovarian cysts (editorial). Am J Dis Child 138:126, 1984.

50. **Sadeghi-Nejad A, Kaplan SL, Grumbach MM,** The effect of medroxyprogesterone acetate on adrenocortical function in children with precocious puberty. J Pediatr 78:616, 1971.

51. **Richman RA, Underwood LE, French FS, Van Wyk JJ,** Adverse effects of large doses of medroxyprogesterone (MPA) in idiopathic isosexual precocity. J Pediatr 79:963, 1971.

52. **Styne DM, Harris DA, Egli CA, Conte FA, Kaplan SL, Rivier J, Vale W, Grumbach MM,** Treatment of true precocious puberty with a potent luteinizing hormone-releasing factor agonist: Effect on growth, sexual maturation, pelvic sonography, and the hypothalamic-pituitary- gonadal axis. J Clin Endocrinol Metab 61:142, 1985.

53. **Mansfield MJ, Beardsworth DE, Loughlin JS, Crawford JD, Bode HH, Rivier J, Vale W, Kushner DC, Crigler JF, Jr., Crowley WF, Jr.,** Long-term treatment of central precocious puberty with a long-acting analogue of luteinizing hormone-releasing hormone. Effects on somatic growth and skeletal maturation. New Eng J Med 309:1286, 1983.

54. **Pescovitz OH, Comite F, Cassorla F, Dwyer AJ, Poth MA, Sperling MA, Hench K, McNemar A, Skerda M, Loriaux DL, Cutler GB, Jr.,** True precocious puberty complicating congenital adrenal hyperplasia: Treatment with a luteinizing hormone-releasing hormone analog. J Clin Endocrinol Metab 58:857, 1984.

55. **Murran D, Dewhurst J, Grant DB,** Precocious Puberty: A follow-up study. Arch Dis Child 59:77, 1984.

56. **Reindollar RH, Byrd JR, McDonough PG,** Delayed sexual development: A study of 252 patients, Am J Obstet Gynecol 140:371, 1981.

57. **Stanhope R, Pringle PJ, Brook CGD, Adams J, Jacobs HS,** Induction of puberty by pulsatile gonadotropin releasing hormone, Lancet ii:552, 1987.

58. **Bayley N, Pinneau SR,** Tables for predicting adult height from skeletal age: Revised for use with the Greulich-Pyle hand standards, J Pediatrics 40:423, 1952.

59. **Pintor C, Loche S, Corda R, Cella SG, Puggioni R, Locatelli V, Muller EE,** Clonidine treatment for short stature, Lancet i:1226, 1987.

60. **Schoen EJ, Solomon IL, Warner D, Wingerd J,** Estrogen treatment of tall girls, Am J Dis Child 125:71, 1973.

61. **Norman H, Wettenhall B, Cahill C, Roche AF,** Tall girls: A survey of 15 years of management and treatment, Adolesc Med 86:602, 1975.

Bayley-Pinneau Table for Average Girls
(J. Pediat. 40:423, 1952)

To predict height, find vertical column corresponding to skeletal age and horizontal row for the present height. The number at the intersection is the predicted height in inches. If figures do not fall at the whole inch or 6-month intervals, the predicted height must be extrapolated.

Skeletal age		6/0	6/6	7/0	7/6	8/0	8/6	9/0	9/6	10/0	10/6	11/0	11/6	12/0
Height	37	51.4												
in inches	38	52.8	51.5											
	39	54.2	52.8	51.5										
	40	55.6	54.2	52.8	51.8									
	41	56.9	55.6	54.2	53.1	51.9								
	42	58.3	56.9	55.5	54.4	53.2	51.9							
	43	59.7	58.3	56.8	55.7	54.4	53.1	52.0						
	44	61.1	59.6	58.1	57.0	55.7	54.3	53.2	52.1	51.0				
	45	62.5	61.0	59.4	58.3	57.0	55.6	54.4	53.3	52.2				
	46	63.9	62.3	60.8	59.6	58.2	56.8	55.6	54.5	53.4	52.0			
	47	65.8	63.7	62.1	60.9	59.5	58.0	56.8	55.7	54.5	53.2	51.9	51.4	51.0
	48	66.7	65.0	63.4	62.2	60.8	59.3	58.0	56.9	55.7	54.3	53.0	52.5	52.1
	49	68.1	66.4	64.7	63.5	62.0	60.5	59.3	58.1	56.8	55.4	54.1	53.6	53.1
	50	69.4	67.8	66.1	64.8	63.3	61.7	60.5	59.2	58.0	56.6	55.2	54.7	54.2
	51	70.8	69.1	67.4	66.1	64.6	63.0	61.7	60.4	59.2	57.7	56.3	55.8	55.3
	52	72.2	70.5	68.7	67.4	65.8	64.2	62.9	61.6	60.3	58.8	57.4	56.9	56.4
	53	73.6	71.8	70.0	68.7	67.1	65.4	64.1	62.8	61.5	60.0	58.5	58.0	57.5
	54		73.2	71.3	69.9	68.4	66.7	65.3	64.0	62.6	61.1	59.6	59.1	58.6
	55		74.5	72.7	71.2	69.6	67.9	66.5	65.2	63.8	62.2	60.7	60.2	59.7
	56			74.0	72.5	70.9	69.1	67.7	66.4	65.0	63.3	61.8	61.3	60.7
	57				73.8	72.2	70.4	68.9	67.5	66.1	64.5	62.9	62.4	61.8
	58					73.4	71.6	70.1	68.7	67.3	65.6	64.0	63.5	62.9
	59					74.7	72.8	71.3	69.9	68.4	66.7	65.1	64.6	64.0
	60						74.1	72.6	71.1	69.6	67.9	66.2	65.6	65.1
	61							73.8	72.3	70.8	69.0	67.3	66.7	66.2
	62								73.5	71.9	70.1	68.4	67.8	67.2
	63								74.6	73.1	71.3	69.5	68.9	68.3
	64									74.2	72.4	70.6	70.0	69.4
	65										73.5	71.7	71.1	70.5
	66										74.7	72.9	72.2	71.6
	67											74.0	73.3	72.7
	68												74.4	73.8
	69													74.8
	70													
	71													
	72													
	73													
	74													

438

12/6	13/0	13/6	14/0	14/6	15/0	15/6	16/0	16/6	17/0	17/6	18/0	
												37
												38
												39
												40
												41
												42
												43
												44
												45
												46
												47
51.0												48
52.1	51.1											49
53.1	52.2	51.3	51.0									50
54.2	53.2	52.4	52.0	51.7	51.5	51.4	51.2	51.2	51.1	51.0	51.0	51
55.3	54.3	53.4	53.1	52.7	52.5	52.4	52.2	52.2	52.1	52.0	52.0	52
56.3	55.3	54.4	54.1	53.8	53.5	53.4	53.2	53.2	53.1	53.0	53.0	53
57.4	56.4	55.4	55.1	54.8	54.5	54.4	54.2	54.2	54.1	54.0	54.0	54
58.4	57.4	56.5	56.1	55.8	55.6	55.4	55.2	55.2	55.1	55.0	55.0	55
59.5	58.5	57.5	57.1	56.8	56.6	56.4	56.2	56.2	56.1	56.0	56.0	56
60.6	59.5	58.5	58.2	57.8	57.6	57.4	57.2	57.2	57.1	57.0	57.0	57
61.6	60.5	59.5	59.2	58.8	58.6	58.4	58.2	58.2	58.1	58.0	58.0	58
62.7	61.6	60.6	60.2	59.8	59.6	59.4	59.2	59.2	59.1	59.0	59.0	59
63.8	62.6	61.6	61.2	60.9	60.6	60.4	60.2	60.2	60.1	60.0	60.0	60
64.8	63.7	62.6	62.2	61.9	61.6	61.4	61.2	61.2	61.1	61.0	61.0	61
65.9	64.7	63.7	63.3	62.9	62.6	62.4	62.2	62.2	62.1	62.0	62.0	62
67.0	65.8	64.7	64.3	63.9	63.6	63.4	63.3	63.2	63.1	63.0	63.0	63
68.0	66.8	65.7	65.3	64.9	64.6	64.4	64.3	64.2	64.1	64.0	64.0	64
69.1	67.8	66.7	66.3	65.9	65.7	65.5	65.3	65.2	65.1	65.0	65.0	65
70.1	68.9	67.8	67.3	66.9	66.7	66.5	66.3	66.2	66.1	66.0	66.0	66
71.2	69.9	68.8	68.4	68.0	67.7	67.5	67.3	67.2	67.1	67.0	67.0	67
72.3	71.0	69.8	69.4	69.0	68.7	68.5	68.3	68.2	68.1	68.0	68.0	68
73.3	72.0	70.8	70.4	70.0	69.7	69.5	69.3	69.2	69.1	69.0	69.0	69
74.4	73.1	71.9	71.4	71.0	70.7	70.5	70.3	70.2	70.1	70.0	70.0	70
	74.1	72.9	72.4	72.0	71.7	71.5	71.3	71.2	71.1	71.0	71.0	71
		73.9	73.5	73.0	72.7	72.5	72.3	72.2	72.1	72.0	72.0	72
		74.9	74.5	74.0	73.7	73.5	73.3	73.2	73.1	73.0	73.0	73
					74.7	74.5	74.3	74.2	74.1	74.0	74.0	74

Bayley-Pinneau Table for Accelerated Girls

To predict height, find vertical column corresponding to skeletal age and horizontal row for the present height. The number at the intersection is the predicted height in inches. If figures do not fall at the whole inch or 6-month intervals, the predicted height must be extrapolated.

Skeletal age		7/0	7/6	8/0	8/6	9/0	9/6	10/0	10/6	11/0	11/6	12/0
Height	37	52.0										
in inches	38	53.4	51.9									
	39	54.8	53.3	52.0								
	40	56.2	54.6	53.3	51.9							
	41	57.6	56.0	54.7	53.2	51.9						
	42	59.0	57.4	56.0	54.5	53.2	51.9					
	43	60.4	58.7	57.3	55.8	54.4	53.2	51.9				
	44	61.8	60.1	58.7	57.1	55.7	54.4	53.1	51.4			
	45	63.2	61.5	60.0	58.4	57.0	55.6	54.3	52.6	54.0		
	46	64.6	62.8	61.3	59.7	58.2	56.9	55.6	53.7	52.1	51.6	51.1
	47	66.0	64.2	62.7	61.0	59.5	58.1	56.8	54.9	53.2	52.7	52.2
	48	67.4	65.6	64.0	62.3	60.8	59.3	58.0	56.1	54.4	53.9	53.3
	49	68.8	66.9	65.3	63.6	62.0	60.6	59.2	57.2	55.5	55.0	54.4
	50	70.2	68.3	66.7	64.9	63.3	61.8	60.4	58.4	56.6	56.1	55.5
	51	71.6	69.7	68.0	66.1	64.6	63.0	61.6	59.6	57.8	57.2	56.6
	52	73.0	71.0	69.3	67.4	65.8	64.3	62.8	60.7	58.9	58.4	57.7
	53	74.4	72.4	70.7	68.7	67.1	65.5	64.0	61.9	60.0	59.5	58.8
	54		73.8	72.0	70.0	68.4	66.7	65.2	63.1	61.2	60.6	59.9
	55			73.3	71.3	69.6	68.0	66.4	64.3	62.3	61.7	61.0
	56			74.7	72.6	70.9	69.2	67.6	65.4	63.4	62.8	62.2
	57				73.9	72.2	70.5	68.8	66.6	64.6	64.0	63.3
	58					73.4	71.7	70.0	67.8	65.7	65.1	64.4
	59					74.7	72.9	71.3	68.9	66.8	66.2	65.5
	60						74.2	72.5	70.1	68.0	67.3	66.6
	61							73.7	71.3	69.1	68.5	67.7
	62							74.9	72.4	70.2	69.6	68.8
	63								73.6	71.3	70.7	69.9
	64								74.8	72.5	71.8	71.0
	65									73.6	72.9	72.1
	66									74.7	74.1	73.3
	67											74.4
	68											
	69											
	70											
	71											
	72											
	73											
	74											

12/6	13/0	13/6	14/0	14/6	15/0	15/6	16/0	16/6	17/0	17/6	
											37
											38
											39
											40
											41
											42
											43
											44
											45
											46
											47
51.9											48
53.0	51.9	50.9									49
54.1	52.9	51.9	51.4	51.0							50
55.2	54.0	53.0	52.5	52.0	51.7	51.5	51.4	51.3	51.1	51.0	51
56.3	55.0	54.0	53.5	53.1	52.7	52.5	52.4	52.3	52.1	52.0	52
57.4	56.1	55.0	54.5	54.1	53.8	53.5	53.4	53.3	53.1	53.0	53
58.4	57.1	56.1	55.6	55.1	54.8	54.5	54.4	54.3	54.1	54.0	54
59.5	58.2	57.1	56.6	56.1	55.8	55.5	55.4	55.3	55.1	55.0	55
60.6	59.3	58.2	57.6	57.1	56.8	56.5	56.4	56.3	56.1	56.0	56
61.7	60.3	59.2	58.6	58.2	57.8	57.6	57.4	57.3	57.1	57.0	57
62.8	61.4	60.2	59.7	59.2	58.8	58.6	58.4	58.3	58.1	58.0	58
63.9	62.4	61.3	60.7	60.2	59.8	59.6	59.4	59.3	59.1	59.0	59
64.9	63.5	62.3	61.7	61.2	60.9	60.6	60.4	60.3	60.1	60.0	60
66.0	64.6	63.3	62.8	62.2	61.9	61.6	61.4	61.3	61.1	61.0	61
67.1	65.6	64.4	63.8	63.3	62.9	62.6	62.4	62.3	62.1	62.0	62
68.2	66.7	65.4	64.8	64.3	63.9	63.6	63.4	63.3	63.1	63.0	63
69.3	67.7	66.5	65.8	65.3	64.9	64.6	64.4	64.3	64.1	64.0	64
70.3	68.8	67.5	66.9	66.3	65.9	65.7	65.5	65.3	65.1	65.0	65
71.4	69.8	68.5	67.9	67.3	66.9	66.7	66.5	66.3	66.1	66.0	66
72.5	70.9	69.6	68.9	68.4	68.0	67.7	67.5	67.3	67.1	67.0	67
73.6	72.0	70.6	70.0	69.4	69.0	68.7	68.5	68.3	68.1	68.0	68
74.7	73.0	71.7	71.0	70.4	70.0	69.7	69.5	69.3	69.1	69.0	69
	74.1	72.7	72.0	71.4	71.0	70.7	70.5	70.3	70.1	70.0	70
		73.7	73.0	72.4	72.0	71.7	71.5	71.4	71.1	71.0	71
		74.8	74.1	73.5	73.0	72.7	72.5	72.4	72.1	72.0	72
				74.5	74.0	73.7	73.5	73.4	73.1	73.0	73
						74.4	74.5	74.4	74.1	74.0	74

Bayley-Pinneau Table for Retarded Girls

To predict height, find vertical column corresponding to skeletal age and horizontal row for the present height. The number at the intersection is the predicted height in inches. If figures do not fall at the whole inch or 6-month intervals, the predicted height must be extrapolated.

Skeletal age		6/0	6/6	7/0	7/6	8/0	8/6	9/0	9/6	10/0	10/6	11/0	11/6
Height	38	51.8											
in inches	39	53.2	51.9										
	40	54.6	53.3	51.9									
	41	55.9	54.6	53.2	52.0								
	42	57.3	55.9	54.5	53.3	52.2	51.0						
	43	58.7	57.3	55.8	54.6	53.5	52.2	51.1					
	44	60.0	58.6	57.1	55.8	54.7	53.5	52.3	51.3				
	45	61.4	59.9	58.4	57.1	56.0	54.7	53.5	52.4	51.5			
	46	62.8	61.3	59.7	58.4	57.2	55.9	54.7	53.6	52.6	51.3		
	47	64.1	62.6	61.0	59.6	58.5	57.1	55.9	54.8	53.8	52.5	51.2	
	48	65.5	63.9	62.3	60.9	59.7	58.3	57.1	55.9	54.9	63.6	52.3	51.8
	49	66.9	65.2	63.6	62.2	60.9	59.5	58.3	57.1	56.1	54.7	53.4	52.9
	50	68.2	66.6	64.9	63.5	62.2	60.8	59.5	58.3	57.2	55.8	54.5	54.0
	51	69.6	67.9	66.2	64.7	63.4	62.0	60.6	59.4	58.4	56.9	55.6	55.1
	52	70.9	69.2	67.5	66.0	64.7	63.2	61.8	60.6	59.5	58.0	56.6	56.2
	53	72.3	70.6	68.8	67.3	65.9	64.4	63.0	61.8	60.6	59.2	57.7	57.2
	54	73.7	71.9	70.1	68.5	67.2	65.6	64.2	62.9	61.8	60.3	58.8	58.3
	55		73.2	71.4	69.8	68.4	66.8	65.4	64.1	62.9	61.4	59.9	59.4
	56		74.6	72.7	71.1	69.7	68.0	66.6	65.3	64.1	62.5	61.0	60.5
	57			74.0	72.3	70.9	69.3	67.8	66.4	65.2	63.6	62.1	61.6
	58				73.6	72.1	70.5	69.0	67.6	66.4	64.7	63.2	62.6
	59				74.9	73.4	71.7	70.2	68.8	67.5	65.8	64.3	63.7
	60					74.6	72.9	71.3	69.9	68.7	67.0	65.4	64.8
	61						74.1	72.5	71.1	69.8	68.1	66.4	65.9
	62							73.7	72.3	70.9	69.2	67.5	67.0
	63							74.7	73.4	72.1	70.3	68.6	68.0
	64								74.6	73.2	71.4	69.7	69.1
	65									74.4	72.5	70.8	70.2
	66										73.7	71.9	71.3
	67										74.8	73.0	72.4
	68											74.1	73.4
	69												74.5
	70												
	71												
	72												
	73												
	74												

12/0	12/6	13/0	13/6	14/0	14/6	15/0	15/6	16/0	16/6	17/0	
											40
											41
											42
											43
											44
											45
											46
											47
51.5											48
52.6	51.6										49
53.6	52.7	51.9	51.2								50
54.7	53.7	52.9	52.2	51.9	51.6	51.3	51.2	51.1	51.1	51.0	51
55.8	54.8	53.9	53.2	52.9	52.6	52.3	52.2	52.1	52.1	52.0	52
56.9	55.8	55.0	54.2	53.9	53.6	53.3	53.2	53.1	53.1	53.0	53
57.9	56.9	56.0	55.3	54.9	54.6	54.3	54.2	54.1	54.1	54.0	54
59.0	58.0	57.1	56.3	56.0	55.6	55.3	55.2	55.1	55.1	55.0	55
60.1	59.0	58.1	57.3	57.0	56.6	56.3	56.2	56.1	56.1	56.0	56
61.2	60.1	59.1	58.3	58.0	57.6	57.3	57.2	57.1	57.1	57.0	57
62.2	61.1	60.2	59.4	59.0	58.6	58.3	58.2	58.1	58.1	58.0	58
63.3	62.2	61.2	60.4	60.0	59.7	59.4	59.2	59.1	59.1	59.0	59
64.4	63.2	62.2	61.4	61.0	60.7	60.4	60.2	60.1	60.1	60.0	60
65.5	64.3	63.3	62.4	62.1	61.7	61.4	61.2	61.1	61.1	61.0	61
66.5	65.3	64.3	63.5	63.1	62.7	62.4	62.2	62.1	62.1	62.0	62
67.6	66.4	65.3	64.5	64.1	63.7	63.4	63.3	63.1	63.1	63.0	63
68.7	67.4	66.4	65.5	65.1	64.7	64.4	64.3	64.1	64.1	64.0	64
69.7	68.5	67.4	66.5	66.1	65.7	65.4	65.3	65.1	65.1	65.0	65
70.8	69.5	68.5	67.6	67.1	66.7	66.4	66.3	66.1	66.1	66.0	66
71.9	70.6	69.5	68.6	68.2	67.7	67.4	67.3	67.1	67.1	67.0	67
73.0	71.7	70.5	69.6	69.2	68.8	68.4	68.3	68.1	68.1	68.0	68
74.0	72.7	71.6	70.6	70.2	69.8	69.4	69.3	69.1	69.1	69.0	69
	73.8	72.6	71.6	71.2	70.8	70.4	70.3	70.1	70.1	70.0	70
	74.8	73.6	72.7	72.2	71.8	71.4	71.3	71.1	71.1	71.0	71
		74.7	73.7	73.3	72.8	72.4	72.3	72.1	72.1	72.0	72
			74.7	74.3	73.8	73.4	73.3	73.1	73.1	73.0	73
					74.8	74.4	74.3	74.1	74.1	74.0	74

14 Obesity

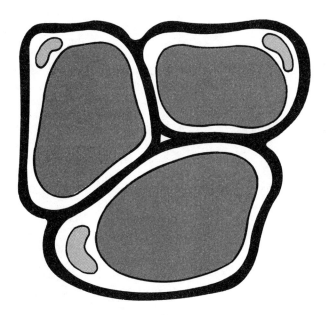

One of the least rewarding experiences in clinical medicine is treating obesity. Because from 25 to 45% of American adults over 30 years old are more than 20% overweight, the unrewarding fight against obesity is all too common, not only with our patients, but also with ourselves. Unfortunately, for over 100 years the incidence of obesity has been increasing in the United States, a reflection of an increasingly sedentary life in an affluent society.(1)

The lack of success in treating obesity is not due to an unawareness of the implications of obesity; there is a clear-cut relationship between mortality and weight. The death rate from diabetes mellitus, for example, is approximately 4 times higher among obese diabetics than among those who control their weight. Also higher among obese individuals is the incidence of gallbladder disease, cardiovascular disease, renal disease, and cirrhosis of the liver. The death rate from appendicitis is double, presumably from anesthetic and surgical complications. Even the rate of accidents is higher, perhaps because fat people are awkward or because their view of the ground or floor is obstructed. When the personal and social problems encountered by obese persons are also considered, it is no wonder that a physician without a weight problem cannot comprehend why fat individuals remain overweight.

The frequency with which a practitioner encounters the obese patient whose weight does not decrease despite a sworn adherence to a limited-calorie diet makes one question if there is something physiologically different about this patient. Is the problem due to lack of discipline and cheating on a diet, or does it also involve a pathophysiologic factor? Is the physiology of obese people unusual, or are they simply gluttons?

As a basis for a more understanding approach to obesity this chapter reviews the physiology of adipose tissue, discusses differences between normal and obese people, and comments on treatment.

Definition of Obesity

There is a difference between obesity and overweight. (2) Obesity is an excess of body fat. Overweight is a body weight in excess of some standard or ideal weight. The ideal weight for any adult is believed to correspond to his or her ideal weight from age 20 to 30. The following formulas give ideal weight in pounds:

Women: $100 + (4 \times (\text{height in inches minus } 60))$

Men: $120 + (4 \times (\text{height in inches minus } 60))$

At a weight close to ideal weight, individuals may be overweight, but not over fat. This is especially true of individuals engaged in regular exercise. An estimate of body fat, therefore, rather than a measurement of height and weight, is more significant.

The most accurate method of determining body fat is to determine the density of the body by underwater measurement. It certainly is not practical to measure density by submerging individuals in water in our offices, therefore skinfold measurements with calipers have become popular as an index of body fat. The skinfold measurement is also not necessary for clinical practice. It is far simpler to utilize the body mass index nomogram, a method which has been found to correspond closely to densitometry measurements.(3)

The body mass index is the ratio of weight divided by the height squared (in metric units). To read the central scale, align a straight edge between height and body weight. A body mass index of about 30 is roughly equivalent to 30% excess body weight, the point at which excess mortality begins. Above 40, the risk from obesity itself is comparable to that associated with major health problems such as hypertension and heavy smoking.

A person is obese when the amount of adipose tissue is sufficiently high (20% or more over ideal weight) to detrimentally alter biochemical and physiologic functions and to shorten life expectancy. Obesity is associated with four major risk factors for atherosclerosis: hypertension, diabetes, hypercholesterolemia, and hypertriglyceridemia. Overweight individuals have a higher prevalence of hypertension at every age, and the risk of developing hypertension is related to the amount of weight gain after age 25.(4) The two in combination (hypertension and obesity) increase the risk of heart disease, cerebrovascular disease, and death.

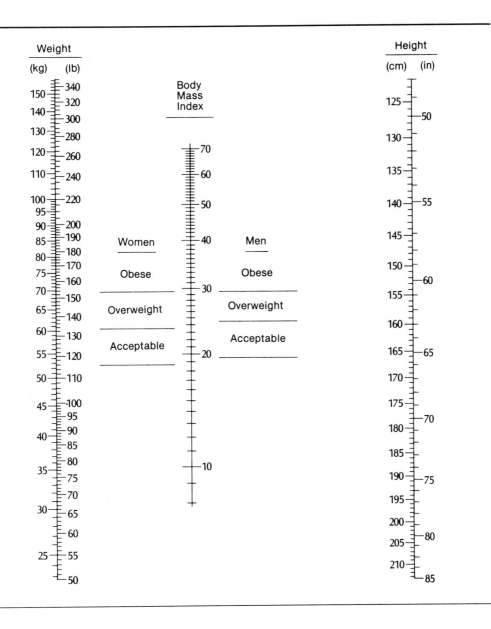

Unfortunately the basal metabolic rate decreases with age. After age 18, the resting metabolic rate declines about 2% per decade. A 30-year-old individual will inevitably gain weight if there is no change in caloric intake or exercise level over the years. The middle aged spread is both a biological and a psychosociological phenomenon. It is therefore important for both our patients and ourselves to understand adipose tissue and the problem of obesity.

Physiology of Adipose Tissue

Adipose tissue serves three general functions:

1. Adipose tissue is a storehouse of energy.

2. Fat serves as a cushion from trauma.

3. Adipose tissue plays a role in the regulation of body heat.

Each cell of adipose tissue may be regarded as a package of triglyceride, the most concentrated form of stored energy. There are 8 calories per gram of triglyceride as opposed to 1 calorie per gram of glycogen. The total store of tissue and fluid carbohydrate in adults (about 300 calories) is inadequate to meet between-meal demands. The storage of energy in fat tissue allows us to do other things beside eating.

The mechanism for mobilizing energy from fat involves various enzymes and neurohormonal agents. Following ingestion of fat and its breakdown by gastric and pancreatic lipases, absorption of long-chain triglycerides and free fatty acids takes place in the small bowel. Chylomicrons (microscopic particles of fat) transferred through lymph channels into the systemic venous circulation are normally removed by hepatic parenchymal cells where a new lipoprotein is released into the circulation. When this lipoprotein is exposed to adipose tissue, lipolysis takes place through the action of lipoprotein lipase, an enzyme derived from the fat cells themselves. The fatty acids that are released then enter the fat cells where they are reesterified with glycerophosphate into triglycerides.

Glucose serves three important functions:

1. Glucose supplies carbon atoms in the form of acetyl coenzyme A (acetyl CoA).

2. Glucose provides hydrogen for reductive steps.

3. Glucose is the main source of glycerophosphate.

The production and availability of glycerophosphate (required for reesterification of fatty acids and their storage as triglycerides) are considered rate-limiting in lipogenesis, and this process depends on the presence of glucose.

After esterification, subsequent lipolysis results in the release of fatty acids and glycerol. In the cycle of lipolysis and reesterification, energy is freed as heat. A low variable level of lipolysis takes place continuously; its basic function may be to provide body heat.

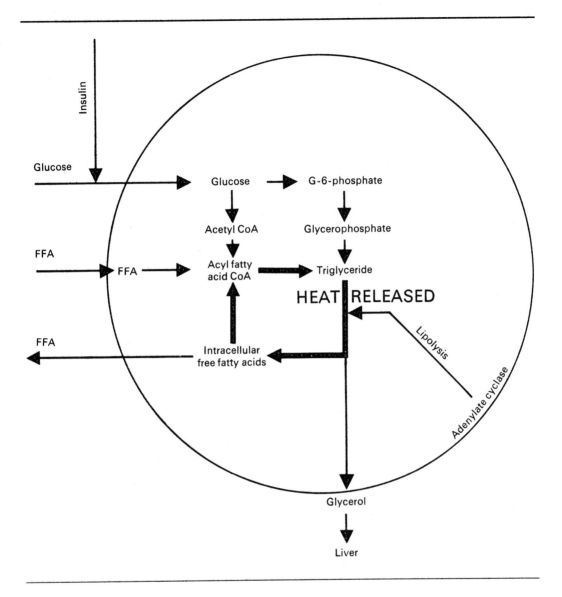

The chief metabolic products produced from fat are the circulating free fatty acids. Their availability is controlled by adipose tissue cells. When carbohydrate is in short supply, a flood of free fatty acids can be released. The free fatty acids in the peripheral circulation are almost wholly derived from endogenous triglyceride that undergoes rapid hydrolysis to yield free fatty acid and glycerol. The glycerol is returned to the liver for resynthesis of glycogen.

Free fatty acid release from adipose tissue is stimulated by physical exercise, fasting, exposure to cold, nervous tension, and anxiety. The release of fatty acids by lipolysis varies from one anatomic site to another. Omental, mesenteric, and subcutaneous fat are more labile and easily mobilized than fat from other sources. Areas from which energy is not easily mobilized are retrobulbar and perirenal fat where the tissue serves a structural function. Adipose tissue lipase is sensitive to stimulation by both epinephrine and norepinephrine. Other hormones that activate lipase are ACTH, thyroid stimulating hormone (TSH), growth hormone, thyroxine (T_4), 3,5,3'-

449

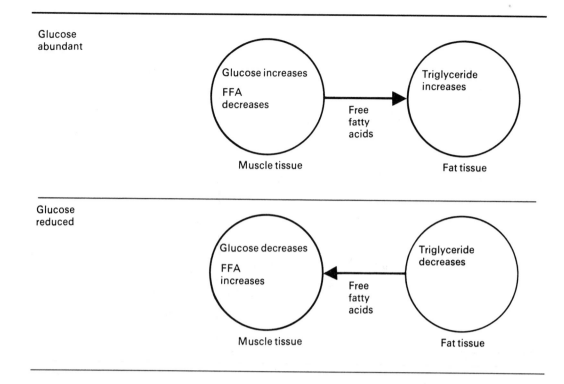

Glucose abundant

Glucose increases

FFA decreases

Muscle tissue

Free fatty acids

Triglyceride increases

Fat tissue

Glucose reduced

Glucose decreases

FFA increases

Muscle tissue

Free fatty acids

Triglyceride decreases

Fat tissue

triiodothyronine (T_3), cortisol, glucagon, as well as vasopressin and human placental lactogen (HPL).

Lipase enzyme activity is inhibited by insulin, which appears to be alone as the major physiologic antagonist to the array of stimulating agents. When both glucose and insulin are abundant, transport of glucose into fat cells is high, and glycerophosphate production increases to esterify fatty acids.

The carbohydrate and fat composition of the fuel supply is constantly changing, depending upon stresses and demands. Since the central nervous system and some other tissues can utilize only glucose for energy, a homeostatic mechanism for conserving carbohydrate is essential. When glucose is abundant and easily available, it is utilized in adipose tissue for producing glycerophosphate to immobilize fatty acids as triglycerides. The circulating level of free fatty acids in muscle will, therefore, be low, and glucose will be used by all of the tissues.

When carbohydrate is scarce, the amount of glucose reaching the fat cells declines and glycerophosphate production is reduced. The fat cell releases fatty acids, and their circulating levels rise to a point where glycolysis is inhibited. Thus, carbohydrate is spared in those tissues capable of using lipid substrates. If the rise of fatty acids is great enough, the liver is flooded with acetyl CoA. This is converted into ketone bodies, and clinical ketosis results.

In the simplest terms, when a person eats, glucose is available, insulin is secreted, and fat is stored. In starvation, the glucose level falls, insulin secretion decreases, and fat is mobilized.

If only single large meals are consumed, the body learns to convert carbohydrate to fat very quickly. Epidemiologic studies on school children demonstrate a positive correlation between fewer meals and a greater tendency toward obesity.(5) The person who does not eat all day and then stocks up at night is perhaps doing the worst possible thing.

Clinical Obesity

Obesity and the Brain

The hypothalamic location of the appetite center was established in 1940 by the demonstration that bilateral lesions of the ventromedial nucleus produce experimental obesity in rats. Such lesions lead to hyperphagia and decreased physical activity. Interestingly, this pattern is similar to that seen in human beings—the pressure to eat is reinforced by the desire to be physically inactive. The ventromedial nucleus was thought to represent an integrating center for appetite and hunger information. Destruction of the ventromedial nucleus was believed to result in a loss of satiety signals, leading to hyperphagia.

Overeating and obesity, however, may not be due to ventromedial nucleus damage but rather to destruction of the nearby ventral noradrenergic bundle.(6) Hypothalamic noradrenergic terminals are derived from long fibers ascending from hindbrain cell bodies. Lesions of the ventromedial nucleus produced by radiofrequency current fail to cause obesity. These lesions lead to overeating and obesity only when they extend beyond the ventromedial nucleus. Selective destruction of the ventral noradrenergic bundle results in hyperphagia. The lesions that produce hyperphagia also reduce the potency of amphetamine as an appetite suppressant. This noradrenergic bundle may function as a satiety system and be the site of amphetamine action.

Signals arriving at these centers originate in peripheral tissues. Opiates, substance P, and cholecystokinin play a role in mediating taste, the gatekeeper for feeding, while peptides released from the stomach and intestine act as satiety signals.(7)

There may be two kinds of obesity: obesity stemming from a CNS regulatory defect, or obesity due to a metabolic problem occurring despite a normal central mechanism.

Psychologic Factors

Obese and lean people respond differently to their environments.(8) Obese people appear to regulate their desire for food through external signals. Lean people, on the other hand, regulate their intake by endogenous signals of hunger and satiety.

Fear does not inhibit gastrointestinal activity and dull the appetite in obese persons as it does in others. Fat people eat because it is mealtime, and food looks, smells, and tastes good. They also eat because other people are eating, but not necessarily because they themselves are hungry.

Obese people are also less physically active than are people of normal weight. The obese person will drive a car around the block repeatedly until a parking space is available, rather than walk a few

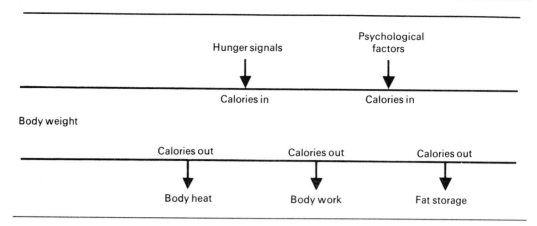

Body weight

blocks. Time-lapse photography studies show that obese people when in a swimming pool spend most of their time floating; lean people move around actively.(9) An obese baby is more willing than is a normal baby to take formula after it has been sweetened, but will take less formula, even though it is sweetened, if the work of eating is increased by a nipple with a smaller hole.

There may be two classes of obesity: one class may include those individuals who clearly eat too much. The other class would be composed of individuals who eat relatively normal diets, but who are extremely inactive.

Fat Cells

Fat cells develop from connective tissue early in fetal life. An important question is whether new fat cells are produced by metaplasia in the adult, or whether an individual achieves a total complement during a certain period of life. In other words is excess fat stored by increasing the size of the fat cell, or by increasing the number of cells? The possibility arises that there is an increase in the total number of fat cells, which just wait to be packed full of storage fat. Furthermore, the total number of fat cells may depend upon an infant's nutritional state during the neonatal period, and perhaps in utero as well.

Studies of fat obtained at surgery indicate that the mean fat cell volume is increased threefold in obese people, but an increase in the number of fat cells is seen only in the grossly obese.(10) When patients diet, the fat cells decrease in size, but not in number. Hypercellular obesity may be a more difficult problem to overcome, since an individual may be saddled with a permanent increase in fat cells.

Some researchers think that, at some period in a person's life, a fixed number of fat cells is obtained. Adolescence, infancy, and intrauterine life seem particularly critical.(11,12) This premise is not solidly established, because there is no certain way to identify an empty fat cell, and potential fat cells cannot be recognized. Nevertheless, a hyperplastic type of obesity (more fat cells) may be associated with childhood and have a poor prognosis; a hypertrophic type (enlarged fat cells) that is responsive to dieting may occur in adults. There certainly appears to be a genetic component. The weights of adopted children in Denmark correlated with the body weights of their biologic parents, but not with their adoptive

452

parents.(13) This would suggest that the genetic influence is even more important in childhood than environmental factors. Other work suggests that the familial occurrence of obesity can be attributed in part to a genetically related reduced rate of energy expenditure.(14)

Some argue that each individual has a setpoint, a level regulated by signals between the fat cells and the brain. According to this argument, previously obese people who have successfully lost weight have to maintain themselves in a state of starvation (at least as far as their fat cells are concerned).

Genetics and biochemistry are against many obese people. It is best to recognize that an obese individual who has suffered with the problem lifelong does have a disorder, a disorder which is not well understood.

Endocrine Changes

The most important endocrine change in obesity is elevation of the basal blood insulin level. Increases in body fat change the body's secretion and sensitivity to insulin. There is a decrease in the number of insulin receptor sites at a cellular level, most significantly in fat, liver, and muscle tissue. The key factors which affect insulin resistance are the amount of fat tissue in the body, the caloric intake per day, the amount of carbohydrates in the diet, and the amount of daily exercise. The mechanism for the increased resistance to insulin observed with increasing weight may be down-regulation of insulin receptors brought about by the increase in insulin secretion. The increase in insulin resistance affects the metabolism of carbohydrate, fat and protein. Circulating levels of free fatty acids increase as a result of inadequate insulin suppression of the fat cell.

Genetics plays a greater role in the development of maturity onset diabetes than juvenile onset.(15) It is impossible to predict exactly who eventually will develop diabetes as the tendency is recessive and it will not develop in every generation in a family. But weight is a good tip-off. As weight increases, the frequency of occurrence of diabetes increases. Both gestational diabetes and insulin-dependent diabetes are more common in overweight pregnant patients.

Contrary to popular misconception, hypothyroidism does not cause obesity. Weight gain due to hypothyroidism is confined to the fluid accumulation of myxedema. There is no place, therefore, for thyroid hormone administration in the treatment of obesity when the patient is euthyroid.

Other endocrine changes associated with obesity include decreased growth hormone secretion, and increased cortisol production and metabolic clearance rates (thus, plasma and urinary cortisol are relatively normal). The fasting level of growth hormone is decreased as well as the response to insulin, arginine, starvation, and sleep. There is evidence of decreased pancreatic alpha cell function in obese non-diabetic people.(16) Glucagon secreted by the α cells acutely raises blood glucose levels by stimulating hepatic glycogenolysis and the production of new glucose from amino acids in the liver. Glucagon also activates lipolysis in the fat cell and stimulates insulin secretion. The basal levels of glucagon are equal in obese and nonobese patients, but the glucagon response to alanine is reduced by 50% in the obese group.

453

Obese people are relatively unable to excrete both salt and water, especially while dieting. During dieting this seems to be mediated by increased output of aldosterone and vasopressin. Since water produced from fat outweighs the fat, people on diets often show little initial weight loss. The early use of a diuretic may encourage a patient to persist with dieting.

The basic question is whether metabolic changes observed in obesity represent adaptive responses to a markedly enlarged fat organ, or whether they are representative of a metabolic or hormonal defect. It appears that the former is true. These changes are secondary responses; they are totally reversible with weight loss. Four-year follow-up in a group of patients who did not regain their weight after dieting revealed persistently normal insulin and glucose responses; patients who regained their weight showed further deterioration in these metabolic factors. (17)

Anatomic Obesity

Gynoid obesity refers to fat distribution in the lower body (femoral and gluteal regions), while android obesity refers to upper body distribution. Gynoid fat is more resistant to catecholamines and more sensitive to insulin than abdominal fat; thus extraction and storage of fatty acids easily occur and fat is accumulated more readily in the thighs and buttocks. This fat is associated with minimal fatty acid flux, and therefore, the negative consequences of fatty acid metabolism are less. Gynoid fat is principally stored fat. The clinical meaning of all this is that women with gynoid obesity are less likely than women with android obesity to develop diabetes mellitus and hypertriglyceridemia.

During pregnancy, lipoprotein lipase activity increases in gynoid fat, further promoting fat storage, and explaining the tendency for women to gain thigh and hip weight during pregnancy. Also because this fat is more resistant to mobilization, it is harder to get rid of. This difficulty is related to the adrenergic receptor concentration in the fat cells, the regulation of which remains a mystery.

Android obesity refers to fat located in the abdominal wall and visceral-mesenteric locations. This fat is more sensitive to catecholamines and less sensitive to insulin, and thus more active metabolically. It more easily delivers triglyceride to other tissues to meet energy requirements. This fat distribution is associated with hyperinsulinemia, impaired glucose tolerance, and diabetes mellitus, largely because of decreased hepatic extraction of insulin.(18) It is upper body obesity that is associated with hypertension, and there is reason to believe that the hypertension is directly linked to the hyperinsulinemia. Weight loss in women with lower body obesity is mainly cosmetic, whereas loss of upper body weight is more important for general health.

The waist:hip ratio is a means of estimating the degree of upper to lower body obesity. The ratio is obtained by measuring the body diameters at the levels of the umbilicus and the anterior iliac crests. Interpretation is as follows:

Greater than 1.2 — Android Obesity

From 0.6 to 1.2 — Normal

Less than 0.6 — Gynoid Obesity

Experimental Obesity

In a Vermont study, 28 male volunteers in the state prison underwent induced weight gain to about 20% above their basal weights.(19) Subjective changes were noted that correlate with the behavior of obese patients. The volunteers experienced increased appetite late in the day and decreased desire for physical activity. Once the weight gain was achieved, these normal people required about twice as many calories to maintain their obesity as did spontaneously obese people; there was no difficulty in returning to normal weight. These results suggest that there is something different about obese people.

With the gain in weight, the subjects showed an increase in fasting plasma insulin levels, decreased glucose tolerance, and decreased responses of adipose tissue to insulin stimulation of lipolysis. There was no increase in adipose cell number. These metabolic changes reverted to normal when the gained weight was lost. Hence, the hyperinsulinemia of obesity does not seem to be an etiologic, primary response, but rather a secondary change.

Management of Obesity

Aside from not smoking cigarettes, weight reduction is the most important health measure available for reducing the risk of cardiovascular disease.(20) For most patients, after a routine evaluation to rule out pathology such as diabetes mellitus, the physician is left with the frustrating task of prescribing a diet. But it is not enough to just prescribe a diet or prescribe an anorectic drug. An effective weight loss program requires commitment from both patient and physician.

Physician and patient should agree on the goal of a diet program. While the physician may wish the patient to reach ideal weight, the patient may be satisfied with less. Motivation is improved when the goals meet both personal and medical objectives. It is realistic to lose 4-5 pounds in the first month and 20-30 pounds in 4-5 months.

Despite various fads and diet books, the best diet continues to be a limitation of calories to between 900 and 1200 calories per day, the actual amount depending on what the individual patient will accept and pursue.

Ideal Diet: Carbohydrates — 40-45%
Protein — 20%
Fat — 35-40%

The discouraging aspect is that to lose a pound of fat, the equivalent to a 3500 calorie intake must be expended. Dieting has to be slow and steady to be effective. Successful programs include behavior modification, frequent visits to the physician, and involvement of family members. Behavior modification starts with daily recording of activity and behavior related to food intake, followed by the elimination of inappropriate cues (other than hunger) which lead to eating.

Careful studies (performed in hospitalized subjects on metabolic wards) have indicated that the carbohydrate and fat composition of the diet has no effect on the rate of weight loss.(8) Restriction of calories remains the important principle. Substituting one of the liquid formulas for meals has been successful in many individuals. Unbalanced formulations, however, have the same side effects as seen with total starvation (carbohydrate-deprived regimens). Adequate carbohydrate is necessary for utilization of amino acids. In addition, electrolyte problems have been encountered, and there is an initial diuretic phase that can lead to postural hypotension.

The protein sparing modified fast is a ketogenic regimen providing approximately 800 calories per day. The liquid protein diets have been associated with deaths due to cardiac arrhythmias. The low-calorie diets which utilize protein and carbohydrate supplemented with minerals and vitamins as the sole source of nutrition should be used only for severe obesity and under medical supervision. (21) These diets are still potentially dangerous. The other disadvantage to the semistarvation diet is that short-term success does not guarantee long-term weight maintenance. It is reported that at best only one-fourth to one-third of individuals who lose weight by a semi-starvation ketogenic regimen plus behavior modification therapy will have significant long-term weight reduction.(22) On the other hand, for that one-fourth to one-third, this represents a major accomplishment and is worth doing. Unfortunately, repeated dieting and recidivism have a negative impact. With each episode, the body learns to become more efficient, so that with each diet, weight comes off more slowly and is regained more rapidly.

As an index of the general lack of success with diets, a summary of 10 studies (approximately 1200 patients) revealed that only 30% lose 20 pounds or more, only 4% lose 40 pounds or more. (10) Commercial organizations are no more successful than physician-directed programs or non-profit self-help groups.(23) Thus, it is obvious why gimmicks abound in this area of patient management.

Anorectics are useful as short-term therapy to control hunger, especially at the beginning of a diet and at a plateau or relapse stage. Compared to amphetamines, there is less abuse associated with the amphetamine congeners (diethylpropion, fenfluramine, methamphetamine, and phentermine). Other non-amphetamine anorectics are phendimetrazine and mazindol. All of these agents act on the central nervous system to depress appetite.

Over-the-counter products contain phenylpropanolamine as the active ingredient. This drug is a sympathomimetic derived from ephedrine, and can act synergistically with caffeine to produce amphetamine-like reactions. *It should be noted that phenylpropanolamine taken in combination with bromocriptine or a monoamine oxidase inhibitor can precipitate a hypertensive crisis.*

Surgical treatment and starvation should be reserved for patients who are morbidly obese. Both methods involve many potential problems and require close monitoring.

Controlled studies have not demonstrated the effectiveness of thyroid preparations or human chorionic gonadotropin (HCG).(24) Indeed, adding thyroid hormone increases the loss of lean body mass rather than fat tissue. It is clear that adjunctive drug measures are not successful unless the patient is also motivated either to limit caloric intake or to increase the exercise level in what will be a lifelong battle.

A regular pattern of physical exercise reduces the risk of myocardial infarction in all people.(25) Both weight loss and increased physical activity, through an unknown mechanism, lower the level of low-density lipoprotein (LDL), and increase the level of high-density lipoprotein (HDL).(26) A further benefit of strenuous or prolonged exercise is an inhibition of appetite which lasts many hours, and which is associated with an increase in the resting metabolic rate for 24-48 hours. There is one study, however, that indicates a rebound increase in appetite 1-2 days after exercise.(27) The optimal program includes, therefore, a *daily* period of exercise.

Unfortunately one cannot burn up significant calories quickly; it takes 18 minutes of running to compensate for the average hamburger.(28)

Activity	Calories per Hour
Sleeping	90
Office work	240
Walking	240
Golf	300
Housework	300
Bicycling	360
Swimming	360
Tennis	480
Bowling	510
Running slowly	750 (ca. 120/mile)
Cross country skiing	840
Running fast	960 (ca. 160/mile)

Most frustrating is the problem of some patients who limit caloric intake, yet do not lose weight. In fact, as the weights of certain patients increase, the number of calories required to remain in equilibrium decreases, probably due to a combination of reduced activity and a change in metabolism. The Vermont study demonstrated that the normal person with induced obesity requires 2700 calories to remain in equilibrium; spontaneously obese patients require only about 1300 calories.(19) Others argue that virtually everyone can lose weight on a diet of 1000 calories per day in that the maintenance requirement for a sedentary adult is about 1.5 times the resting metabolic rate (about 1000-1500 calories per day).(29) The physician must be careful to avoid a condemning or punitive attitude, and understand that it is possible to significantly restrict caloric intake and not lose weight.

Patients appear doomed to frustration and despair unless the physician can motivate them to increase physical activity. In all individuals dieting is more effective when combined with physical exercise, but this is especially true in chronically obese patients. In other words, the life-style of an obese person must be changed to overcome the desire to be inactive (walk instead of riding). Only by significantly increasing caloric expenditure will the input-output equilibrium be disturbed.

The obese person feels trapped. Obesity leads to characteristic behavioral manifestations, including passive personality, frequent periods of depression, decreased self-respect, and a sense of being hopelessly overwhelmed by problems. But just as the endocrine and metabolic changes seem to be secondary to obesity, many of the psychosocial attributes surrounding obesity may also be secondary.(30)

Motivation to change and emotional support during the change are important. They can be provided by friends, relatives, physicians, or self-help organizations. If the vicious circle of failed diets, resignation to fate, guilt, and shame can be broken, a more effective, happier person will emerge.

References

1. **Van Itallie JB, Hirsch J,** Appraisal of excess calories as a factor in causation of disease, Am J Clin Nutr 32:2648, 1979.

2. **Powers PS,** *Obesity, the Regulation of Weight,* Williams & Wilkins, Baltimore, 1980.

3. **Thomas AE, McKay DA, Cutlip MB,** A nomograph method for assessing body weight, Am J Clin Nutr 29:302, 1976.

4. **Stamler R, Stamler J, Riedlinger WF, Algera G, Roberts RH,** Weight and blood pressure: findings in hypertension screening of 1 million Americans, JAMA 240:1607, 1978.

5. **Fabry P, Hejda S, Cerny K,** Effects of meal frequency in school children. Changes in weight-height proportion and skinfold thickness, Am J Clin Nutr 18:358, 1966.

6. **Gold RM,** Hypothalamic obesity: the myth of the ventromedial nucleus, Science 182:488, 1973.

7. **Morley JE,** Neuropeptide regulation of appetite and weight, Endocrin Rev 8:256, 1987.

8. **Gordon ES,** Metabolic aspects of obesity, Adv Metab Disord 4:229, 1970.

9. **Mayer J,** Inactivity as a major factor in adolescent obesity, Ann NY Acad Sci 131:502, 1965.

10. **Bray GA, Davidson MB, Drenick EJ,** Obesity: a serious symptom, Ann Intern med 77:787, 1972.

11. **Ravelli G, Stein ZA, Susser MW,** Obesity in young men after famine exposure in utero and early infancy, New Eng J Med 295:349, 1976.

12. **Charney E, Goodman HC, McBride M, Lyon B, Pratt R,** Childhood antecedents of adult obesity, New Eng J Med 295:6, 1976.

13. **Stunkard AJ, Sorensen TIA, Teasdale TW, Chakraborty R, Schull WJ, Schulsinger F,** An adoptive study of human obesity, New Eng J Med 314:193, 1986.

14. **Ravussin E, Lillioja S, Knowler WC, Christin L, Freymond D, Abbott WGH, BoyceV, Howard BV, Bogardus C,** Reduced rate of energy expenditure as a risk factor for body-weight gain, New Eng J Med 318:467, 1988.

15. **Fanda OP, Soeldner SS,** Genetic, acquired, and related factors in the etiology of diabetes mellitus, Arch Intern Med 137:461, 1977.

16. **Wise JK, Hendler R, Felig P,** Obesity: evidence of decreased secretion of glucagon, Science 178:513, 1972.

17. **Hewing R, Liebermeister H, Daweke H, Gries FA, Gruneklee D,** Weight regain after low calorie diet: long term pattern of blood sugar, serum lipids, ketone bodies, and serum insulin levels, Diabetologia 9:197, 1973.

18. **Stern MP, Haffner SM,** Body fat distribution and hyperinsulinemia as risk factors for diabetes and cardiovascular disease, Arteriosclerosis 6:123, 1986.

19. **Sims EAH, Danforth E Jr, Horton ES, Bray GA, Glennon JA, Salans LB,** Endocrine and metabolic effects of experimental obesity in man, Recent Prog Hor Res 29:457, 1973.

20. **Gordon T, Kannel WB,** Obesity and cardiovascular disease: the Framingham study, Clin Endocrinol Metab 5:367, 1976.

21. **Bistrian BR,** The medical treatment of obesity, Arch Intern Med 141:429, 1981.

22. **Bistrian BR, Sherman M,** Results of the treatment of obesity with a protein-sparing modified fast, Int J Obes 2:143, 1978.

23. **Volkmar FR, Stunkard AJ, Woolston J, Bailey RA,** High attrition rates in commercial weight reduction programs, Arch Intern Med 141:426, 1981.

24. **Rivlin RS,** Drug therapy: therapy of obesity with hormones, New Eng J Med 292:26, 1975.

25. **Paffenbarger RS Jr, Wing AL, Hyde RT,** Physical activity as an index of heart attack risk in college alumni, Am J Epidemiol 108:161, 1978.

26. **Weisweiler P,** Plasma lipoproteins and lipase and lecithin: Cholesterol acyltransferase activities in obese subjects before and after weight reduction, J Clin Endocrinol Metab 65:969, 1987.

27. **Edholm OG, Fletcher JG, Widdowson EM, McCance RA,** The energy expenditure and food intake of individual men, Brit J Nutr 9:286, 1955.

28. **Konishi F,** Food energy equivalents of various activities, J Am Diet Assoc 46:186, 1965.

29. **Welle SL, Amatruda JM, Forbes GB, Lockwood DH,** Resting metabolic rates of obese women after rapid weight loss, J Clin Endocrinol Metab 59:41, 1984.

30. **Solow C, Siberfarb PM, Swift K,** Psychosocial effects of intestinal bypass surgery for severe obesity, New Eng J Med 290:300, 1974.

15   Steroid Contraception

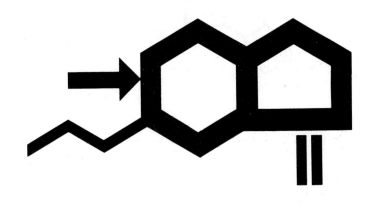

The new birth control pills are extremely safe. The reason for this safety is the now clearly demonstrated dose-response relationship between the steroid components and side effects. The clinical trials with steroids for contraception started with combination pills in 1952, and they were first commercially available in 1960. However, it was not until 1968 that the first reliable prospective studies were initiated, and it was not until the late 1970s that a dose-response relationship between problems and the amount of steroids in the pill was appreciated. As a result, health care providers and patients are confronted by a bewildering array of different products and formulations. The solution to this clinical dilemma is relatively straightforward: use the safest but still effective lowest dose oral contraceptives.

Contraceptive steroids are not natural hormones and should not be so considered, i.e. a woman on the pill is not the same as a pregnant woman in more ways than the obvious one, nor can the effects be equated with the phases of the menstrual cycle. Contraceptive steroids induce a pharmacologic state, not a physiologic one. *This chapter will survey those physiologic mechanisms under stress in the woman receiving steroid contraception and review our methods for patient management. The major theme of this chapter is the relationship between steroid dose and side effects, emphasizing the safety of the low dose birth control pills.*

Pharmacology of Steroid Contraception

The Estrogen Component

The major obstacle to the use of steroids for contraception was inactivity of the compounds when given orally. A major breakthrough occurred in 1938 when it was discovered that the addition of an ethinyl group at the 17 position made estradiol orally active. Ethinyl estradiol is a very potent oral estrogen and is one of the two forms of estrogen in every oral contraceptive. The other estrogen is the 3-methyl ether of ethinyl estradiol, mestranol.

461

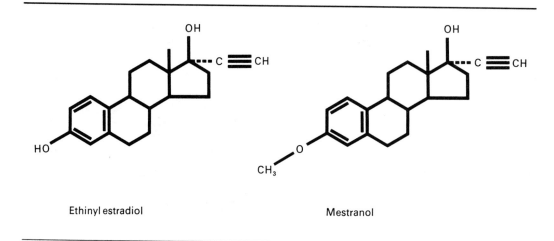

Ethinyl estradiol	Mestranol

Mestranol and ethinyl estradiol are different from natural estradiol and must be regarded as pharmacologic drugs. Animal studies have suggested that mestranol is weaker than ethinyl estradiol, because mestranol must first be converted to ethinyl estradiol in the body. Indeed, mestranol will not bind to the cellular estrogen receptor. Therefore, unconjugated ethinyl estradiol is the active estrogen in the blood for both mestranol and ethinyl estradiol. In the human body, differences in potency between ethinyl estradiol and mestranol do not appear to be significant, certainly not as great as indicated by assays in rodents. This is now a minor point since all of the low dose pills contain ethinyl estradiol.

The estrogen content (dosage) of the pill is of major clinical importance. Thrombosis is one of the most serious side effects of the pill, playing a key role in the increased risk of death from a variety of circulatory problems. This side effect is related to estrogen, and it is dose related. Therefore, the dose of estrogen is a critical issue in selecting a birth control pill.

The Progestin Component

The discovery of ethinyl substitution and oral potency led to the preparation of ethisterone, an orally active derivative of testosterone. In 1951, it was demonstrated that removal of the 19 carbon from ethisterone to form norethindrone did not destroy the oral activity, and most importantly, it changed the major hormonal effect from that of an androgen to that of a progestational agent. Accordingly, the progestational derivatives of testosterone were designated as 19-nortestosterones (denoting the missing 19 carbon). The androgenic properties of these compounds, however, were not totally eliminated and minimal anabolic and androgenic potential remains within the structure.

The "impurity" of the 19-nortestosterone, i.e. androgenic as well as progestational effects, was further complicated in the past by a mistaken belief that they were metabolized within the body to estrogenic compounds. This question was restudied, and it was discovered that the previous evidence for metabolism to estrogenic compounds was due to an artifact in the laboratory analysis. Any estrogenic activity, therefore, would have to be due a direct effect. In animal and human studies, however, only norethindrone, norethynodrel, and ethynodiol diacetate have estrogen activity and it is

462

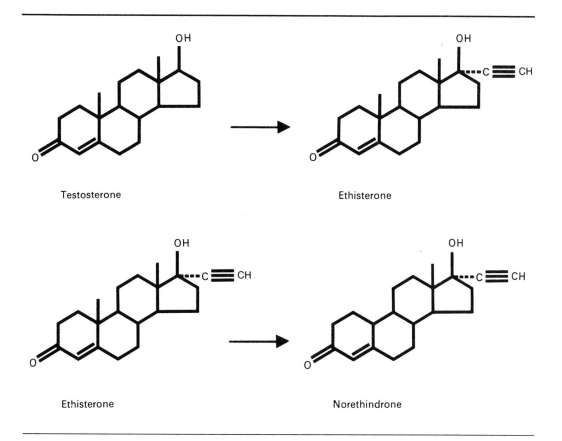

Testosterone → Ethisterone

Ethisterone → Norethindrone

very slight due to weak binding to the estrogen receptor. (1) Clinically androgenic and estrogenic activities of the progestin component are insignificant due to the low dosage in the new birth control pills. As with the estrogen component, serious side effects are related to the progestin dose, and routine use of oral contraceptives should now be limited to the low dose formulations.

Norethindrone is the prototype of this family of compounds, and for many years the patent (now expired) for norethindrone was held by the Syntex Corporation. The formation of the Syntex Corporation, a significant force in American steroid pharmacology, is a fascinating story.(2) This episode in steroid history begins with Russell Marker, a chemist who never received his Ph.D. degree. After leaving school, Marker worked with the Ethyl Gasoline Corporation, and in 1926, developed the process of octane rating, based on the discovery that knocking in gasoline was due to hydrocarbons with an uneven number of carbons.

From 1927 to 1935, Marker worked at the Rockefeller Institute, publishing a total of 32 papers on configuration and optical rotation as methods of identifying compounds. In 1935, he moved to Pennsylvania State University where he trained himself in steroid chemistry and became interested in solving the problem of producing abundant and cheap amounts of progesterone. At that time it required the ovaries from 2,500 pregnant pigs to produce 1 mg of progesterone. In 1939, Marker became convinced that the solution to the problem of obtaining large quantities of steroid hormones was to find plants which contained sufficient amounts of sapogenin, a plant steroid which could be used as a starting point for steroid hormone biosynthesis. This conviction was strengthened with his discovery that a species of *Trillium,* known locally as Beth's root, was collected in North Carolina and used in the preparation of Lydia Pinkham's Compound, popular at the time to relieve menstrual troubles. The active ingredient in Beth's root was diosgenin, a plant steroid.

Marker organized extensive botanical expeditions. In 1942, he collected the roots of the Mexican yam, and back in Pennsylvania, he worked out the degradation of diosgenin to progesterone. United States pharmaceutical companies refused to back Marker, and even refused to patent the process at Marker's urging.

In 1943, Marker resigned from Pennsylvania State University and went to Mexico where he prepared several pounds of progesterone (worth $600,000). This progesterone gained him entry to Hormone Laboratories in Mexico City. The 2 partners in Hormone Laboratories and Marker formed a company which they called Syntex. The price of progesterone fell from $200 to $2 a gram.

In 1947, the 3 partners had a falling out, and Marker sold his share of the company and retired to the Pennsylvania State University campus. However, he took his knowhow with him. Fortunately for Syntex, he had published a scientific description of his process, and there still was no patent on his discoveries. Syntex recruited George Rosenkranze to reinstitute the commercial manufacture of progesterone, a task which took him 2 years.

In 1949, it was discovered that cortisone relieved arthritis, and the race was on to develop an easy and cheap method to synthesize cortisone. Dr. Carl Djerassi joined Syntex to work on this synthesis using the Mexican yam plant steroid diosgenin as the starting point. This accomplishment was reported in 1951, but soon after an even better method of cortisone production was discovered at Upjohn, using microbiologic fermentation. This latter method used progesterone as the starting point, and therefore, Syntex found itself as the key supplier to other companies for this important process, at the rate of 10 tons of progesterone per year and a price of 48 cents per gram.

The Syntex chemists then turned their attention to the sex steroids. They discovered that the removal of the 19 carbon from progesterone increased the progestational activity of the molecule. Ethisterone, prepared a dozen years earlier, was available, and the Syntex chemists reasoned that removal of the 19 carbon would increase the progestational potency of this orally active compound. In 1951, norethindrone was synthesized, and the patent for this drug is the only patent for a drug listed in the National Inventor's Hall of Fame in Washington. Shortly after, the Searle Company filed a patent for norethynodrel.

Both the Syntex and Searle compounds were tested by Gregory Pincus and colleagues in 1953-1954. Pincus had been a consultant for Searle for quite some time, and therefore, he picked the Searle compound for extended use. Syntex, a wholesale drug supplier,

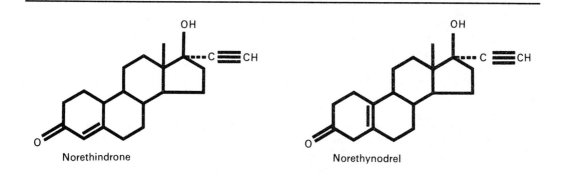

Norethindrone

Norethynodrel

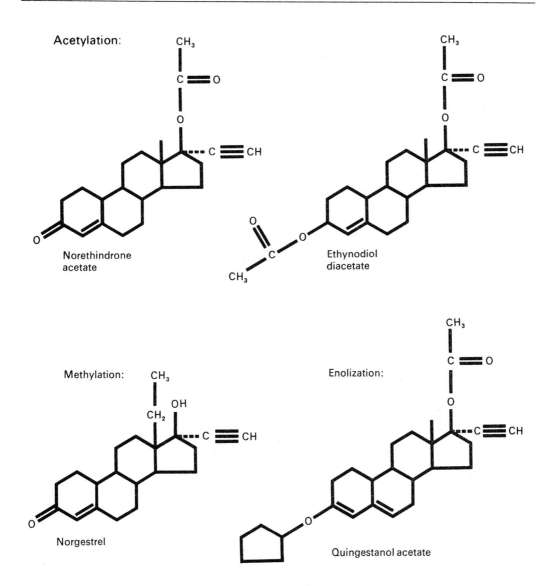

Acetylation:

Norethindrone acetate

Ethynodiol diacetate

Methylation:

Norgestrel

Enolization:

Quingestanol acetate

was without marketing expertise and organization. Pincus convinced Searle that the commercial potential of an oral contraceptive warranted the risk of possible negative consumer reaction. By the time Syntex had secured arrangements with Ortho for a marketing outlet, Searle marketed Enovid in 1960. Ortho-Novum using norethindrone from Syntex appeared in 1962.

The norethindrone family contains the following 19-nortestosterone progestins: norethindrone, norethynodrel, norethindrone acetate, ethynodiol diacetate, norgestrel, desogestrel, and gestodene. Levonorgestrel is the active isomer of norgestrel. Desogestrel undergoes two metabolic steps before the progestational activity is expressed as 3-keto-desogestrel. This metabolite differs from levonorgestrel only by a methylene group in the 11 position. Gestodene differs from levonorgestrel by the presence of a double bond between carbons 15 and 16, thus it is delta 15 gestodene.

A second group of progestins became available for use when it was discovered that acetylation of the 17-hydroxy group of 17-hydroxyprogesterone produced oral potency. Acetylation at the 17 position gives oral potency, but an addition at the 6 position is necessary to give sufficient progestational strength for human use, probably by inhibiting metabolism. Derivatives of progesterone with substituents at the 17 and 6 positions include the widely used medroxyprogesterone aceate.

New Formulations

The latest development in oral contraceptive technology is the multiphasic preparation, altering the dosage of both the estrogen and progestin components, periodically throughout the pill-taking schedule. The future will bring even more products and different formulations. The aim of these new formulations is to alter steroid levels in an effort to achieve lesser metabolic effects and minimize the occurrence of breakthrough bleeding and amenorrhea, while maintaining efficacy. We are probably at or very near the lowest dose levels which can be achieved without sacrificing efficacy. Metabolic studies with the multiphasic preparations indicate no differences or slight improvements over the metabolic effects of low dose monophasic products. Physicians and patients are urged to choose a new multiphasic preparation or to use the low dose (30 and 35 μg estrogen) monophasic pills. The use of higher dose pills should be discontinued, and all women on higher dose pills should be stepped down to low dose preparations. Stepping down can be safely accomplished with absolutely no decrease in efficacy. The therapeutic principle remains: utilize the pills which give effective contraception and the greatest margin of safety.

Mechanism of Action

The combination pill, consisting of the estrogen and progestin components, is given daily for 3 out of every 4 weeks. The combination pill prevents ovulation by inhibiting gonadotropin secretion via an effect on both pituitary and hypothalamic centers. The progestational agent in the pill primarily suppresses luteinizing hormone (LH) secretion, while the estrogenic agent suppresses follicle-stimulating hormone (FSH) secretion. Therefore, the estrogenic component significantly contributes to the contraceptive efficacy. The estrogen in the pill serves two other purposes. It provides stability to the endometrium so that irregular shedding and unwanted breakthrough bleeding can be avoided; and the presence of estrogen is

466

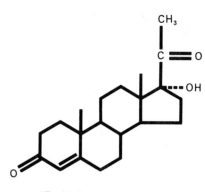

17α-Hydroxyprogesterone

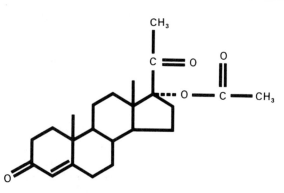

17-Acetoxy progesterone

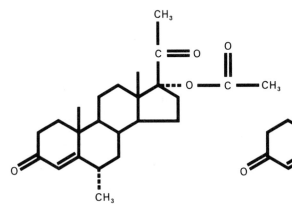

Medroxyprogesterone acetate
(Provera)

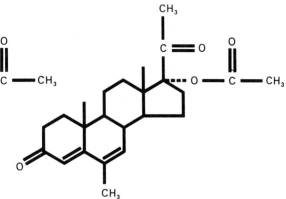

Megestrol acetate

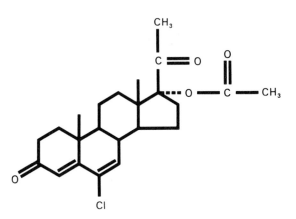

Chlormadinone acetate

467

required to potentiate the action of the progestational agents. The latter function of estrogen has allowed reduction of the progestational dose in the pill. The mechanism for this action is probably the effect (an increase) on the concentration of intracellular progestational receptors by estrogen. Therefore, a certain pharmacologic level of estrogen is necessary to maintain the potency of the combination pill.

Since the effect of a progestational agent will always take precedence over estrogen (unless the dose of estrogen is increased many, many fold), the endometrium, cervical mucus, and perhaps tubal function reflect progestational stimulation. The progestin in the combination pill produces an endometrium which is not receptive to ovum implantation, a decidualized bed with exhausted and atrophied glands. The cervical mucus becomes thick and impervious to sperm transport. It is possible that further contraceptive effects are obtained by progestational influences on secretion and peristalsis within the fallopian tubes.

With this variety of contraceptive actions, it is hard to understand how the omission of a pill or two can result in a pregnancy. Indeed, careful review of pill failures reveals that pregnancies usually occur because initiation of the next cycle is delayed a few days allowing escape from ovarian suppression. Strict adherence to only 7 pill-free days is most critical in order to obtain reliable, effective contraception, and this is probably even more important with the new low dose pills. For this reason, the 28 day pill package, incorporating 7 pills which do not contain steroids, is a very useful aid to assure adherence to the proper schedule.

The contraceptive effectiveness of the multiphasic formulations are unequivocally comparable to low dose (less than 50 μg estrogen) and higher dose monophasic combination birth control pills.

Failure Rates per Year:		
	Optimal	Usual Use
Oral contraceptives	0.1%	2.5%
IUD	1.5%	4.0%
Condoms	3.0%	10.0%
Diaphragm	3.0%	18.0%
Foam/Cream/Jelly	10.0%	20.0%
Rhythm	10.0%	24.0%

Metabolic Effects

Cardiovascular Disease

There are 2 on-going major British prospective studies which continue to provide us with solid clinical information upon which reasonable decisions can be based. (3-10) The Royal College of General Practitioners (RCGP) study began in 1968 with 23,000 pill users matched with 23,000 non-users. The Oxford/Family Planning Association (OFPA) study involves 17,032 women. There was a third prospective study, an American study (the Walnut Creek Study), which unfortunately is no longer on-going. It enrolled 16,638 women between 1968 and 1972.(11) An additional resource which continues to help clinicians and patients is the Centers for Disease Control cancer and steroid hormone study, a case-control study which involves 8 geographic areas throughout the United States.

Venous thromboembolism is believed to be an effect of estrogen, limited to current users only, with a disappearance of the risk by 4-6 weeks after discontinuing oral contraception as the coagulation factors rapidly return to normal. The British data indicated that the risk of deep thrombosis in the leg is 4 times greater in oral contraceptive users than nonusers, and that of superficial thrombosis in the leg, 2 times greater. There is no evidence that varicose veins have any influence on deep thrombosis associated with pill use.

These conclusions, however, were based on data derived from higher dose pills. As long ago as 1974, the RCGP noted that reducing the estrogen dose to 50 μg significantly lowered the risk of thrombosis. (3) Since then, Swedish and RCGP reports indicated that women who use 50 μg estrogen pills have a higher incidence of thrombosis and arterial disease than those who use 30 and 35 μg estrogen pills.(12,13) One explanation for this dose-response relationship is the finding that the impact of estrogen on various clotting factors is related to dose, with little, if any, impact at doses less than 50 μg of ethinyl estradiol.(14) Studies of the blood coagulation system have concluded that both monophasic and multiphasic low dose birth control pills achieve homeostasis. Slight increases in thrombin formation are offset by increased fibrinolytic activity. Thus there is no increase in platelet activation and clotting.(15) It is not surprising that with the growing use of low dose formulations, the risk of venous thrombosis has decreased.(16)

The first public awareness of an increased risk for myocardial infarction followed the reports of 2 retrospective studies in England.(17,18) The increased risk was noted especially in older women, and consideration of other risk factors (hypertension, hypercholesterolemia, cigarette smoking, obesity, and diabetes mellitus) indicated that oral contraceptives acted synergistically with these factors, rather than additively.(19-22) Indeed, it is now apparent that the majority of women who develop myocardial infarction are smokers. In the 1983 RCGP report, only older (over age 35) smokers currently using oral contraceptives had a statistically significant increased risk of ischemic heart disease compared to controls.(7) The Walnut Creek study and a case-control report (the Puget Sound study) in the United States did not find an increased risk of myocardial infarction with use of oral contraceptives.(11,23) These later findings probably reflect to a significant degree the avoidance of

469

prescribing oral contraception to women with risk factors for cardiovascular disease.

The British data have also indicated a relationship between progestin levels and the risk of cardiovascular disease.(13,24) The RCGP study found an increased rate of all arterial diseases with increasing doses of norethindrone acetate in 50 μg pills, and a 50% higher rate with 0.25 mg of norgestrel compared to 0.15 mg in a 30 μg pill.(24) *It is important to note that the British studies found an increased risk only with progestin doses no longer utilized.* Because these older high dose pills were used by older women in the British studies, the results are further confounded by the factor of age.

Clinical reports have been consistent with an association between the use of oral contraceptives and neurovascular accidents in otherwise healthy young women. According to retrospective studies, pill use increases the risk of thrombotic stroke 3-fold, and that of hemorrhagic stroke, 2-fold.(25) The RCGP 1983 report and the 1984 OFPA report indicated that the increased risk of stroke was approximately doubled.(7,10) However, when healthy patients on low dose pills were studied (Walnut Creek by its study population and Puget Sound by design), no significant association between stroke and oral contraceptives was observed.(11,23) The most recent OFPA report emphasized that after 9100 women years of use, not a single patient on the low dose (less than 50 μg estrogen) pills had suffered a stroke.(10)

Despite the comfort of these more recent reports, and because of the seriousness of this potential complication, the onset of visual symptoms or severe headaches should be considered as indications for discontinuation of the pill. Rather than immediately discontinuing the pill, however, the clinician and patient should consider switching to another brand within the same low dose range (less than 50 μg estrogen), and certainly if the patient is at a higher dose, a move to the low dose pill often relieves the symptoms.

Clues to vascular headaches:

-Headaches which last a long time.
-Dizziness, nausea, or vomiting with headaches.
-Scotomata or blurred vision.
-Episodes of blindness.
-Unilateral headaches.
-Headaches which continue despite medication.

In summary, the relationship between cardiovascular disease and pill use is significantly affected by risk factors (especially smoking) and age. The risk for a young (under 35) healthy woman may be negligible with the new low dose pills. Beginning at age 35, and certainly after age 40, the risk increases, but mortality is largely confined to smokers over age 35.

Analyses of vital statistics data in the United States and in 21 countries in Europe, Asia, and North America failed to reveal the high levels of death from cardiovascular diseases associated with pill use which the early British data appeared to indicate.(26,27) In December of 1980, the Walnut Creek study reported no significant differences in mortality rates between ever and never users of oral contraceptives.(11) A short time later, the RCGP and OFPA updated their ongoing studies and supported the favorable conclusions of the Walnut Creek study.(6,9) The important observations reported in 1981 included the following:

-Duration of oral contraceptive use had no effect on mortality when age was controlled.

-The effect of age was less than previously thought. The increased mortality in users was concentrated in smokers over the age of 35. Users under the age of 35 (smokers and nonsmokers) had minimally increased mortality risks that could have arisen by chance.

-For women age 35 to 44, the major risk is in smokers, and nonsmokers without risk factors for vascular disease can expect the benefits of oral contraceptive use to outweigh the risks.

-Deaths from cerebral vascular disease and heart disease accounted for most of the increased mortality, with pulmonary embolism accounting for only 10%.

Observations that the risk of death is higher among former users do not establish that this is due to a residual effect of oral contraception.(28) The women reported to have the greatest residual effect are women who smoked heavily and used oral contraception while they were in their 30s. Former users may have stopped taking the pill because of health problems which later led to circulatory death. In addition, these results are derived from women who took pills of high estrogen content, and they indicate a greater relative risk, which, in terms of actual numbers of cases attributable to use of the pill, is very small. For all of these reasons, there should be only limited concern over any lingering risks to past users of oral contraceptives, especially to past users of the low dose pills.

Both the RCGP and OFPA studies indicated, therefore, that women under the age of 35, regardless of smoking status, are at no significantly increased risk of death when taking oral contraceptives. Mortality data using the new low dose pills (less than 50 μg estrogen) do support this favorable outlook. In 54,971 woman-years of oral contraceptive use in the Seattle area, there were no cardiovascular deaths among users compared with 11 cardiovascular deaths in the nonuser group.(23)

471

The increased safety of the low dose pills may be explained by their effects on high-density and low-density lipoprotein carriers of cholesterol. The significant lipoproteins are the following:

VLDL: Very low-density lipoproteins, which carry triglycerides (mainly) and cholesterol.

LDL: Low-density lipoproteins, which carry cholesterol in plasma; the levels of LDL are directly associated with the incidence of coronary heart disease.

HDL: High-density lipoproteins, which also carry cholesterol in plasma and are inversely associated with the risk of coronary heart disease. Weight reduction and exercise increase HDL levels.

Only a small increase in HDL-cholesterol is significantly associated with a reduction in coronary heart disease. (29) A weaker relationship exists for heart disease risk and LDL, but in general, as LDL-cholesterol increases, one's risk increases. The risk associated with a low HDL-cholesterol is exaggerated when combined with other atherosclerotic risk factors such as hypertension and elevated LDL-cholesterol. Estrogens and progestins have different effects on lipoprotein levels. Estrogen in relatively low doses generally increases HDL-cholesterol and decreases LDL-cholesterol, a protective effect against atherosclerosis, while progestins decrease HDL-cholesterol and increase LDL-cholesterol, an effect which promotes heart disease. The importance of these effects on the lipoprotein profile in young women should not be underestimated. Atherogenesis begins early in life.

The balance of estrogen and progestin potency in a given oral contraceptive formulation can determine cardiovascular risk by its overall effect on lipoprotein levels. Oral contraceptives with relatively high doses of progestins (doses not used in today's low dose formulations) do produce unfavorable lipoprotein levels. (30) A modern view of the serious side affects associated with oral contraceptives, supported by the recent epidemiologic data, attributes venous thromboembolism to the estrogen component and an arteriosclerotic process responsible for heart attacks and strokes to the progestin component.(31) This is not without dispute; cardiovascular complications could have been mediated by high dose estrogen-stimulated thrombosis.

The levonorgestrel triphasic exerts no significant changes on HDL-cholesterol, LDL-cholesterol, apoprotein B, and no change or an increase in apoprotein A, while the levonorgestrel monophasic combination has a tendency to increase LDL-cholesterol and apoprotein B, and to decrease HDL-cholesterol and apoprotein A.(32-35) In one study, however, the levonorgestrel triphasic was associated with an increase in LDL-cholesterol values after 6 and 12 months of use (although in this particular study, the triphasic contained the racemic mixture in a higher dose.(36) The bulk of the evidence indicates that the levonorgestrel triphasic appears to have no significant impact on the lipoprotein profile in contrast to an adverse effect of the levonorgestrel monophasic pill. The monophasic desogestrel pill has a favorable effect on the lipoprotein profile, while the triphasic gestodene pill produces only slight changes, although these are beneficial alterations in the LDL/HDL and apoprotein B/apoprotein A ratios.(32-35,37) Like the triphasic levonorgestrel pills, norethindrone multiphasic pills have no significant impact on the lipoprotein profile over 6-12 months.(36,38)

There is experimental evidence in monkeys to suggest that the combination of estrogen and progestin in oral contraceptives directly correlates with a lesser amount of atherosclerosis in the coronary arteries despite an adverse impact (decrease) on HDL-cholesterol levels.(39) Thus the risk of the new formulations has been reduced tremendously, now possibly at the level of no significant clinical impact.

There currently is no statistically significant evidence that any specific oral contraceptives containing different progestational components in the low doses have a major advantage or disadvantage when side effects are compared. Furthermore, it should be recognized that the clinical relevance of the lipid modifications remains to be substantiated by epidemiologic data. It is appropriate to question the clinical and biological significance of the reported changes because the great majority of the changes have still been within the physiological ranges for age and sex. The strong relationship between coronary artery disease and lipoprotein concentrations, however, leads one to support and advocate pill formulations which minimize the adverse effects of lipid alterations.

In conclusion, the low dose pills are safer than the pills previously used. The overall risk is very close to minimal in healthy women under the age of 40 who do not smoke, and under the age of 35 the synergistic effect of smoking appears to be negligible. Only smokers 35 and older have a significantly increased risk of dying from circulatory diseases.

Hypertension

Oral contraceptive pill-induced hypertension was observed in approximately 5% of users of higher dose pills.(3) More recent evidence indicates that small increases in blood pressure can be observed even with 30 μg estrogen, monophasic pills, (40-43) however an increased incidence of clinically significant hypertension has not been reported. No significant changes in blood pressure have been noted with any of the multiphasic formulations. This is another reason to limit routine use to low dose pills; however, an annual assessment of blood pressure is still an important element of clinical surveillance, even when low dose oral contraceptives are used.

The mechanism for an effect on blood pressure is thought to involve the renin-angiotensin system. The most consistent finding is a marked increase in plasma angiotensinogen, the renin substrate, up to 8 times normal values. In the majority of women, excessive vasoconstriction is prevented by a compensatory decrease in plasma renin concentration. If hypertension does develop, the renin-angiotensinogen changes take 3-6 months to disappear after stopping the pill.

473

Variables such as previous toxemia of pregnancy or previous renal disease do not predict whether a woman will develop hypertension on the pill. In addition, women who have developed hypertension on the pill are not more predisposed to develop toxemia of pregnancy.

One must also consider the effects of oral contraceptives in patients with pre-existing hypertension or cardiac disease. A judgment is necessary regarding the importance of 100% contraception. Studies in the literature indicate that pre-existing hypertension does increase the risk of thrombosis, but with medical control of the blood pressure and close follow-up, the patient and her clinician may choose the low dose pill for contraception. Close follow-up is also indicated in women with a history of pre-existing renal disease or a strong family history of hypertension and cardiovascular disease. One consideration is the effect of the oral contraceptive on cardiac work. Significant increases in cardiac output and plasma volume have been recorded, probably a result of fluid retention. It seems prudent to suggest that patients with marginal cardiac reserve should utilize other means of contraception.

Oncogenic Potential

A major concern about the impact of the pill on human health is whether steroid contraception causes cancer. The concern in this area has been directed toward the uterus (corpus and cervix) and the breast. It must be acknowledged that the duration of use of steroids has not been long enough to permit absolute statements on this critical issue. Nevertheless, reasonably secure judgments can be made on the basis of a large body of epidemiologic work.

Estrogen not only supports normal endometrium, but prolonged unopposed estrogen is associated with a progression of histologic change from hyperplasia to adenomatous hyperplasia to atypia. As currently constituted, one would expect the combination of progestin and estrogen to have a protective effect on the endometrium. Indeed, the use of oral contraceptives for at least 12 months reduces the risk of developing endometrial cancer by 50%, with the greatest protective effect gained by use greater than 3 years.[44] This protection persists for 15 or more years after discontinuation (the actual length of duration of protection is unknown). This protection is equally protective for all 3 major histological subtypes of endometrial cancer: adenocarcinoma, adenoacanthoma, and adenosquamous cancers. Finally, protection is seen with all monophasic formulations of oral contraceptives, including pills with less than 50 μg of estrogen. (There are no data as of yet with multiphasic preparations). The protective effect depends upon the balance of the steroidal components; too much estrogen or too little progestin would not confer the safety seen with current formulations.

The risk of developing epithelial ovarian cancer in users of birth control pills is reduced by 40% compared to that of nonusers.[45] Again this protective effect increases with duration of use (taking 5-10 years to become apparent) and continues for at least 10-15 years after stopping the medication. This protection is seen in women who use oral contraceptives for as little as 3 to 6 months, and it is a benefit associated with all monophasic formulations. Again, the multiphasic pills have not been in use long enough to yield any data on this issue. Approximately 2000 cases of endometrial cancer

474

and 1700 cases of ovarian cancer are averted annually by past and current users of oral contraceptives.

Early studies suggested that the risk for dysplasia and carcinoma-in-situ of the uterine cervix increased with the use of birth control pills for 5 or more years. It is well-recognized, however, that the number of partners a woman has had and age at first coitus are the most important risk factors for cervical neoplasia. When differences in sexual activity are controlled, apparent increases in the incidence of cervical neoplasia among pill users are no longer statistically significant. (46,47) At least one study, however, has claimed a link between long-term pill use and cervical cancer even when data analysis accounts for the confounding factors.(48) On the other hand, an excellent CDC study concluded there is no increased risk of invasive cervical cancer in users of oral contraception, and an apparent increased risk of carcinoma in situ is due to enhanced detection of disease.(49) These considerations obviously constitute important reasons for annual Pap smear surveillance. Fortunately, steroid contraception does not mask abnormal cervical changes, and the necessity for prescription renewals offers the opportunity for improved screening for cervical disease (the very reason why studies on this subject find links between cervical neoplasia and oral contraceptive use).

While there is not a major concern in regard to uterine cancer, there are fears of the effects of estrogen on breast tissue. Worth emphasizing is a protective effect on benign disease of the breast associated with the progestin component of the pill, an effect which becomes apparent after 2 years of continuous usage. After 2 years of usage there is a progressive reduction in the incidence of fibrocystic disease of the breast with increasing duration of use. Women who take the pill are one-fourth as likely to develop benign breast disease as nonusers.

The RCGP, OFPA, and Walnut Creek studies have indicated no significant differences in breast cancer rates between users and nonusers. However patients were enrolled in these studies at a time when oral contraceptives were used primarily by married couples spacing out their children. Because this population may not reflect use by younger women delaying their first pregnancy, several case-control studies focused on the use of oral contraceptives before the age of 25.(50-52) All reported an increased risk of breast cancer in early users of oral contraceptives. Another case-control study suggested that the risk of premenopausal breast cancer is increased by long-term use (12 or more years) in young women.(53)

These reports prompted the Centers for Disease Control in Atlanta to review information from its on-going case-control study on steroid use and cancer. No increased risk of breast cancer was found in women using oral contraceptives before the age of 20 with a duration of use greater than 4 years, or before the age of 25 with a duration of use greater than 6 years, or with greater than 4 years use before a first pregnancy.(54) In addition, no increased risk of breast cancer was found among any subgroups of users including women with benign breast disease or a family history of breast cancer.

In a further analysis of the CDC study, the largest on the subject, there was no increased risk associated with any specific type of oral contraceptive, progestin only pills, or the use of 2 or more types.(55) In addition, there was no increased risk associated with any specific progestin or estrogen component, and most importantly, it was demonstrated that long-term use (15 or more years) was not associated with an increased risk of breast cancer. The reliability of the CDC study is reinforced by the fact that the data confirmed the previously identified risk factors, such as nulliparity, late age at first birth, history of benign breast disease, and a family history of breast cancer. Finally, the CDC conclusions are supported by a significant national study from New Zealand.(56)

The results of the CDC study, because of its large size, are very reassuring. However, the data reflect only the use of monophasic formulations. In addition, because the population at risk for breast cancer is the age group over 45 years old, and because of the long latent phase for breast cancer, data in the 1990's and 2000's will be required to answer one last very important question: the possibility of very late effects of use. Thus far the CDC Cancer and Steroid Hormone Study has found no evidence for a latent effect on breast cancer risk through age 54.(57)

Progestational agents have been implicated as causal factors for breast cancer. The situation is a very special one, being limited only to experiments with beagle dogs. Mammary tumors in the beagle dog are increased as a result of prolonged stimulation with large doses (up to 25 times human luteal phase levels) of progesterone or 17-hydroxyprogesterone derivatives (such as medroxyprogesterone acetate). This has not been reported in any other species, and there is no clinical evidence for a relationship between progestin use and breast cancer in women. Indeed, World Health Organization follow-up of women using Depo-Provera for contraception indicates that exposure to Depo-Provera protects women against breast cancer.(58)

The Walnut Creek Study suggested in 1977 that another cancer linked to pill usage is melanoma. However, the major risk factor for melanoma is exposure to sunlight, and this was not controlled. More recent and accurate evaluation has not indicated a significant difference in melanoma in oral contraceptive users.(59)

Adrenal Gland

For some time it has been known that estrogen increases the cortisol-binding globulin, transcortin. It had been thought that the increase in plasma cortisol while on the pill was due to increased binding by the globulin and not an increase in free active cortisol. Now it is apparent that free and active cortisol levels are also elevated. Estrogen decreases the ability of the liver to metabolize cortisol, and in addition, progesterone and related compounds can displace cortisol from transcortin, and thus contribute to the elevation of unbound cortisol. The effects of these elevated levels over prolonged periods of time are unknown. To put this into perspective, the increase is not as great as that which occurs in pregnancy, and, in fact, it is within the normal range for nonpregnant women.

476

The adrenal gland responds to ACTH normally in women on oral contraceptives, therefore there is no suppression of the adrenal gland itself. Initial studies showed that the response to metyrapone (a 11 hydroxylase blocker) was abnormal, suggesting that the pituitary was suppressed. However estrogen accelerates the conjugation of metyrapone by the liver, and therefore the drug has less effect, thus explaining the subnormal responses initially reported. The pituitary-adrenal reaction to stress is normal in women on oral contraceptive pills.

Thyroid

As with transcortin, estrogen increases thyroxine-binding globulin, Prior to the introduction of new methods for measuring free thyroxine levels, evaluation of thyroid function was a problem. Measurement of TSH (thyroid stimulating hormone) and the free thyroxine level in a woman on oral contraception provides an accurate assessment of a patient's thyroid state. Birth control pills affect the total thyroxine level in the blood as well as the amount of binding globulin, but the free thyroxine level is unchanged.

Carbohydrate Metabolism

An impaired glucose tolerance test is present in up to 40% of women using birth control pills with 50 μg or more of estrogen. In these women, plasma levels of insulin as well as the blood sugar are elevated. Generally the effect of the pill is to produce an increase in peripheral resistance to insulin action, probably by lowering concentrations of insulin receptors. Most women can meet this challenge by increasing insulin secretion, and there is no change in the glucose tolerance test. Individuals who cannot respond with an appropriate increase in insulin will have an abnormal glucose tolerance.

Carbohydrate metabolism is affected mainly by the progestin component of the pill. The derangement of carbohydrate metabolism may also be affected by estrogen influences on lipid metabolism, hepatic enzymes, and elevation of unbound cortisol. The glucose intolerance is dose-related, and once again effects are less with the low dose formulations. *Insulin and glucose changes with the low dose monophasic and multiphasic pills are so minimal, that it is now believed that they are of no clinical significance.*(37,60-62) This includes long-term evaluation with hemoglobin A1c. The one exception is the claim that the levonorgestrel monophasic pill is too strongly progestational, leading over 3 years to progressive deterioration of glucose tolerance.(63)

It can be stated definitively that birth control pill use does not produce an increase in diabetes mellitus.(64) The hyperglycemia associated with oral contraception is not deleterious and is completely reversible. Even women who have risk factors for diabetes in their history do not seem to be affected.

There is some controversy regarding the response of women with previous gestational diabetes mellitus. Kung et al report higher plasma insulin levels and a deterioration of glucose tolerance (interpreted as the presence of peripheral resistance to insulin) after 6 months of the levonorgestrel triphasic.(65) On the other hand, Skouby et al reported no effect over 6 months on either glucose tolerance or lipids.(66,67) It should be noted that the abnormal results reported

477

by Kung et al are due to abnormal data in 4 of 11 women. It will take larger numbers and accumulated data to determine whether Kung's results reflect the natural course of diabetes in that small series, or a true consequence of multiphasic oral contraception.

In clinical practice, it may, at times, be necessary to prescribe oral contraception for the overt diabetic. The effect on insulin requirement is neither consistent nor predictable, but one would expect little, if any, change with low dose pills. According to the epidemiologic data, the use of oral contraceptives increases the risk of thrombosis in women with insulin-dependent diabetes mellitus; therefore, women with diabetes should be encouraged to use other forms of contraception. However this effect in women under age 35 who are otherwise healthy is probably very minimal with the low dose pills, and reliable protection against pregnancy is a benefit for these patients that outweighs the small risk.

Liver

The liver is affected in more ways and with more regularity and intensity by the sex steroids than any other extragenital organ. Estrogen influences the synthesis of hepatic DNA and RNA, hepatic cell enzymes, serum enzymes formed in the liver, and plasma proteins. Estrogenic hormones also affect hepatic lipid and lipoprotein formation, the intermediary metabolism of carbohydrates, and intracellular enzyme activity.

The active transport of biliary components is impaired by a large number of estrogens as well as some progestins. The mechanism is unclear, but cholestatic jaundice and pruritus are occasional complications of the birth control pill, and are similar to the recurrent jaundice of pregnancy, i.e. benign and reversible.

The only absolute hepatic contraindication to pill use is acute or chronic cholestatic liver disease. Cirrhosis and previous hepatitis are not aggravated. Once recovered from the acute phase of liver disease, a woman can take oral contraceptive pills.

Liver Adenomas

Hepatocellular adenomas can be produced by steroids of both the estrogen and androgen families. Actually, there are two different lesions, peliosis and adenomas. Peliosis is characterized by dilated vascular spaces without endothelial lining, and may occur in the absence of adenomatous changes. The adenomas are not malignant; their significance lies in the potential for hemorrhage. The most common presentation is acute right upper quadrant or epigastric pain. The tumors may be asymptomatic, or they may present suddenly with hematoperitoneum. There is some evidence that the tumors regress when the pill is stopped. Epidemiologic data have not support the contention that mestranol increased the risk more than ethinyl estradiol.

The risk appears to be related to duration of pill use and to the steroid dose in the pills. This is reinforced by the rarity of the condition ever since low dose pills became available. The ongoing prospective studies have accumulated many women years of use and have not identified a single case of such a tumor. In our view it isn't even worth mentioning during the informed consent process. Nevertheless, there continues to be concern, and recent studies implicate a risk for hepatocellular carcinoma with long-term pill use.

478

(68) However, the incredibly small number of cases and thus the difficulties in study design require great caution in interpretation.

No reliable screening test or procedure is currently available. Routine liver function tests are normal. CT scanning may be the best means of diagnosis; angiography and ultrasonography are not reliable. Palpation of the liver should be part of the periodic evaluation in pill users. If an enlarged liver is found, the pills should be stopped, and regression should be evaluated and followed by CT scan.

Gallbladder Disease

The incidence of gallstones in early reports from Britain indicated an increased incidence after the first 2 years of use, with a return to the level of the control group after 4 years. The latest British data, however, have indicated that this apparent increase was due to an acceleration of gallbladder disease in women already susceptible.(69) In other words, the overall risk of gallbladder disease is not increased, but in the first years of use, disease is activated or accelerated in women who are vulnerable because of asymptomatic disease or a tendency toward gallbladder disease. The mechanism appears to be induced alterations in the composition of gallbladder bile, specifically a rise in cholesterol saturation that is presumably an estrogen effect.(70) One anticipates a lesser effect in the forthcoming reports describing the effects of low dose pills.

Other Metabolic Effects

Gastrointestinal disorders, breast discomfort, and weight gain continue to be disturbing effects, but the incidence is significantly less with low dose pills. Fortunately, these effects are most intense in the first few months of use, and in most cases, gradually disappear. Weight gain which takes place rarely usually responds to dietary restriction, but for some patients, the weight gain is an anabolic response to the sex steroids, and discontinuation of oral contraception is the only way that weight loss can be achieved.

Chloasma, a patchy increase in facial pigment, was at one time found to occur in approximately 5% of pill users. It is now an infrequent problem due to the increasing use of low dose oral contraceptives. Unfortunately, once chloasma appears, it fades only gradually following discontinuation of the pill, and may never disappear completely. Skin blanching medications may be useful.

In the British prospective studies, urinary tract infections were increased by 20%, and a correlation was noted with estrogen dose. An increased incidence of cervicitis was also reported, an effect related to the progestin dose. The incidence of cervicitis increased with the length of time the pill was used, from no higher after 6 months to 3 times higher by the 6th year of use. A significant increase in a variety of viral diseases, e.g. chickenpox, was observed, suggesting steroid effects on the immune system. The prevalence of these effects with low dose pills is yet unknown.

Hematologic effects include an increased sedimentation rate due to increased levels of fibrinogen, increased total iron binding capacity due to the increase in globulins, and a decrease in prothrombin time. The cyclic use of the pill may prevent the appearance of symptoms in porphyria precipitated by menses. On the other hand, porphyria may be worsened. Changes in vitamin metabolism have been noted: a small nonharmful increase in Vitamin A, decreases in blood levels of pyridoxine (B_6) and the other B vitamins, folic acid, and ascorbic acid. Despite these changes, routine vitamin supplements have not been shown to be of benefit for women eating adequate, normal diets.

In well-controlled studies, no increases in eye abnormalities have been detected in pill users (contrary to early anecdotal reports). Rarely, mental depression is associated with oral contraceptives. In some cases, the effect is due to estrogen interference with the synthesis of tryptophan and can be reversed with pyridoxine treatment. It seems wiser, however, to discontinue the pill if depression is encountered. Though infrequent, a reduction in libido is occasionally a problem, and may be a cause for seeking an alternative method of contraception.

Useful side effects include relief of dysmenorrhea, improvement of premenstrual tension, a decrease (two-thirds less) in menstrual bleeding and iron deficiency anemia, and improvement in hirsutism. The RCGP reported a 50% decrease in rheumatoid arthritis, but a large case-control study concluded that there was no association between oral contraceptives and rheumatoid arthritis.(71)

Because estrogen is known to stimulate prolactin secretion and to cause hypertrophy of the pituitary lactotrophs, it was appropriate to be concerned over a possible relationship between oral contraception and prolactin-secreting pituitary adenomas. Several case-control studies have uniformly concluded that no such relationship exists. There is insufficient information regarding the effect of oral contraceptives on existing prolactinomas, although at least one study demonstrated that previous use of oral contraceptives had no effect on the size of prolactinomas.(72) We have routinely prescribed birth control pills to patients with pituitary microadenomas and have never observed evidence of tumor growth.

The Pill and PID

The use of oral contraceptives reduces the risk of contacting pelvic inflammatory disease as well as the degree of severity. This protection may not extend, however, to chlamydial tubal infections.(73) On the other hand, this latter conclusion is based on vaginal culture results, and there is no information available regarding upper genital tract chlamydial infection. Furthermore, a study specifically addressing the relationship of tubal infertility to oral contraceptive use has failed to find evidence of either an increased risk or a decreased risk, although women who used a low dose pill early in life had a decreased risk for tubal infertility which was of borderline statistical significance.(74) The usual surveillance for pelvic infection is sufficient.

Postpill Amenorrhea

The approximate incidence of "postpill amenorrhea" is 0.7-0.8%, but there is no evidence to support the idea that oral contraception causes secondary amenorrhea. Most women (80%) resume normal ovarian function in 3 months after discontinuing the pill, and 95-98% are ovulating in 1 year. If a cause and effect relationship exists between the pill and subsequent amenorrhea, one would expect the incidence of infertility to be increased after a given population discontinues use of the pill. In those women who discontinue the pill in order to get pregnant, 50% conceive by 3 months, and after 2 years, a maximum of 15% of nulliparous women and 7% of parous women fail to conceive (75), figures comparable to those quoted for the prevalence of spontaneous infertility. Attempts to document a cause and effect relationship between pill use and secondary amenorrhea have failed. While patients with this problem come more quickly to our attention because of previous pill use and follow-up, there is no cause and effect relationship. Women who have not resumed menstrual function within 12 months should be evaluated as any other patient with secondary amenorrhea.

An important related question is: should birth control pills be advised for a young woman with irregular menses and oligoovulation or anovulation? The fear of subsequent infertility should not be a deterrent to providing appropriate contraception. Women who have irregular menstrual periods are more likely to develop secondary amenorrhea whether they take the pill or not. The possibility of subsequent secondary amenorrhea is less of a risk and a less urgent problem for a young woman than leaving her unprotected. The need for contraception takes precedence.

Evaluation of Patient
and Choice of Pill

ABSOLUTE CONTRAINDICATIONS TO THE USE OF THE PILL

1. Thrombophlebitis, thromboembolic disorders, cerebral vascular disease, coronary occlusion, or a past history of these conditions, or conditions predisposing to these problems.

2. Markedly impaired liver function. Steroids are contraindicated in patients with hepatitis until liver function tests return to normal.

3. Known or suspected carcinoma of the breast.

4. Known or suspected estrogen-dependent neoplasia, especially carcinoma of the endometrium.

5. Undiagnosed abnormal genital bleeding (requires diagnostic evaluation).

6. Known or suspected pregnancy.

7. Congenital hyperlipidemia.

8. Smokers (over 15 cigarettes per day) who are over age 35.

RELATIVE CONTRAINDICATIONS REQUIRING CLINICAL JUDGMENT AND INFORMED CONSENT

1. Migraine headaches. In retrospective studies, migraine headaches have been associated with an increased risk of stroke. However, some younger (under 30) women report an improvement in their headaches.

2. Hypertension. A woman under 30 who is otherwise healthy and whose blood pressure is controlled by medication can elect to use the pill.

3. Uterine leiomyoma. This is no longer a problem with the low dose formulations. Indeed, there is evidence that the risk of leiomyomas is decreased by 31% in women who use the pill for 10 years.(76)

4. Gestational diabetes. Low dose formulations do not affect glucose tolerance in women with previous gestational diabetes, and there is no evidence that pill use increases the incidence of overt diabetes mellitus, but these women should have periodic tests of glucose tolerance.

5. Elective surgery. The pill should be discontinued, if possible, 1 month prior to elective surgery to avoid an increased risk of post-operative thrombosis.

6. Epilepsy. Despite the warning in the package inserts, oral contraceptives do not exacerbate epilepsy, and in some women, improvement in seizure control has occurred. (77)

7. Obstructive jaundice in pregnancy (not all patients with this history will develop jaundice on the pill).

8. Sickle cell disease or sickle C disease, but not sickle cell trait.

9. Diabetes mellitus.

10. Gallbladder disease.

Clinical Management

Previously, patients have been monitored every 6 months while on oral contraception. In view of the increased safety of low dose pills for healthy young women with no risk factors, patients need be seen only every 12 months for exclusion of problems by history, palpation of the liver, urinalysis, measurement of the blood pressure, breast examination, and pelvic examination with Pap smear. Women with risk factors (such as smoking) can be seen every 6 months by appropriately trained paramedical personnel for screening of problems by history and blood pressure measurements (breast and pelvic examinations are necessary only yearly). It is worth emphasizing that better compliance is achieved by reassessing new pill users within 6 months. It is at this time that subtle fears and unvoiced concerns need to be confronted and resolved.

Laboratory surveillance should be used only when indicated. Routine biochemical measurements fail to yield sufficient information to warrant the expense. There is one exception. All adults should have at least one screening lipid profile to detect subclinical hyperlipidemia which in young people can be present in the absence of a family history of premature coronary artery disease. The following is a useful guide as to who should be monitored with blood screening tests for glucose, lipids, and lipoproteins:

Young women, at least once.
Women 35 years or older.
Women with a strong family history of heart disease, diabetes mellitus, or hyperlipidemia.
Women with gestational diabetes mellitus.
Women with xanthomatosis.
Obese women.
Diabetic women.

The therapeutic principle remains: utilize the pill which gives effective contraception and the greatest margin of safety. The multiphasic preparations do have a reduced progestin dosage compared to some of the existing monophasic products, and this may manifest itself in improved metabolic effects. Based on currently available information, there is little difference between the low dose monophasics and the multiphasics. Thus the argument in favor of multiphasic use is at this time a theoretical argument, but it makes good clinical sense: use the lowest dose pills which produce good results with the greatest possible safety margin.

You and your patients are urged to choose a new multiphasic preparation or the low dose (30 and 35 μg estrogen) monophasic pills. The current evidence supports the view that there is greater safety with pills containing less than 50 μg of estrogen. The arguments in this chapter indicate that all patients should begin oral contraception with the new low dose pills, and that patients on higher dose pills should be stepped down to the low dose preparations. Stepping down to a lower dose can be made immediately with no adverse reactions such as increased bleeding or failure of contraception.

Anecdotal reports have suggested that ovarian cysts are encountered more frequently and suppress less easily with multiphasic formulations. This remains to be seen and reminds one of many early observations linked to combination pills which failed to withstand careful scrutiny. Certainly functional ovarian cysts occur less frequently in women taking combination formulations, although this beneficial effect is not seen with the progestin-only minipill.(78)

The pharmacologic effects in animals of various birth control pills have been used as a basis for therapeutic recommendations in selecting the optimal oral contraceptive pill. All too often this leads to the prescribing of a pill of excessive dosage with its attendant increased risk of serious side effects. In addition, it is by no means established that you can project potency data in animals to the clinical situation.(79) The validity of this approach, so-called tailor-making the pill to the patient, is not supported by appropriately controlled clinical trials. It is far more prudent to be guided by the principles of effectiveness and safety.

The obstetrical tradition of scheduling the postpartum visit at 6 weeks should be changed. A 3-week visit would be more productive in avoiding postpartum surprises, since the first ovulation essentially never occurs prior to the 3rd postpartum week. There is one possible exception: if bromocriptine is used to suppress prolactin and lactation promptly after delivery, ovulation may occur earlier. After the termination of a pregnancy of less than 12 weeks, oral contraception can be started immediately. After a pregnancy of 12 or more weeks, oral contraception should not be started until 2 weeks after delivery to avoid the increased risk of thrombosis during the postpartum period.

Combination pill contraception has been shown to diminish the quantity and quality of lactation in postpartum women. In adequately nourished women, no impairment of infant growth can be detected; presumably compensation is achieved either through supplementary feedings or increased suckling.(80) Also of concern is the potential hazard of crossover of steroids to the infant (a significant amount of the progestational component is transferred into breast milk)(81), however no adverse effects have thus far been identified. For these reasons oral contraception is best deferred until lactation is discontinued. A good alternative, however, is the progestin-only minipill which has no impact on breast milk. Although the minipill has a failure rate of 2-3%, when it is combined with the contraceptive action of prolactin due to lactation, highly effective protection can be achieved.

Effective contraception is present during the first cycle of pill use, provided the pills are started no later than the 5th day of the cycle, and no pills are missed. If a woman misses 1 pill she should take that pill as soon as she remembers and take the next pill as usual. If she misses 2 pills, she should immediately begin using another form of contraception, stop taking the pills, wait 7 days and start a new cycle. The 7-day interval between pill cycles is crucial; extending this duration of time is probably the most important factor for contraceptive failure during pill usage. This is the major reason for the growing popularity of the 28-day package which contains a terminal 7 days of nonsteroid pills to enhance accurate adherence to the schedule. The importance of this 7-day interval has led many to advise their patients to decrease the pill-free interval to 5 days.

There is no rationale for recommending a pill-free interval of a few months. The serious side effects are not eliminated by pill-free intervals. In addition, this practice all too often results in unwanted pregnancies.

There is no evidence that the use of oral contraceptives in the pubertal, sexually active girl impairs growth and development of the reproductive system. Again, the most important concern is and should be the prevention of an unwanted pregnancy. For most teen-agers the pill is the contraceptive method of choice, dispensed in the 28-day package for better compliance.

There are many anecdotal reports of patients who conceived on oral contraceptives while taking antibiotics. There is good reason to believe that rifampin decreases the efficacy of oral contraceptives by stimulating the liver's metabolic capacity. There is little evidence, however, that antibiotics such as ampicillin and tetracycline, which reduce the bacterial flora of the gastrointestinal tract, affect pill efficacy. Indeed, studies indicate that while antibiotics can alter the excretion of steroids, plasma levels are unchanged. To be cautious, patients on medications that affect liver metabolism (rifampin, coumadin, phenobarbital, phenytoin, primidone, and carbamazepine) should choose an alternative contraceptive, and women requiring antibiotics (including griseofulvin) should be advised to practice additional contraception.

Oral contraception is safer than we thought it was, and the low dose birth control pills are extremely safe. Health care providers should make a significant effort to get this message to both our colleagues and our patients. It is important that professionals be more involved with the media, providing accurate, balanced information to counteract misinformation and hype. In addition, we should make sure our patients receive adequate counseling, either from ourselves or our professional staff. Put the risks into proper perspective, and take time to emphasize the benefits as well as the risks.

Major Benefits of Oral Contraception
Hospitalizations Prevented Annually in the U.S.A. (82)

Condition	Hospitalizations
Iron-deficiency anemia	27,200
Benign breast disease	23,000
Pelvic inflammatory disease	15,595
Ectopic pregnancy	11,695
Ovarian cysts	3,500
Endometrial cancer	2,000
Ovarian cancer	1,700

Major Problems with Low Dose Pills

Amenorrhea on the Pill

The low estrogen content is not of sufficient potency in some women to stimulate endometrial growth. The progestational effect dominates to such a degree that a shallow atrophic endometrium is produced, lacking sufficient tissue to yield withdrawal bleeding. It should be emphasized that permanent atrophy of the endometrium does not occur, and resumption of normal ovarian function will restore endometrial growth and development.

The major problem with amenorrhea while on the pill is the anxiety produced in both patient and health professional because the lack of bleeding may be an early sign of pregnancy. The patient is anxious because of the uncertainty regarding pregnancy, and the clinician is anxious because of the medical-legal concerns stemming from the retrospective studies which indicated an increased risk of congenital malformations of the VACTERL group (vertebral, anal,

485

cardiac, tracheoesophageal, renal, and limb) among the offspring of women who inadvertently used oral contraception in early pregnancy. These initial positive reports have not been substantiated. Simpson, in a careful review, examined the literature on hypospadias, cardiac malformations, limb reduction deformities, neural tube defects, and the VACTERL group, and concluded that there was no association between oral contraceptive use and these malformations.(83)

The only noteworthy association is a greater frequency of dizygous twinning when oral contraceptives are used within 1 month of conception.(84) No other effects on fetal health or on the gender of the offspring have been noted. (85) Furthermore, no adverse effects on subsequent births have been noted in women who discontinue oral contraception, including no increase in chromosomal anomalies and no increase in the spontaneous abortion rate.(75) Indeed, the only reason (and it's a good one) to recommend that women defer attempts to conceive for a month or two after stopping the pill is to improve the accuracy of gestational dating.

The incidence of amenorrhea in the first year of use with both multiphasic and monophasic pills is less than 1%. Information on the incidence with long-term use is not available, but there is a clinical impression that it can reach 5-6% after several years of use. Thus it is important to alert patients upon starting the pill that diminished bleeding and possibly no bleeding may ensue.

Amenorrhea is a difficult management problem. The use of a pregnancy test for the beta subunit of human chorionic gonadotropin (HCG) will allow reliable testing for pregnancy even at this early stage. However, routine repeated use of such testing is expensive and annoying, and may lead to discontinuation of oral contraception. A simple test for pregnancy is to assess the basal body temperature during the 7 days off of steroids; a basal body temperature less than 98 degrees (36.6 C) is inconsistent with pregnancy and the pills may be continued. Some women are reassured with an understanding of why there is no bleeding and are able to continue on the pill despite the amenorrhea. Some women cannot reconcile themselves to a lack of bleeding, and this is an indication for trying other formulations. Some clinicians have observed that the addition of extra estrogen for 1 month (1.25 mg conjugated estrogens daily throughout the 21 days of the steroid-containing pills) will rejuvenate the endometrium, and withdrawal bleeding will resume, persisting for many months.

Breakthrough Bleeding

The major deterrent to the use of the lower dose pills is breakthrough bleeding. It is not surprising that the incidence of this problem increased as the estrogen dose of the pill was decreased. There are two characteristic breakthrough bleeding problems: irregular bleeding in the first few months after starting the pills, and unexpected bleeding after many months on the pills. Effort should be made to manage the bleeding problem in a way that allows the patient to remain on the low dose pill.

Breakthrough bleeding which occurs in the first few months of use is best managed by encouragement and reassurance. This bleeding usually disappears by the third cycle in the majority of women. If necessary, even this early pattern of breakthrough bleeding can be treated as outlined below. It is helpful to explain to the patient that this bleeding represents tissue breakdown as the endometrium adjusts from its usual thick state to the relatively thin state allowed by the hormones in the pill.

Breakthrough bleeding which occurs after many months of pill use is a consequence of the progestin-induced decidualization. This endometrium is shallow and tends to be fragile and prone to breakdown and asynchronous bleeding. The incidence of breakthrough bleeding with the multiphasic formulations is comparable to the monophasic low dose combination pills.

If bleeding occurs just before the end of the pill cycle, it can be managed by having the patient stop the pills, wait 7 days and start a new cycle. If breakthrough bleeding is prolonged or if it is aggravating for the patient, regardless of the point in the pill cycle, control of the bleeding can be achieved with a short course of exogenous estrogen. Conjugated estrogens, 2.5 mg, or ethinyl estradiol, 20 μg, are administered daily for 7 days when the bleeding is present, no matter where the patient is in her pill cycle. The patient continues to adhere to the schedule of pill taking. Usually one course of estrogen solves the problem, and recurrence of breakthrough bleeding is unusual (but if it does recur, another 7-day course of estrogen is effective).

Responding to irregular bleeding by having the patient take 2 or 3 pills daily is not effective. The progestin component of the pill will always dominate, hence doubling the number of pills will also double the progestational impact with its decidualizing, atrophic effect on the endometrium. The addition of extra estrogen while keeping the progestin dose unchanged is logical and effective. This allows the patient to remain on the lowest dose pill with its advantage of greater safety. Any bleeding which is not handled by this routine requires investigation for the presence of pathology.

Should the Older Woman Use the Pill?

Some means of contraception is necessary for many women until the age of 50. If an older woman elects to utilize oral contraception, she should be aware of the higher risk involved with increasing age; however, it is appropriate to emphasize several considerations.

1. The risk of death for a woman in good health is less than what we had been led to believe by the early British reports. With avoidance of risk factors and use of low dose pills, the risk may be negligible for healthy women.

2. Even though the risk increases with age, the risk of death is still lower than that associated with pregnancy itself (especially after the age of 40).

3. The risk to life increases rapidly for pill users who smoke and are over the age of 35. In addition to smoking, predisposing risk factors include: hypertension, diabetes mellitus, obesity, elevated lipids and lipoproteins, and a strong family history of coronary heart disease.

The birth control pill is virtually contraindicated for women over the age of 35 who smoke more than 15 cigarettes per day or have any of the following high risk factors: hypertension, prior thromboembolism, grossly abnormal carbohydrate or lipid laboratory values.

Nonsmokers ages 36 to 50 who are in good health can continue oral contraception utilizing low dose formulations. Women over 35, who are potentially at high risk because of obesity or a strong family history of diabetes mellitus, hyperlipidemia, or cardiovascular disease should be encouraged to seek other methods. If these high risk women insist on the use of oral contraception, they must agree to being followed closely, with laboratory surveillance of cholesterol, triglycerides, HDL-cholesterol, LDL-cholesterol, and an occasional glucose screen. After a repeat of these tests at 6 months, surveillance can be spaced at a yearly interval.

The risk for healthy, nonsmoking, older women is minimal, if any, with low dose formulations. Although the extent of this risk has not been documented, it is an acceptable, reasonable choice. An alternative approach is to urge surgical sterilization for one of the partners.

An Alternative to the Pill

A useful alternative to the pill, especially in those women in whom estrogen is contraindicated, is Depo-Provera. Two observations are important: first, it requires 6-8 months for the drug to totally clear from the average woman, and second, the effective contraception level is maintained for 4 months. Therefore, 150 mg given intramuscularly every 3 months assures 100% contraception.

The progestin in depot form effectively blocks the LH surge, and in addition, affects the endometrium and cervical mucus. The suppression of gonadotropins is not as complete as with the pill. This is an advantage, since follicular growth is maintained at a sufficient level to produce estrogen levels comparable to those in the follicular phase of a normal cycle. In other words, Depo-Provera does not produce a hypoestrogenic state.

This progestin, in large continuous doses, produced breast tumors in beagle dogs. This appears to be an effect unique to the beagle dog, and has not appeared in other animals or in women after years of use. Indeed, follow-up studies of women indicate that exposure to Depo-Provera offers significant protection against breast cancer.(58)

Major problems with Depo-Provera are breakthrough bleeding, breast tenderness, weight gain, and depression. Breakthrough bleeding can be treated with exogenous estrogen as noted above. The incidence of breakthrough bleeding is 30% in the first year, and 10% thereafter. The majority of women become totally amenorrheic. Serious weight gain and depression (less than 5% incidence) are not relieved until the drug clears the body 6-8 months after the last injection. Depo-Provera has cortisol-like effects, and in larger doses, suppresses adrenal function. This is not a significant clinical problem in contraceptive doses. It is important to note that the long-term impact of Depo-Provera on the lipoprotein profile is uncertain.

488

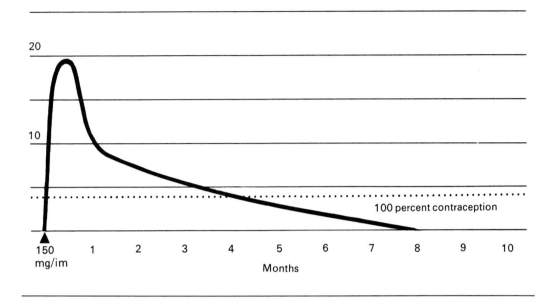

Provera Blood Level
ng/ml

20

10

100 percent contraception

150
mg/im

Months

1   2   3   4   5   6   7   8   9   10

Women embarking on this method of contraception should be screened and followed at least yearly to detect adverse effects, especially on HDL-cholesterol levels.

The major advantage to the use of Depo-Provera is its freedom from the side effects of estrogen. Hence, it can be considered for patients with congenital heart disease, sickle cell anemia, patients with a previous history of thromboembolism, and women over 30 who smoke or have other risk factors. *However, the absolute safety in regard to thrombosis has not been proven in a controlled study.*

A further advantage in patients with sickle-cell disease is evidence indicating an inhibition of in vivo sickling with hematologic improvement during treatment with Depo-Provera. (86) Depo-Provera is also useful for cases where compliance is a problem, e.g. mentally retarded young women. Another advantage is the finding that Depo-Provera increases the quantity of milk in nursing mothers, a direct contrast to the effect seen with combination pills. The concentration of the drug in the breast milk is very small, and no effects of the drug on infant growth and development have been observed.(87) A final benefit of Depo-Provera is its ability to exert a modest improvement in seizure control in epileptics. (88)

The belief that infertility with suppressed menstrual function may be caused by Depo-Provera is not borne out by epidemiologic data. The pregnancy rate in women discontinuing the injections because of a desire to become pregnant is normal.(89) The delay to conception is about 9 months after the last injection, and the delay does not increase with increasing duration of use. Thus, suppressed menstrual function persisting beyond 12 months after the last injection is not due to the drug and deserves evaluation.

489

In many parts of the world, a variety of injectable contraceptives are being developed and utilized. These include norethindrone enanthate, long-acting esters of norgestrel, and biodegradable microcapsules which release progestational agents over a period of 3-6 months. The major compliance problem is irregularity of bleeding. Dosage and type of progestin as well as combinations with estrogen are being investigated for better bleeding control.

Other Methods

The minipill is the continuous daily use of a low dose of a potent progestational agent. The contraceptive effect is more dependent upon endometrial and cervical mucus effects, since LH is not consistently suppressed. Tubal physiology may also be affected, but ectopic pregnancy is not prevented as effectively as intrauterine pregnancy.

The main disadvantages are incomplete contraception and breakthrough bleeding. The use-pregnancy rate is 2-3%. Breakthrough bleeding (30-40% incidence) is so unexpected, irregular, and occasionally heavy that extreme patient dissatisfaction is common. Nevertheless, certain clinical situations warrant consideration of the minipill: older women who smoke or have risk factors and postpartum lactating women—in general, those women in whom estrogen is hazardous.

Available minipills:

Micronor	Norethindrone	0.35 mg
Nor-Q-D	Norethindrone	0.35 mg
Ovrette	Norgestrel	0.075 mg

Steroids diffuse through the walls of silastic capsules at a rate controlled by the thickness of the walls and the surface area. A large dose of a potent progestin inside of a silastic capsule implanted under the skin will give highly effective (less than 1% pregnancy rate) contraception for several years. However, the capsules must be removed through an incision. Bleeding problems are similar to the use of Depo-Provera, since the principle is the same. Currently available in many parts of the world is a system of 6 subdermal capsules (Norplant) which release levonorgestrel over a period of 6-7 years, providing effective contraception for a minimum of 5 years. Equally effective, but easier to insert and remove, is Norplant 2, two small rods containing levonorgestrel.

Another approach is the use of vaginal silastic rings impregnated with progestational compounds. One advantage is the ability to leave the ring in for several years, or to remove it on a monthly basis. The problem of side effects can be further reduced using low dose progestin-impregnated silastic devices near the cervix.

Postcoital Contraception

Estrogen in large doses is effective in preventing conception after midcycle coital exposure.(90) The mechanism for this "morning after" technique remains to be determined, but its effectiveness has been confirmed in large clinical studies. The failure rate is approximately 1%. Treatment should be initiated as soon after exposure as possible, but no later than 72 hours. Side effects reflect the high doses used: nausea, vomiting, headache, dizziness. Various estrogens can be used, and even a combination birth control pill, as follows:

Conjugated estrogens, 30 mg per day for 5 days, or 50 mg iv on each of 2 consecutive days.
Ethinyl estradiol, 5 mg per day for 5 days.
Ovral, 4 tablets (2 given 12 hours apart).

In view of the fact that treatment with a high dose combination birth control pill achieves the same results as estrogen, this method is preferred. The total amount of steroid administered is significantly less, and a reduction in the total number of doses limits the side effects to a much shorter time period.

Because of possible harmful effects to a fetus, an already existing pregnancy should be ruled out prior to use of postcoital hormones. Furthermore, the patient should be offered therapeutic abortion if the drug fails.

The Medicated IUD

The intrauterine device (IUD) does not require continued motivation, and is easily reversible. There are significant drawbacks, however, including bleeding, pain, expulsion of the device, perforation, and unplanned pregnancies either with the device in situ or after unnoticed expulsion or perforation. The number of ectopic pregnancies is not absolutely increased in IUD wearers; however, the risk of ectopic pregnancy is increased in comparison to users of oral contraceptives, although it is actually less when compared to non-contraceptors.

If pregnancy occurs with an IUD in place, the greatest risk of spontaneous or septic abortion is in the second trimester. If the IUD is not removed, there is, in addition, a greater risk for premature labor. An IUD should be removed as soon as possible when pregnancy occurs.

The continuous release of small amounts of the hormone in the progesterone T is associated with a local effect on the uterus without systemic effects. Sustained continuous release allows the use of progesterone itself rather than one of the synthetic progestins. Even though progesterone has a short half-life, the steady release allows maintenance of a constant and effective local level of the hormone.

The mechanism of action is unknown, although it is believed that it is the local effect of the progesterone on the endometrium which renders it incapable of sustaining an implantation. The local progesterone also affects the cervical mucus, thus making passage of sperm difficult. There is a reduction in the incidence of cramping and bleeding due to a decrease in endometrial production of prostaglandins. For the same reason, there is a beneficial effect of the local progesterone on dysmenorrhea and menorrhagia. The pregnancy rates are approximately 1.9 and 2.5 per 100 women-years in parous and nulliparous women, respectively. Currently, the device must be replaced every year.

Contraception and GnRH Agonists and Antagonists

Administration of GnRH agonists or antagonists can have contraceptive effects by lowering gonadotropin stimulation of ovarian function. The key to the action of the agonist is the achievement of down regulation of GnRH receptors in the anterior pituitary gland.

At first glance, these applications of the GnRH-related compounds offer hope for a specific method of contraception which would be effective but free of side effects. However, the application of such methods carries with it many practical problems. Any method which depends upon short-term interruption of the menstrual cycle requires absolutely accurate timing. A very difficult problem with long-term administration is the production of a hypoestrogenic state, or irregular, unacceptable patterns of bleeding. For these reasons, this method is not around the corner.

Progesterone Antagonism

Antagonism of progesterone is both a logical and attractive idea for contraception. RU 486 is a 19-norsteroid derivative that binds to the progesterone receptor and prevents or interrupts progestational action. It has been studied as both an abortifacient and as a contraceptive agent.(91,92) A single dose given in the midluteal phase induces menses in about 72 hours, an effect which cannot be overcome with HCG. This appears to be due to a direct effect on the endometrium because when HCG is added, the luteolytic action of RU 486 on the corpus luteum is prevented, yet vaginal bleeding still ensues. Menses are not induced by RU 486 unless luteal phase levels of progesterone are present, or more specifically, secretory phase endometrium must be in place. The availability of this substance as a once-a-month form of fertility control awaits further clinical studies.

In addition to its direct anti-progesterone activity, there is evidence that RU 486 can induce endometrial prostaglandin secretion which in turn can contribute to its efficacy as an abortifacient agent. In Europe, the combination of RU 486 and prostaglandin administration has been demonstrated to be a very effective and safe method for inducing abortion in early pregnancy, with a low incidence of side effects.(93)

To Keep Up-To-Date

A monthly newsletter is available which reviews the latest information, and highlights current problems and questions:

Contraceptive Technology Update
67 Peachtree Drive N.E.
Atlanta, GA 30309

492

References

1. **Edgren RA,** Progestagens, *Clinical Uses of Steroids,* Givens J, editor, Yearbook, Chicago, 1980, pp 1-29.

2. **Goldzieher JW,** Hormonal Contraception—whence, how, and whither? *Clinical Uses of Steroids,* Givens J, editor, Yearbook, Chicago, 1980, pp 31-43.

3. **Royal College of General Practitioners,** *Oral Contraceptives and Health,* Pitman Publishing, New York, 1974.

4. **Royal College of General Practitioners,** Oral contraception study: mortality among oral contraceptive users, Lancet ii:727, 1977.

5. **Royal College of General Practitioners,** Oral contraceptive study: oral contraceptives, venous thrombosis, and varicose veins, J Roy Coll Gen Pract 28:393, 1978.

6. **Royal College of General Practitioners Oral Contraceptive Study,** Further analyses of mortality in oral contraceptive users, Lancet i:541, 1981.

7. **Royal College of General Practitioners Oral Contraceptive Study,** Incidence of arterial disease among oral contraceptive users, J Roy Coll Gen Pract 33:75, 1983.

8. **Vessey MP, McPherson K, Johnson B,** Mortality among women participating in the Oxford/Family Planning Association contraceptive study, Lancet ii:731, 1977.

9. **Vessey MP, McPherson K, Yeates D,** Mortality in oral contraceptive users, Lancet i:549, 1981.

10. **Vessey MP, Lawless M, Yeates D,** Oral Contraceptives and stroke: findings in a large prospective study, Brit Med J 289:530, 1984.

11. **Ramcharan S, Pellegrin FA, Ray RM, Hsu J-P,** The Walnut Creek Contraceptive Drug Study. A prospective study of the side effects of oral contraceptives, J Reprod Med 25:366,360, 1980.

12. **Bottinger LE, Boman G, Eklund G, Westerholm B,** Oral contraceptives and thromboembolic disease: effects of lowering oestrogen content, Lancet i:1097, 1980.

13. **Meade TW, Greenburg G, Thompson SG,** Progestogens and cardiovascular reactions associated with oral contraceptives and a comparison of the safety of 50- and 30- μg estrogen preparations, Brit Med J 280:1157, 1980.

14. **Beller FK, Ebert C,** Effects of oral contraceptives on blood coagulation, a review, Obstet Gynecol Survey 40:425, 1985.

15. **Bonnar J,** Coagulation effects of oral contraception, Am J Obstet Gynecol 157:1042, 1987.

16. **Porter JB, Hunter JR, Jick H, Stergachis A,** Oral contraceptives and nonfatal vascular disease, Obstet Gynecol 66:1, 1985.

17. **Mann JI, Vessey MP, Thorogood M, Doll R,** Myocardial infarction in young women with special reference to oral contraceptive practice, Brit Med J 2:241, 1975.

493

18. **Mann JI, Inman WHW,** Oral contraceptives and death from myocardial infarction, Brit Med J 2:245, 1975.

19. **Ory HW,** Association between oral contraceptives and myocardial infarction, JAMA 237:2619, 1977.

20. **Shapiro S, Slone D, Rosenberg L, Kaufman DW, Stolley PD, Miettinen OS,** Oral contraceptive use in relation to myocardial infarction, Lancet i:743, 1979.

21. **Hennekens CH, Evans D, Peto R,** Oral contraceptive use, cigarette smoking and myocardial infarction, Brit J Fam Plann 5:66, 1979.

22. **Rosenberg L, Hennekens CH, Rosner B, Belanger C, Rothman KH, Speizer FE,** Oral contraceptive use in relation to nonfatal myocardial infarction, Am J Epidemiol 11:59, 1980.

23. **Porter JB, Hershel J, Walker AM,** Mortality among oral contraceptive users, Obstet Gynecol 70:29, 1987.

24. **Kay CR,** The happiness pill, J Roy Coll Gen Pract 30:8, 1980.

25. **Collaborative Group for the Study of Stroke in Young Women,** Oral contraceptives and stroke in young women, JAMA 231:718, 1975.

26. **Tietze C,** The pill and mortality from cardiovascular disease: another look, Fam Plann Perspect 11:80, 1979.

27. **Belsey MA, Russel Y, Kinnear K,** Cardiovascular disease and oral contraceptives: a reappraisal of vital statistics data, Fam Plann Perspect 11:84, 1979.

28. **Slone D, Shapiro S, Kaufman DW, Rosenberg L, Miettinen OS, Stolley PD,** Risk of myocardial infarction in relation to current and discontinued use of oral contraceptives, New Eng J Med 305:420, 1981.

29. **Lipid Research Clinics Program: The Lipid Research Clinics Coronary Primary Prevention Trial Results,** II. The relationship of reduction in incidence of coronary heart disease to cholesterol lowering, JAMA 251:365, 1984.

30. **Wahl P, Walden C, Knopp R, Hoover J, Wallace R, Heiss G, Refkind B,** Effect of estrogen/progestin potency on lipid/lipoprotein cholesterol, New Eng J Med 308:862, 1983.

31. **Knopp RH,** Arteriosclerosis risk: the roles of oral contraceptives and postmenopausal estrogen, J Reprod Med 31:913, 1986.

32. **Kloosterboer HJ, van Wayjen RGA, van den Ende A,** Comparative effects of monophasic desogestrel plus ethinyloestradiol and triphasic levonorgestrel plus ethinyloestradiol on lipid metabolism, Contraception 34:135, 1986.

33. **Fotherby K,** Effect of oral contraceptives on lipid metabolism, in Genazzani AR, Volpe A, Facchinetti F, editors, *Gynecological Endocrinology*, The Parthenon Publishing Group, New Jersey, 1987, pp. 393-398.

34. **Gaspard U,** Metabolic effects of oral contraceptives, Am J Obstet Gynecol 157:1029, 1987.

35. **Burkman RT, Robinson JC, Kruszon-Moran D, Kimball AW, Kwiterovich P, Burford RG,** Lipid and lipoprotein changes associated with oral contraceptive use: A randomized clinical trial, Obstet Gynecol 71:33, 1988.

36. **Percival-Smith RKL, Morrison BJ, Sizto R, Abercrombie B,** The effect of triphasic and biphasic oral contraceptive preparations on HDL-cholesterol and LDL-cholesterol in young women, Contraception 35:179, 1987.

37. **Bertolini S, Capitanio GL, Terrile E, Cuzzolaro S, Cossom, Daroda P, Croce S,** Effects of gestodene on lipoprotein metabolism, in Genazzani AR, Volpe A, Facchinetti F, editors, *Gynecological Endocrinology,* The Parthenon Publishing Group, New Jersey, 1987, pp. 533-535.

38. **Rabe T, Runnebaum B, Kohlmeyer M, Weicker H,** Lipid, carbohydrate, and androgen metabolism in women using a triphasic oral contraceptive containing norethindrone for one year, Int J Fertil, Supplement, 1986, pp. 46-52.

39. **Adams MR, Clarkson TB, Koritnik DR, Nash HA,** Contraceptive steroids and coronary artery atherosclerosis in cynomolgus macaques, Fertil Steril 47:1010, 1987.

40. **Meade TW, Haines AP, North WRS, Chakrabarti R, Howarth DI, Stirling Y,** Haemostatic, lipid, and blood pressure profiles of women on oral contraceptives containing 50 mcg or 30 mcg oestrogen, Lancet ii:948, 1977.

41. **Khaw K-T, Peart WS,** Blood pressure and contraceptive use, Brit Med J 285:403, 1982.

42. **Wilson E, Cruickshank I, McMaster M, Weir RJ,** A prospective controlled study of the effect on blood pressure of contraceptive preparations containing different types and dosages of progestogen, Brit J Obstet Gynaecol 91:1254, 1984.

43. **Kovacs L, Bartfai G, Apro G, Annus J, Bulpitt C, Belsey E, Pinol A,** The effect of the contraceptive pill on blood pressure: a randomized controlled trial of three progestogen-oestrogen combinations in Szeged, Hungary, Contraception 33:69, 1986.

44. **The Cancer and Steroid Hormone Study of the CDC and NICHD,** Combination oral contraceptive use and the risk of endometrial cancer, JAMA 257:796, 1987.

45. **The Cancer and Steroid Hormone Study of the CDC and NICHD,** The reduction in risk of ovarian cancer associated with oral-contraceptive use, New Eng J Med 316:650, 1987.

46. **Clarke EA, Hatcher J, McKeown-Eyssen GE, Lickrish GM,** Cervical dysplasia: association with sexual behavior, smoking, and oral contraceptive use, Am J Obstet Gynecol 151:612, 1985.

47. **Hellberg D, Valentin J, Nilsson S,** Long term use of oral contraceptives and cervical neoplasia: an association confounded by other risk factors, Contraception 32:337, 1985.

48. **Brinton LA, Huggins GR, Lehman HF, Mallin K, Savitz DA, Trapido E, Rosenthal J, Hoover R,** Long-term use of oral contraceptives and risk of invasive cervical cancer, Internat J Cancer 38:339, 1986.

49. **Irwin KL, Rosero-Bixby L, Oberle MW, Lee NC, Whatley AS, Fortney JA, Bonhomme MG,** Oral contraceptives and cervical cancer risk in Costa Rica: Detection bias or causal association? JAMA 259:59, 1988.

50. **Pike MC, Krailo MD, Henderson BE, Duke A, Roy S,** Breast cancer in young women and use of oral contraceptives: possible modifying effect of formulation and age at use, Lancet ii:926, 1983.

51. **Olsson H, Landin-Olsson M, Moller TR, Ranstam J, Holm P,** Oral contraceptive use and breast cancer in young women in Sweden, Lancet i:748, 1985.

52. **McPherson K, Vessey MP, Neil A, Doll R, Jones L, Roberts M,** Early oral contraceptive use and breast cancer: Results of another case-control study, Brit J Cancer 56:653, 1987.

53. **Meirik O, Dami H, Christoffersen T, Lund E, Bergstrom R, Bergsjo P,** Oral contraceptive use and breast cancer in young women, Lancet ii:650, 1986.

54. **Stadel BV, Rubin GL, Webster LA, Schlesselman JJ, Wingo PA,** Oral contracpetives and breast cancer in young women, Lancet ii:970, 1985.

55. **Cancer and Steroid Hormone Study, CDC and NICHD,** Oral contraceptive use and the risk of breast cancer, New Eng J Med 315:405, 1986.

56. **Paul C, Skegg DCG, Spears GFS, Kaldor JM,** Oral contraceptives and breast cancer: a national study, Brit Med J 2923:723, 1986.

57. **Schlesselman JJ, Stadel BV, Murray P, Lai S,** Breast cancer in relation to early use of oral contracpetives. No evidence of a latent effect, JAMA 259:1828, 1988.

58. **W.H.O. Collaborative Study of Neoplasia and Steroid Contraceptives,** Breast cancer, cervical cancer, and depot medroxyprogesterone acetate, Lancet ii:1207, 1984.

59. **Helmrich SP, Rosenberg L, Kaufman DW, Miller DR, Schottenfeld D, Stolley PD, Shapiro S,** Lack of an elevated risk of malignant melanoma in relation to oral contraceptive use, J Nat Ca Inst 72:617, 1984.

60. **Gaspard UJ, Buret J, Gillain DJ, Romus MA, Lambotte R,** Serum lipid and lipoprotein changes induced by new oral contraceptives containing ethinylestradiol plus levonorgestrel or desogestrel, Contraception 31:295, 1985.

61. **Runnebaum B, Rabe T,** New progestogens in oral contraceptives, Am J Obstet Gynecol 157:1059, 1987.

62. **van der Vange N, Kloosterboer HJ, Haspels AA,** Effect of seven low-dose combined oral contraceptive preparations on carbohydrate metabolism, Am J Obstet Gynecol 156:918, 1987.

63. **Wynn V, Godsland I,** Effects of oral contraceptives on carbohydrate metabolism, J Reprod Med 31:892, 1986.

64. **Duffy TJ, Ray R,** Oral contraceptive use: prospective follow-up of women with suspected glucose intolerance, Contraception 30:197, 1984.

65. **Kung AWC, Ma JTC, Wong VCW, Li DFH, Ng MMT, Wang CCL, Lam KSL, Young RTT, Ma HK,** Glucose and lipid metabolism with triphasic oral contraceptives in women with history of gestational diabetes, Contraception 35:257, 1987.

66. **Skouby SO, Kuhl C, Molsted-Pedersen L, Petersen K, Christensen MS,** Triphasic oral contraception: metabolic effects in normal women and those with previous gestational diabetes, Am J Obstet Gynecol 153:495, 1985.

67. **Skouby SO, Andersen O, Saurbrey N, Kuhl C,** Oral contraception and insulin sensitivity: *In vivo* assessment in normal women and women with previous gestational diabetes, J Clin Endocrinol Metab 64:519, 1987.

68. **Neuberger J, Forman D, Doll R, Williams R,** Oral contraceptives and hepatocellular carcinoma, Brit Med J 292:1355, 1986.

69. **Royal College of General Practitioners' Oral Contraception Study,** Oral contraceptives and gallbladder disease, Lancet ii:957, 1982.

70. **Bennion LJ, Ginsberg RL, Garnick MB, Bennett PH,** Effects of oral contraceptives on the gallbladder bile of normal women, New Eng J Med 294:189, 1976.

71. **del Junco DJ, Annegers JF, Luthra HS, Coulam CB, Kurland LT,** Do oral contraceptives prevent rheumatoid arthritis? JAMA 254:1938, 1985.

72. **Hutting AL, Werner S, Hagenfeldt K,** Oral contraceptive steroids do not promote the development or growth of prolactinomas, Contraception 27:69, 1982.

73. **Washington AE, Gove S, Schachter J, Sweet R,** Oral contraceptives, chlamydial trachomatis infection, and pelvic inflammatory disease, JAMA 253:2246, 1985.

74. **Cramer DW, Goldman MB, Schiff I, Belisle S, Albrecht B, Stadel B, Gibson M, Wilson E, StillmanR, Thompson I,** The relationship of tubal infertility to barrier method and oral contraceptive use, JAMA 257:2446, 1987.

75. **Royal College of General Practitioners,** Oral contraception study, the outcome of pregnancy in former oral contraceptive users, Brit J Obstet Gynaecol 83:608, 1976.

76. **Ross RK, Pike MC, Vessey MP, Bull D, Yeates D, Casagrande, JT,** Risk factors for uterine fibroids: Reduced risk associated with oral contraceptives, Brit J Med 293:359, 1986.

77. **Mattson RH, Cramer JA, Darney PD, Naftolin F,** Use of oral contraceptives by women with epilepsy, JAMA 256:238, 1986.

78. **Vessey M, Metcalfe A, Wells C, McPherson K, Westhoff C, Yeates D,** Ovarian neoplasms, functional ovarian cysts, and oral contraceptives, Brit Med J 294:1518, 1987.

79. **Gillmer MDG,** Progestogen potency in oral contraceptive pills, Am J Obstet Gynecol 157:1048, 1987.

80. **W.H.O. Task Force on Oral Contraceptives,** Effects of hormonal contraceptives on milk volume and infant growth, Contraception 30:505, 1984.

81. **Betrabet SS, Shikary ZK, Toddywalla VS, Toddywalla SP, Patel D, Saxena BN,** Transfer of norethisterone (NET) and levonorgestrel (LNG) from a single tablet into the infant's circulation through the mother's milk, Contraception 35:517, 1987.

82. **Ory HW,** The noncontraceptive health benefits from oral contraceptive use, Fam Plann Persp 14:4, 1982.

83. **Simpson JL,** Relationship between congenital anomalies and contraception, Adv Contraception 1:3, 1985.

84. **Rothman K,** Fetal loss, twinning, and birth weight after oral contraceptive use, New Eng J Med 297:468, 1977.

85. **Rothman K, Liess J,** Gender of offspring after oral contraceptive use, New Eng J Med 295:859, 1976.

86. **DeCeular K, Gruber C, Hayes R, Serjeant GR,** Medroxyprogesterone acetate and homozygous sickle-cell disease, Lancet ii:229, 1982.

87. **Jimenez J, Ochoa M, Soler MP, Portales P,** Long-term follow-up of children breast-fed by mothers receiving depot-medroxyprogesterone acetate, Contraception 30:523, 1984.

88. **Mattson RH, Cramer JA, Caldwell BV, Siconolfi BC,** Treatment of seizures with medroxyprogesterone acetate: preliminary report, Neurology 34:1255, 1984.

89. **Pardthaisong T,** Return of fertility after use of the injectable contraceptive Depo Provera: up-dated data analysis, J Biosoc Sci 16:23, 1984.

90. **Yuzpe AA,** Postcoital contraception, *Fertility Control,* Corson SL, Derman RJ, Tyrer LB, editors, Little, Brown and Company, Boston, 1985, pp 289-298.

91. **Couzinet B, LeStat N, Ulmann A, Baulieu E, Schaison G,** Termination of early pregnancy by the progesterone antagonist RU 486 (Mifepristine), New Eng J Med 315:1565, 1986.

92. **Nieman LK, Choate RM, Chrousos GP, Healy DL, Morin M, Renquist D, Merriam GR, Spitz IM, Bardin CW, Baulieu E, Loriaux DL,** The progesterone antagonist RU 486, a potential new contraceptive agent, New Eng J Med 316:187, 1987.

93. **Cameron IT, Michie AF, Baird DT,** Therapeutic abortion in early pregnancy with antiprogestogen RU486 alone or in combination with prostaglandin analogue (Gemeprost), Contraception 34:459, 1986.

16 Sperm and Egg Transport, Fertilization, and Implantation

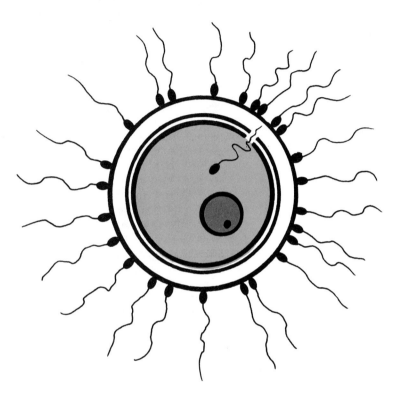

Knowledge of the interactions that take place between sperm and the female reproductive tract can aid the physician in making rational clinical judgments. *Therefore, prior to reviewing the clinical problem of infertility, this chapter will briefly examine the mechanisms involved in sperm and egg transport, fertilization, and implantation.*

Sperm Transport

Semen forms a gel almost immediately following ejaculation, but then is liquefied in 20-30 minutes by enzymes derived from the prostate gland. The alkaline pH of semen provides protection for the sperm from the acid environment of the vagina. This protection is transient, and most sperm left in the vagina are immobilized within 2 hours. The more fortunate sperm, by their own motility, gain entrance into the tongues of cervical mucus that layer over the ectocervix. It is the sperm that enter the uterus; the seminal plasma is left behind in the vagina. This entry is rapid, and sperm have been found in mucus within 90 seconds of ejaculation.(1) Bedford demonstrated that destruction of all sperm in the vagina 5 minutes after ejaculation does not interfere with fertilization in the rabbit, further attesting to the rapidity of transport.(2)

Uterine contractions propel the sperm upward, and in the human they can be found in the tube 5 minutes after insemination.(3) It is possible that the first sperm to enter the tube are at a disadvantage. In the rabbit these early sperm have only poor motility, and there is frequent disruption of the head membranes.(4) The sperm in this vanguard are unlikely to achieve fertilization. Other sperm that have colonized the cervical mucus, the cervical crypts, and the portion of the tubal isthmus nearest the uterus then make their way more slowly to the ampulla of the tube in order to meet the egg. Human sperm have been found in the fallopian tube as long as 85 hours after intercourse, but it is not known whether these sperm have retained their fertilizing ability.(5) In animals, the fertilizable life-span is usually one half the motile life-span.

The attrition in sperm numbers from vagina to tube is substantial. Of an average of 200 million to 300 million sperm deposited in the vagina, less than 200 achieve proximity to the egg. The major loss occurs in the vagina, with expulsion of semen from the introitus playing an important role. Other causes for loss are digestion of sperm by vaginal enzymes, phagocytosis of sperm along the reproductive tract, and, to a limited extent, movement of sperm through the fallopian tube into the peritoneal cavity. There are also reports of sperm burrowing into or being engulfed by endometrial cells.

Capacitation

The discovery in 1951 that rat and rabbit spermatozoa must spend some hours in the female tract before acquiring the capacity to penetrate ova stimulated intensive research efforts to delineate the environmental conditions required for this change in the sperm to occur. The process by which the sperm were transformed was called capacitation. Attention was focused upon the hormonal and time requirements, and the potential for in vitro capacitation.

An important finding was that capacitation changes the surface characteristics of sperm, as exemplified by removal of seminal plasma antigens, modification of their surface charge, and restriction of receptor mobility. This is associated with decreased stability of the plasma membrane and the membrane lying immediately under it, the outer acrosomal membrane. The membranes undergo further, more striking, modifications when capacitated sperm reach the vicinity of an ovum or when they are incubated in follicular fluid. There is a breakdown and merging of the plasma membrane and the outer acrosomal membrane. (6,7) This allows egress of the enzyme contents of the acrosome, the cap-like structure that covers the sperm nucleus. These enzymes, which include hyaluronidase, a neuraminidase-like factor, corona-dispersing enzyme, and a protease called acrosin, are all thought to play roles in sperm penetration of the egg investments. The changes in the sperm head membranes also prepare the sperm for fusion with the egg membrane. In addition, capacitation endows the sperm with hypermotility, and the increased velocity of the sperm may be the most critical factor in mediating zona penetration.(8)

Although capacitation classically has been defined as a change sperm undergo in the female reproductive tract, it is now apparent that sperm of some species, including the human, can acquire the ability to fertilize after a short incubation in defined media and without residence in the female reproductive tract. Therefore, in vitro fertilization is possible.

Egg Transport

Egg transport encompasses the period of time from ovulation to the entry of the egg into the uterus. The egg can be fertilized only during the early stages of its sojourn in the fallopian tube.

In rats and mice the ovary and distal portion of the tube are covered by a common fluid-filled sac. Ovulated eggs are carried by fluid currents to the fimbriated end of the tube. By contrast, in primates, including humans, the ovulated eggs adhere with their cumulus mass of follicular cells to the surface of the ovary. The fimbriated end of the tube sweeps over the ovary in order to pick up the egg. Entry into the tube is facilitated by muscular movements that bring the fimbriae into contact with the surface of the ovary. Variations in this pattern surely exist, as evidenced by women who achieve pregnancy despite having only one ovary, and a single tube located on the contralateral side. Furthermore, eggs deposited in the cul-de-sac by transvaginal injection are picked up by the tubes.(9)

Although there can be a small negative pressure in the tube in association with muscle contractions, ovum pickup is not dependent upon a suction effect secondary to this negative pressure. Ligation of the tube just proximal to the fimbriae does not interfere with pickup.(10) The cilia on the surface of the fimbriae have adhesive sites, and these seem to have prime responsibility for the initial movement of the egg into the tube. This movement is dependent upon the presence of follicular cells surrounding the egg, because removal of these cells prior to egg pickup prevents effective egg transport. In the ampulla of the tube the cilia beat in the direction of the uterus. In man and monkey this unidirectional beat is also found in the isthmus of the tube, whereas in the rabbit there are additional rows of cilia that beat in the direction of the ovary. The specific contribution of the cilia to egg transport in the ampulla and isthmus is an unresolved question. Most investigators have credited muscular contractions of the tubes as the primary force for moving the egg. Halbert et al showed in the rabbit, however, that interference with muscle contractility did not block egg transport.(11) They concluded that, in this species, cilia play a major role. Reversing a segment of the ampulla of the tube so that the cilia in this segment beat toward the ovary interferes with pregnancy in the rabbit without blocking fertilization. The fertilized ova are arrested when they come in contact with the transposed area.(12) This again suggests that ciliary beat is crucial for egg transport. Cilia play, in all likelihood, a less important role in the human. There are *fertile* women who have Kartagener's syndrome in which there is a congenital absence of dynein arms in cilia and, thus, the cilia do not beat. This deficiency in the cilia is found in the fallopian tubes as well as in the respiratory tract.(13)

Muscular contractions of the tube are associated with a to-and-fro movement of the eggs rather than with a continuous forward progression. In most species transport of the ovum through the tube requires approximately 3 days.(14) The time spent within the various parts of the tube varies from one species to another. Transport through the ampulla is rapid in the rabbit, whereas in women it requires 30 hours for the egg to reach the ampullary-isthmic junction. The egg remains at this point another 30 hours, at which time it begins rapid transport through the isthmus of the tube.

Attempts to modify tubal function as a method for understanding its physiology have involved three major pharmacologic approaches. These are: 1) altering levels of steroid hormones, 2) the interference with or supplementation of adrenergic stimuli, and 3) treatment with prostaglandins. Although there is an abundant literature on the effects of estrogen and progesterone on tubal function, it is clouded by the use of different hormones, different doses, and different timing of injections. Because of these variations it is difficult to obtain a coherent picture and to relate the experimental results to the in vivo situation. In general, pharmacologic doses of estrogen favor retention of eggs in the tube. This ''tube locking'' effect of estrogen can be partially reversed by treatment with progesterone.

The isthmus of the tube has an extensive adrenergic innervation. Surgical denervation of the tube, however, does not disrupt ovum transport. Prostaglandins (PG) of the E series relax tubal muscle, whereas those of the F series stimulate muscle activity of the tube. Although $PGF_{2\alpha}$ stimulates human oviductal motility in vivo, it does not cause acceleration of ovum transport.

The effect on fertility of removal of different segments of the tube has been reviewed by Pauerstein and Eddy, who noted that excision of the ampullary-isthmic junction in rabbits did not block fertility.(15) This is equally true if small segments of the ampulla are removed, and pregnancy can occur even if the entire isthmus and uterotubal junction are excised. Although the fimbriae are thought to play a crucial role in fertility, spontaneous pregnancies have been reported following sterilization by fimbriectomy or following surgical repair of tubes whose fimbriated ends had been excised. (16,17)

In most species, a period of residence in the tube appears to be a prerequisite for full development. Rabbit eggs can be fertilized in the uterus, but they do not develop unless transferred to the tubes within 3 hours of fertilization.(18) This and other work imply that there may be a component in uterine fluid during the first 48 hours following ovulation that is toxic to the egg.(18) Indirect evidence of an inhospitable environment is also provided by studies indicating that there must be synchrony between development of the endometrium and the egg for successful pregnancy to occur.(19) If the endometrium is in a more advanced stage of development than the egg, fertility is compromised. These studies, done in animals, may not be relevant to the human.

Successful pregnancies have occurred in the human following the Estes procedure, in which the ovary is transposed to the uterine cornua.(20) Eggs are ovulated directly into the uterus, completely bypassing the tube. Moreover, when fertilized donor eggs are transferred to women who are on hormone supplementation, there are a number of days during the treatment cycle when the blastocysts will

502

implant.(21) This crucial difference between animal and human physiology is of more than academic importance. There has been speculation concerning the use of drugs that could accelerate tubal transport, as a means of providing contraception by ensuring that the egg would reach the uterus when it was in an unreceptive state. Although this may work in animals, it is of doubtful value in the human because perfect synchrony is not required.

Animal and human reproduction also differ in the occurrence of ectopic pregnancy. Ectopic pregnancies are rare in animals, and in rodents they are not induced even if the uterotubal junction is occluded immediately following fertilization. The embryos reach the blastocyst stage and then degenerate.

Fertilization

Following ovulation, the fertilizable life-span of the rabbit egg is between 6 and 8 hours. The fertilizable life of the human ovum is unknown, but most estimates range between 12 and 24 hours. However, immature human eggs recovered for in vitro fertilization can be fertilized even after 36 hours of incubation. Equally uncertain is knowledge of the fertilizable life-span of human sperm. The most common estimate is 48 hours, although motility can be maintained after the sperm have lost the ability to fertilize. Contact of sperm with the egg, which occurs in the ampulla of the tube, appears to be random, and there is no current evidence that the egg lures sperm to its surface.

Despite the evolution from external to internal fertilization over a period of about 100 million years, many of the mechanisms have remained the same.(22) The acellular zona pellucida that surrounds the egg at ovulation and remains in place until implantation, has two major functions in the fertilization process:

1. It contains receptors for sperm which are, with some exceptions, relatively species-specific; and

2. It undergoes the *zona reaction* in which the zona becomes impervious to other sperm once the fertilizing sperm penetrates, and thus it provides a bar to polyploidy. (23)

Penetration through the zona is rapid and possibly is mediated by acrosin, a trypsin-like proteinase which is bound to the inner acrosomal membrane of the sperm.(24) The pivotal role assigned to acrosin has been disputed. For example, manipulations that increase the resistance of the zona to acrosin do not interfere with sperm penetration and thus, sperm motility may be the critical factor.

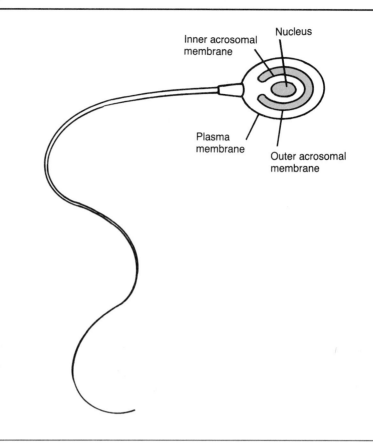

The acrosome is a lysosome-like organelle in the anterior region of the sperm head, lying just beneath the plasma membrane. The acrosome contains a variety of enzymes which are exposed by the *acrosome reaction*. This reaction is characterized by the influx of sodium and calcium ions, the efflux of hydrogen ion, an increase in pH, and fusion of the plasma membrane with the outer acrosomal membrane, leading to the exposure of the enzymes contained on the inner acrosomal membrane. Binding to the zona pellucida is required to permit a component of the zona to induce the acrosomal reaction. This component is believed to be a glycoprotein sperm receptor, which thus serves a dual function.

The initiation of the block to penetration of the zona (and the vitellus) by other sperm is mediated by the *cortical reaction*, a release of materials from the cortical granules, lysosome-like organelles which are found just below the egg surface.(25) As with other lysosome-like organelles, these materials include various hydrolytic enzymes. Changes brought about by these enzymes lead to the *zona reaction*, the hardening of the extracellular layer and inactivation of sperm receptors. Thus the zona block to polyspermy is accomplished.

The second polar body is released at the time of fertilization and leaves the egg with a haploid complement of chromosomes. The addition of chromosomes from the sperm restores the diploid number to the now fertilized egg.

The postacrosomal region of the sperm head makes initial contact with the vitelline membrane (the egg plasma membrane). At first the egg membrane engulfs the sperm head, and subsequently there is fusion of egg and sperm membranes. This fusion will occur only with sperm which have undergone the acrosome reaction. The chromatin material of the sperm head decondenses and the male pronucleus is formed. The male and the female pronuclei migrate toward each other, and as they move into close proximity the limiting membranes break down, and a spindle is formed on which the chromosomes become arranged. Thus, the stage is set for the first cell division.

The clinician is interested not only in how normal fertilization takes place, but also in the occurrence of abnormal events that can interfere with pregnancy. It is worthwhile, therefore, to consider the failures that occur in association with in vivo fertilization. Studies in the nonhuman primate have involved monkeys and baboons. A surgical method was used to flush the uterus of regularly cycling rhesus monkeys, and 9 preimplantation embryos and 2 unfertilized eggs were recovered from 22 flushes. Two of the 9 embryos were morphologically abnormal and probably would not have implanted.[26] Hendrickx and Kraemer used a similar technique in the baboon and recovered 23 embryos, of which 10 were morphologically abnormal.[27] This suggests that in nonhuman primates some ovulated eggs are not fertilized and that many early embryos are abnormal and, in all likelihood, will be aborted. Similar findings have been reported in the human in the classic study of Hertig et al.[28] They examined 34 early embryos recovered by flushing and examination of reproductive organs removed at surgery. Ten of these embryos were morphologically abnormal, including 4 of the 8 preimplantation embryos. Because the 4 preimplantation losses would not have been recognized clinically, there would have been 6 losses recorded in the remaining 30 pregnancies.

Using sensitive pregnancy tests, it has been suggested that approximately 25-40% of conceptions may be lost before they are clinically perceived. There is evidence for biologic selection against abnormal gametes and embryos throughout the reproductive process. Morphologically abnormal sperm are less successful than normal sperm in penetrating cervical mucus and in negotiating the uterotubal junction.[29] This selection does not seem to be operative against chromosomally abnormal sperm that are morphologically normal. Another protective mechanism is the attrition of sperm numbers that occurs between the vagina and the area of the tube that contains the egg. With only a small number of sperm making contact with the egg, there may be a decreased chance for penetration of the egg by more than one sperm.

In the postimplantation period, if only clinically diagnosed pregnancies are considered, the generally accepted figure for spontaneous abortion in the first 4–20 weeks is 15%. Approximately 50-60% of these abortions have chromosome abnormalities.[30] This suggests that a minimum of 7.5% of all human conceptions are chromosomally abnormal. The fact that only 1 in 200 newborns has a chromosome abnormality attests to the powerful selection mechanisms operating in early human gestation.

| In Vitro Fertilization and Embryo Loss | A number of the in vivo protective mechanisms are not present during in vitro fertilization. The filtering effect of the cervical mucus and the uterotubal junction is not available to remove grossly abnormal sperm. In most in vitro experiments, relatively large numbers of sperm are placed in the vicinity of the egg, and this may increase the risk for penetration of the egg by more than one sperm. The zona blocking mechanisms are efficient enough, however, to prevent this from becoming a serious clinical problem. |

The relatively low percentage of pregnancies achieved with in vitro fertilization to date is explainable to some extent by the high rate of embryo loss associated even with in vivo fertilization. This alone, however, does not completely account for the current results. Many of the losses result following transfer of embryos, and in some animals, this process is associated with a 50% embryo mortality. With increased experience the results should improve. It is clear, however, that there is a need for further understanding of the fertilization process and of implantation, before we can feel confident that the in vitro environment is as physiologic as possible.

Implantation

Implantation is defined as the process by which an embryo attaches to the uterine wall and penetrates first the epithelium and then the circulatory system of the mother. It is a process that is limited in both time and space. Implantation begins 2-3 days after the fertilized egg enters the uterus, and is marked initially by apposition of the blastocyst to the uterine epithelium. A prerequisite for this contact is a loss of the zona pellucida, which, in vitro, can be ruptured by contractions and expansions of the blastocyst. In vivo this activity is less critical, as the zona can be lysed by components of the uterine fluid. The exact nature and function of these components and related proteins which are thought to mediate the implantation process (implantation-initiating factor, uteroglobin and blastokinin) are uncertain. Their production is, however, known to be dependent upon secretion of ovarian steroid hormones.(31) Even if the hormonal milieu and protein composition of the uterine fluid are hospitable to the implantation, it may not occur if the embryo is not at the proper stage of development. It has been inferred from this information that there must be developmental maturation of the surface of the embryo before it is able to achieve attachment and implantation.

Reports on changes in the surface charge of preimplantation embryos differ in their findings and it is unlikely that changes in surface charge are solely responsible for adherence of the embryo to the surface of epithelial cells. Binding of the lectin concanavalin A to the embryo changes during the preimplantation period, an indication that the surface glycoproteins of the embryo are in transition.(32) It is reasonable to assume that these changes in configuration on the surface occur in order to enhance the ability of the embryo to adhere to the maternal surface.

As the embryo comes into close contact with the endometrium, the microvilli on the surface flatten and interdigitate with those on the luminal surface of the epithelial cells. A stage is reached where the cell membranes are in very close contact and junctional complexes are formed. The embryo can no longer be dislodged from the surface of the epithelial cells by flushing the uterus with physiological solutions. Schlafke and Enders described 3 types of subsequent interactions between the implanting trophoblast and the uterine epithelium.(33) In the first, trophoblast cells intrude between uterine epithelial cells on their path to the basement membrane. In the second type of interaction, the epithelial cells lift off the basement membrane, an action which allows the trophoblast to insinuate itself underneath the epithelium. Lastly, fusion of trophoblast with individual uterine epithelial cells has been identified by electron microscopy in the rabbit.(34) This latter method of gaining entry into the epithelial layer raises interesting questions concerning the immunologic consequences of mixing embryonic and maternal cytoplasm.

Trophoblast has the ability to phagocytose a variety of cells, but in vivo this activity seems largely confined to removal of dead endometrial cells, or cells that have been sloughed from the uterine wall. Similarly, despite the invasive nature of the trophoblast, destruction of maternal cells by enzymes secreted by the embryo does not seem to play a major role in implantation. The embryo does secrete a variety of enzymes, and these may be important for digesting the intercellular matrix that holds the epithelial cells together. Studies in vitro have demonstrated the presence of plasminogen activator in mouse embryos, and its activity is important in the attachment and early outgrowth stages of implantation. (35)

The embryo at a somewhat later stage of implantation can digest, in vitro, a complex matrix composed of glycoproteins, elastin and collagen, all of which are components of the normal intercellular matrix.(36) Additional studies in vitro have shown that cells move away from trophoblast in a process called ''contact inhibition.''(37) Trophoblast then spreads to fill the spaces vacated by the co-cultured cells. Once the intracellular matrix has been lysed, this movement of epithelial cells away from trophoblast would allow space for the implanting embryo to move through the epithelial layer. Trophoblast movement is aided by the fact that only parts of its surface are adhesive, and the major portion of the surface is nonadhesive to other cells.

Invasion by the trophoblast is limited by the formation of the decidual cell layer in the uterus. Fibroblast-like cells in the stroma are transformed into glycogen and lipid-rich cells. In the human, decidual cells surround blood vessels late in the nonpregnant cycle, but extensive decidualization does not occur until pregnancy is established. Ovarian steroids govern decidualization, and in the human a combination of estrogen and progesterone is critical. In animals, implantation is preceded by an increase in uterine stromal capillary permeability at the precise site where the blastocyst will attach. The localized nature of this reaction and of decidualization in rodents raises the possibility that a signal from the embryo might be an important triggering stimulus. Thus, maternal recognition of and preparation for pregnancy may depend upon receiving signals released by the embryo.

Boving suggested that the release of CO_2 by the embryo in the form of bicarbonate raises the pH of the embryo surface, which, in turn, increases its stickiness.(38) CO_2 may also act as a signal to induce a decidual response in the mother.

507

Another role for the embryo in initiating implantation has been demonstrated in pigs.(39) The pig blastocyst synthesizes estrogen starting on day 12 of pregnancy, which is 6 days before definitive attachment to the uterine wall occurs. The estrogen can feedback on the pituitary to promote LH secretion, which is essential for maintenance of the corpus luteum.

The human conceptus produces HCG about the time of implantation on day 6 of pregnancy. The exact timing of the release in terms of whether it begins before or after the embryo enters the epithelium is uncertain. Function of the corpus luteum is crucial during the first 7-9 weeks of pregnancy, and luteectomy early in pregnancy can precipitate abortion.(40) Similarly, early pregnancy loss in primates can be induced by injections of anti-HCG serum.(41)

In rodents, implantation can be interrupted by injection of prostaglandin inhibitors. Kennedy showed that indomethacin prevented the increase in endometrial vascular permeability normally seen just prior to implantation.(42) Additional evidence for a role by prostaglandins in the earliest stages of implantation is the finding of increased concentrations of the drug at prospective implantation sites. The source or sources of the prostaglandins is not known. Rabbit blastocysts contain prostaglandins, but there is no evidence of significant prostaglandin production by rat blastocysts in vitro. The endometrial cells are a likely source of prostaglandin, and its synthesis may be stimulated by the tissue damage that accompanies implantation.

Shelesnyak suggested that histamine initiated the decidual response.(43) He found that antihistamines given systemically or directly into the uterus prevented the decidual response in rats. This was disputed when other workers found that systemic antihistamines were not effective in preventing the decidual response. However, it has been shown that there are two different receptors for histamines, H1 and H2. These are not blocked by the same agents, and early experiments demonstrating a lack of effect of antihistamines may have utilized only a block to one receptor. Brandon and Wallis blocked both receptors in rats and found a decrease in the number of implantation sites.(44) Mast cells in the uterus are a major source of histamine, but it is possible that the embryo can also synthesize histamine.(45) This would explain why the increase in capillary permeability and decidualization in the endometrium is localized to areas near the implanting embryo.

One of the great mysteries associated with implantation is the mechanism by which the mother rejects a genetically abnormal embryo or fetus. It is possible that the abnormal embryo cannot produce a signal in early pregnancy that can be recognized by the mother.

The embryonic signals will be effective only in a proper hormone milieu. Much of the knowledge concerning the hormone requirements for implantation in animals has been gained from studies of animals in delayed implantation. In a number of species, preimplantation embryos normally lie dormant in the uterus for periods of time which may extend for as long as 15 months before implantation is initiated. In other species, delayed implantation can be imposed by postpartum suckling or by performing ovariectomy on day 3 of pregnancy. This produces a marked decrease in synthesis of DNA and protein by the blastocyst. The embryo can be maintained at the blastocyst stage by injecting the mother with progesterone. Using this model, hormonal requirements for implantation have been determined. In mice there is a requirement for estrogen and progesterone followed by estrogen, which initiates implantation. In other species the nidatory stimulus of estrogen is not required, and progesterone alone is sufficient.

Although it is known that the the hormone milieu of delayed implantation renders the embryo quiescent, it is not known whether this represents a direct effect on the embryo or whether there is a metabolic inhibitor present in uterine secretions that acts upon the embryo. Removal of the embryo from the uterus in delay to culture dishes allows rapid resumption of normal metabolism, suggesting that there has, in fact, been a release from the inhibitory effects of a uterine product.(46)

Unanswered Questions

Why is gamete production so wasteful? Billions of sperm are produced, but only a few are ever successful in fertilizing an egg. Does it relate to early forms of reproduction—for example, those in fish, where the sperm are released into the sea and large numbers are needed to assure that a few reach the egg? Does the overpopulation of sperm allow selection processes to take place ensuring that the more abnormal sperm are filtered out before the tube is reached? In the female approximately 350 ova are ovulated during a woman's life, yet the ovaries contain over a million eggs at birth.

What is the purpose of capacitation? Is it needed to overcome the protective mechanisms that have been built into the sperm, specifically those that prevent premature release of acrosomal enzymes. Penetration by sperm of the egg is desirable, but invasion of other maternal cells might trigger immunologic reactions against sperm. Does capacitation free the sperm from some inhibitors, thus allowing the hypermotility that may be needed for zona penetration?

Why are there so many abnormal embryos? Current estimates are that 50% of embryos do not survive to term. Why is there a high rate of embryo loss, and, specifically, why is there a high selection against abnormal embryos? Is it because of intrinsic programming defects within the embryo, or to an inability of the embryo to produce a signal recognized by the mother; or does the maternal organism in some way recognize abnormality and react against it?

Why has embryo transfer in the human following in vitro fertilization resulted in a low number of takes? Can the uterine environment be manipulated in such a way as to increase successful implantation of in vitro fertilization eggs?

References

1. **Sobrero AJ, MacLeod J,** The immediate postcoital test, Fertil Steril 13:184, 1962.

2. **Bedford JM,** The rate of sperm passage into the cervix after coitus in the rabbit, J Reprod Fertil 25:211, 1971.

3. **Settlage DSF, Motoshima M, Tredway DR,** Sperm transport from the external cervical os to the fallopian tubes in women: a time and quantitation study, Fertil Steril 24:655, 1973.

4. **Overstreet JW, Cooper GW,** Rabbit sperm do not survive rapid transport through the female reproductive tract, Ninth Annual Meeting of the Society for the Study of Reproduction, Philadelphia, August 10-13, 1976, (abstract).

5. **Ahlgren M,** Sperm transport to and survival in the human fallopian tube, Gynecol Invest 6:206, 1975.

6. **Bedford JM,** Sperm capacitation and fertilization in mammals, Biol Reprod Suppl 2:128, 1970.

7. **Yanagimachi R,** Fertilization in *In Vitro fertilization and embryo transfer,* Crosignani PG, Rubin BL, editors, Academic Press, London, 1983.

8. **Overstreet J,** Transport of gametes in the reproductive tract of the female mammal, in *Mechanism and Control of Animal Fertilization,* Hartmann, JF, editor, Academic Press, New York, 1983.

9. **Sharma V, Mason B, Riddle A, Campbell S,** Peritoneal oocyte and sperm transfer, Fifth World Congress on In Vitro Fertilization and Embryo Transfer, Norfolk, Virginia, April 5-10, 1987, (abstract).

10. **Clewe TH, Mastroianni L,** Mechanisms of ovum pickup: I. Functional capacity of rabbit oviducts ligated near the fimbriae, Fertil Steril 9:13, 1958.

11. **Halbert SA, Tam PY, Blandau RJ,** Egg transport in the rabbit oviduct: the roles of cilia and muscle, Science 191:1052, 1976.

12. **Eddy CA, Flores JJ, Archer DR, Pauerstein CJ,** The role of cilia in infertility: an evaluation by selective microsurgical modification of the rabbit oviduct, Am J Obstet Gynecol 132:814, 1978.

13. **Jean Y, Langlais J, Roberts KD, Chapdelaine A, Bleau G,** Fertility of a woman with nonfunctional ciliated cells in the fallopian tubes, Fertil Steril 31:349, 1979.

14. **Croxatto HB, Ortiz MS,** Egg transport in the fallopian tube, Gynecol Invest 6:215, 1975.

15. **Pauerstein CJ, Eddy CA,** The role of the oviduct in reproduction; Our knowledge and our ignorance, J Reprod Fertil 55:223, 1979.

16. **Tompkins P,** Letter to the editor, Fertil Steril 31:696, 1979.

17. **Novy MJ,** Reversal of Kroener fimbriectomy sterilization, Am J Obstet Gynecol 137:198, 1980.

18. **Glass RH,** Fate of rabbit eggs fertilized in the uterus, J Reprod Fertil 31:139, 1972.

19. **Adams CE,** Consequences of accelerated ovum transport, including a re-evaluation of Estes' operation, J Reprod Fertil 55:239, 1979.

20. **Ikle FA,** Pregnancy after implantation of the ovary into the uterus, Gynaecologia 151:95, 1961.

21. **Rosenwaks Z,** The donor oocyte program in Norfolk, Fifth World Congress on In Vitro Fertilization and Embryo Transfer, Norfolk, Virginia, April 5-10, 1987, (abstract).

22. **Wassarman PM,** The biology and chemistry of fertilization, Science 235:553, 1987.

23. **Hartmann JF, Gwatkin RBL,** Alteration of sites on the mammalian sperm surface following capacitation, Nature 234:479, 1971.

24. **Zaneveld LJD, Polakoski KL, Williams WL,** Properties of a proteolytic enzyme from rabbit sperm acrosomes, Biol Reprod 6:30, 1972.

25. **Barros C, Yanagimachi R,** Induction of zona reaction in golden hamster eggs by cortical granule material, Nature 233:2368, 1971.

26. **Hurst PR, Jefferies K, Eckstein P, Wheeler AG,** Recovery of uterine embryos in rhesus monkeys, Biol Reprod 15:429, 1976.

27. **Hendrickx AG, Kraemer DC,** Preimplantation stages of baboon embryos Anat Rec 162:111, 1968.

28. **Hertig AT, Rock J, Adams EC, Menkin MC,** Thirty-four fertilized ova, good, bad and indifferent from 210 women of known fertility, Pediatrics 23:202, 1959.

29. **Krzanowska H,** The passage of abnormal spermatozoa through the uterotubal junction of the mouse, J Reprod Fertil 38:81, 1974.

30. **Short RV,** When a conception fails to become a pregnancy, in *Maternal Recognition of Pregnancy*, Whelan J, editor, *Ciba Foundation Symposium 64* (NS), Excerpta Medica, Amsterdam, 1979.

31. **Beier HM, Mootz U,** Significance of Maternal Uterine Proteins in the Establishment of Pregnancy, in *Material Recognition of Pregnancy*, Whelan J, editor, *Ciba Foundation Symposium 64* (NS), Excerpta Medica, Amsterdam, 1979.

32. **Sobel JS, Nebel L,** Changes in concanavalin A agglutinability during development of the inner cell mass and trophoblast of mouse blastocyst in vitro, J Reprod Fertil 52:239, 1978.

33. **Schlafke S, Enders AC,** Cellular basis of interaction between trophoblast and uterus at implantation, Biol Reprod 12:41, 1975.

34. **Larsen JF,** Electron microscopy of the implantation site in the rabbit, Am J Anat 109:319, 1961.

35. **Strickland S, Reich E, Sherman MI,** Plasminogen activator in early embryogenesis: enzyme production by trophoblast and parietal endoderm, Cell 9:231, 1976.

36. **Glass RH, Aggeler J, Spindle A, Pedersen RA, Werb Z,** Degradation of extracellular matrix by mouse trophoblast outgrowths: A model for implantation, J Cell Biol 96:1108, 1983.

511

37. **Glass RH, Spindle AI, Pedersen RA,** Mouse embryo attachment to substratum and the interaction of trophoblast with cultured cells, J Exp Zool 203:327, 1979.

38. **Boving BG,** Implantation, Ann NY Acad Sci 75:700, 1959.

39. **Heap RB, Flint AP, Gadsby JE,** Embryonic signals that establish pregnancy, Brit Med Bull 35:129, 1979.

40. **Csapo AI, Pulkkinen MO, Wiest WO,** Effects of luteectomy and progesterone replacement therapy in early pregnant patients, Am J Obstet Gynecol 115:759, 1973.

41. **Stevens VC,** Potential control of fertility in women by immunization with HCG, Res Reprod 7:1, 1975.

42. **Kennedy TG,** Evidence for a role for prostaglandins in the initiation of blastocyst implantation in the rat, Biol Reprod 16:286, 1977.

43. **Shelesnyak MC,** Inhibition of decidual cell formation in the pseudopregnant rat by histamine antagonists, Am J Physiol 170:522, 1952.

44. **Brandon JM, Wallis RM,** Effect of mepyramine, a histamine H_1-, and burimamide, a histamine H_2- receptor antagonist, on ovum implantation in the rat, J Reprod Fertil 50:251, 1977.

45. **Dey SK, Johnson DC, Santos JG,** Is histamine production by the blastocyst required for implantation in the rabbit? Biol Reprod 21:1169, 1979.

46. **Psychoyos A,** Hormonal requirements for egg implantation, in *Advances in the Biosciences 4,* Raspe G, editor, Pergamon Press, Oxford, 1970.

17 Investigation of the Infertile Couple

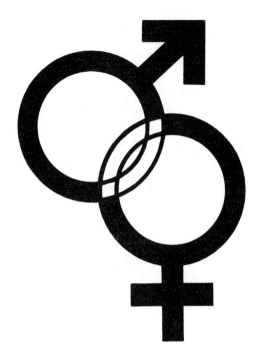

Infertility is defined as 1 year of unprotected coitus without conception. It affects approximately 10-15% of couples which makes it an important component of the practices of many physicians.(1) Infertile couples are older, more likely to be black, and to have had no previous children. The risk is doubled for women 35-44 compared to women 30-34.

The Epidemiology of Infertility

During 1982, nearly one in 5 ever-married women of reproductive age reported that they had sought professional help during their lifetimes because of infertility.(2) A sharp escalation of demand for infertility services began in 1981.(3) From approximately 600,000 visits in 1968, the total increased to nearly 1 million in the early 70's, then in the early 80's, the total went over 2 million.

An appreciation for the change in the demography of infertility only can be gained by understanding the changes taking place in fertility.(4) The first U.S. census was in 1790. At that time, the birth rate was 55 per 1,000 population, almost 8 births per woman. Two hundred years later, it is 15.5 per 1,000 population, 1.8 births per woman. Post World War II, the total fertility rate increased, reaching a high of 3.8 births per woman, the so-called baby boom.

513

In the United States, women now are likely to have 2 children as compared with 3 or more for their mothers, but about the same as their grandmothers. Women now complete their families in about 7 years as compared to 10 years for their mothers.

This change in fertility has a significant impact on our future. Improvements in mortality will have little impact on our population, because this effect on our older population will not balance the changes taking place with the reproductive potential of our country. Immigration does have an effect. Currently 500,000 people legally immigrate to the U.S. per year, while 100,000 people leave.

Our population will become stable in the middle of the next century. Without immigration, our population would decline. With our current situation, the percent of people over age 65 will grow from 12% in 1985 to 23.5% over the next 100 years. It is highly probable that fertility is destined to remain low, and therefore, our major problems will include dealing with aging and a decreasing work force.

There are some obvious and some speculative explanations for the decline in U.S. fertility.(5,6)

POPULAR EXPLANATIONS FOR THE DECLINE IN U.S. FERTILITY

—Changing roles and aspirations for women
—Postponement of marriage
—Delayed age of childbearing
—Increasing use of contraception
—Liberalized abortion
—Concern over environment
—Unfavorable economic conditions

Results from the 1980 U.S. Current Population Survey indicate that the factors which emerged in the 70's and affected the level of fertility continue to be important. (7) The deferment of marriage is a significant change in our society. In 1960, 28% of women 20-24 were single; in 1985, 58.5%. In 1960, 10% of women 25-29 were single; in 1985, 26%. But only 16% of the decline in the total fertility rate is accounted for by the increase in the average age at first marriage; 83% of the decline in total fertility rate is accounted for by changes in marital fertility rates. In other words, postponement of pregnancy in marriage is the more significant change. (4-6) The mean age at first birth is now 3 years older than that for women born 2 decades earlier.

Aging and Fertility

Deferment of marriage and first birth means that the factor of age must be considered. The classic study is that of the Hutterites.(8) The Hutterites live in the Dakotas, Montana, and the adjacent parts of Canada. The sect originated in Switzerland in 1528, and practically all of the living Hutterites came to South Dakota in the 1870's. From 4 colonies of 443 Hutterites in 1880, by 1950, there were 93 colonies containing 8,542 Hutterites. Contraception is condemned, and because of the communal arrangement of their society, there is no incentive to limit the size of their families—all families are provided for equally.

In the 1950's, Joseph Eaton of Western Reserve University studied the Hutterites, focusing on the incidence of mental disorders. He provided his demographic data to Tietze who analyzed the fertility rates.(8) Only 5 of 209 women had no children for an infertility rate of 2.4%, BUT IT TOOK 20.7 YEARS OF MARRIAGE TO ACHIEVE THIS LOW INCIDENCE. The average age of the last pregnancy was 40.9 years, and there was a definite increase in the infertility rate with age.

Pregnancies averaged 9.8 per mother. There were 22 pregnancies in the 45-49 age group, and 117 pregnancies during ages 40-44. The fertility of the Hutterites has become a living legend in its own demographic time. The total fertility rate of the Hutterites is used as an example of how high fertility can be when a population is healthy, stable, and not using contraception. Using their data, it can be concluded that a population which marries relatively late, has some lactational amenorrhea, and some age-related and parity-related decline in coitus, can produce 11 live births per married woman. If marriage were early, there were no lactational amenorrhea, and no sterilization or decline in coitus, the total fertility rate would be about 15 live births per woman.(9)

The oldest pregnancy in modern times (according to The Guinness Book of World Records) occurred in a woman from Portland, Oregon, who delivered when she was 57 years and 120 days old. In older times, a Scottish woman was reported to have delivered 6 children after the age of 47, the last at age 62!(10)

Recent American data support evidence for a decline of fecundity with advancing age.(11) In data from 1976, 34-46% of women age 35 and older were unable to become pregnant. Unfortunately, there are demographic data to support the contention that one contributing factor to this decline is a decrease with aging in the frequency of sexual intercourse.(12)

The French studied the pregnancy rate in a donor insemination program, including only women with azoospermic husbands. The decrease in conception rate per cycle was not great, but it was significant after 30 years of age, and then it accelerated after age 35.(13) Below the age of 31 the pregnancy rate was 74%; this decreased to 62% at ages 31 to 35 and to 54% when the women were older than 35. An American study with artificial insemination with donors also documented a decreasing conception rate with increasing maternal age. (14)

In at least 10 different populations, the decline of fertility among married couples with advancing age has been repeatedly documented. *It is safe to say that about one-third of women who defer pregnancy until the mid to late 30's will have an infertility problem.*

The mechanisms for decreased fertility with aging are not clear. The increased incidence of anovulation associated with age and the effects of aging on oocytes could act synergistically with uterine factors to cause a decline in fertility. In addition, as women enter their 30's, there is a greater likelihood of being affected by a number of diseases, for example endometriosis, that can interfere with

515

fertility. Cumulative exposures to occupational or environmental hazards also could lessen fertility as a woman ages. Additional factors that have contributed to an increase in infertility at all ages are the spread of sexually transmitted diseases with their damaging effect on the fallopian tube, and pelvic inflammation secondary to IUD use.

Certainly the aging of the reproductive system plays a role, but spontaneous abortion is a major factor. The majority of early abortions after age 35 are due to autosomal trisomies, the incidence of which increases with maternal age. Indeed, spontaneous abortion related just to age is the most outstanding risk for an older woman who becomes pregnant, increasing from about 10% until age 30, to 18% in the late 30's, and 34% in the early 40's.(15)

The impact of this decline in fertility with age is best appreciated by relating it to the changing demography of our country. The highest ever number of births in the U.S. occurred between 1947 and 1965—the baby boom. Women born in this period won't be reaching their 45th birthday until around 2010. For approximately a 30 year period, therefore, there will be an unprecedented number of women in the later child-bearing years. It is estimated that the number of women ages 35-49 will increase 61% between 1982 and 1995. The proportion of births accounted for by this group of women will increase by about 72%, from 5% in 1982 to 8.6% in 2000.(16)

Concern with Infertility

The percent of married couples who were infertile increased significantly among women 20-24, from 3.6% in 1965 to 10.6% in 1982, probably a reflection, at least in part, of increases in sexually transmitted diseases, but the percentage did not change significantly in the other age groups.(17)

Thus there have been no dramatic changes in the proportion of infertile couples since 1965. About 1 in 7 couples are infertile at age 30-34; about 1 in 5 at age 35-39; and about 1 in 4 at age 40-44. In 1982, 8.5% of all currently married couples in the United States with a wife in childbearing age were considered infertile. Eliminating those who were surgically sterile, the percentage was 13.9%.(18)

Why then is there this increasing concern for infertility? First, although the proportion of married couples considered infertile has shown no recent dramatic change, there is an increasing number of infertile couples. The aging of the baby boom generation is yielding a greater number of women who are delaying marriage and childbirth. The decision to defer childbearing has several important impacts: the problem of achieving a pregnancy later in life, the problem of being pregnant later in life, and the need for effective contraception. Combine this with the increase in sexually transmitted diseases, the possible exposure to toxins in work and the environment, and we have an increase in age-specific infertility rates. Furthermore, these couples, pressed for time, have a desire to get pregnancies accomplished in a shorter period of time.

There is a greater awareness of modern treatments and a greater ability to afford health care. The impact of widespread publicity is significant. Furthermore, the current effectiveness of the control of fertility allows more attention to be given to infertility. Also to be considered is the decreased supply of infants for adoption.

There is an increased availability of services. Membership in the American Fertility Society increased from 3,600 in 1974 to over 10,000 in 1988. The creation of the subspecialty of Reproductive Endocrinology by the American Board of Obstetrics and Gynecology has filled the country with expertise. There is a greater knowledge of the diagnosis and management of infertility among physicians.

Finally, infertility is now more socially acceptable as a problem. Consider the number of books available to the public, as well as the proliferation of self-help groups in this area.

The post World War II baby boom generation has faced an unique evolutionary change. They were the first to be able to exercise control over their fertility, and then as they aged and deferred pregnancy, they had to deal with the problem of unintended infertility. Because many American couples defer pregnancy and then desire their families within a condensed interval of time, there is a growing demand for infertility services.

When is a medical success really a success? There is an incidence of spontaneous pregnancy. About one-half of couples presenting after one year of infertility can be expected to become pregnant spontaneously in the following year. In an English study, only 20% of women who had failed to have a birth within the first 2 years of marriage never had a child.[19] In a life-table analysis of 58 untreated apparently normal infertile couples, 74% were pregnant by 2 years; however normal couples achieve this rate in 9 months.[20]

One of the important missions for the infertility physician is not necessarily to take credit for achieving a pregnancy, but to speed up the period of time required for that achievement. For couples in their 30's, the recommendation to seek help promptly is valid—the sooner a problem is detected, the better.

The Role of the Physician

In response to this need physicians should have four goals in mind:

1. The first goal is to seek out and to correct the causes of infertility. With proper evaluation and therapy, the majority of the women attending an infertility clinic will become pregnant.

2. The second goal is to provide accurate information for the couple and to dispel the misinformation commonly gained from friends and mass media. A few of the myths concerning infertility are detailed at the end of this chapter.

3. The third goal is to provide emotional support for the couple during a trying period. The inability to conceive generates a feeling in many couples that they have lost control over a very significant segment of their lives. That burden is aggravated by the additional impositions generated by the manipulations that couples have to undergo during the infertility investigation, including the need to have intercourse on schedule. Couples need to have an opportunity to ventilate their concerns and dispel some of their fears. A valuable adjunct to the efforts of the physician are support groups for infertile couples such as those organized by RESOLVE:

> Resolve National Headquarters
> 5 Water Street
> Arlington, MA 02174

Meeting in groups allows individuals to realize that their problem is not unique, and it enables them to obtain information on how others cope with infertility. It must be emphasized that, while severe anxieties can interfere with ovulation and frequency of intercourse, there is no evidence that infertility is caused by the usual anxieties besetting a couple trying to conceive.

4. An often neglected goal is that of counseling a couple concerning the proper time to discontinue investigation and treatment. This is especially important in the 10% of couples with no known cause for their infertility. Despite the absence of pathology, couples with 4 years or more of infertility have a poor prognosis.

The Female Infertility Investigation

There are advantages to having the male present during the initial interview. He may contribute valuable historical information. It also gives the physician the opportunity to emphasize that both partners are involved in the infertility investigation. A male who has been acquainted at its inception with the physician's treatment of the infertility problem will be less reluctant, as time progresses, to ask for clarification of any aspect of the testing. This can prevent misunderstandings engendered when the male partner's only source of information is the woman. Early in the physician-couple interaction, frequency of coitus and possible sexual problems should be ascertained.

An excellent modern study in England indicated the following causes and frequencies of infertility in couples (these percentages may not be completely applicable to infertility in other countries): (21)

Unexplained	**—28% of infertile couples**
Sperm problem	**—21%**
Ovulatory failure	**—18%**
Tubal damage	**—14%**
Endometriosis	**— 6%**
Coital problems	**— 5%**
Cervical mucus	**— 3%**
Other male problems	**— 2%**

Failure to ovulate is the major problem in approximately 40% of women with infertility, another 30-50% have tubal pathology, and 10% or less have a cervical barrier to fertility. It should be noted that induced abortions do not influence subsequent pregnancy rates.(22) Fetal wastage is definitely higher in DES exposed women, and while there is still some uncertainty, evidence suggests that primary infertility is also more common.(23) Besides the well-known impact of smoking on pregnancy, there is a growing story that fecundity is reduced in men and women who smoke.(24)

Couples sometimes need to be aware that there is a normal time requirement. In each ovulatory cycle normal couples have only about a 25% chance of becoming pregnant. Guttmacher's classic table has been a standard since 1956.

Time Required for Conception (25)	
Months of Exposure	*% Pregnant*
3 months	57%
6 months	72%
1 year	85%
2 years	93%

Because the male factor accounts for approximately 40% of infertility in the United States, the examination of the semen should be an early diagnostic step in the investigation. (See Chapter 19) If abnormal, further diagnostic procedures in the woman should be deferred until decisions are reached regarding the man. If normal, attention is directed to the woman.

Postcoital Test

The postcoital test provides information both as to the receptivity of cervical mucus and the ability of sperm to reach and survive in the mucus. Estrogen levels peak just prior to ovulation and this provides maximal stimulation of the cervical glands. An outpouring of clear, watery mucus is fostered which may be of sufficient quantity to be noted by the woman. Earlier in the cycle when estrogen output is lower, and starting 2 to 3 days after ovulation when progesterone levels increase and counteract the estrogen, the mucus is thick, viscid, and opaque.

The postcoital test is performed around the time of the expected LH surge as determined by previous basal body temperature charts or by the length of prior cycles. Timing also can be obtained with ultrasound and LH monitoring but this is usually not necessary. Between 2 and 8 hours after coitus, cervical mucus is removed with a nasal polyp forcep or tuberculin syringe and examined for macroscopic and microscopic characteristics. A less than 2 hour interval between coitus and examination has been recommended as giving maximal information, but this early evaluation may be deceptive because complement dependent reactions in mucus which can immobilize sperm may not be apparent for a few hours. Others have suggested that a 16 to 24 hour interval provides a better assessment of sperm longevity and a study has indicated that there is no drop in the number of sperm at any time during the first 24 hours.(26) There are other indications, however, that the number of sperm does decrease after 8 hours, and this is more in keeping with our

519

experience. Therefore, we suggest that the couple have coitus in the morning or late at night, and that the test be performed 2 to 8 hours later. It is also suggested that the couple abstain from intercourse for 48 hours prior to the postcoital test.

The stretchability (spinnbarkeit) of the mucus at midcycle should be 8-10 cm or more. This characteristic can be assessed as the mucus is pulled from the cervix, or alternatively, by placing the mucus on a slide, covering it with a coverslip and then lifting the coverslip. At midcycle the mucus contains 95-98% water and should be watery, thin, clear, acellular, and abundant. When dried on a slide it should form a distinct fern pattern.

Fern Pattern

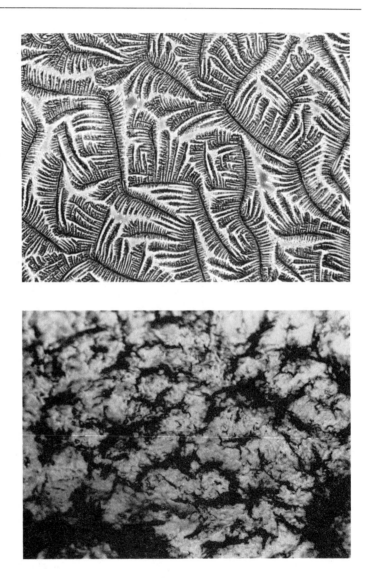

Lack of Fern

If the mucus is thick rather than thin, opaque instead of clear, the proximity of the test to ovulation should be determined by the onset of the next period (or by the temperature chart if one is being taken during that cycle). If poor mucus quality is related to inaccurate timing, the test should be repeated in the subsequent cycle. Poor mucus at midcycle is a physical barrier that decreases sperm penetration and requires alteration to enhance fertility. In one study 54% of women with good mucus became pregnant, compared to 37% with poor mucus, a statistically significant difference.(27) In all likelihood some of these poor tests were reflections of inaccurate timing, and pregnancies do occur even with poor mucus at ovulation time. Moreover, one study showed no difference in pregnancy rates between individuals with good or poor mucus.(28) It remains our impression, however, that poor mucus is associated with a decreased chance for fertility.

Treatment of poor mucus can be accomplished by giving 0.625 mg of conjugated estrogen daily for the 8 or 9 days preceding the expected time of ovulation. In a 28 day cycle that would be between days 5 and 13. There is no advantage to continuing the hormone treatment through the luteal phase of the cycle. If the initial treatment with estrogen fails to produce a change in the mucus, the dose is increased to 1.25 mg/day. In refractory cases 5 mg of conjugated estrogen has been given in conjunction with HCG. Guaifenesin, a mucolytic agent found in some over-the-counter cough syrups, also has been used to treat thick mucus. If there is evidence of chronic cervicitis with thick yellowish mucus, culture for chlamydia is important, and, where appropriate, systemic antibiotics should be used. On rare occasions the cervix is treated with electrocautery or cryosurgery.

Another tactic to overcome the barrier of thick cervical mucus is intrauterine insemination of sperm. (See Chapter 19) Normally, after coitus only the sperm enter the uterine cavity and semen remains in the vagina. Intrauterine insemination of even small amounts of semen can stimulate strong uterine contractions and produce an anaphylactic type reaction. For this reason the sperm should be washed and separated by the swimup method. The concentration and motility of the sperm should be rechecked prior to insemination. The intrauterine method allows direct introduction of bacteria into the uterus but with the use of the swimup technique overt tubal infections have not been a problem.

An alternative treatment for mucus utilizes stimulation with human menopausal gonadotropins (Pergonal) to enhance estrogen production, and, as a result, increased mucus formation occurs. This treatment is seldom warranted for this purpose because it is expensive and entails the risk of multiple births and ovarian hyperstimulation.

What constitutes a normal number of sperm in a postcoital test has been a matter of dispute. The estimates range from 1 to over 20/ high power field (HPF) and the majority of writers on the subject use 5 motile sperm/HPF as the lower limit of normal. In a study of the relationship between the postcoital test and the sperm penetration assay, it was found that for 0 to 4, 5 to 9, 10 to 19, or 20 or more motile sperm/HPF the sperm penetration assay means were 22.9, 30.6, 37.5, and 30.4% respectively.(29) One wonders if the individuals with 0 sperm per HPF had been excluded from the 0 to 4 sperm per HPF category, whether the difference between it and the 5 to 9 group would have been even less. This study does not provide convincing support for the use of 5 motile sperm/HPF as a cutoff.

More critical than the controversy over theoretical normal values is the question of what prognostic value the postcoital test has for the infertile couple. Collins et al could find no difference in the pregnancy rates between groups having no sperm, no motile sperm, 1 to 5 motile sperm, 6 to 10 motile sperm, and 11 or more motile sperm/HPF.(28) Another study showed that there was a statistically significant increase in the percentage of pregnancies only when there were more than 20 sperm/HPF.(27) There was no statistically significant difference in percentage of pregnancies between groups having 0, 1 to 5, 6 to 10, or 11 to 20 sperm/HPF. It would obscure the issue to call a postcoital test with 21 or more sperm/HPF "normal", suggesting that fewer than 21 is somehow abnormal. The former gives a better prognosis for pregnancy, but a substantial number of pregnancies occur even when no sperm are found in the postcoital test. This finding was substantiated by the results of a study of postcoital tests in *fertile* couples. Twenty percent had either no sperm or less than 1 sperm/HPF. (30)

Because of these findings and an observation that the number of sperm in the cervical mucus correlates with total motile sperm count some have questioned whether the PCT is of any value. Hull et al, however, reported that individuals with progressively motile sperm in the postcoital test had significantly higher pregnancy rates than those with no progressively motile sperm.(31) Another study found that intrauterine insemination enhanced the chances for pregnancy when there were 3 or less sperm/HPF but not when there were 5 or more sperm/HPF.(32) Thus a postcoital test can be of value in determining therapy.

In view of the somewhat contradictory findings, what useful information can be gleaned from the postcoital test? If the mucus is clear and abundant with good spinnbarkeit, the patient has a better chance for pregnancy than if it is thick and sparse. If sperm are found in the mucus it is reasonable assurance that coital technique is adequate. Normally sperm rapidly leave the semen pool and enter the cervical mucus. The semen is lost through the vaginal introitus or is broken down by vaginal enzymes. Women should be told that loss of semen is a normal occurrence and not a cause for infertility. If live sperm are found in the cervical mucus, the pH is not hostile and the pregnancy rate is higher than if the sperm are all immotile. If there are more than 20 sperm/HPF, the male, in all likelihood, has a sperm count above 20 million/ml and the couple has a significantly better chance for pregnancy than if the postcoital test contains fewer than 20 sperm/HPF. A poor result in the postcoital test can raise a suspicion of an immunologic problem and this is discussed below. A poor result also can suggest the need for intrauterine inseminations. Beyond this basic information little more can be obtained from the postcoital test. In our view, there is little advantage in having, for example, 10 sperm/HPF compared to having 1 sperm/HPF, although the former may be associated with a shorter time to conception.(31)

Attempts to refine the postcoital test by studying individual fractions from different levels in the cervical canal, with emphasis on the sample from the internal os, have not produced convincing evidence of value. Drake, Tredway, and Buchanan showed that sperm distribution is uniform throughout the cervical canal and that selective sampling at the level of the internal os is not necessary.(33)

One of the most difficult problems in infertility is the postcoital test which repeatedly shows no sperm or only dead sperm despite good mucus. The patient should be cautioned that lubricants such as K-Y Jelly and Surgilube have a spermicidal effect in vitro and should not be used by infertile couples. If lubrication is necessary, vegetable oil can be used without interfering with sperm movement. As noted earlier, re-examination of the husband's semen to check sperm count and motility is a necessity if the postcoital test is poor.

If the semen is normal, the pH of the cervical mucus at midcycle should be determined. Ansari, Gould and Ansari reported good results using a precoital douche of 1 tablespoon of sodium bicarbonate in 1 quart of water when a poor postcoital test was associated with a pH below 7. (34) Cervical cultures should be obtained for chlamydia if the mucus is yellowish and sperm antibody testing should be done in cases where there are no sperm or mostly nonmotile sperm without explanation. In addition, sperm antibody testing is mandatory when, in a postcoital test with good mucus, the sperm are found shaking in place but not moving progressively. This shaking movement is a common finding in immunologic infertility.

In vitro crosstesting utilizing donor or bovine mucus and donor sperm can help to determine whether the poor postcoital test is due to factors in the mucus or to defects in the sperm. A drop of the consort's sperm and a drop of donor sperm separately are placed in contact with the patient's mucus on a slide, and penetration of the mucus by the two specimens compared under a microscope. A similar test can be performed with donor mucus. A commercially available test, consisting of bovine cervical mucus in capillary tubes, can be substituted for donor mucus. In this test the sperm are allowed to swim into the capillary and the depth of penetration measured. Lastly, intrauterine inseminations can be offered for treatment.

A postcoital test cannot be considered a substitute for a semen analysis. While 21 or more sperm/HPF is almost always associated with a sperm count above 20 million/ml, the postcoital test gives little information concerning the morphology of sperm in the ejaculate. There are considerably fewer abnormal forms in the cervical mucus compared to the ejaculate. This may represent a filtering effect of the cervical mucus or may indicate that abnormal forms do not have the motility to penetrate the cervical mucus.

In addition to providing an evaluation of the mucus, the postcoital test also gives information concerning the male. Absence of sperm requires a review of the couple's coital technique. Repeated cancellations of appointments for the postcoital test may be a clue that there are sexual problems that have not been uncovered by the interview. More importantly, absence of sperm necessitates a detailed review of the semen specimen.

The need for scheduling the postcoital test at precise times in the cycle may produce problems for the couple who cannot have sex on demand. This may further burden a couple already troubled by the need to cope with their infertility and the loss of control involved in the infertility investigation. A physician must be sympathetic to this problem, and on occasion, precise timing must be sacrificed and the woman told to come into the office following unscheduled intercourse.

Hysterosalping-
ography

A history of pelvic inflammatory disease, septic abortion, intrauterine device (IUD) use, ruptured appendix, tubal surgery or ectopic pregnancy alerts the physician to the possibility of tubal damage. Almost one-half of patients who are eventually found to have tubal damage and/or pelvic adhesions, however, have no history of antecedent disease. There have been a few reports of damaged tubes showing histologic evidence of viral infection which could explain the absence of traditional causes of tubal damage.

The convenience of performing a Rubin's test with CO_2 in the office and the avoidance of radiation are outweighed by the discomfort of the test and the high percentage of false readings which suggest tubal occlusion. This test is now only of historical interest.

The hysterosalpingogram (HSG) has replaced the Rubin's test. The x-ray study is performed 2 to 5 days after cessation of a menstrual flow. If there is a history suggestive of pelvic inflammatory disease, a sedimentation rate is first obtained and, if elevated, antibiotic therapy is given. The procedure is then postponed for a month when a repeat sedimentation rate is obtained. Only if this is normal is the HSG scheduled. If masses or tenderness are revealed by the pelvic examination at any time, the HSG should be bypassed and the pelvis evaluated by laparoscopy. If there is a documented history of pelvic inflammatory disease, the risk of a serious reinfection following HSG is too high and it should be replaced by laparoscopy. If an HSG is done in a patient who is at questionable risk for infection, a water-soluble rather than an oil dye should be used because of the faster absorption. The antibiotics commonly employed for prophylaxis, tetracyclines and ampicillin, are relatively ineffective against the anaerobic bacteria which can be a major cause of the infrequent infections that can follow an HSG. The overall risk of infection with HSG is probably less than 1%, although in a high-risk population serious infection can occur in approximately 3% of cases.(35)

HSG should be done under image intensification fluoroscopy and a minimal number of films taken. Too often, multiple oblique views are taken to delineate minimal filling defects in the uterus which are of no clinical significance. In our experience the oblique films are of little help even in diagnosing tubal patency. Only 3 films are usually required—a preliminary before dye is injected, a film showing spill of dye from one or both tubes, and a delayed film to show spread of dye through the peritoneal cavity. It is advantageous if the gynecologist does the actual injection of the dye, but in most instances this is now done by the radiologist. The dye can be injected either using a classic Jarcho cannula with a single-tooth tenaculum, or a suction apparatus appended to the cervix and dye injected through a contained cannula. A third technique involves threading a pediatric Foley catheter through the cervix into the uterus. This is a relatively atraumatic method. The balloon on the catheter does, however, obscure portions of the uterine cavity. Use of a prostaglandin inhibitor which can be purchased over the counter and taken 30 minutes prior to the procedure can decrease the pain which many women experience with HSG.

The dye should be injected slowly so that abnormalities of the uterine cavity are not missed. This is of special importance in DES daughters, many of whom have abnormalities of uterine contour. Usually no more than 3 to 6 ml of dye are required to fill the uterus and tubes. If the patient complains of cramping, the injection of dye should be stopped for a few minutes and fluoroscopy temporarily discontinued. Spasm is rare with Ethiodol, an oil dye which is our preferred medium; if it does occur, slow injection with pauses may be helpful. If the tubes fill but dye droplets do not spill from the ends of the tubes, the uterus should be pushed up in the abdomen by means of the tenaculum or suction cup. This puts the tubes on stretch and may help to release dye from the fimbriated end. The droplets seen coming from the tube are the result of mixing of the oil dye and peritoneal fluid. On occasion, injection of dye into a hydrosalpinx will produce a similar pattern, and a delayed film to show loculation of dye is crucial in differentiating this condition from normal spill where the dye is distributed throughout the pelvis. If dye does not pass into the tubes, changing the woman to a prone position will sometimes facilitate passage of dye. (36)

If dye goes through one tube rapidly and fails to enter the other tube, it usually means that the dye-containing tube presents the path of least resistance. In this situation, the nonfilling tube is usually normal. When both tubes were patent on x-ray, the pregnancy rate in our own series was only slightly higher (58%) than when there was unilateral patency and nonfilling of the other tube (50%).

While the diagnostic usefulness of the HSG is established, its value as a therapeutic procedure in infertility is a subject of some controversy. Whitelaw et al (37) found no increase in the pregnancy rate following hysterosalpingography, whereas Palmer (38) reported that 75% of patients having an HSG showing tubal patency, and whose husbands had normal sperm counts, became pregnant within 1 year of the procedure. This was 3 times the pregnancy rate found by the same author among patients who had not had an HSG. Speculation concerning the precise mode of therapeutic action of the procedure has included the following:

1. It may effect a mechanical lavage of the tubes, dislodging mucus plugs.

2. It may straighten the tubes and thus break down peritoneal adhesions.

3. It may provide a stimulatory effect for the cilia of the tube.

4. It may improve the cervical mucus.

5. The iodine may exert a bacteriologic effect on the mucous membranes.

6. Ethiodol decreases in vitro phagocytosis by peritoneal macrophages.(39) If the same effect occurs in vivo it could decrease phagocytosis of sperm and thus aid fertility.

If an HSG does enhance fertility, is the effect seen with both oil and water-soluble dyes? Gillespie reported a conception rate of 41.3% within 1 year of an HSG with oil media, whereas the rate was only 27.3% when water-soluble agents were employed.(40) This is in accord with other reports where the great majority of pregnancies which followed HSG occurred within 7 months of the procedure. (41,42) A review of the question of oil versus aqueous dye noted that in every retrospective study in which increased pregnancy rates were noted after HSG, an oil dye was used.(43) Similarly, a prospective, controlled study showed oil contrast media was followed by a higher pregnancy rate (7 of 9 patients) compared to water dye (1 of 10 patients) when the cause of the infertility was unknown.(44) With known infertility factors, there was no difference in groups having oil or water based HSG. Whereas the case for a fertility enhancing effect for Ethiodol seems strong, one group recently has found, in a prospective study, no difference in pregnancy rates between those individuals having HSG with oil or with water dye.(45) Beyond its possible value in enhancing fertility, Ethiodol produces a better film image and a lower incidence of pain on injection compared to water-soluble dyes.

The use of an oil medium has been criticized on grounds that it is only slowly absorbed and may cause granuloma formation. Granulomas are found very infrequently and they also may follow the use of water dyes. An additional fear with oil dye is embolization. Bateman et al reported that there were 13 cases of dye intravasation in 533 HSG's performed with Ethiodol.(46) Six of these women had embolization of the dye but there were no symptoms and no morbidity was noted. The authors emphasized that when fluoroscopy is used, venous or lymphatic intravasation can be detected immediately and injection of dye halted.

Hysteroscopy

Hysteroscopy is a technique which complements hysterosalpingography. The hysteroscope is good for differentiating between endometrial polyps and submucous leiomyomas, the definitive diagnosis and treatment of intrauterine adhesions, and for the diagnosis and treatment of intrauterine congenital anomalies. One can argue from a cost-effective point of view that hysterosalpingography is the more useful screening procedure, and the hysteroscope should be reserved to pursue abnormalities identified on the hysterogram.(47) For the surgical management of recurrent abortions secondary to a septate uterus, hysteroscopy is now the method of choice.(48)

Disorders of Ovulation

Disorders of ovulation account for approximately 20% of all infertility problems. These may be anovulation or severe oligoovulation. In the latter cases, even though ovulation does occur, its relative infrequency decreases the woman's chances for pregnancy. If periods occur only every 3 or 4 months, for practical purposes it matters little whether these are ovulatory or anovulatory. This situation should be treated with clomiphene citrate to increase the frequency of, or to initiate, ovulation (see Chapter 20), and this can be started immediately, even before other areas have been investigated.

Basal Body Temperature

Women who have menstrual periods at monthly intervals marked by premenstrual symptoms and dysmenorrhea are almost always ovulatory. Indirect confirmatory evidence of ovulation is obtained by use of basal body temperature (BBT) charts. The temperature can be taken either orally or rectally, with a regular thermometer or with special instruments that show a range of only a few degrees and thus are easier to read. It is worth emphasizing that the temperature must be taken immediately upon awakening and before any activity. The woman may be surprised to find that the basal temperatures are substantially lower than the usual 98.6°F. Days when intercourse takes place should be noted on the chart, and this may give the physician an indication that coital frequency is a problem.

Use of the BBT chart has been criticized because a small percentage of women who ovulate have monophasic graphs and there is often disagreement among physicians concerning interpretation of individual charts. Moreover, the time of ovulation predicted by the BBT does not always correlate well with measurements of the LH surge or with perceptions of maximal cervical mucus production. There is a relationship between a nadir in the BBT and the LH surge, but the BBT is reliable in predicting the day of the LH surge only within 2-3 days. (49) Although the nadir is believed to represent the beginning of the LH surge, the occurrence of a nadir is variable and often is not detected. To be used prospectively to predict ovulation, nearly absolute cycle regularity is required.

Nevertheless, we still find it helpful as a preliminary indicator of ovulation and as a tool for examining with patients the timing of intercourse. Even using temperature charts, though, no one can pinpoint the exact day of ovulation. A significant increase in temperature is not noted until 2 days after the LH peak, coinciding with a rise in peripheral levels of progesterone to greater than 4 ng/ml. Physical release of the ovum probably occurs on the day prior to the time of the first temperature elevation. The temperature rise should be sustained for 11 to 16 days and it will then drop at the time of the subsequent menstrual period.

If an approximate time of ovulation can be determined by temperature charts, a sensible schedule for coitus is every 36 to 48 hours in a period encompassed by 3 to 4 days prior to and 2 days after expected ovulation. It is unwise, however, to demand rigid adherence to a schedule. This may produce psychologic stress sufficient to inhibit sexual relations. In discussing coital timing, the patient will usually want to know the fertilizable life of the sperm and the egg. The information on human gametes is speculative. Cases have been reported in which isolated coitus even up to 7 days prior to the rise in basal body temperature has resulted in pregnancy, but this probably represents the limits of biologic variation. It is estimated that sperm retain their ability to fertilize for 24 to 48 hours and that the human egg is fertilizable for 12 to 24 hours. Immature human eggs aspirated from follicles for in vitro fertilization can be fertilized, however, after incubation in vitro for even as long as 36 hours.

Endometrial Biopsy

The most reliable assessment of ovulation and the luteal phase requires endometrial biopsy. Endometrial biopsy is performed 2 to 3 days prior to the expected period and the histology is read by the criteria outlined by Noyes, Hertig and Rock.(50) While premenstrual biopsy could interrupt a pregnancy if performed in a conception cycle, the danger is minimal.(51) An alternative, taking the biopsy on the first day of menses has three disadvantages:

1. Inconvenient time for patient and physician.

2. The tissue is disrupted and often more difficult to interpret.

3. A slight amount of bleeding can occur at the time of the expected period even if the patient is pregnant.

We recommend the use of the plastic endometrial suction curette (Pipelle from Unimar, Wilton, Connecticut, or the Z-Sampler from Zinnanti, Chatsworth, California). It is easy to use, requires no cervical dilatation (3 mm diameter), and is virtually painless.

Progesterone

A serum progesterone level of less than 3 ng/ml is identical with follicular phase levels.(52) To confirm ovulation, values at the mid-luteal phase, just at the midpoint between ovulation and the onset of the subsequent menstrual period, should be 6.5 ng/ml and preferably 10 ng/ml or more. The consensus of opinion is that a mid-luteal phase progesterone level is insufficient evidence upon which to judge the adequacy of the luteal phase. The progesterone level is subject to the variation associated with pulsatile secretion, but more importantly, there is poor correlation with the histologic state of the endometrium.

Inadequate Luteal Phase

An inadequate luteal phase occurs when there is deficient progesterone secretion by the corpus luteum. The term has been applied to both a short interval (less than 11 days) between ovulation and menstruation with relatively normal peak values of progesterone, and, more commonly, to a luteal phase of normal length with lower than normal progesterone levels. A related, but rare condition is the absence of progesterone receptors in the endometrium. An inadequate luteal phase can be found in up to 30% of isolated cycles of normal women and only if the defect is found in 2 cycles is it thought to be a significant factor in infertility. Approximately 3 to 4% of infertile women will be diagnosed as having an inadequate luteal phase and the incidence may be higher in women with a history of recurrent abortion.

Although an inadequate luteal phase is a direct result of decreased hormone production by the corpus luteum, the underlying causes of this dysfunction can be multiple. Decreased levels of FSH in the

528

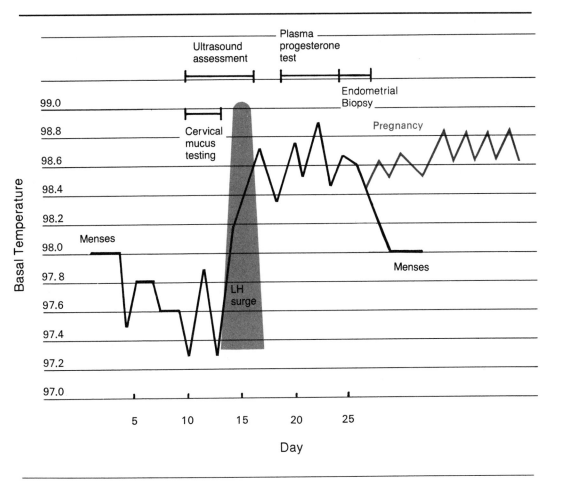

follicular phase of the cycle, abnormal patterns of LH secretion, and decreased levels of LH and FSH at the time of the ovulatory surge have been implicated. Elevated prolactin levels also may be associated with an inadequate luteal phase. The preponderance of evidence supports a preovulatory cause. Nuclear progesterone receptor concentrations are normal in luteal phase endometrial samples from women with inadequate luteal phases, but the concentration is reduced during the proliferative phase (suggesting an alteration, such as lesser estrogen stimulation, during the proliferative phase).(53)

The diagnosis should be considered in women with normal cycles and unexplained infertility, women with a short luteal phase demonstrated by basal temperature charts, and women with a history of recurrent abortion. The diagnosis can be approached in a number of ways. The basal body temperature chart may be biphasic, but the duration of the rise is less than 11 days. A diagnosis made on the basis of basal temperature charts should be corroborated by endometrial biopsy. Even with a normal temperature chart an endometrial biopsy taken 2 to 3 days prior to menstruation can indicate that the development of the endometrium lags behind the cycle day (in relation to the onset of the subsequent menstrual period) by more than 2 days. A discrepancy between the development of the glands and the stroma also may be indicative of an inadequate luteal phase. Making a diagnosis based on the histologic appearance of a biopsy specimen can be difficult. The endometrial sample can show varying patterns and there may be differing interpretations by different observers. Despite these drawbacks, endometrial biopsy remains the classical way to diagnose an inadequate luteal phase.

Because of the discomfort and expense associated with endometrial biopsy, attention has turned to direct measurements of serum progesterone levels as a means of diagnosing the adequacy of luteal phase. Exact values of progesterone that are needed to rule out an inadequate luteal phase are in dispute. Many physicians believe that a value of 12 to 15 ng/ml a week prior to the onset of menstruation is a good indication of the adequacy of the luteal phase. This has been disputed, and the histologic diagnosis of an inadequate luteal phase has been documented in women who had progesterone levels in excess of 15 ng/ml.(54) For now, the majority opinion favors biopsy as the more accurate method for diagnosis.

Based on findings that low FSH values prior to ovulation can be associated with an inadequate luteal phase, it would seem reasonable, in selected cases, to use human menopausal gonadotropin (Pergonal) or clomiphene citrate. Pergonal has the potential for causing severe hyperstimulation of the ovaries and it creates an increased risk of multiple births. Because of these effects Pergonal is seldom used for this indication. Clomiphene citrate is the first choice of many physicians for the treatment of an inadequate luteal phase. Its risks, other than multiple births, are small. The initial dose is 50 mg a day for 5 days starting on day 5 of the cycle. (See Chapter 20)

Because there is a deficiency of progesterone in the inadequate luteal phase, replacement by exogenous progesterone has been utilized with success. A vaginal suppository containing 25 mg of progesterone is inserted twice a day starting approximately 3 days after ovulation. Treatment is maintained until menstruation occurs or until a pregnancy is diagnosed. If the latter, a switch is made to weekly injections of 17-hydroxyprogesterone caproate through the 10th week of pregnancy. Using this therapy, success rates of approximately 50% have been achieved, but good control studies are lacking. Balasch et al used biopsy in 2 consecutive cycles to diagnose a luteal phase inadequacy in women with normal levels of progesterone and prolactin.(55) Significantly better results in terms of improvement in endometrial morphology (greater than 60%) were obtained when progesterone vaginal suppositories or dehydrogesterone were used compared to a nontreated group (17%). The percentage of pregnancies was also higher in the treated groups but the numbers were very small.

In studies comparing pregnancy rates with clomiphene versus progesterone treatment, there is no difference. (56,57) In our view, this is an argument in favor of clomiphene because of a significant disadvantage associated with progesterone therapy. Progesterone supplementation prolongs the luteal phase, which is not a problem for the physician, but for the couple the disappointment at the time of menses or a negative pregnancy test is even more profound.

Bromocriptine has been reported to correct luteal phase defects associated with hyperprolactinemia, but its value in women with normal prolactin levels has not been demonstrated. In a subgroup of patients with unexplained infertility, high normal prolactin levels but expressible galactorrhea, treatment with bromocriptine enhanced fertility compared to similar women treated with pyridoxine.(58) Even if the prolactin is normal, if galactorrhea is present, ovulatory dysfunction responds well to bromocriptine.(59) In the absence of galactorrhea, the prolactin elevation may be subtle (such as an increase in nocturnal peaks), explaining good responses to bromocriptine. (See Chapter 20) In evaluating any therapy it is important to recognize that pregnancies occur without treatment in some women who are diagnosed as having an inadequate luteal phase.(60)

Mycoplasma

Mycoplasma, a pleuropneumonia-like organism, has been implicated as a possible cause of recurrent abortion and salpingitis. Gnarpe and Friberg reported that infertile couples had a markedly higher prevalence of T mycoplasma (now called Ureaplasma urealyticum) in cervical mucus and semen than did a group of fertile women and men.(61) Treatment with doxycycline decreased the numbers of couples with mycoplasma and also was associated with pregnancy in 15 of 52 couples (29%), all of whom had had primary infertility of at least 5 years duration. However, a series of reports from England agreed with these findings in only one respect.(62,63) They confirmed that treatment with doxycycline could eliminate mycoplasma from the genital tract of the majority of individuals. There was no difference, however, in the frequency of either T strain or Mycoplasma hominis between infertile and fertile couples. In a double-blind study, treatment with doxycycline for 28 days had no effect on the rate of conception, and the English group suggested that culturing for mycoplasma in the routine investigation of infertility was unrewarding.

Since those publications, a number of studies have established the widespread distribution of ureaplasma urealyticum in both fertile and infertile populations. Some have found higher colonization in infertile couples, whereas others have found no relationship between the organisms and infertility. In a study that received a great deal of media attention, it was reported that 60% of males who were culture positive for ureaplasma urealyticum and were cleared of infection by antibiotic treatment achieved a pregnancy.(64) Failure to clear the infection resulted in a 5% pregnancy rate. This study suffers from lack of clarity on the criteria for entry into treatment and from any mention of individuals lost to follow-up. Cassell and coworkers found that the incidence of ureaplasma infection was only significantly higher in those women whose male partners had semen abnormalities.(65)

It can be concluded that culturing for ureaplasma may be reasonable with male infertility but is not worthwhile in cases of unexplained infertility, and indiscriminate treatment with antibiotics is not warranted.(66)

531

Sperm Allergy

Sperm are very antigenic, and are normally isolated by a blood-testes barrier. This is an anatomic and functional barrier in the seminiferous tubules (perhaps a function of the Sertoli Cells). Disruption in this barrier can lead to antibodies; hence antibodies can follow vasectomy, testicular torsion, infections or trauma.

It has been over 2 decades since Franklin and Dukes sparked interest in the role of sperm antibodies in infertility.(67) Despite intensive investigation since that time there remain considerable areas of ambiguity. There is a developing consensus, however, that a small percentage of infertility can be explained on an immunologic basis. Older studies have concerned themselves with the role of agglutinating antibodies found in serum. In men there is a good correlation between the titer of agglutinating antibodies and the prognosis for fertility.(68) In women the correlation is not as clear. In addition, agglutinating antibodies can be found in nonimmunologic components of the serum.

A complement-dependent sperm immobilization test is a more precise method for determining immunologic infertility in women. It is positive in 5 to 10% of women with unexplained infertility. Jones suggested that sperm immobilization tests be performed on both serum and cervical mucus because antibodies have been found in the cervix in individuals who do not have circulating antibodies.(69) Working with mucus may be difficult for a clinical laboratory and such testing may be suitable only in laboratories with a special interest in the area.

Our approach to diagnosing sperm antibodies utilizes immunobeads with anti-IgG, anti-IgA and anti-IgM specificities.(70,71) Localization of antibody, for example, to the sperm head or tail, can be obtained with this method. The exact roles for IgG and IgA are not known, but attachment of the zona pellucida is affected only by head-directed antibodies. In in vitro fertilization, fertilization rates are not reduced unless antibodies of both IgG and IgA classes are present.

To test the male, the sperm are incubated with immunobeads. To test the female, her serum or cervical mucus is used to treat antibody free sperm which then, in turn, are incubated with immunobeads. The normal result in a particular laboratory depends upon the correlation of results with other parameters of sperm capability, such as the sperm penetration test and ultimately achievement of pregnancy. In some laboratories, binding of less than 50% of the sperm population has no effect on sperm penetration of cervical mucus and this is considered the percentage that separates positive (>49% of sperm bound) from negative tests.(72) Ayvaliotis et al noted that only 15.3% of partners of untreated males with greater than 50% of their sperm antibody-bound achieved a pregnancy compared to 66.7% of the partners of untreated males with less than 50% of sperm antibody-bound.(73) In our own laboratory, greater than 10% is regarded as a positive result. Each laboratory must correlate the percentage of sperm antibody-bound with other parameters of fertility, such as the hamster penetration test.

532

Interestingly, antibodies which interfere with penetration of human cervical mucus do not prevent penetration of bovine cervical mucus. This indicates that bovine cervical mucus is not a good screen for sperm antibodies.

A crucial but unresolved question is whether all couples with unexplained infertility should be tested for sperm antibodies or whether it should be restricted only to those couples with "poor" postcoital tests. Our current practice is to test when repetitive postcoital tests show all immobilized sperm, sperm with shaking tails but no progressive motility, or no sperm despite a normal semen analysis and adequate coital technique. Bronson et al also use the postcoital test as a screen but included for antibody testing those couples who have less than 5 motile sperm/HPF.(72) We also test for antibodies in men who have less than normal results with the sperm penetration assay.

Treatment has been the subject of controversy. Occlusive condom therapy has been used in the presence of agglutinating antibodies in women. The results, however, are uncertain and there is a reasonable pregnancy rate even without treatment. In addition, there is no evidence that the pregnancy rate is increased when occlusive therapy is used to treat immobilizing antibodies. The use of high-dose corticosteroids (methylprednisolone 96 mg/day for 7 days) has been suggested for both males and females with positive antibody tests but benefits must be weighed against the risks, including aseptic necrosis of the femoral head. Alexander et al showed that prednisone, 60 mg daily, for 7 days can decrease the titer of sperm antibodies, and that this is associated with higher pregnancy rates, compared to the results in untreated individuals.(74) Hendry et al treated males with sperm antibodies with prednisolone 40 mg daily from day 1 to 10 of their partner's menstrual cycle.(75) The dose was increased to 80 mg daily if the antibody titer did not fall. The pregnancy rate was 33%, but 53% of the subjects experienced some side effects. Mood changes were the most troubling of these side effects.

There is some reason to believe that men with oligospermia with antisperm antibodies respond better to long-term low-dose steroid treatment rather than to the short-term method timed to the woman's menstrual cycle. We have encountered men with poor to zero performance on sperm penetration assays (with antibodies) who have improved the sperm penetration and achieved pregnancy with treatment consisting of prednisone, 5 mg tid.

It is still not known whether sperm become coated with antibody in the epididymis or at the time of ejaculation. If the antibodies are applied after ejaculation then perhaps attempts to promptly remove the antibodies might yield good results. Thus efforts have been made to rapidly dilute and wash the sperm and to pass the semen through separation columns.(76) Sperm washing does not do a good job of removing antibodies and there is poor performance during swim-up. Passing the semen through columns improves the sperm penetration assay, but there are no data regarding pregnancy rates. Thus most attention has been directed to treatment of the man with steroids. Treatment of genitourinary infection in the male is also worthwhile.

**Luteinized
Unruptured Follicle**

Because many infertility investigations do not reveal a cause for the failure to conceive, there has been a search for abnormalities that are not elucidated by the usual diagnostic approaches. The increasing use of ultrasound monitoring has focused attention on follicular development.

On occasion, a corpus luteum will form despite the failure of release of the oocyte. Initially it was thought that this problem could be identified at laparoscopy by noting an absence of the ovulatory stigma, but now it is apparent that the stigma can be epithelialized rapidly and thus obscured from view.(77) Currently, clinical diagnosis of a luteinized unruptured follicle (LUF) is made on the basis of ultrasound monitoring. The preovulatory growth of the follicle usually is normal but the follicle does not collapse following the LH surge and there may be increased growth in the luteal phase. The interior of the follicle lacks the echoes often seen in corpora lutea. Whereas these criteria seem straightforward, establishing the diagnosis of LUF is often difficult. Even if ultrasound is done daily the collapse of the follicle can be missed and a corpus luteum refilled with blood can be mistaken for a persistent follicle. Failure of ovulation can be associated with lower levels of estradiol and progesterone in peritoneal fluid compared to controls, but this too may not be absolutely diagnostic.(78) One study suggested that recurrent LUF is seen only in association with pelvic adhesions or the use of ovulation inducing drugs.(79) Therefore, routine ultrasound screening of women with unexplained infertility is of questionable value. It is doubtful that LUF is a significant cause of infertility. It may be worthwhile, however, to do peri and postovulatory ultrasound monitoring in cases of ovulation induction.

Serial ultrasound observation of ovarian cycles has raised many questions. Alleged asynchronies have been identified involving the estradiol surge, the gonadotropin surge, deficient luteinization, and the growth and disappearance of follicles. (See Chapter 19 for monitoring follicular growth and development with ultrasound) Another diagnosis that can be made by ultrasound is ovulation from a lead follicle that is smaller than normal (less than 18 mm). While its meaning is uncertain, it has been suggested that this, too, can be a cause for infertility.

Endoscopy

Laparoscopy is the final diagnostic procedure of any infertility investigation. If the HSG is normal, the endoscopic procedure is done after an interval of 6 months from the x-ray. This allows time for the fertility-enhancing effect of the x-ray procedure. Because of the possible benefit from the HSG, we disagree with physicians who bypass it and go directly to laparoscopy. An exception would be made for the woman who is at high risk for pelvic infection. Obviously, if the HSG shows tubal occlusion or other major abnormalities, we do not hold to the 6 month delay. The findings at laparoscopy agree with those of HSG in approximately two-thirds of the cases. The major area of disagreement is the failure of the HSG to detect pelvic adhesions or endometriosis. Approximately 50% of patients undergoing laparoscopy will have pelvic pathology, usually endometriosis (see Chapter 18) or pelvic adhesions. With due care in selection of cases, many of these abnormalities can be treated through the laparoscope either by lysis of adhesions or fulguration of implants of endometriosis. If manipulation through the laparoscope is not possible, alternative approaches include laparotomy or hormone therapy.

When findings at laparoscopy are combined with those of the other test procedures, the majority of couples will have a discoverable cause for their inability to conceive. Still there will be a significant number of couples in whom no abnormality is found.

Recurrent Abortion

Abortion is defined as the termination of pregnancy before 20 weeks of gestation or below a fetal weight of 500 gm. Approximately 15% of all pregnancies between 4-20 weeks of gestation will undergo spontaneous abortion. The true abortion rate is closer to 50% because of the high rate of abortion in the weeks immediately following conception. The majority of these cases are caused by chromosomal abnormalities in the sperm or the egg.

Habitual abortion classically has been defined as 3 or more consecutive abortions. In 1938, Malpas, using theoretical calculations, stated that a woman with a history of 3 consecutive abortions had a 73% chance of aborting in the next pregnancy.(80) In 1946 Eastman presented statistical calculations indicating that after 3 abortions the risk was 83.6%.(81) These early papers, based primarily upon intuition rather than clinical studies, established the notion that the chance for a subsequent abortion increases dramatically with each successive abortion and that after 3 abortions the chances for a successful pregnancy are very low. Studies on the efficacy of many types of treatments used these pessimistic figures for comparison rather than containing their own controls. If treatment increased the salvage rate to 70% it was considered curative. However, clinical studies have indicated that the risk of abortion after 3 successive abortions is in fact only 30-55%. (82-84) The chance of a successful live birth after 3 consecutive abortions without a live birth is 40-50%; with at least one previous normal pregnancy in addition to the repetitive abortions, the chance is 70%.

The projections by Malpas and Eastman were theoretical exercises which were not confirmed when appropriate data were collected. Thus, it is not surprising that treatment with a wide range of approaches, including vitamins and psychotherapy, produced successful pregnancies in a reasonable percentage of women with habitual abortion. These cures were not due to the therapy but, rather, the claims for success were based on a comparison with the discredited statistics of Malpas and Eastman.

The reproductive loss between conception and clinically recognizable pregnancy is significant and just now becoming apparent.(85,86) The use of sensitive assays for HCG suggests that 15-20% of pregnancies are lost between implantation and the 6th week. It is important for physicians and their patients to be aware of the high degree of reproductive loss, especially in older women due in part to the increasing frequency of trisomies with advancing age.

Despite the knowledge that the spontaneous salvage rate is 45-70%, it is still worth trying to uncover causes for repetitive first trimester pregnancy losses. A recognized cause of the problem is a genetic abnormality, and karyotyping of couples will reveal that 8% have some abnormality, most frequently a translocation.(87) Karyotyp-

535

ing is especially vital if the couple has had a malformed infant or fetus in addition to abortions. It is important to emphasize that karyotyping uncovers only a percentage of those pregnancies lost due to genetic abnormalities. There may be single gene defects which are not manifested by chromosomal abnormalities, and it is very likely that a percentage of those patients now considered to have unexplained repetitive pregnancy loss have this type of genetic defect. In addition, karyotyping of blood cells misses abnormalities of meiosis, which can be found in sperm cell lines. If the karyotype is abnormal, nothing can be done to lessen the chances for another abortion. Amniocentesis should be offered, however, in any pregnancy that goes beyond the first trimester, because of the risk of an abnormal child.

According to McDonough, treatment of endocrine factors yields a 90% normal child rate, correction of anatomic factors, a 60-70% rate, but known genetic factors are associated with only a 32% expectation for a normal child.(88)

It is helpful to have a karyotype on a previous abortion, to determine aneuploidy or euploidy. Once determined, there is a high likelihood that subsequent abortions will be the same, although there is still a chance for a normal pregnancy. If aneuploidy is documented, based on animal studies relating aneuploidy to aging of ovum and sperm, accurately timed inseminations could be considered, otherwise the choice is between hoping for the best or donor insemination. Once pregnant, chorionic villus sampling should be considered. If euploidy is documented previously, anatomic and endocrine factors should be corrected.

Diabetes mellitus (with relatively good control) and thyroid problems are no longer considered reasons for recurrent abortions.

Approximately 12-15% of women with habitual abortion have a uterine malformation, and this can be diagnosed by HSG. Surgical repair of these defects is rewarded with salvage rates in the 70-80% range. The septate uterus is most frequently responsible for recurrent early abortions.

Hormonal Treatment

A study of the role of hormonal deficiency as a cause of habitual abortion has largely focused on deficiencies of progesterone or its metabolites. Attempts to implicate low pregnanediol levels in early pregnancy as a cause for abortion, and, as a corollary, to treat with exogenous progesterone or progestins, have been shown to be fruitless.(89) A second approach has been to diagnose an inadequate luteal phase during the nonpregnant state and to initiate treatment with progesterone a few days after ovulation. Jones and Delfs (90) claimed that 30% of women with pregnancy wastage had an inadequate luteal phase, whereas Tho et al (87) found that 23% of the women in their group of 100 couples with recurrent abortion had an inadequate luteal phase. In this latter study it was unclear whether the diagnosis was made on the basis of only one endometrial biopsy. If this were so, their report over-diagnoses the frequency of inadequate luteal phase. Botella-Llusia found that 38% of women with 3 or more consecutive abortions had poorly developed secretory endometrium compared with only 6% of infertile women, and others estimate a 28% prevalence of inadequate luteal phase in patients with recurrent abortions.(91,92)

Two studies dealt with serum progesterone levels of women who had had 3 consecutive abortions. One study indicated that 10 such women had abnormally low levels of progesterone during the luteal phase, and all 10 women subsequently aborted again.(93) The authors neglected to indicate how the women were selected for the study, although all were said to have progestational deficiency on biopsy. The second study found that 6 habitual aborters had a mid-luteal serum progesterone concentration of greater than 4 ng/ml and 5 had full-term pregnancies. (94) The fate of the 6th woman was not specified. Four other women did not become pregnant again. Three of them had progesterone values below 4 ng/ml. Interestingly, there were no subsequent abortions in this latter study. Hensleigh and Fainstat treated women who had a history of recurrent abortion and a serum progesterone level below 10 ng/ml, with progesterone suppositories.(95) In addition, they treated women with a similar history who had serum progesterones below 15 ng/ml during the first trimester of pregnancy. While their results were good in terms of pregnancy outcome, the study contained no controls, and for that reason can be judged only as an interesting observation. One study found increased salvage in women with a history of habitual abortion when they were treated with human chorionic gonadotropin. All had demonstrable fetal heart activity at the initiation of therapy. The surprise is not that salvage was so good in the HCG group (10 of 10) but that it was so poor (3 of 10) in the placebo group despite fetal heart activity. (96)

The uncertainty that plagues physicians in dealing with the inadequate luteal phase in infertility is also apparent when considering habitual abortion. If repetitive endometrial biopsies or progesterones are abnormal or if the BBT chart shows a luteal phase of less than 11 days, it is reasonable to treat with clomiphene or progesterone suppositories as described in the section on the inadequate luteal phase. Progesterone should be used only if these criteria are met; it should not be used empirically. Placebo treatment may be useful in maintaining a physician/patient relationship in which the patient derives needed psychologic sustenance. It seems to us, however, that the use of hormones for placebo effect on the basis of no known harmful effect denies the important lesson learned in the discovery of the relationship between DES treatment and genital abnormalities. Reputed harmlessness is a potential dangerous approach based on negative data. It must be remembered that there is a reasonable cure rate in unexplained habitual abortion, even without treatment.

Other causes

Autoimmunity. In autoimmunity, a humoral or cellular response is directed against a specific component of the host. The lupus anticoagulant is an antibody against thromboplastin, present in a variety of clinical conditions and not just with lupus erythematosus. In one series, 10% of women with recurrent abortions had the lupus anticoagulant.(97) This antithromboplastin anticoagulant is associated with fetal growth retardation and fetal death in addition to recurrent abortion, and there is a high rate of second trimester fetal deaths. The mechanism of pregnancy loss is probably decidual and placental insufficiency due to the thrombotic tendency. The lupus

537

anticoagulant prolongs the prothrombin time and the partial thromboplastin time. The activated partial thromboplastin time is the most sensitive screening test. Patients also may have antibodies against cardiolipin.

Patients with recurrent abortions should be screened with the activated partial thromboplastin time, antinuclear antibodies, and the anticardiolipin antibody. Therapy consists of aspirin, 40 mg daily, and prednisone in a dose to restore the thromboplastin time to the normal range.(98) Treatment is not always successful; therapy with glucocorticoids is not very effective in eliminating the anticardiolipin antibody. Virtually all patients develop pre-eclampsia, often very severe.

Alloimmmunity. Alloimmunity includes all causes of recurrent abortion related to an abormal maternal immune response to antigens on placental or fetal tissues.(97) Normally, maintenance of pregnancy requires the formation of blocking factors (probably complexes of antibody and antigen) which prevent maternal rejection of fetal antigens. It has been argued that couples with repetitive abortion have an increased sharing of human lymphocte antigens (HLA), a condition which would not allow the mother to make blocking antibodies.

Immunotherapy has been offered to produce a favorable maternal immune response in order to protect the developing embryo. Women with recurrent abortions have been treated with infusions of their partner's lymphocytes; 77% receiving their husband's cells gave birth compared to 37% receiving their own cells.(99) Others have claimed good results with transfusion of leukocyte-rich, erythrocyte-rich donor blood (3 transfusions every 4-8 weeks).(100)

Women have been selected for immunotherapy by HLA typing, but HLA typing is controversial. Some investigators have failed to confirm that sharing of HLA antigens is found in couples with recurrent abortions.(101) This agrees with experiments in animals where sharing of HLA antigens has not been found to affect reproduction. There is also concern that immunization of mothers may affect placenta and fetus. Critics contend that success in the control group (99) points out that even in the absence of treatment, positive results are achieved, raising the question of the adequacy of matching in the selection of control groups. This approach remains experimental with potential risk of adverse consequences on the immune systems of mother and child.

The patient with recurrent abortions usually presents as an anxious, frustrated individual on the verge of despair. Evaluation should be spaced over several visits, allowing the physician to establish communication and rapport with the patient. The emotional support that the physician can bring to this interaction will be most useful, and in some cases may be therapeutic.(102) It should be emphasized that continued attempts at conception are rewarded with success in the majority of women labeled as habitual aborters.

When Should Adoption Be Advised?	With proper evaluation and therapy, the majority of couples attending an infertility clinic will become pregnant. Of those who do not achieve a pregnancy, the group most in need of counseling are those with unexplained infertility. Despite the absence of pathology, couples with 4 or more years of infertility have a poor prognosis and for these patients, as well as those who have exhausted their treatment options, the physician should encourage consideration of either in vitro fertilization or adoption. The former offers pregnancy rates of approximately 20% per cycle in which eggs are transferred. The success is somewhat lower in those individuals with unexplained infertility.

People who turn to the social agencies involved with adoption may be accorded a bleak picture of their prospects for adoption. This can compound the depression that the individuals may already feel from their inability to conceive. An alternative is private adoption, which can provide babies more rapidly, at reasonable cost, and without resort to foreign countries. In private adoption a fee should not be paid to the biologic mother for giving up the baby. In most cases the biologic mother will know who adopted the child and this lack of anonymity may direct some couples away from private adoption. In addition, there is a short time period during which the biologic mother can reclaim the baby. In our experience this occurs in approximately 5% of private adoptions.

Patients should be encouraged to "spread the word" that they are interested in adoption. In addition, letters can be directed to obstetricians throughout the country describing the couple and their desires for adoption. Consultation with a lawyer is necessary to obtain information concerning the adoption laws in the individual states because a number of states do not allow private adoption. An excellent review of private adoption, including the legal aspects, can be found in Friedman and Gradstein's book, *Surviving Pregnancy Loss*, (103) and another superb resource is the book, *Beating the Adoption Game*, by Martin.(104)

Myths

It is important for physicians and other health care professionals to dispel the myths that are associated with infertility. Women should not be told that they are infertile because they are too nervous. Unless anxiety interferes with ovulation or coital frequency, there is no present evidence that infertility is caused by the usual anxieties besetting a couple attempting to conceive. Despite many anecdotes to the contrary, adoption does not increase a couple's fertility.(105) The treatment of euthyroid infertile women with thyroid has been shown repeatedly to be worthless. A dilatation and curettage (D and C) is not a legitimate part of a routine infertility investigation. It provides minimal information beyond that obtained by endometrial biopsy and is both expensive and potentially hazardous because it subjects the woman to the risk of general anesthesia. There is also no evidence to support the old belief that a woman becomes more fertile following D and C. Quite the contrary, one study indicates a decreased fertility potential for those women undergoing D and C.(106)

A retroverted uterus is not a cause for infertility although it can be found in association with pelvic adhesions or endometriosis that do influence infertility.

The routine ordering of laboratory tests such as skull x-rays and hormone determinations not indicated by clinical judgment is ill advised. These may be of value in selected cases but certainly not in every case.

The physician should try to avoid the philosophy "try it, it might just work." There are many disillusioned couples who, without any indication, have been given clomiphene citrate, progestational agents, and low-dose estrogen, and then have been treated with husband inseminations. A substantial number of pregnancies occur in infertile couples without treatment, irrespective of the diagnosis.(107) Thus, the physician should not feel obligated to render a treatment just to do something. The goals of the practitioner should be to accomplish a thorough investigation, to treat any abnormalities that are uncovered, to educate the couple in the workings of the reproductive system, to give the couple some estimate of their fertility potential, to counsel for adoption where appropriate, and to provide emotional support. If these goals are achieved by a sympathetic, understanding physician, they will satisfy most couples who suffer from infertility.

References

1. **Pratt WF, Mosher WD, Bachrach C, Horn MC,** Infertility—United States, 1982, MMWR 34:197, 1985.

2. **Horn MC, Mosher WD,** Use of services for family planning and infertility: United States, 1982, Advance data from vital and health statistics, No. 103, U.S. Public Health Service, Department of Health and Human Services, Hyattsville, Maryland, 1984.

3. **Hirsch MB, Mosher WD,** Characteristics of infertile women in the United States and their use of infertility services, Fertil Steril 47:618, 1987.

4. **Westoff CF,** Fertility in the United States, Science 234:554, 1986.

5. **Gibson C,** The U.S. fertility decline, 1961-1975: The contribution of changes in marital status and marital fertility, Fam Plann Persp 8:249, 1976.

6. **Rindfuss RR, Bumpass LL,** How old is too old? Age and the sociology of fertility, Fam Plann Persp 8:226, 1976.

7. **Wineberg H, McCarthy J,** Differential fertility in the United States, 1980: Continuity or change? J Biosoc Sci 18:311, 1986.

8. **Tietze C,** Reproductive span and rate of reproduction among Hutterite women, Fertil Steril 8:89, 1957.

9. **Robinson WC,** Another look at the Hutterites and natural fertility, Soc Biol 33:65, 1982.

10. **Kennedy WJ,** Edinburgh Med J 27:1086, 1882.

11. **Mosher WD,** Infertility trends among U.S. couples: 1965-1976, Fam Plann Persp 14:22, 1982.

12. **James WH,** The causes of the decline in fecundability with age, Soc Biol 26:330, 1979.

13. **Federation CECOS, Schwartz D, Mayaux JM,** Female fecundity as a function of age: Results of artificial insemination in 2193 nulliparous women with azoospermic husbands, New Eng J Med 306:404, 1982.

14. **Virro MS, Shewchuk AB,** Pregnancy outcome in 242 conceptions after artificial insemination with donor sperm and effects of maternal age on the prognosis for successful pregnancy, Am J Obstet Gynecol 148:518, 1984.

15. **Warburton D, Kline J, Stein Z, Strobino B,** Cytogenetic abnormalities in spontaneous abortions of recognized conceptions, in Porter IH, editor, *Perinatal Genetics: Diagnosis and Treatment,* Academic Press, New York, 1986, p. 133.

16. **Spencer G,** Projections of the population of the United States, by age, sex, and race: 1983-2080, *Current Population Reports—Population Estimates and Projections,* U.S. Department of Commerce, May, 1984, Series P-25, No. 952.

17. **Mosher WD, Aral SO,** Factors related to infertility in the United States, 1965-1976, Sexually Transmitted Diseases 12:117, 1985.

18. **Mosher WD,** Reproductive impairments in the United States, 1965-1982, Demography 22:415, 1985.

19. **Menken J, Trussell J, Larsen U,** Age and infertility, Science 233:1389, 1986.

20. **Barnea ER, Holford TR, McInnes DRA,** Long-term prognosis of infertile couples with normal basic investigations: A life-table analysis, Obstet Gynecol 66:24, 1985.

21. **Hull MGR, Glazener CMA, Kelly NJ, Conway DI, Foster PA, Hinton RA, Coulson C, Lambert PA, Watt EM, Desai KM,** Population study of causes, treatment, and outcome of infertility, Brit Med J 291:1693, 1985.

22. **Stubblefield PG, Monson RR, Schoenbaum SC, Wolfson CE, Cookson DJ, Ryan KJ,** Fertility after induced abortion: A prospective follow-up study, Obstet Gynecol 63:186, 1984.

23. **Senekjian EK, Potkul RK, Frey K, Herbst A,** Infertility among daughters either exposed or not exposed to diethylstilbestrol, Am J Obstet Gynecol 158:493, 1988.

24. **Stillman RJ, Rosenberg MJ, Sachs BP,** Smoking and reproduction, Fertil Steril 46:545, 1986.

25. **Guttmacher AF,** Factors affecting normal expectancy of conception, JAMA 161:855, 1956.

26. **Gibor Y, Garcia CJ, Cohen MR, Scommegna A,** The cyclical changes in the physical properties of the cervical mucus and the results of the postcoital test, Fertil Steril 21:20, 1970.

27. **Jette NT, Glass RH,** Prognostic value of the postcoital test, Fertil Steril 23:29, 1972.

28. **Collins JA, So Y, Wilson EH, Wrixon W, Casper RF,** The postcoital test as a predictor of pregnancy among 355 infertile couples, Fertil Steril 41:703, 1984.

541

29. **Soules MR, Moore DE, Spadoni LR, Stenchever MA,** The relationship between the postcoital test and the sperm penetration assay, Fertil Steril 38:384, 1982.

30. **Kovacs GT, Newman GB, Henson GL,** The postcoital test: What is normal? Brit Med J 1:818, 1978.

31. **Hull MGR, Savage PE, Bromham DR,** Prognostic value of the postcoital test: Prospective study based on time-specific conception rates, Brit J Obstet Gynaecol 89:299, 1982.

32. **Quagliarello J, Arny M,** Intracervical versus intrauterine insemination: Correlation of outcome with antecedent postcoital testing, Fertil Steril 46:870, 1986.

33. **Drake TS, Tredway DR, Buchanan GC,** A reassessment of the fractional postcoital test, Am J Obstet Gynecol 133:382, 1979.

34. **Ansari AH, Gould KG, Ansari VM,** Sodium bicarbonate douching for improvement of the postcoital test, Fertil Steril 33:608, 1980.

35. **Stumpf PG, March CM,** Febrile morbidity following hysterosalpingography: Identification of risk factors and recommendations for prophylaxis, Fertil Steril 33:487, 1980.

36. **Spring D,** Prone hysterosalpingography, Radiology 136:235, 1980.

37. **Whitelaw MJ, Foster TN, Graham WH,** Hysterosalpingography and insufflation, J Reprod Med 4:56, 1970.

38. **Palmer A,** Ethiodol hysterosalpingography for the treatment of infertility, Fertil Steril 11:311, 1960.

39. **Boyer P, Territo MC, de Ziegler D, Meldrum DR,** Ethiodol inhibits phagocytosis by pelvic peritoneal macrophages, Fertil Steril 46:715, 1986.

40. **Gillespie HW,** The therapeutic aspect of hysterosalpingography, Brit J Radiol 38:301, 1965.

41. **Mackey RA, Glass RH, Olson LE, Vaidya RA,** Pregnancy following hysterosalpingography with oil and water soluble dye, Fertil Steril 22:504, 1971.

42. **DeCherney AH, Kort H, Barney JB, DeVore GR,** Increased pregnancy rate with oil soluble hysterosalpingography dye, Fertil Steril 33:407, 1980.

43. **Soules MR, Spadoni LR,** Oil versus aqueous media for hysterosalpingography: A continuing debate based on many opinions and few facts, Fertil Steril 38:1, 1982.

44. **Schwabe MG, Shapiro SS, Haning RV Jr,** Hysterosalpingography with oil contrast medium enhances fertility in patients with infertility of unknown etiology, Fertil Steril 40:604, 1983.

45. **Alper MM, Garner PR, Spence JEH, Quarrington AM,** Pregnancy rates after hysterosalpingography with oil- and water-soluble contrast media, Obstet Gynecol 68:6, 1986.

46. **Bateman BG, Nunley WC Jr, Kitchin JD,** Intravasation during hysterosalpingography using oil-base contrast media, Fertil Steril 34:439, 1980.

542

47. **Fayez JA, Mutie G, Schneider PJ,** The diagnostic value of hysterosalpingography and hysteroscopy in infertility investigation, Am J Obstet Gynecol 156:558, 1987.

48. **March CM, Israel,** Hysteroscopic management of recurrent abortion secondary to septate uterus, Am J Obstet Gynecol 156:834, 1987.

49. **Quagliarello J, Arny M,** Inaccuracy of basal body temperature charts in predicting urinary luteinizing hormone surges, Fertil Steril 45:334, 1986.

50. **Noyes RW, Hertig AT, Rock J,** Dating the endometrial biopsy, Fertil Steril 1:3, 1950.

51. **Wentz AC, Herbert CM III, Maxon WS, Hill GA, Pittaway DE,** Cycle of conception endometrial biopsy, Fertil Steril 46:196, 1986.

52. **Wathen NC, Perry L, Lilford RJ, Chard T,** Interpretaton of single progesterone measurement in diagnosis of anovulation and defective luteal phase: Observations on analysis of the normal range, Brit Med J 288:7, 1984.

53. **Jacobs MH, Balasch J, Gonzalez-Merlo JM, Vanrell JA, Wheeler C, Strauss JF III, Blasco L, Wheeler JE, Lyttle CR,** Endometrial cytosolic and nuclear progesterone receptors in the luteal phase defect, J Clin Endocrinol Metab 64:472, 1987.

54. **Jones GE, Aksel S, Wentz AC,** Serum progesterone values in the luteal phase defects: Effect of chorionic gonadotropin, Obstet Gynecol 56:26, 1974.

55. **Balasch J, Vanrell JA, Marquez M, Burzaco I, Gonzalez-Merlo J,** Dehydrogesterone versus vaginal progesterone in the treatment of the endometrial luteal phase deficiency, Fertil Steril 37:751, 1982.

56. **Huang K-E,** The primary treatment of luteal phase inadequacy: Progesterone versus clomiphene citrate, Am J Obstet Gynecol 155:824, 1986.

57. **Murray D, Reich L, Adashi EY,** Clomiphene citrate and progesterone suppositories in the treatment of luteal phase dysfunction: A comparative study, American Fertility Society, Abstract 216, 1986.

58. **DeVane GW, Guzick DS,** Bromocriptine therapy in normoprolactinemic women with unexplained infertility and galactorrhea, Fertil Steril 46:1026, 1986.

59. **Padilla SL, Person GK, McDonough PG, Reindollar RH,** The efficacy of bromocriptine in patients with ovulatory dysfuntion and normoprolactinemic galactorrhea, Fertil Steril 44:695, 1985.

60. **Driessen F, Holwerda PJ, Putte SCJ, Kremer J,** The significance of dating an endometrial biopsy for the prognosis of the infertile couple, Int J Fertil 25:112, 1980.

61. **Gnarpe H, Friberg J,** T-mycoplasmas as a possible cause for reproductive failure, Nature 242:120, 1973.

62. **de Louvois J, Blades M, Harrison RF, Hurley R, Stanley VC,** Frequency of mycoplasma in fertile and infertile couples, Lancet i:1073, 1974.

63. **Harrison RF, de Louvois J, Blades M, Hurley R,** Doxycycline treatment and human infertility, Lancet i:605, 1975.

543

64. **Toth A, Lesser ML, Brooks C, Labriola D,** Subsequent pregnancies among 161 couples treated for T-mycoplasma genital tract infection, New Eng J Med 308:505, 1983.

65. **Cassell GH, Younger JB, Brown MB, Blackwell RE, Davis JK, Marriott P, Stagno S,** Microbiologic study of infertile women at the time of diagnostic laparoscopy, New Eng J Med 308:502, 1983.

66. **Gump DW, Gibson M, Ashikaga T,** Lack of association between genital mycoplasmas and infertility, New Eng J Med 310:937, 1984.

67. **Franklin RR, Dukes CD,** Further studies on sperm agglutinating antibody and unexplained infertility, JAMA 190:682, 1964.

68. **Rumke P, Van Amstel N, Messer EN, Bezemer PD,** Prognosis of fertility of men with sperm agglutins in the serum, Fertil Steril 25:393, 1974.

69. **Jones WR,** Immunological infertility, fact or fiction? Fertil Steril 33:577, 1980.

70. **Bronson R, Cooper RG, Rosenfeld D,** Sperm antibodies: Their role in infertility, Fertil Steril 42:171, 1984.

71. **Clarke GN, Elliott PJ, Smaila C,** Detection of sperm antibodies in semen using the immunobead test: A survey of 813 consecutive patients, Am J Reprod Immunol Microbiol 7:118, 1985.

72. **Bronson RA, Cooper GW, Rosenfeld DL,** Autoimmunity to spermatozoa: Effect on sperm penetration of cervical mucus as reflected by postcoital testing, Fertil Steril 41:609, 1984.

73. **Ayvaliotis B, Bronson R, Rosenfeld D, Cooper G,** Conception rates in couples where autoimmunity to sperm is detected, Fertil Steril 43:739, 1986.

74. **Alexander NJ, Sampson JH, Fulgham DL,** Pregnancy rates in patients treated for antisperm antibodies with prednisone, Int J Fertil 28:63, 1983.

75. **Hendry WF, Treehuba K, Hughes L, Stedronska J, Parslow JM, Wass JAH, Besser GM,** Cyclic prednisolone therapy for male infertility associated with autoantibodies to spermatozoa, Fertil Steril 45:249, 1986.

76. **Kiser CG, Alexander NJ, Fuchs EF, Fulgham DL,** In vitro immune absorption of antisperm antibodies with immunobead-rise, immunomagnetic, and immunocolumn separation techniques, Fertil Steril 47:466, 1987.

77. **Dhont M, Serreyn R, Duvivier P, Vanluchene E, DeBoever J, Vandekerckhove D,** Ovulation stigma and concentration of progesterone and estradiol in peritoneal fluid: Relation with fertility and endometriosis, Fertil Steril 41:872, 1984.

78. **Janssen-Caspers HAB, Kruitwagen RFPM, Wladimiroff JW, deJong FH, Drogendijk AC,** Diagnosis of luteinized unruptured follicle by ultrasound and steroid hormone assays in peritoneal fluid: A comparative study, Fertil Steril 46:823, 1986.

79. **Hamilton CJCM, Wetzels LCG, Evers JLH, Hoogland HJ, Muijtjens A, deHaan J,** Follicle growth curves and hormonal patterns in patients with the luteinized unruptured follicle syndrome, Fertil Steril 43:541, 1985.

80. **Malpas P,** A study of abortion sequence, J Obstet Gynaecol Brit Emp 45:932, 1938.

81. **Eastman NJ,** Habitual abortion, in Meigs JV, Sturgis S, editors, *Progress in Gynecology,* Vol 1, Grune & Stratton, New York, 1946.

82. **Warburton D, Fraser FS,** Spontaneous abortion risks in man: Data from reproductive histories collected in a medical genetics unit, Am J Hum Genet 16:1, 1964.

83. **Poland BJ, Miller JR, Jones DC, Trimble BK,** Reproductive counseling in patients who have had a spontaneous abortion, Am J Obstet Gynecol 127:685, 1977.

84. **Roman E,** Fetal loss rates and their relation to pregnancy order, J Epidemiol Community Health 38:29, 1984.

85. **Wramsby H, Fredga K, Liedholm P,** Chromosome analysis of human oocytes recovered from preovulatory follicles in stimulated cycles, New Eng J Med 316:121, 1987.

86. **Warburton D,** Reproductive loss: How much is preventable? New Eng J Med 316:158, 1987.

87. **Tho PT, Byrd Jr, McDonough PG,** Etiologies and subsequent reproductive performance of 100 couples with recurrent abortion, Fertil Steril 32:389, 1978.

88. **McDonough PG,** Repeated first-trimester loss: Evaluation and management, Am J Obstet Gynecol 153:1, 1985.

89. **Sherman RP, Garrett WJ,** Double blind study of effect of 17-hydroxy-progesterone caproate on abortion rate, Brit Med J 1:292, 1963.

90. **Jones GES, Delfs E,** Endocrine patterns in term pregnancies following abortion, JAMA 146:1212, 1951.

91. **Botella-Llusia J,** The endometrium in repeated abortion, Int J Fertil 7:147, 1962.

92. **Balasch J, Vanrell JA,** Corpus luteum insufficiency and fertility: A matter of controversy, Human Reprod 2:557, 1987.

93. **Hernanez Horta JL, Gordillo Fernandez J, Soto de Leon B, Cortez-Gallegos V,** Direct evidence of luteal insufficiency in women with habitual abortion, Obstet Gynecol 49:705, 1977.

94. **Yip SK, Sung ML,** Plasma progesterone in women with a history of recurrent early abortions, Fertil Steril 28:151, 1977.

95. **Hensleigh PA, Fainstat T,** Corpus luteum dysfunction: Serum progesterone levels in diagnosis and assessment of therapy for recurrent and threatened abortion, Fertil Steril 32:396, 1979.

96. **Harrison RF,** Treatment of habitual abortion with human chorionic gonadotropin: Results of open and placebo-controlled studies, Europ J Gynecol Reprod Biol 20:491, 1985.

97. **Scott JR, Rote NS, Branch DW,** Immunologic aspects of recurrent abortion and fetal death, Obstet Gynecol 70:645, 1987.

98. **Edelman PH, Rouquette AM, Verdy E, Elias A, Cabane J, Cornet D, Barate J, Chavinie J, Salat-Baroux J, Sureau Cl,** Autoimmunity, fetal losses, lupus anticoagulant: Beginning of systemic lupus erythematosus or new autoimmune entity with gynaeco-obstetrical expression? Human Reprod 1:295, 1986.

99. **Mowbray JF, Gibbings C, Liddell H, Reginald PW, Underwood JL, Beard RW,** Controlled trial of treatment of recurrent spontaneous abortion by immunization with paternal cells, Lancet i:941, 1985.

100. **Unander AM, Lindholm A,** Transfusions of leukocyte-rich erythrocyte concentrates: A successful treatment in selected cases of habitual abortion, Am J Obstet Gynecol 154:516, 1986.

101. **Adinolfi M,** Recurrent habitual abortion, HLA sharing and deliberate immunization with partner's cells: A controversial topic, Human Reprod 1:45, 1986.

102. **Stray-Pedersen B, Stray-Pedersen S,** Etiologic factors and subsequent reproductive performance in 195 couples with a prior history of habitual abortion, Am J Obstet Gynecol 148:140, 1984.

103. **Friedman RR, Gradstein BD,** *Surviving Pregnancy Loss,* Little, Brown and Co., Boston, 1982.

104. **Martin CB,** *Beating the Adoption Game,* Oak Tree Publications, Inc., San Diego, 1980.

105. **Lamb EJ, Leurgans S,** Does adoption affect subsequent fertility? Am J Obstet Gynecol 134:138, 1979.

106. **Taylor PJ, Graham G,** Is diagnostic curettage harmful in women with unexplained infertility? Brit J Obstet Gynaecol 89:296, 1982.

107. **Collins JA, Wrixon W, Janes LB, Wilson EH,** Treatment independent pregnancy among infertile couples, New Eng J Med 309:1201, 1983.

18 Endometriosis and Infertility

Endometriosis is a term indicating ectopic endometrial glands and stroma. Very few problems in infertility have as many unresolved questions as endometriosis. Does mild endometriosis cause infertility? If so, is the mechanism increased concentrations of prostaglandins in peritoneal fluid, the activation of peritoneal macrophages, or some unknown factor? What is the proper treatment of mild or moderate endometriosis—surgery, drugs, or expectant management? If a drug is used, should it be the birth control pill, progestins alone, or danazol? What is the minimal effective dose of danazol? If surgery is performed, should it be accompanied by preoperative or postoperative use of medical treatment?

Studies are providing information that can allow the clinician to provide reasonably educated answers to some of the perplexing problems involved in the management of endometriosis. *This chapter will review the more recent information, as well as what is known about the etiology and pathophysiology of endometriosis.*

Etiology

Endometriosis was described in the medical literature in the 1800's, but it was not until this century that its common occurrence was appreciated. Based on clinical observation and examination of histopathologic specimens, John Sampson of Albany, in 1921, suggested that peritoneal endometriosis in the pelvis arose from seedings from ovarian endometriosis. Subsequently, in 1927, he published his classic paper, ''Peritoneal Endometriosis Due to Menstrual Dissemination of Endometrial Tissue Into the Peritoneal Cavity'', which introduced the term ''endometriosis'' and established retrograde flow of endometrial tissue through the fallopian tubes and into the abdominal cavity as the primary cause of the disease.(1) The conclusions of Sampson have been validated by the following observations:

547

1. During laparoscopy, flow of blood from the fimbriated end of the tube has been noted in menstruating women.

2. Endometriosis is most commonly found in dependent portions of the pelvis.

3. Endometrial fragments from the menstrual flow can grow both in tissue culture and following injection beneath the abdominal skin.

4. Endometriosis developed when the cervices of monkeys were transposed so that menstruation occurred into the peritoneal cavity.(2)

5. The risk of endometriosis is increased in women with shorter menstrual cycles and longer flows, characteristics that give greater opportunity for ectopic endometrial implantation.(3)

Endometriosis at sites distant from the pelvis may be due to vascular or lymphatic transport of endometrial fragments. Endometriosis can occur in almost every organ of the body.(4) For example, pulmonary endometriosis occurs and can be manifested by asymptomatic nodules or as pneumothrorax, hemothorax, or hemoptysis during menses. Urologic endometriosis is of importance because of the possiblity for ureteral obstruction.

There are even case reports of endometriosis in men who received treatment with estrogen, and therefore, another possible cause of endometriosis is the transformation of coelomic epithelium into endometrial-type glands as a result of unspecified stimuli.(5,6)

Because many women have reflux seeding of menstrual debris into the peritoneal cavity, and not all develop endometriosis, there may be genetic or immunologic factors that influence the susceptibility of a woman to the disease. Simpson and co-workers reported 6.9% of first-degree relatives of patients with endometriosis had the disease, compared with 1.0% in a control group.(7) Dmowski and co-workers demonstrated that monkeys with endometriosis had decreased cellular immunity to endometrial tissue, suggesting that specific immunologic defects can render some individuals susceptible to endometriosis.(8) Others have found an increased prevalence of humoral antibodies directed against endometrial and ovarian tissue in the sera of women with endometriosis.(9)

Prevalence

Widely varying figures for the prevalence of endometriosis have been published, and a rough estimate is that 10% of women in the reproductive age group and 25-35% of infertile women have endometriosis.(10) About 4 per 1000 women age 15-64 are hospitalized with endometriosis each year, slightly more than those admitted with breast cancer. The common perceptions that endometriosis only occurs in goal-oriented women over the age of 30 and is not found often in black women have now been discredited. Whereas endometriosis does not occur before menarche, there are increasing reports of its occurrence in the teen years.(11) A number of these cases involve anatomic abnormalities that obstruct the outflow tract. Endometriosis is not confined to nulliparous women, and physicians should be alert to the presence of endometriosis in cases of secondary infertility.

Diagnosis of Endometriosis	Endometriosis should be suspected in any woman complaining of infertility. Suspicion is heightened when there are also complaints of dysmenorrhea and dyspareunia.
Symptoms and Signs	Dysmenorrhea is even more suggestive of endometriosis if it begins after years of relatively pain-free menses. It should be recognized, however, that many women who have endometriosis are asymptomatic. A common observation is that some women with extensive endometriosis have little or no pain, whereas others with only minimal endometriosis complain of severe pain. Pain can be diffuse in the pelvis or it can be more localized, often in the area of the rectum. Symptoms also can arise from rectal, ureteral or bladder involvement with endometriosis, and can be present throughout the month. Low back pain, too, may be due to endometriosis. An association of endometriosis and premenstrual spotting has been suggested, but in most cases menstrual dysfunction is not increased with endometriosis. An association between galactorrhea and endometriosis has been claimed, but baseline elevations of prolactin are not higher in women with endometriosis compared to controls.

The CA-125 Assay. CA-125 is a cell surface antigen found on derivatives of the coelomic epithelium (which includes endometrium). Serum CA-125 levels are elevated in patients with endometriosis and correlate with both the degree of disease and the response to treatment.(12,13) The sensitivity of this assay is too low to use it as a screening test, but it can be a marker of response to treatment and for recurrence. In addition, serum CA-125 determinations can differentiate endometriotic from nonendometriotic benign adnexal cysts.(14)

Examination	The uterus is often in fixed retroversion and the ovaries may be enlarged. However, retroversion of the uterus is not an etiologic factor and prophylactic uterine suspension is no longer recommended. Nodularity (which is usually tender) of the uterosacral ligaments and cul-de-sac can be found in one-third of patients with endometriosis. The diagnosis almost always should be confirmed by laparoscopy before treatment is initiated. Minimal findings such as a slight beading of the uterosacral ligaments in the young, asymptomatic patient can be treated, however, by cyclic use of birth control pills.

The appearance of endometriosis is quite varied. All too often the clinician fails to observe endometrial lesions because of a preconceived expectation limited to the classic blue or black powder burn appearance. Lesions can be red, black, blue, or white and nonpigmented.(15) Adhesions and tan, creamy, fresh-appearing endometrium can also be observed. The dark pigmented lesions are later consequences of tissue bleeding responses to cyclic hormones. The ovary is the most common site for both implants and adhesions, followed by widespread distribution, anteriorly and posteriorly, over the broad ligament and cul-de-sac.

The AFS Classification System. Because both treatment and prognosis are determined to some extent by the severity of the disease, it is desirable to have a uniform system of classification that takes into account both the extent and severity of the disease. A uniform classification is also crucial for comparing the results of different treatments. The American Fertility Society has developed a classification system based on findings at laparoscopy or laparotomy, and forms are available from the Society.(16)

Endometriosis and Infertility

When endometriosis involves the ovaries and causes adhesions that block tubal motility and pickup of the egg from the ovarian surface, there is no question of its role in causing mechanical interference with fertility. Less secure is the information on the role of peritoneal endometriosis on fertility. Many physicians believe that even minimal endometriosis can cause infertility. Dyspareunia secondary to endometriosis could play a role.

Another mediator could be prostaglandins produced by the implants, which could, in turn, affect tubal motility, or folliculogenesis and corpus luteum function. Meldrum et al first noted increased levels of prostaglandin $F_{2\alpha}$ in the peritoneal fluid of patients with endometriosis.(17) Drake and co-workers found that patients with endometriosis had an increase in both the volume of peritoneal fluid and the concentration of thromboxane B_2 and 6-keto-prostaglandin $F_{1\alpha}$ in the fluid.(18,19) Rock and colleagues, however, found neither an increase in peritoneal fluid nor an increase in concentration of peritoneal fluid prostaglandin E_2, prostaglandin $F_{2\alpha}$, 15-keto-13,14-dihydroprostaglandin $F_{2\alpha}$, and thromboxane B_2.(20,21)

Subsequent studies also have provided contradictory information. Sgarlatta et al could find no elevation in prostanoid levels during the proliferative phase in women with endometriosis and Mudge et al noted no elevation in 6-keto prostaglandin $F_{1\alpha}$ levels in the luteal phase. (22,23) However, others have reported elevated concentrations of prostanoids in the peritoneal fluid of women with endometriosis.(24) These differences may be accounted for by differing levels of prostaglandin synthesis according to different morphologic characteristics of the lesions.(25) In summary, it has not been established that women with endometriosis have higher levels of prostanoids in peritoneal fluid compared to other infertile women. Even if higher levels were found consistently, their role in infertility still would be speculative.

Peritoneal macrophages have been suggested as possible mediators of infertility, and increased activation of macrophages has been found in association with endometriosis.(26,27) Phagocytosis of sperm by macrophages could be one mechanism of action.(28) However, patients with and without endometriosis have the same number of motile sperm recoverable from the peritoneal cavity.(29) To date, the role of macrophages in endometriosis-associated infertility has not been established, but it remains an interesting area for study.

The question of how mild endometriosis can affect fertility, which is addressed by the above studies, now has been superseded by the question of whether there is *any* effect of mild endometriosis on fertility. Many articles purporting to show that therapy overcomes endometriosis-associated infertility are flawed by lack of control

American Fertility Society Classification of Endometriosis

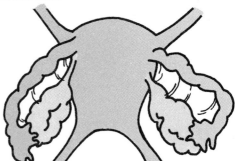

Patient's Name_____

Stage I (Minimal)   —1–5
Stage II (Mild)   —6–15
Stage III (Moderate)—16–40
Stage IV (Severe)   —>40

Total_____

*If the fimbriated end of the fallopian tube is completely enclosed, change the point assignment to 16.

	ENDOMETRIOSIS	<1cm	1-3cm	>3cm
PERITONEUM	Superficial	1	2	4
	Deep	2	4	6
OVARY	R Superficial	1	2	4
	Deep	4	16	20
	L Superficial	1	2	4
	Deep	4	16	20
	ADHESIONS	<1/3 Enclosure	1/3-2/3 Enclosure	>2/3 Enclosure
OVARY	R Filmy	1	2	4
	Dense	4	8	16
	L Filmy	1	2	4
	Dense	4	8	16
TUBE	R Filmy	1	2	4
	Dense	4*	8*	16
	L Filmy	1	2	4
	Dense	4*	8*	16

POSTERIOR CULDESAC OBLITERATION	Partial	Complete
	4	40

groups and the failure to use life table analyses.(30) Moreover, expectant management of mild endometriosis is rewarded with reasonable pregnancy rates.(31-36)

These latter reports force a reassessment of our thinking concerning the role of mild endometriosis in infertility. Specifically, should peritoneal implants be treated if the only complaint is infertility? Whereas the studies cited above (31-36) strongly suggest that medical or surgical treatment of mild endometriosis may not be worthwhile, there are those who champion fulguration treatment under laparoscopic visualization.(37-39) Because of lack of proof of its efficacy, the occasional report of ureteral injury occurring during fulguration of endometrial implants on the uterosacral ligaments, and the suspicion of some clinicians that burned areas may become a nidus for adhesion formation, we would reserve laparoscopic fulguration of minimal endometrial implants for those patients who have significant pelvic pain. This conservative approach may become outmoded as the use of laser provides precise destruction of implants with less risk than cautery of extending damage to normal tissue. Furthermore, an argument can be made that active treatment of even mild endometriosis can slow progression of the disease.

Not everyone agrees with this hands-off approach. An aggressive method was used by Buttram and Betts (40) who noted that of 56 women with mild endometriosis and an average duration of infertility of 37 months, 73.2% were pregnant within 15 months of conservative surgery by laparotomy. Of those who conceived, 36.6% did so in 3 months and 55.7% within 6 months. *It should be emphasized, however, that based on monthly fecundity rates and life table analyses, no study has shown an advantage for conservative surgery as opposed to expectant management.*(41)

Surgical Treatment of Endometriosis

In contrast to the dispute over the proper treatment of mild endometriosis, there is little doubt that adhesive disease associated with endometriosis, or large (>1 cm) endometriomas, is best treated by surgery. The object of surgery should be to restore normal anatomical relationships and to excise or fulgurate as much of the endometriosis as possible. A moderate approach that emphasizes avoiding the creation of large areas that cannot be reperitonealized and not risking damage to blood vessels and vital organs has been rewarded with a higher pregnancy rate in women with moderate or severe endometriosis than an aggressive approach that attempts to remove every vestige of the disease. Similarly, removal of severely diseased adnexa when the other side is more normal produces better results than attempts to do major repairs. The text by Buttram and Reiter is recommended for a description of surgical techniques. (42)

Because of the propensity for adhesion formation at the site of ovarian surgery, great care must be taken in approximating the edges of the ovary if an endometrioma is removed. A fine running suture of 6-0 Dexon, or Vicryl of similar size, should be used. The use of 32% Dextran-70 to prevent adhesions is now controversial because of lack of proof of efficacy; however, we continue to instill approximately 200 ml into the pelvis prior to closing the peritoneum. Suspension of a retroverted uterus may be a useful adjunct to prevent further adhesion formation by preventing the ovaries from adhering to raw areas in the cul-de-sac. Plication of the uterosacral ligaments

552

following excision of endometrial implants will aid in keeping the uterus in anterior position. Presacral neurectomy does not enhance fertility, although many surgeons advocate it to alleviate dysmenorrhea. This may be less compelling now that prostaglandin inhibitors are available to accomplish the same purpose.

The success of surgery in relieving infertility is directly related to the severity of endometriosis. Patients with moderate disease can expect a pregnancy success of approximately 60%, whereas the comparable figure is 35% in those with severe disease.(39) There is support for selective use of danazol for 2-3 months following laparoscopy and prior to conservative surgery. (43) Preoperative treatment aids surgery by softening endometrial implants. Postoperative use of hormones has been the subject of greater controversy. The highest pregnancy rates following conservative surgery occur in the first year after surgery, and most physicians have been reluctant to use hormones that prevent pregnancy even for a few months. Wheeler and Malinak, however, treated 19 women with 400-800 mg/day of danazol for 3-6 months following surgery for *severe* endometriosis.(44) All became amenorrheic for at least 3 months. Fifteen (79%) of these women conceived. By contrast, only 36 of 199 (30%) women with severe endometriosis treated by surgery alone conceived. While on the basis of this report, danazol appears to be a useful postoperative adjunct to surgery for severe endometriosis, conflicting findings have been reported by Buttram et al.(45)

If pregnancy does not occur within 2 years of surgery for endometriosis, the chances are poor that it will occur. The recurrence rates reported for endometriosis after surgery are usually below 20%, but when it does recur, second surgeries to aid fertility have only a limited chance for success.

The type of surgery that we have been discussing is labeled "conservative" to indicate that reproductive function is maintained. When endometriomas are removed a vigorous attempt should be made to leave behind any normal ovarian tissue. Even 1/10 of an ovary can be enough to preserve function and fertility. Increasingly, conservative surgery is being accomplished by laser laparoscopy which decreases costs and morbidity, yet provides results that are as efficacous in all stages of disease as other forms of therapy.(46)

"Conservative" surgery is in contradistinction to "radical" surgery, which involves hysterectomy and usually bilateral salpingo-oophorectomy. When radical surgery is performed, an uninvolved ovary can be preserved in some cases if all of the nonovarian endometriosis is removed by fulguration or excision. This does provide a risk for recurrent disease, but the risk seems to be small.

Hormonal Treatment of Endometriosis

Medical therapy for dysmenorrhea, dyspareunia, and pelvic pain associated with endometriosis is very successful, and the various agents used are comparable in terms of efficacy. Implants of endometriosis react to steroid hormones in a manner somewhat similar to normally stimulated endometrium. Thus, estrogen stimulates growth of the implants.

553

Hormone therapy is designed to interrupt the cycle of stimulation and bleeding. An early approach was the use of massive doses of diethylstilbestrol (DES), which, because of variable success, the risk of affecting a female fetus, and side effects of severe bleeding and nausea, is now of only historical interest. Treatment with androgens (methyltestosterone linguets 5-10 mg/day) can provide temporary relief of the pain of endometriosis, but its effect on infertility appears to be negligible. In addition, ovulation can occur while on treatment, and there is a risk of exposure of the fetus to the androgen.

Until the late 1970's the most important alternative to conservative surgery was the use of combination birth control pills taken in a continuous fashion.(47) It seems to matter little which preparation is used to accomplish the conversion of endometrial implants into decidualized cells associated with a few inactive endometrial glands. At this time the efficacy of the multiphasic formulations is unknown. The usual dose of the combination birth control pills is one pill per day continuously for 6-12 months. Conjugated estrogens (2.5 mg daily for 1 week) are added if breakthrough bleeding occurs. The treatment with birth control pills was called pseudopregnancy because of the amenorrhea and the decidualization of the endometrial tissue induced by the estrogen-progestin combination. It also reflected the commonly held belief that pregnancy can improve endometriosis, a belief that has been disputed. The side effects of treatment are those associated with birth control pills (Chapter 15), but some, e.g., weight gain, are more common with continuous as opposed to cyclic use. Pregnancy rates after stopping medication are reported to be in the 40-50% range. Whereas published recurrence rates are not excessive, this therapy, as with all hormone treatment for endometriosis, must be viewed as suppressive rather than curative.

Danazol

In distinction to the pseudopregnancy induced by birth control pills, danazol produces what has been incorrectly termed as pseudomenopause. Danazol is an isoxazole derivative of the synthetic steroid 17α-ethinyltestosterone.(48) It originally was thought to exert its effect solely by inhibition of pituitary gonadotropins. Although danazol can decrease follicle-stimulating hormone (FSH) and luteinizing hormone (LH) in castrated individuals, it does not alter basal gonadotropin concentrations in premenopausal women. It does, however, eliminate the midcycle surge of FSH and LH. Asch et al demonstrated a shortening of the luteal phase in monkeys treated with danazol, an effect that was not reversed by injections of human chorionic gonadotropin (HCG), suggesting a direct effect on the ovary.(49) Similarly, danazol inhibits steroidogenesis in the human corpus luteum.(50) Danazol is metabolized to at least 60 different products, some of which may contribute to its many effects. The multiple actions of danazol include:(51)

1. Binding to androgen, progesterone, and glucocorticoid receptors, producing both agonistic and antagonistic actions.

2. No binding to intracellular estrogen receptors.

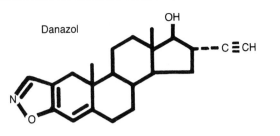

Danazol

3. Binding to sex hormone binding globulin (displacing testosterone and thus increasing free testosterone) and to corticosteroid binding globulin (with a small increase in free cortisol).

4. Decrease in sex hormone binding globulin production by the liver as well as an increase in a host of other liver proteins.

5. Prevention of the midcyle surge of FSH and LH, but no significant suppression of basal FSH or LH (mainly an androgen agonistic action).

6. No effect on aromatization.

7. Inhibition of the following enzymes involved in steroidogenesis:
   cholesterol cleavage enzyme
   3β-hydroxysteroid dehydrogenase
   17β-hydroxysteroid dehydrogenase
   17,20-desmolase
   17α-hydroxylase
   11β-hydroxylase
   21-hydroxylase

The multiple effects of danazol produce a high androgen, low estrogen environment that does not support the growth of endometriosis, and the amenorrhea that is produced prevents new seeding from the uterus into the peritoneal cavity.

The side effects of danazol are related both to the hypoestrogenic environment it creates and to its androgenic properties. The most common side effects are weight gain, fluid retention, fatigue, decreased breast size, acne, oily skin, growth of facial hair, atrophic vaginitis, hot flushes, muscle cramps, and emotional lability. Some of these side effects occur in approximately 80% of women who are taking danazol, but less than 10% find the side effects sufficiently troublesome to warrant discontinuation of the drug. An occasional skin rash may be an allergic response to the red dye contained in the capsule. Because danazol has been associated with the development *in utero* of female pseudohermaphroditism, it should not be given if there is the possibility of pregnancy.(52) The androgenic action of danazol can irreversibly deepen the voice.(53) It is worth enquiring whether singing is an important part of your patient's life.

Danazol is metabolized largely in the liver, and in some patients it causes hepatocellular damage. Its use, therefore, is contraindicated in women with liver disease. The fluid retention that is often associated with danazol makes it dangerous to use when there is severe hypertension, congestive heart failure, or impaired renal function. It may produce increased cholesterol levels and decreased high-density lipoproteins. It is uncertain how this relatively short-term effect should influence the use of danazol. The drug has been used to treat autoimmune disease, but it is not known if this action plays a role in its effects on endometriosis.

It should be noted again that treatment of mild endometriosis associated with infertility has been called into question because women with untreated mild endometriosis have pregnancy rates equal to women who have received treatment for the endometriosis. Garcia and David reported that 11 of 17 (64.7%) women with mild endometriosis became pregnant without treatment within two years of laparoscopy.(31) These 17 women had had a mean duration of infertility of 3.3 years. Schenken and Malinak found that 12 of 16 (75%) patients with mild endometriosis conceived within a year without treatment compared with a conception rate of 72.4% (21 of 29) in women with similar disease who had conservative surgery. (32) In a prospective study, Seibel et al reported 13 of 19 (68%) women with minimal endometriosis became pregnant during 1 year of observation.(33) This compared with 5 pregnancies in 13 women (38%) with minimal endometriosis who were treated with danazol for 6 months and then observed for 6 months. Others have made similar observations.(34-36) Thus, treatment of mild endometriosis either with danazol or by laparotomy has little scientific support.

On the other hand, danazol is useful to relieve the pain of endometriosis, to treat infertility due to moderate endometriosis, and to prevent progression of the disease. Pain relief is obtained in 90% of patients. The usual dose is two 200 mg tablets twice a day (although some claim that spacing the drug at 6 hour intervals may be more effective) for 6 months. Dmowski and Cohen reviewed 99 women who completed danazol treatment for a period of 3-18 months (average 6 months) and who were reevaluated an average of 37 months later.(54) During the course of treatment all the patients had symptomatic improvement and the majority (85%) were clinically improved. At the time of the reevaluation, however, approximately one-third were symptomatic and had clinical findings suggestive of recurrent endometriosis. In the majority of these patients, the symptoms recurred within the first year after discontinuation of the drug. Of the 84 patients who desired pregnancy after treatment with danazol, 39 (46.5%) conceived. The authors claimed that if couples with other causes of infertility, in addition to endometriosis, were excluded, the corrected pregnancy rate was 72.2%.

The success of danazol treatment is greatest in cases of peritoneal endometriosis or those with small lesions of the ovary. Endometriomas larger than 1.0 cm are less likely to respond to danazol, although quite surprising regression of endometriomas larger than 1.0 cm are sometimes seen.

Because of the significant side effects encountered with danazol, and its cost, there has been a trend toward the use of lower doses than the usual 800 mg daily. Dmowski et al feel, however, that doses below 800 mg are less effective.(55) They also imply that the occurrence of amenorrhea is correlated with improved outcome and that this is more consistently obtained at the 800 mg level. Others, however, do not believe that amenorrhea is an important consideration because many of the patients will bleed from an atrophic endometrium.

Biberoglu and Behrman compared women receiving 100, 200, or 600 mg daily of danazol.(56) Patients receiving 100 mg of danazol required 2 months to gain considerable relief of symptoms, whereas relief came in the 1st month for those using higher doses. By the 6th month of treatment, the percentages of patients with amenorrhea were 29% with 100 mg, 38% with 200 mg, 86% with 400 mg, and 88% with 600 mg. These figures correlated roughly with laparoscopically determined freedom from endometriosis, which was 14.2% with 100 mg, 62.5% with 200 mg, 57.1% with 400 mg, and 87.5% with 600 mg. These latter figures did not take into consideration endometriomas, because the authors believed that ovarian endometriomas greater than 1.0 cm are relatively unresponsive to danazol. The numbers of pregnancies were too small to compare for the different groups.

Gambrell and Greenblatt reported a double blind study that utilized daily doses of 0.2, 6.25, 25 and 100 mg of danazol in 27 infertile women with laparoscopically proven endometriosis.(57) The results were compared with 37 women treated with either 400 or 800 mg of danazol. Amenorrhea occurred in all 41 patients treated with the 2 higher doses but only 3 (11.1%) of those treated with doses below 400 mg. When patients with other infertility factors were eliminated from consideration, pregnancy rates were 69.2% when 0.2-100 mg of danazol were used, compared to 81.8% in those women treated with 400-800 mg of danazol. One drawback to the use of very low doses of danazol is that pregnancy may occur while the patient is taking the medication, thus entailing a risk of genitourinary abnormalities in the fetus. Buttram and co-workers found that cumulative pregnancy rates were similar with 400 mg/day and 800 mg/day of danazol.(45)

Our approach is to start with 400 mg/day on day 1 of menses and continue at that dose if the patient becomes amenorrheic after the subsequent menses. If bleeding recurs after that time, the dose is increased to 600 mg per day or 800 mg per day. Therapy usually is continued for 6 months although shorter periods (3-4 months) may be appropriate.

There is a general perception, but only limited experimental evidence, that danazol is more effective than birth control pills for the treatment of endometriosis.(58) Noble and Letchworth compared danazol with a high dose estrogen-progestin combination (Enovid). (59) The dose of both danazol and the birth control pill was increased until the patients became amenorrheic. One of 25 patients taking danazol could not complete 5 months of treatment, whereas 7 of 17 (41%) of the group taking birth control pills dropped out because of side effects. Danazol was more effective than estrogen-progestin in relieving symptoms, and laparoscopic assessment showed much better results with danazol. Seven of 12 danazol-treated patients became pregnant compared with 4 of the 10 women who had taken birth control pills. Unfortunately, the study size was too small to allow statistical analysis.

To date it has not been established whether danazol or surgery is the better treatment for moderate endometriosis that is not associated with pelvic adhesions.

Provera

Both oral Provera (medroxyprogesterone acetate, 30 mg/day) and injectable Depo-Provera have been effective in treating endometriosis. *In a comparison study, oral medroxyprogesterone acetate was found to be as effective as danazol.*(36) For this reason and because it is more cost-effective and there are fewer side effects, medroxyprogesterone acetate is the first choice for medical treatment of endometriosis. Breakthrough bleeding is a common occurrence although it is usually cleared by short-term (7 days) administration of estrogen. Depression is a significant problem, and both patient and physician should be alert for its development. The usefulness of Depo-Provera in infertile patients is limited by the varying length of time it takes for ovulation to resume after discontinuation of therapy. This is not a major problem with oral administration.

GnRH Agonist

A long-acting GnRH agonist delivered intranasally or subcutaneously can create a pseudomenopause for the treatment of endometriosis.(60,61) At the end of 2-4 weeks of daily administration of the agonist, estrogen levels will decrease to those found in oophorectomized women. Thus, the "medical oophorectomy" caused by the continuous use of a GnRH agonist adds a new approach to the treatment of endometriosis. An excellent, large, well-designed study (with advanced disease in nearly 50% of the patients) compared a GnRH agonist by nasal spray with danazol.(62) The results in terms of reduction of disease (as demonstrated by post-treatment laparoscopies) and pregnancy rates (39%) were the same with either treatment. In addition, an experimental comparison of agonist and progestin treatment in monkeys concluded that the progestin was just as effective as the agonist.(63)

As with all other drug therapies of endometriosis, the GnRH agonist provides suppression rather than cure of the disease. The long-term consequences on calcium metabolism and bone are of concern and still uncertain. Nevertheless, the GnRH agonist provides an equally effective alternative when side effects prevent the use of danazol or progestin treatment.

Recurrence

Endometriosis tends to recur unless definitive surgery is performed. The recurrence rate is approximately 5-20% per year (reaching a cumulative rate at 5 years as much as 40%). Speculation regarding the reason for recurrence focuses on endometriosis (perhaps microscopic) which escaped detection, incomplete treatment, or reestablishment of primary disease by whatever mechanism is responsible. The treatment choices and results are no different than when originally confronted. Therefore it is not surprising that patients and physicians ultimately may choose in vitro fertilization or intrafallopian tube transfer to achieve fertility or definitive surgery to achieve relief.

Hormone Replacement after Surgery	Definitive surgery for severe endometriosis, which includes abdominal hysterectomy and bilateral salpingo-oophorectomy as well as resection of all endometriosis, is the only cure for the disease. If oophorectomy is performed, estrogen-progestin replacement at usual doses can be used with an almost negligible risk of inciting growth of residual endometriosis.
Long-Term Hormonal Therapy	Long-term hormonal therapy without surgery is useful in patients with severe symptoms but with little in the way of palpable findings. Before undertaking prolonged therapy, diagnosis should be established by laparoscopy. Prolonged therapy also is indicated if symptoms recur after conservative surgery.
Prevention of Infertility	A common clinical problem is the finding at surgery of mild endometriosis in a young woman who has no immediate interest in pregnancy. Cyclic birth control pills to prevent further seeding are appropriate for treatment of very mild disease, for example a few implants in the cul de sac. More advanced disease should be treated with 6 months of danazol or medroxyprogesterone acetate, followed by cyclic birth control pills to decrease the risks of further seeding.
Endometriosis and Spontaneous Abortion	Endometriosis has been purported to be associated with an increased risk of spontaneous abortion, a risk that is said to be substantially lessened by either hormonal or surgical treatment.[64] In appropriately controlled studies, however, the abortion rate was in the normal range in women with endometriosis who were not treated, and it is likely that previous studies were flawed by their choice of control figures.[65,66]
Endometriosis and Ovulation	The frequency of anovulation and luteal phase defects is similar in women with and without endometriosis.[67] Thus, a woman need not be ovulating in order to have endometriosis. One report has suggested, however, that the success of ovulation induction in women with endometriosis is enhanced by prior treatment with danazol.[68]
Endometriosis and In Vitro Fertilization	Use of in vitro fertilization to treat infertility associated with mild or moderate endometriosis is rewarded with pregnancy rates comparable to those achieved when IVF is used in women with tubal disease. By contrast, the results with severe endometriosis are exceedingly poor. This reflects not only a greater difficulty in exposing follicles for aspiration but some unspecified deficiency in embryo survival.[69,70]

References	1. **Sampson JA,** Peritoneal endometriosis due to the menstrual dissemination of endometrial tissue into the peritoneal cavity, Am J Obstet Gynecol 14:422, 1927.
	2. **Scott RB, TeLinde RW, Wharton LR Jr,** Further studies on experimental endometriosis, Am J Obstet Gynecol 66:1082, 1953.
	3. **Cramer DW, Wilson E, Stillman RJ, Berger MJ, Belisle S, Schiff I, Albrecht B, Gibson M, Stadel BV, Schoenbaum SC,** The relation of endometriosis to menstrual characteristics, smoking and exercise, JAMA 355:1904, 1986.

4. **Rock JA, Markham SM,** Extra pelvic endometriosis, in Wilson EA, editor, *Endometriosis,* Alan R. Liss, Inc., New York, 1987, pp 185-206.

5. **Oliker AJ, Harris AE,** Endometriosis of the bladder in a male patient, J Urol 106:858, 1971.

6. **Merrill JA,** Endometrial induction of endometriosis across millipore filters, Am J Obstet Gynecol 94:780, 1966.

7. **Simpson JL, Elias J, Malinak LR, Buttram VC,** Heritable aspects of endometriosis. I. Genetic studies, Am J Obstet Gynecol 137:327, 1980.

8. **Dmowski WP, Steele RW, Baker GF,** Deficient cellular immunity in endometriosis, Am J Obstet Gynecol 141:377, 1981.

9. **Mathur S, Peress MR, Williamson HO, Youmans CD, Maney SA, Garvin AJ, Rust PF, Fudenberg HH,** Autoimmunity to endometrium and ovary in endometriosis, Clin Exp Immunol 50:259, 1982.

10. **Cramer DW,** Epidemiology of endometriosis, in Wilson EA, editor, *Endometriosis*, Alan R. Liss, Inc., New York, 1987, pp 5-22.

11. **Sanfillippo JS,** Endometriosis in adolescents, in Wilson EA, editor, *Endometriosis,* Alan R. Liss, Inc., New York, 1987, pp 161-172.

12. **Barbieri RL, Niloff JM, Bast RC Jr, Schaetzl E, Kistner RW, Knapp RC,** Elevated serum concentrations of CA-125 in patients with advanced endometriosis, Fertil Steril 45:630, 1986.

13. **Pittaway DE, Fayez JA,** The use of CA-125 in the diagnosis and management of endometriosis, Fertil Steril 46:790, 1986.

14. **Pittaway DE, Fayez JA,. Douglas JW,** Serum CA-125 in the evaluation of benign adnexal cysts, Am J Obstet Gynecol 157:1426, 1987.

15. **Jansen RPS, Russell P,** Nonpigmented endometriosis: Clinical, laparoscopic and pathologic definition, Am J Obstet Gynecol 155:1154, 1986.

16. **Revised American Fertility Society Classification of Endometriosis,** Fertil Steril 43:351, 1985.

17. **Meldrum DR, Shamonki IM, Clark KE,** Prostaglandin content of ascitic fluid in endometriosis: A preliminary report, Program, Twenty-Fifth Annual Meeting, Pacific Coast Fertility Society, October 1977.

18. **Drake TS, Metz SA, Grunert GM, O'Brien WF,** Peritoneal fluid volume in endometriosis, Fertil Steril 34:280, 1980.

19. **Drake TS, O'Brien WF, Ramwell PW, Metz SA,** Peritoneal fluid thromboxane B_2 and 6-keto-prostaglandin $F_{1\alpha}$ in endometriosis, Am J Obstet Gynecol 140:401, 1981.

20. **Rock JA, Dubin NH, Ghodgaonkar RB, Berquist CA, Erozan YS, Kimball AW Jr,** Cul-de-sac fluid in women with endometriosis: Fluid volume and prostanoid concentration during the proliferative phase of the cycle—days 8 to 12, Fertil Steril 37:747, 1982.

21. **Rezai N, Ghodgaonkar RB, Zacur HA, Rock JA, Dubin NH,** Cul-de-sac fluid in women with endometriosis: Fluid volume, protein and prostanoid concentration during the periovulatory period—days 13 to 18, Fertil Steril 48:29, 1987.

22. **Sgarlatta CS, Hertelendy F, Mikhail G,** The prostanoid content in peritoneal fluid and plasma of women with endometriosis, Am J Obstet Gynecol 147:563, 1983.

23. **Mudge TJ, James MJ, Jones WR, Walsh JA,** Peritoneal fluid 6-keto-prostaglandin $F_{1\alpha}$ levels in women with endometriosis, Am J Obstet Gynecol 152:901, 1985.

24. **DeLeon FD, Vijayakumar R, Brown M, Rao CV, Yussman MA, Schultz G,** Peritoneal fluid volume, estrogen, progesterone, prostaglandin, and epidermal growth factor concentrations in patients with and without endometriosis, Obstet Gynecol 68:189, 1986.

25. **Vernon MW, Beard JS, Graves K, Wilson EA,** Classification of endometriotic implants by morphologic appearance and capacity to synthesize prostaglandin F, Fertil Steril 46:801, 1986.

26. **Halme J, Becker S, Wing R,** Accentuated cyclic activation of peritoneal macrophages in patients with endometriosis, Am J Obstet Gynecol 148:85, 1984.

27. **Chacho KJ, Chacho MS, Andresen PJ, Scommegna A,** Peritoneal fluid in patients with and without endometriosis: Prostanoids and macrophages and their effect on the spermatozoa penetration assay, Am J Obstet Gynecol 154:1290, 1986.

28. **Muscato JJ, Haney AF, Weinberg JB,** Sperm phagocytosis by human peritoneal macrophages: A possible cause of infertility and endometriosis, Am J Obstet Gynecol 144:503, 1982.

29. **Stone SC, Himsl K,** Peritoneal recovery of motile and nonmotile sperm in the presence of endometriosis, Fertil Steril 46:338, 1986.

30. **Olive DL, Haney AF,** Endometriosis-associated infertility: A critical review of therapeutic approaches, Obstet Gynecol Surv 41:538, 1986.

31. **Garcia CF, David SS,** Pelvic endometriosis: Infertility and pelvic pain, Am J Obstet Gynecol 129:740, 1977.

32. **Schenken RS, Malinak LR,** Conservative surgery versus expectant management for the infertile patient with mild endometriosis, Fertil Steril 37:183, 1982.

33. **Seibel M, Berger MJ, Weinstein FG, Taymor ML,** The effectiveness of danazol on subsequent fertility in minimal endometriosis, Fertil Steril 38:534, 1982.

34. **Portuondo JA, Echanojauregui AD, Herran C, Alijarte I,** Early conception in patients with untreated mild endometriosis, Fertil Steril 39:22, 1983.

35. **Olive DL, Stohs GF, Metzger DA, Franklin RR,** Expectant management and hydrotubations in the treatment of endometriosis-associated infertility, Fertil Steril 44:35, 1985.

36. **Hull ME, Moghissi KS, Magyar DF, Haves MF,** Comparison of different treatment modalities of endometriosis in infertile women, Fertil Steril 47:40, 1987.

37. **Hasson HM,** Electrocoagulation of pelvic endometriotic lesions with laparoscopic control, Am J Obstet Gynecol 135:115, 1979.

561

38. **Sulewski JM, Curcio FD, Bronitsky C, Stenger VG,** The treatment of endometriosis at laparoscopy for infertility, Am J Obstet Gynecol 138:128, 1980.

39. **Martin DC,** CO_2 laser laparoscopy for endometriosis associated with infertility, J Reprod Fertil 31:1089, 1986.

40. **Buttram VC Jr, Betts JW,** Endometriosis, Curr Probl Obstet Gynecol 11:No. 11, 1979.

41. **Olive DL, Lee KL,** Analysis of sequential treatment protocols for endometriosis-associated infertility, Am J Obstet Gynecol 154:613, 1986.

42. **Buttram VC Jr, Reiter RC,** *Surgical Treatment of the Infertile Female,* Williams & Wilkins, Baltimore, 1985.

43. **Donnez J, Lemaire-Rubbers M, Karaman Y, Nisolle-Pochet M, Casanas-Roux F,** Combined (hormonal and microsurgical) therapy in infertile women with endometriosis, Fertil Steril 48:239, 1987.

44. **Wheeler JM, Malinak LR,** Postoperative danazol therapy in infertility patients with severe endometriosis, Fertil Steril 36:460, 1981.

45. **Buttram VC Jr, Reiter RC, Ward S,** Treatment of endometriosis with danazol: Report of a six year prospective study, Fertil Steril 43:353, 1985.

46. **Olive DL, Martin DC,** Treatment of endometriosis-associated infertility with CO_2 laser laparoscopy: The use of one- and two-parameter exponential models, Fertil Steril 48:18, 1987.

47. **Kistner RW,** Management of endometriosis in the infertile patient, Fertil Steril 26:1151, 1975.

48. **Dmowski WP,** Endocrine properties and clinical application of danazol, Fertil Steril 31:237, 1979.

49. **Asch RH, Fernandez EO, Siler-Khodr TM, Bartke A, Pauerstein CJ,** Mechanism of induction of luteal phase defects by danazol, Am J Obstet Gynecol 136:932, 1980.

50. **Barbieri RL, Osathanondh R, Ryan KJ,** Danazol inhibition of steroidogenesis in the human corpus luteum, Obstet Gynecol 57:722, 1981.

51. **Barbieri RL, Hornstein MD,** Medical therapy for endometriosis, in Wilson EA, editor, *Endometriosis,* Alan R. Liss, Inc., New York, 1987, pp 111-140.

52. **Quagliarello J, Alba Greco M,** Danazol and urogenital sinus formation in pregnancy, Fertil Steril 43:939, 1985.

53. **Wardle PG, Whitehead MI, Mills RP,** Nonreversible and wide ranging vocal changes after treatment with danazol, Brit Med J 287:946, 1983.

54. **Dmowski WP, Cohen MR,** Antigonadotropin (danazol) in the treatment of endometriosis: Evaluation of post-treatment fertility and three-year follow-up data, Am J Obstet Gynecol 130:41, 1978.

55. **Dmowski WP, Kapetanakis E, Scommegna A,** Variable effects of danazol on endometriosis at 4 low-dose levels, Obstet Gynecol 59:408, 1982.

56. **Biberoglu KO, Behrman SJ,** Dosage aspects of danazol therapy in endometriosis: Short-term and long-term effectiveness, Am J Obstet Gynecol 139:645, 1981.

57. **Gambrell RD Jr, Greenblatt RB,** Treatment of infertility due to endometriosis with low dosages of danazol, Fertil Steril 37:304, 1982.

58. **Barbieri RL, Evans S, Kistner RW,** Danazol in the treatment of endometriosis: Analysis of 100 cases with a 4-year follow-up, Fertil Steril 37:737, 1982.

59. **Noble AD, Letchworth AT,** Medical treatment of endometriosis : A comparative trial, Postgrad Med J 55 (Suppl 5):37, 1979.

60. **Meldrum DR,** Clinical management of endometriosis with luteinizing hormone-releasing hormone analogues, Seminars Reprod Endocrinol 3:371, 1985.

61. **Lemay A, Sandow J, Bureau M, Maheux R, Fontaine J-Y, Merat P,** Prevention of follicular maturation in endometriosis by subcutaneous infusion of luteinizing hormone-releasing hormone agonist started in the luteal phase, Fertil Steril 49:410, 1988.

62. **Henzl MR, Corson SL, Moghissi K, Buttram VC, Berqvist C, Jacobson J,** Administration of nasal nafarelin as compared with oral danazol for endometriosis, New Eng J Med 318:485, 1988.

63. **Mann DR, Collins DC, Smith MM, Kessler MJ, Gould KG,** Treatment of endometriosis in monkeys: Effectiveness of continuous infusion of a gonadotropin-releasing hormone agonist compared to treatment with a progestational steroid, J Clin Endocrinol Metab 63:1277, 1986.

64. **Groll M,** Endometriosis and spontaneous abortion, Fertil Steril 41:933, 1984.

65. **Metzger DA, Olive DL, Stohs GF, Franklin RR,** Association of endometriosis and spontaneous abortion: Effect of control group selection, Fertil Steril 45:18, 1986.

66. **FitzSimmons J, Stahl R, Gocial B, Shapiro SS,** Spontaneous abortion and endometriosis, Fertil Steril 47:696, 1987.

67. **Pittaway DE, Maxson W, Daniell J, Herbert C, Wentz AC,** Luteal phase defects in infertility patients with endometriosis, Fertil Steril 39:712, 1983.

68. **Dmowski WP, Radwanska E, Binor Z, Rana N,** Mild endometriosis and ovulatory dysfunction: Effect of danazol treatment on success of ovulation induction, Fertil Steril 46:784, 1986.

69. **Chillik CF, Acosta AA, Garcia JE, Perera S, VanUem JFHM, Rosenwaks Z, Jones HW Jr,** The role of in vitro fertilization in infertile patients with endometriosis, Fertil Steril 44:56, 1985.

70. **Matson PL, Yovich JL,** The treatment of infertility associated with endometriosis by in vitro fertilization, Fertil Steril 46:432, 1986.

19   Male Infertility

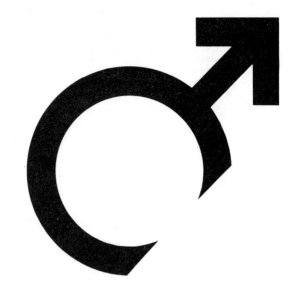

The perception of the degree of male involvement in infertility has undergone a number of revisions during the past 50 years. Initially, infertility was considered primarily a female problem. This notion gave way to the realization that 40% of infertility is wholly or in part due to a male factor. More recently, there have been attempts to redefine, in a downward direction, the lower limit of "normal" for a sperm count. Thus, many men who in the past would have been categorized as subfertile now are considered normal, and the focus has turned to their female partners.

Despite these recent changes, there is no doubt that a substantial percentage of infertility is due to deficiencies in the semen. For that reason it is important to be knowledgeable concerning male infertility. After initial evaluation, it is our responsibility to determine whether urologic consultation is required. *This chapter will consider the analysis of semen, indicate factors responsible for abnormalities in the semen, and consider available treatment for problems of male infertility, including artificial insemination.*

Regulation of the Testes

The testes have 2 distinct components, the seminiferous tubules (site of spermatogenesis) and the Leydig cells (source of testosterone). The function of these 2 components requires both pituitary gonadotropins, follicle-stimulating hormone (FSH) and luteinizing hormone (LH). The primary effect of LH is to stimulate the synthesis and secretion of testosterone by Leydig cells, an effect that is enhanced by FSH which also binds to Leydig cells and increases the number of LH receptors on the cells. Increasing levels of testosterone, in turn, inhibit LH secretion, acutely through the hypothalamus and chronically at the pituitary level. This negative feedback action does not require aromatization to estrogen. In men virtually all of the estrone and estradiol present is derived from androstene-dione and testosterone; there is essentially no direct secretion of estrogen.

Leydig cells contain receptors for prolactin. Prolactin at normal levels stimulates testosterone secretion, whereas hypersecretion of prolactin leads to reduced testosterone secretion. Although studies suggest that prolactin synergises with LH and testosterone in the testes, a role for prolactin has not been established for normal testicular function.

FSH, in conjunction with testosterone, acts on the seminiferous tubules to stimulate spermatogenesis. This effect may be mediated by activation of Sertoli cell function. In other words, the Sertoli cells are controlled by 2 hormones, FSH and testosterone. FSH binds to Sertoli cells and stimulates the production of several proteins, chief of which is ABP, the androgen binding protein. Spermatogenesis requires a very high local concentration of testosterone and dihydrotestosterone, higher than that present in the circulation, and greater than can be administered exogenously. The ABP is secreted into the tubule lumen and binds testosterone and dihydrotestosterone as they diffuse into the lumen, concentrating the androgens in the seminiferous epithelium for spermatogenesis and in the epididymis for sperm maturation.

In contrast to the effects of testosterone on LH, steroid hormones at physiologic levels do not suppress FSH secretion. Orchiectomy is followed, however, by a rise in FSH levels. This phenomenon led to the discovery of inhibin, a polypeptide that is synthesized in the Sertoli cells in response to FSH and specifically inhibits FSH secretion. Inhibin has been found in seminal fluid, spermatozoa, testes and Sertoli cells.

The seminiferous tubules and the intraluminal environment are controlled by the Sertoli cells. Tight junctions beween the Sertoli cells effectively seal off the tubules, creating the blood-testis barrier. The Leydig cells are in the connective tissue between the seminiferous tubules.

Developing sperm are enveloped by Sertoli cells which influence the sequential process of spermatogenesis. Spermatogonia undergo mitotic division to form the primary spermatocytes, which in turn form the haploid secondary spermatocytes (23 chromosomes) by meiotic division. The secondary spermatocytes proceed through a maturation process to the spermatid stage, ultimately becoming the spermatozoa. Most of the testis is composed of the tightly coiled seminiferous tubule, which, if uncoiled, would reach a length of 70 cm. Approximately 74 days are required to produce spermatozoa, about 50 days of which are spent in the tubule.

After leaving the testes, sperm take 12-26 days to travel the epididymis and appear in the ejaculate. Sperm are stored in the epididymis, where they undergo a process of maturation before they are capable of progressive motility and fertilization. The semen is composed of secretions contributed in a sequential fashion, first the prostatic fluid and contents of the distal vas deferens, followed by seminal vesicular secretions. Keep in mind that the semen analysis can reflect events which occurred days or weeks earlier.

Semen Analysis

Dissatisfaction with the traditional means of assessing male infertility potential has spurred the introduction of newer diagnostic tests. These include measurements of sperm penetration of cervical mucus in vitro, utilization of bovine cervical mucus, and, more importantly, penetration of hamster eggs denuded of their zonae. Before considering these tests and their place in the evaluation of male fertility potential, we will review the major aspects of male infertility starting with the interpretation of the semen analysis.

An abstinence period of 2-3 days prior to semen collection is adequate, although some urologists favor 5 days. Increasing the ejaculatory frequency reduces the volume and count, but it is doubtful whether there is a significant impact on quality (morphology and moltility). The specimen should be protected from the cold and delivered to the laboratory within 1 hour of collection. Semen liquification, which occurs 20-30 minutes after ejaculation, is a necessary prerequisite for doing an accurate analysis. On occasion, a specimen does not undergo normal liquification, and, if this is associated with a poor postcoital test, it may be a factor in infertility. Techniques used to break up a viscid specimen in preparation for doing a sperm count or for artificial insemination include mechanically dispersing the gel by running the semen repeatedly through a number 19 needle, collecting the semen as a split ejaculate because the first part may be less viscid, and treating the semen with proteolytic enzymes. If the postcoital test is normal, however, high viscosity probably is not an infertility factor.

Because of the variability in semen specimens from the same individual, at least 2 and preferably 3 specimens should be evaluated over the course of the infertility investigation. The specimen should be collected directly into a clean container and not into a condom because the latter contains spermicidal agents. Both the Milex Company and the HDC Corporation produce sheathes that do not contain a spermicidal agent, and they can be used if the male cannot or will not obtain a specimen by masturbation. In addition, one report suggests that in oligospermic males better counts are seen following collection in a sheath compared to collection by masturbation.(1) By contrast, collection of a specimen by withdrawal runs the risk of losing the first part of the specimen which contains the highest concentration of sperm.

Interpretation of the semen analysis is hampered by the often erroneous normal values printed on data sheets supplied by many laboratories. They may quote the lower limits of normal as 40 million, 60 million or even 80 million/ml. MacLeod established that the percentage of pregnancy decreases only when the sperm count drops below 20 million/ml.(2)

There is reason to believe that sperm counts are decreasing. In MacLeod's 1951 report, 5% of fertile men had counts below 20 million; today 20-25% of fertile men have counts below 20 million.(3,4) A reasonable argument can be made for an impact due to increased toxins in our environment. Despite evidence that there is a decrease in sperm counts, however, the percent of American married couples who were infertile did not change significantly between 1962 and 1982. Thus the apparent decrease in sperm count is not reflected in a parallel change in the rate of infertility. It is important to keep in mind that even with counts below 20 million/ml, the pregnancy rate without therapy is approximately 20-25%.

For determination of motility, a drop of semen is placed on a slide and looked at initially without a coverslip at 100X magnification. A rough estimate is made of both the percentage of motile sperm and the percentage of sperm that show progressive motility across the field. At least 50% of the sperm should show the latter quality. This can be confirmed by placing a coverslip on the specimen and using both 100X and 400X magnification. More precise quantification can be performed when a Makler chamber (Sefi Medical Instruments, Israel) is used for both evaluation of count and motility. Videomicrography can provide information on sperm velocity and patterns of movement, but its clinical usefulness remains to be determined. In order to compare serial specimens it should be standard procedure to evaluate motility 1-2 hours after ejaculation. There is no evidence that checking motility at more prolonged intervals gives any useful information concerning fertility potential.

Simple staining methods can be used to evaluate sperm morphology. Over 60% of the sperm should have a normal shape. The usual ejaculate volume is between 2 and 6 ml (range 1-7 ml) and it is influenced by the frequency of ejaculation. Low volumes in association with absence of sperm in the postcoital test suggest a need for artificial insemination with the partner's sperm because there may be failure of the small bolus of semen to make contact with the cervix. Higher than normal volumes are often associated with lower concentrations of sperm and this can be treated by use of split ejaculate inseminations, a technique that will be discussed later in this chapter.

Other abnormalities of semen that can contribute to infertility are: (1) infection, manifested by the presence of more than a few white blood cells, and (2) agglutination of sperm. Agglutination occurs on occasion in many individuals, but if present in repeated specimens may represent an autoimmune reaction or may signal the presence of infection.

Normal Values for the Semen Analysis

Volume — **2-6 ml**
Viscosity — **liquefaction in 1 hour**
pH — **7-8**
Count — **20 million/ml or more**
Motility — **50% or more**
Morphology — **60% or more**

Abnormal Sperm Follow-Up

If the laboratory report on the initial semen analysis is abnormal it is reasonable to repeat the analysis. Inquiry should be made concerning the presence of the following factors, any of which can produce abnormal sperm quality and quantity.

1. History of testicular injury, surgery or mumps.

2. Heat. A small rise in scrotal temperature can adversely affect spermatogenesis, and a febrile illness may produce striking changes in sperm count and motility. The effect of the illness can be seen in the sperm count and motility even 2-3 months later. This reflects the 74 days required for a spermatozoan to be generated from a primary germ cell. Environmental sources of heat, such as the use of jockey shorts instead of boxer shorts, excessively hot baths, hot tubs, or occupations that require long hours of sitting, e.g. long distance truck driving, may all decrease fertility potential. Even one visit to a sauna can adversely affect sperm for the subsequent month. Conversely, application of a cooling pouch to the scrotum has been advanced as a treatment for male infertility.(5)

3. Severe allergic reactions.

4. Exposure to radiation, or industrial or environmental toxins. This area has received increasing attention highlighted by studies suggesting a deterioration of semen quality in the population over the past two decades. One hypothesis is that industrial pollution may be responsible, and a study from Scandinavia did show lower sperm counts in males from an urban area compared to males in rural areas.(6) More direct evidence of a deleterious effect of environmental hazards is difficult to obtain because there is a reluctance of workers to produce the serial semen specimens that would be required for a thorough industrial study. In any case, the physician should determine if a male with an abnormal semen specimen has had exposure to industrial or environmental toxins.

5. Heavy marijuana use can depress sperm counts and testosterone levels and there is increasing evidence that cigarette smoking can depress sperm motility.(7) Certain drugs, including cimetidine, spironolactone, Furadantin, sulfasalazine, and chemotherapeutic agents depress sperm quantity and quality. Men with ulcerative colitis should use mesalazine instead of sulfasalazine.

6. Coital timing. Counts at the lower levels of the normal range may be depressed to below normal levels by ejaculations occurring daily or more frequently. Conversely, abstinence for 7 days or more to save up sperm may be counterproductive because the minimal gain in numbers can be offset by the lower motility produced by the increased proportion of older sperm. For most couples, coitus every 36 hours around the time of ovulation will give the optimal chance for pregnancy.

7. Exposure to diethylstilbestrol in utero has been suggested, but not proven, as a cause of male infertility.

Urologic Evaluation

If none of these problems pertain to the male under investigation then referral is made to a urologist in order to look for an anatomic abnormality, an infection, an endocrine disorder, a varicocele, or an immunologic reaction to sperm.

Incidence of Male Disorders (8)

Varicocele	— **37.4%**
Idiopathic	— **25.4%**
Testicular failure	— **9.4%**
Obstruction	— **6.1%**
Cryptorchid	— **6.1%**
Semen volume	— **4.7%**
Agglutination	— **3.1%**
Viscosity	— **1.9%**

Anatomic
Abnormalities

Examination may reveal a physical impairment, such as a marked hypospadias which can cause sperm to be deposited outside the vagina. In rare cases of diabetes, with some neurologic diseases, or occasionally following prostatectomy, there can be retrograde ejaculation into the bladder. Pregnancies have been reported after insemination of sperm obtained by catheterization of the bladder, or following treatment with a variety of drugs. Retrograde ejaculation may be only partial, and some men with this condition have small amounts of ejaculate emitted from the urethra.

Obstruction or absence of the vas deferens is a relatively uncommon cause for male infertility. If the ducts are congenitally absent, fructose which is produced in the seminal vesicles will be absent from the semen. Testicular biopsy can differentiate between a block in the outflow tract or primary damage to the testes. In the latter case, if the biopsy reveals hyalinization and fibrosis of the seminiferous tubules there is very little chance for fertility. Testicular damage or maldevelopment can be found following mumps orchitis, cryptorchidism, or in association with Klinefelter's syndrome. Males with the latter genetic abnormality (XXY) usually have small testes and azoospermia.

It is important that any infection in the genitourinary tract, including those due to mycoplasma and chlamydia, be treated because white cells in the seminal plasma can significantly reduce sperm motility and egg penetration. (9)

Endocrine Disorders

While endocrine disorders are an uncommon cause for infertility, testing for thyroid, gonadotropins, prolactin, and testosterone may uncover unsuspected abnormalities. FSH levels are elevated with germ cell aplasia, whereas testosterone levels are decreased in men who are hypogonadotropic. Hyperprolactinemia is commonly associated with impotence, and, in the absence of impotence, measuring a prolactin level is unlikely to aid in the diagnosis.

Infusion of gonadotropin releasing hormone (GnRH) can stimulate secretion of gonadotropins, and there have been occasional reports of the usefulness of this treatment in those males who have an isolated gonadotropin deficiency. While nonspecific therapy with thyroid, clomiphene citrate, and human chorionic gonadotropin has been used extensively, there is no compelling evidence that it is beneficial. Clomiphene citrate can elevate the sperm count but an associated increase in fertility has not been shown.

A fundamental problem in most studies of the efficacy of drug therapy in male fertility is the lack of a control group for comparison. Investigators make the erroneous assumption that the spontaneous cure rate of male infertility is zero and that any pregnancy that occurs during or following treatment is due solely to that treatment. A number of studies, however, have attested to the spontaneous cure rate of male infertility. In one study, approximately one-third of males with counts below 10 million/ml who were not treated successfully impregnated their partners.(10) In summary, hormonal treatment of infertile males who do not have an endocrine disorder is almost always unrewarding and it does not improve fertility beyond what occurs by chance.

Varicocele

A varicocele is an abnormal tortuosity and dilatation of the veins of the pampiniform plexus within the spermatic cord. Approximately 25% of infertile males have a varicocele, usually on the left side because of the direct insertion of the spermatic vein into the renal vein. Varicoceles, in all likelihood, exert their effects by raising testicular temperature. Besides an anatomical basis, a review of mechanisms suggests a hemodynamic problem due to impaired vasoregulation, which in turn can be responsible for the recognized temperature differences in testes with varicoceles.(11)

A clue to the presence of a varicocele (or other insults to the testes) is the finding of tapering sperm heads. Approximately 10-15% of males in a general population have a varicocele and there is no evidence that males with normal semen characteristics need treatment even if a varicocele is present. They should be checked periodically, however, to be sure that there is no deterioration in their semen characteristics.

Ligation of varicocele results in a 30-50% pregnancy rate, although this response rate is very controversial.(12) While the beneficial effects of treatment of varicocele have been disputed by some investigators,(13) current clinical practice supports the utilization of varicocele ligation in those males who have infertility and an impaired semen specimen. Nevertheless, there has never been a randomized study of varicocele repair. A group from Melbourne, Australia, tried, but failed because of poor compliance.(14) Because the authors told their patients that varicocele repair might make no difference, only 283 of 651 men chose to have it done. In those who had the repair, the only impact on the semen analysis was an improvement in motility from 33.5% to 39.3%, the classically reported finding. *The same change, however, was noted in the nonoperated group, and the pregnancy rates in both the operated and nonoperated groups were the same!*

Recent attention has focused on trying to identify those males with varicocele who have the best chance of benefiting from surgery. Rogers et al found that 24% of males who underwent varicocele ligation had a shift in their hamster penetration test from abnormal to normal. (15) This was not significantly different from the results in a group who did not have surgery. However, a majority of the males (7 of 10) who had surgery and improved hamster tests were

571

able to achieve a pregnancy compared to no pregnancies in 6 who had improved hamster tests without the benefit of surgery. Only one pregnancy occurred in 40 males who showed a continuing abnormality in the hamster test after surgery. A small group of 5 males with normal hamster tests did not achieve a pregnancy after varicocele ligation and Rogers suggested that a normal hamster test should direct attention away from varicocele surgery. It is likely that only a small percent of men with varicoceles will benefit from repair.

Males with counts below 10 million/ml do not respond well to surgical interruption of the internal spermatic vein. Dubin and Amelar reported, however, that they could increase the pregnancy rate in these males after varicocelectomy by treating them with human chorionic gonadotropin.(16)

Some varicoceles only can be diagnosed by ultrasound examination, but it is questionable whether these small varicoceles have any clinical significance. While surgical interruption of the internal spermatic vein is the usual treatment for clinically apparent varicoceles, there is also a nonsurgical approach that utilizes embolization to occlude the vein.

Sperm Penetration
Assay

In the preceding pages there has been occasion to refer to the hamster penetration test, which is also known as the sperm penetration assay (SPA) or the humster (human plus hamster) test. It is based on the relatively unique property of golden hamster eggs, when their zonae are removed, to be penetrated by sperm of other species including the human.(17) Removal of the zona is crucial because foreign sperm are unable to penetrate it.

Eggs are collected from golden hamsters that have been superovulated with gonadotropins. The zonae are removed by enzyme treatment and the denuded eggs cultured for 2 to 3 hours with human sperm that have been washed, resuspended in a physiologic medium, and incubated for a period of time. This incubation allows the acrosome reaction to occur, which prepares the sperm for penetration. The presence of a swollen sperm head in the egg cytoplasm is evidence of penetration and the results are reported as percent of eggs penetrated. Another end point is the average number of sperm penetrations per egg. A positive control semen specimen is run in parallel with each test specimen.

There has been some controversy over what constitutes an abnormal test, with some investigators maintaining zero penetration is the only indicator of abnormality, whereas others use 10% or 14% as the lower limit of normal. Unfortunately, the variability in test conditions from one laboratory to another makes comparisons of their normal values difficult. Rogers cited 4 studies in which SPA's were performed on males who were married to women with proven fertility, or women who had no demonstrable infertility factors.(18) Based on the findings in these studies, where the male is presumably infertile, Rogers has defined an abnormal SPA as less than 10% of eggs penetrated. It must be emphasized that despite this categorization there are instances where partners of males who have a zero SPA achieve pregnancy.

Despite the lack of a complete correlation with human egg fertilization, the SPA is a useful screening procedure in cases of unexplained infertility where 16% of men with normal semen analyses have an abnormal SPA. Donor insemination can be considered in cases of poor SPA's and a normal workup. The SPA can be useful in screening couples with unexplained infertility for in vitro fertilization. In males with normal semen there is a good correlation between positive penetration of hamster eggs and those of the human. Whereas an abnormal test does not preclude fertilization of human eggs by in vitro fertilization, there are indications that the chances for fertilization are decreased.(19) The correlation between the SPA and IVF is not good in cases of male infertility and here a normal SPA does not provide assurance that fertilization of human eggs will occur.(20) The converse is also true. A negative SPA does not mean that human oocyte fertilization cannot occur.

It should be noted that the classic method of sperm preparation for the hamster test involves resuspension of the sperm pellet, in contrast to the swimup technique used in IVF. Increased penetration is seen with specimens prepared by swimup and this may account for some of the discrepancies seen between the hamster test and IVF. Changes in the technique of performing (use of test yolk buffer) and interpreting (number of penetrations per egg) the SPA may increase its correlation with fertilization of the human egg in cases of male infertility.

Therapeutic Insemination

The limited success with treatment for male infertility has prompted attempts to improve the semen specimen by selecting out the best sperm. This approach is a logical consequence of the poor results obtained with therapeutic insemination of whole ejaculates, a technique which is associated with pregnancy rates of approximately 20%. (21) The percentage is similar to the spontaneous pregnancy rate when oligospermia or poor motility is not treated. The indications for therapeutic insemination are therefore few, including when the intravaginal deposition of sperm is impossible, such as with hypospadias or retrograde ejaculation.

The poor response with therapeutic insemination is not universal. Diamond et al achieved a pregnancy rate of 53% when their patients, mostly with compromised semen or poor postcoital tests, used a cervical cup in conjunction with inseminations at home.(22) Its advantages include placement of the entire bolus of semen near the cervix, protection of semen from the hostile environment of the vagina, and elimination of the necessity of transporting a specimen to the physician's office. However others have not found an enhanced pregnancy rate associated with home use of the cervical cup.(23)

Another method of working with the semen is to collect the ejaculate in 2 portions.(24) This splitting of the specimen can be facilitated by taping two cups together. The first portion, which should consist of the first few drops of the ejaculate, contains the sperm-rich fraction and prostatic fluid. The second portion, which usually has lower numbers of sperm, originates in the seminal vesicles. In the majority of cases the first specimen contains not only a greater concentration of sperm, but an improved motility compared to both the second portion and the whole ejaculate. Inseminations with the

573

first part of the split ejaculate provide a better chance for pregnancy for males with poor motility than for those with oligospermia. In cases where split ejaculates are advisable, the couple also can use an in vivo technique. The male withdraws as soon as he feels the ejaculation has started. The success rate with both split ejaculate techniques is modest.

Ericsson and co-workers layered sperm on columns of liquid albumin as a means of separating out the Y chromosome bearing sperm.(25) The albumin column also allows separation of the most vigorous sperm from the dead and poorly moving sperm. The vigorously moving sperm, suspended in physiologic solutions, can be used for intrauterine inseminations. In our experience, the technique provides a specimen with enhanced motility but with no appreciable effect on fertility.(26) Others using the same technique have reported a few successes.

Washed Intrauterine Insemination (IUI). Because only a few thousand sperm normally make it to the uterus, it makes sense that several million sperm placed in the uterus would be better, especially with less than normal sperm. The goals of the washing procedure include: elimination of the seminal fluid, an increase in the sperm concentration, and separation of the best sperm. The optimal method, therefore, incorporates some migration technique which accomplishes all of the above goals.

During the process of preparing sperm for use in in vitro fertilization the semen is washed twice, centrifuged and then overlaid with media. The most motile sperm swim up into the media and these have both a greater motility and a more normal morphology than the sperm found in the ejaculate. The attractiveness of the swimup portion of the specimen has prompted its use for the treatment of infertility.

INDICATIONS FOR INTRAUTERINE INSEMINATION

Male Indications:
>Abnormal anatomy
>Abnormal semen
>Sex selection

Female Indications:
>Cervical mucus problems
>Poor postcoital tests (with good mucus)

The indications for IUI obviously go beyond those for therapeutic insemination, and there is early evidence to support these more liberal indications. The advantages include the concentration of normal sperm, a shorter distance to travel, and placement in time close to ovulation. Because the reservoir effect of sperm in the cervix is lost with IUI, timing of the insemination is very important. There are different methods, and the timing varies with each.

Timing Methods for Intrauterine Insemination

Basal Body Temperature Chart—inseminate twice beginning 1-2 days before the expected rise.

Clomiphene—inseminate on days 16 or 17.

Ultrasound & HCG, 10,000 IU—HCG at 18 mm diameter and inseminate 24-36 hours later.

Urinary LH Detection—inseminate day after color change.

We initially use the Tom Cat catheter (Monoject, St. Louis, MO), putting a curve in its memory about one inch from the end. If this proves unsuccessful, we use the Shepard insemination device (Cook, Bloomington, IN). It may be useful to direct the insemination to the tubal openings. Dye studies indicate that if directed to the tube, 20% of the fluid volume enters the tube directly. (27)

At Yale, an overall pregnancy rate of 24% has been achieved in patients who have had about 5 years of infertility; presumably the time for spontaneous pregnancies had passed.(28) There have been no problems with infection, uterine contractions, increased abortion rates, or fetal abnormalities. By the 5th cycle of treatment, 92% of the couples who eventually achieved pregnancy in the Yale series were pregnant, suggesting that 6 cycles represent an adequate trial.

Results in Israel are similar to Yale's.(29) In general, results were less with abnormal hamster penetration tests. It should be noted that it has been documented that IUI yields fewer pregnancies with sperm penetration tests that are not normal, but whether IUI increases the pregnancy rate for a man with an abnormal penetration test is not known.

The use of IUI has been compared to intercourse, both with LH timing, in couples with oligospermia.(30) Each treatment was in sequence, either a single act of intercourse or a single IUI the day after the LH surge. There were 9 pregnancies in 34 cycles with the insemination technique and none in 32 cycles with intercourse, a statistically significant difference. Criteria for entering into the study required 2 of the following: normal morphology less than 40%, a motility less than 40%, and a sperm count of less than 40 million/ml. The latter value is more liberal than the usual criterion of 20 million/ml as the lower limit of normal, and thus the results may not be directly applicable to males with counts below 20 million/ml. However, in men with severe semen defects, the IUI conception rate was significantly increased: 8.7% pregnancy rate per cycle vs zero.

Despite these optimistic results, the swimup technique has not proven to be a panacea. In most studies, treatment of male infertility with intrauterine insemination of separated specimens has not produced pregnancy rates higher than those reported without treatment.(31-33) This strongly suggests that even the best sperm from a poor specimen may be at a disadvantage. When equal numbers of motile sperm from oligospermic and normospermic specimens were used to inseminate hamster eggs, the sperm from the normal specimens

575

produced higher percentages of penetration.(34) In contrast to the poor results in cases of male infertility, intrauterine inseminations have been useful in cases where there is a poor postcoital test. Wiltbank et al (31) showed that there is a better chance for pregnancy with intrauterine inseminations when a poor postcoital is associated with a normal hamster penetration test (3 of 8 individuals) than when it is associated with a poor hamster test (1 pregnancy in 12 cases). It has been suggested that couples with normal postcoital tests do not benefit from IUI.(35)

It is very difficult to compare the available studies. There is a lack of uniformity in patient selection, timing of inseminations, number of cycles, use of the sperm penetration assay, semen parameters, and semen preparation.

One of the factors to be considered in the results is the age of the female partner. An American study with therapeutic insemination with donors has documented the now-familiar decreasing conception rate with increasing maternal age.(36) Of note was the requirement for more treatment cycles to achieve pregnancy in the older woman: perhaps 9-10 cycles are in order for women over 35 rather than the usual 6.

There is some evidence that results with therapeutic insemination and IUI are better with superovulation.(37) In a study of IUI with normal vs stimulated cycles, a higher pregnancy rate has been found with the stimulated cycles.(38) These suggest that a trial of superovulation and IUI is worthwhile before proceeding to in vitro fertilization or gamete intrafallopian transfer in individuals with patent fallopian tubes (GIFT).

At the present time some believe that IUI can achieve pregnancies in couples with sperm problems, at least to help them get pregnant faster. However, it should be emphasized that whether superovulation is clinically significant in terms of pregnancy rates has not been demonstrated in appropriately randomized and controlled clinical studies.

Other attempts to improve the ejaculate by treating the semen prior to insemination have not been successful. For a time there was enthusiasm for adding caffeine because it stimulates sperm motility. However, this has not resulted in increased pregnancy rates.(39)

Superior pregnancy rates have been achieved when male factor infertility or poor cervical mucus was treated with in vitro fertilization (IVF) or gamete intrafallopian tube transfer (GIFT) compared to intrauterine inseminations, and these offer another option for therapy.(40,41) (Chapter 21)

Whereas IVF has been employed in cases of male factor infertility, some caution is advisable. Despite the insemination of oocytes with higher than the usual number of sperm, failure of fertilization is more common in cases of male infertility. Counts below 10 million/ml or motilities below 30% are associated with lower fertilization rates.(42) The group at Eastern Virginia Medical School has set a minimal requirement of 1.5 million or more rapidly motile sperm in the swimup fraction for specimens to be used in male factor IVF.

(43) Once fertilization does occur, the pregnancy rates following embryo transfer are comparable to those achieved when IVF is done for tubal disease.

Therapeutic Insemination with Donor Sperm

Male infertility and decreased availability of adoptable babies have served to increase the demand for TID, therapeutic insemination with donor sperm. Thousands of babies are born each year in this country as a result of TID.

The procedure raises emotional, ethical, and legal questions. The male may feel that he is devalued and his virility questioned. In a few cases, a woman's ovulation may become abnormal in the cycle where inseminations have been planned. For obvious reasons the physician must never do inseminations without the consent of both partners. Both should be in favor of the procedure. Because there may be emotional or psychological consequences, some couples may require counseling beyond that provided by the physician.

Increasingly, single women are seeking TID. McGuire and Alexander point out that children in single head of household families are as psychologically adjusted as those from 2 parent households and that TID should not be denied to single women solely on the basis of their lack of a husband.(44)

Three points are worth emphasizing:

1. Donor inseminations do not guarantee pregnancy. The success rate with fresh semen is about 70%. The use of frozen semen lowers the success rate unless the post-thaw specimens are of exceptional quality. The fecundability (chance of getting pregnant per cycle) has been reported to be 18.9% with fresh semen and only 5.0% with frozen semen.(45) This difference may be compensated for by more cycles of insemination. It takes approximately 12 cycles with frozen semen to achieve the accumulative pregnancy rate reached at 6 cycles with fresh semen. Because of concerns regarding the transmission of AIDS and the desirability of quarantining semen for at least 6 months it is unlikely that TID in the future with other than frozen semen will be acceptable.

2. How would the couple react if the child were born with a congenital anomaly? This will occur in perhaps 4 to 5% of all pregnancies, irrespective of whether they follow intercourse or therapeutic insemination.

3. Both the man and the woman should sign a consent form. The procedure is covered by law in over 20 states. In California, once the husband signs the consent form, he is the legal father of the baby conceived through TID. In other areas it is worthwhile for the physician to know the legal status of TID in his/her state so that correct information can be conveyed to patients.

As a rule the donor should be unknown to the couple. His health and fertility must be unimpeachable, and there should be no family history of genetic diseases. Lethal genetic diseases have been transmitted by donor insemination.(46) Despite this danger a survey of physicians performing TID has revealed a wide range of criteria for screening donors.(47) The usual genetic screening consists of a family

577

history and only a rare biochemical test. As the compilers of the survey point out, such screening depends on both the awareness of family medical history and the honesty of the donor. In one study in which donors were screened by medical and family histories, fewer than 10% of potential donors were disqualified for genetic reasons.(48) However, despite the low disqualification rate and the absence of karyotyping in this study, the occurrence of congenital malformations following TID was not higher than that in a control population of infertile couples. Jewish donors should be screened for Tay-Sachs heterozygosity. Black donors should be tested for sickle cell anemia, and donors of Greek or Italian extraction for B thalassemia.

Among the problems that can occur with donor insemination are the transmission of venereal disease from donor to recipient. Periodic testing of donors for gonorrhea, syphilis, herpes, chlamydia, and mycoplasma is important. Screening donors for hepatitis-B surface antigen and core antibody, cytomegalovirus, and for acquired immune deficiency syndrome (AIDS) has become accepted medical practice because of reports of transmission of these diseases by donor insemination.(49) A complete guideline for screening donors has been published by the American Fertility Society.(50)

The donor will not be a mirror image of the husband, but an attempt should be made to match physical characteristics. Rh negative sperm donors should be used for Rh negative women. TID is usually a private matter between the physician and the couple. Discussions with friends or relatives should be discouraged. Use of friends or relatives as donors raises the potential for emotional problems in the future, although we have used a relative when requested by a stable, intelligent couple who understood the long-term implications. A request to mix the husband's sperm with the donor's signifies that the couple may not have made the emotional adjustment to the thought of donor insemination. The husband's semen also may be deleterious for the donor's sperm, although this is in dispute.

Donor inseminations are useful in azoospermia, severe oligospermia, or asthenospermia refractory to treatment. They are also useful if the woman has a history of fetal loss due to Rh sensitization. Here an Rh negative donor would be used. Other genetic diseases may, on occasion, be an indication for donor inseminations.

The basal body temperature chart (BBT), the woman's perception of vaginal wetness and ovulatory pain, if present, are useful guides for timing of inseminations. More precise timing can be accomplished by ultrasound visualization of the preovulatory follicle and monitoring of the day of the LH surge either by measurements of LH in serum, or by measurements of LH in urine with any of a number of commercially available kits. In our experience approximately 75% of women can successfully use the kits at home to identify their LH surge. The kits are not inexpensive, and they do not always correlate with the more precise measurements of LH in serum. Insemination is performed the day after the color change is detected, although some find maximal cervical mucus on the day of the color change.

Alternative monitoring and treatment approaches utilize ultrasound to monitor preovulatory follicle growth and an injection of 10,000 IU of human chorionic gonadotropin when the dominant follicle reaches 18 mm or greater in diameter. Inseminations are performed 24-36 hours after the HCG injection. Ultrasound, LH monitoring or HCG injection also can be used to time partner inseminations.

If the BBT alone is used, an attempt is made to inseminate on the day just before the temperature rise with the timing based on reviewing 2 months of charts and/or the day of maximal vaginal wetness. Usually one to two donor inseminations are done each month. Approximately 50% of the successful cases will occur within the first 2 months of treatment. If pregnancy has not occurred by that time, the infertility evaluation is pursued. Over 85% of pregnancies that will occur do so within 6 months with fresh semen and within 12 months with frozen semen. Those who fail should have laparoscopy and perhaps IVF.

We prefer to inseminate at the entrance to the cervical canal by means of a polyethylene catheter. The major portion of the semen overflows into the posterior fornix. The overflow collects on the posterior blade of the speculum, and the cervical os is allowed to dip into this pool while the woman rests for 20 minutes with her hips elevated. If TID is unsuccessful after 3 cycles, consideration can be given to doing intrauterine TID with sperm obtained by the swimup technique.

The Future

In the future, more sophisticated investigative techniques may uncover causes of male infertility not diagnosable by current methods. For example, electron microscopic examination of sperm from a few infertile males has revealed an absence of the acrosome, the enzyme-containing caplike structure that covers the anterior portion of the nucleus, or structural abnormalities of the tail not evident by light microscopy. Assessment of the role of ABP, the androgen binding protein, and the process of spermatogenesis and maturation may uncover specific disorders currently unknown. The genetic analysis of sperm may make it possible to be selective for "good" sperm. It may be possible to measure factors in the sperm required for capacitation and the acrosome reaction. Finally, micromanipulation is now possible, placing a single sperm within an egg.

References

1. **Zavos PM,** Seminal parameters of ejaculates collected from oligospermic and normospermic patients via masturbation and at intercourse with the use of a silastic seminal fluid collection device, Fertil Steril 44:517, 1985.

2. **MacLeod J, Gold RA,** The male factor in fertility and infertility. II. Spermatozoan counts in 1000 cases of known fertility and 1000 cases of infertile marriage, J Urol 66:436, 1951.

3. **Nelson CMK, Bunge RG,** Semen analysis: Evidence for changing parameters of male fertility potential, Fertil Steril 25:503, 1974.

4. **Zukerman Z, Rodriguez-Rigau LJ, Smith KD, Steinberger E,** Frequency distribution of sperm counts in fertile and infertile males, Fertil Steril 28:1310, 1977.

5. **Zorgniotti AW, Sealfon AI, Toth A,** Chronic scrotal hypothermia as a treatment for poor semen quality, Lancet i:904, 1980.

579

6. **Liedholm OP, Ranstam J,** Depressed semen quality: A study over two decades, Arch Androl 12:113, 1984.

7. **Kulikauskas V, Blaustein D, Ablin RJ,** Cigarette smoking and its possible effects on sperm, Fertil Steril 44:526, 1985.

8. **Greenberg SH, Lipshultz LI, Wein AJ,** Experience with 425 subfertile male patients, J Urol 119:507, 1978.

9. **Maruyama DK Jr, Hale RW, Rogers BJ,** Effects of white blood cells on the in vitro penetration of zona-free hamster eggs by human spermatozoa, J Androl 6:127, 1985.

10. **Glass RH, Ericsson RJ,** Spontaneous cure of male infertility, Fertil Steril 31:305, 1979.

11. **Kaufman DG, Nagler HM,** The varicocele: Concepts of pathophysiology—present and future, World J Urol 34:88, 1986.

12. **Crockett ATK, Takihara H, Cosentino MJ,** The varicocele, Fertil Steril 41:5, 1984.

13. **Vermeulen A, Vandeweghe M,** Improved fertility after varicocele correction: Fact or fiction? Fertil Steril 42:249, 1984.

14. **Baker HWG, Burger HG, de Kretser DM, Hudson B, Rennie GC, Straffon WGE,** Testicular vein ligation and fertility in men with varicoceles, Brit Med J 291:1678, 1985.

15. **Rogers BJ, Mygatt GG, Soderdahl DW, Hale RW,** Monitoring of suspected infertile men with varicocele by the sperm penetration assay, Fertil Steril 44:800, 1985.

16. **Dubin L, Amelar RD,** Varicocelectomy as therapy in male infertility: A study of 504 cases, Fertil Steril 26:217, 1975.

17. **Yanagimachi R,** Zona-free hamster eggs: Their use in assessing fertilizing capacity and examining chromosomes of human spermatozoa, Gamete Res 10:187, 1984.

18. **Rogers BJ,** The sperm penetration assay: Its usefulness reevaluated, Fertil Steril 43:821, 1985.

19. **Margalioth EJ, Navot D, Laufer N, Yosef SM, Rabinowitz R, Yarkoni S, Schenker JG,** Zona-free hamster ovum penetration assay as a screening procedure for in vitro fertilization, Fertil Steril 40:386, 1983.

20. **Margalioth EJ, Navot D, Laufer N, Lewin A, Rabinowitz R, Schenker JG,** Correlation between the zona-free hamster egg sperm penetration assay and human in vitro fertilization, Fertil Steril 45:665, 1986.

21. **Nachtigall RD,** Indications, techniques, and success rates for AIH, Seminars Reprod Endocrinol 5:5, 1987.

22. **Diamond MP, Christianson C, Daniell JF, Wentz AC,** Pregnancy following use of the cervical cup for home artificial insemination utilizing homologous semen, Fertil Steril 39:480, 1983.

23. **Corson SL, Batzer FR, Otis C, Fee D,** The cervical cap for home artificial insemination, J Reprod Med 31:349, 1986.

24. **Amelar RD, Hotchkiss RS,** The split ejaculate, Fertil Steril 16:46, 1965.

25. **Ericsson RJ, Langevin CN, Nishino M,** Isolation of fractions rich in human Y sperm, Nature 246:421, 1973.

26. **Glass RH, Ericsson RJ,** Intrauterine insemination of isolated motile sperm, Fertil Steril 29:535, 1978.

27. **DiMarzo SJ, Rakoff JS,** Intrauterine insemination with husband's washed sperm, Fertil Steril 46:470, 1986.

28. **Huszar G, DeCherney A,** The role of intrauterine insemination in the treatment of infertile couples: The Yale experience, Seminars Reprod Endocrinol 5:11, 1987.

29. **Makler A,** Washed intrauterine insemination in the treatment of idiopathic infertility, Seminars Reprod Endocrinol 5:35, 1987.

30. **Kerin JFP, Peek J, Warnes GM, Kirby C, Jeffrey R, Matthews CD, Cox LW,** Improved conception rate after intrauterine insemination of washed spermatozoa from men with poor quality semen, Lancet i:533, 1984.

31. **Wiltbank MC, Kosasa S, Rogers B,** Treatment of infertile patients by intrauterine insemination of washed spermatozoa, Andrologia 17:22, 1985.

32. **Allen NC, Herbert CM, Maxson WS, Rogers BJ, Diamond MP, Wentz AC,** Intrauterine insemination: A critical review, Fertil Steril 44:569, 1985.

33. **Confino E, Friberg J, Dudkiewicz AB, Gleicher N,** Intrauterine inseminations with washed human spermatozoa, Fertil Steril 46:55, 1986.

34. **Syms AJ, Johnson A, Lipshultz LI, Smith RG,** Reduced ability of motile human spermatozoa obtained from oligospermic males to penetrate zona-free hamster eggs, Fertil Steril 41:1055, 1984.

35. **Quagliarello J, Arny M,** Intracervical versus intrauterine insemination: Correlation of outcome with antecedent postcoital testing, Fertil Steril 46:870, 1986.

36. **Virro MS, Shewchuk AB,** Pregnancy outcome in 242 conceptions after artificial insemination with donor sperm and effects of maternal age on the prognosis for successful pregnancy, Am J Obstet Gynecol 148:518, 1984.

37. **Dodson WC, Whitesides DB, Hughes CL Jr, Easley HA III, Haney AF,** Superovulation with intrauterine insemination in the treatment of infertility: A possible alternative to gamete intrafallopian transfer and in vitro fetilization, Fertil Steril 48:441, 1987.

38. **Kemmann E, Bohrer M, Shelden R, Fiasconaro G, Beardsley L,** Active ovulation management increases the monthly probability of pregnancy occurrence in ovulatory women who receive intrauterine insemination, Fertil Steril 48:916, 1987.

39. **Harrison RF,** Insemination of husband's semen with and without the addition of caffeine, Fertil Steril 29:532, 1978.

40. **Hewitt J, Cohen J, Krishnaswamy V, Fehilly CB, Steptoe PC, Walters DE,** Treatment of idiopathic infertility, cervical mucus hostility, and male infertility: Artificial insemination with husband's semen or in vitro fertilization? Fertil Steril 44:350, 1985.

41. **Yovich JL, Matson PL,** Pregnancy rates after high intrauterine insemination of husband's spermatozoa or gamete intrafallopian transfer, Lancet ii:1287, 1986.

42. **Battin DA, Vargyas JM, Sato F, Brown J, Marrs R,** In vitro fertilization rates of male factor patients, Fertil Steril 41:Abstract 42S, 1984.

43. **Acosta AA, Chillik CF, Brugo S, Ackerman S, Swanson RJ, Pleban P, Yuan J, Haque D,** In vitro fertilization and the male factor, Urol 28:1, 1986.

44. **McGuire M, Alexander NJ,** Artificial insemination of single women, Fertil Steril 43:182, 1985.

45. **Richter MA, Haning RV Jr, Shapiro SS,** Artificial donor insemination: Fresh versus frozen semen; the patient as her own control, Fertil Steril 41:277, 1984.

46. **Shapiro DN, Hutchinson RJ,** Familial histocytosis in offspring of two pregnancies after artificial insemination, New Eng J Med 304:757, 1981.

47. **Curie-Cohen M, Luttrell L, Shapiro S,** Current practice of artificial insemination by donor in the United States, New Eng J Med 300:585, 1979.

48. **Verp MS, Cohen MR, Simpson JL,** Necessity of formal genetic screening in artificial insemination by donor, Obstet Gynecol 62:474, 1983.

49. **Mascola L, Guinan ME,** Screening to reduce transmission of sexually transmitted diseases in semen used for artifical insemination, New Eng J Med 3314:1354, 1986.

50. **The American Fertility Society,** New guidelines for the use of semen donor insemination: 1986, Fertil Steril 46:Suppl 2, 1986.

20 Induction of Ovulation

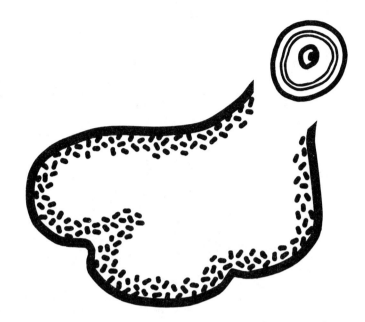

In the past, a woman with an ovulatory dysfunction had little hope of achieving a pregnancy. The successful therapy of this problem is one of the most dramatic advances in gynecologic endocrinology. Today, if lack of ovulation is the only problem causing infertility, a persistent couple can expect their chances of conceiving to match the rate found in the general population.

The physician has available for general clinical use many pharmacologic preparations for the induction of ovulation: clomiphene citrate, bromocriptine (Parlodel), human menopausal gonadotropins (Pergonal), purified FSH (Metrodin), and gonadotropin releasing hormone (GnRH). The programs of clomiphene and Pergonal administration described in this chapter have evolved over the past 2 decades. These methods have reduced side effects to a clinically acceptable frequency and retained a high success rate in terms of induced pregnancies. The other agents are only recent additions to our armamentarium, and an understanding of their use is still evolving. *This chapter will review the principles which guide the use of clomiphene, Pergonal, bromocriptine, purified FSH, and GnRH, and consider the results and complications of the medical induction of ovulation. In addition, ovarian wedge resection will be examined briefly.*

Despite the specificity of the therapy and the promise of successful results, it is incumbent upon the practitioner to perform the appropriate medical evaluation to ensure that a contraindication to therapy is not overlooked. The reader is referred to Chapter 6 and Chapter

583

7 for a consideration of anovulation and hirsutism, Chapter 5 and Chapter 9 for the evaluation of amenorrhea and galactorrhea.

Clomiphene Citrate

Clomiphene citrate was first synthesized in 1956, introduced for clinical trials in 1960, and approved for clinical use in the United States in 1967. Clomiphene citrate is an orally active nonsteroidal agent distantly related to diethylstilbestrol. Its chemical name is 2-[p-(2-chloro-1,2-diphenylvinyl) phenoxy] triethylamine dihydrogen citrate. Clomiphene is a racemic mixture of its 2 stereochemical isomers, originally described as the cis and trans isomers. This designation is now recognized to have been inaccurate, and the isomers have been relabeled as zuclomiphene and enclomiphene citrate.(1) Clomiphene is available in 50 mg tablets, under the trade names of Clomid and Serophene, which contain 38% of the active zuclomiphene form.

The similarity of clomiphene's structure to an estrogenic substance is the clue to its mechanism of action. Clomiphene exerts only a very weak biologic estrogenic effect. The structural similarity to estrogen is sufficient to achieve uptake and binding by estrogen receptors, however there are several important different characteristics.(2,3) Perhaps most importantly, clomiphene occupies the nuclear receptor for long periods of time, for weeks rather than hours. Clomiphene, therefore, does not competitively inhibit the action of estrogen at the receptor level, but rather it modifies hypothalamic activity by affecting the concentration of the intracellular estrogen receptors. Specifically, the concentration of estrogen receptors is reduced by inhibition of the process of receptor replenishment.

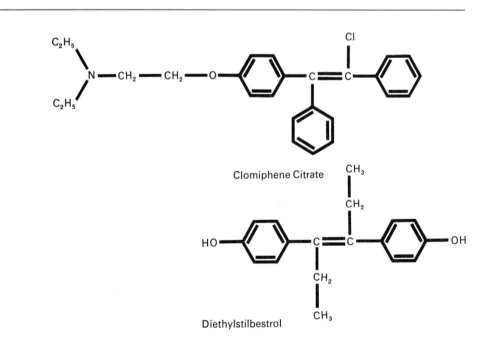

Clomiphene Citrate

Diethylstilbestrol

When exposed to clomiphene, the hypothalamic-pituitary axis cannot perceive or act upon the true endogenous estrogen level in the circulation. Thinking that the estrogen level in the circulation is low because perception is obscured, the neuroendocrine mechanism for GnRH secretion is activated. Follicle-stimulating hormone (FSH) and luteinizing hormone (LH) pulse frequency (but not amplitude) is increased, suggesting an increase in GnRH pulse frequency.(4,5) Further evidence that clomiphene works in the hypothalamus can be found in experiments utilizing hypothalamic in vitro preparations in which clomiphene increases GnRH secretion in the presence of estradiol.(6)

During the period of clomiphene administration, peripheral serum levels of FSH and LH rise. The subsequent ovulation which occurs after clomiphene therapy is a manifestation of the hormonal and morphologic changes produced by the growing follicles. Clomiphene therapy does not directly stimulate ovulation, but it supports a sequence of events that are the physiologic features of a normal cycle. The effectiveness of the drug, however, may not be restricted to its ability to cause an appropriate GnRH discharge.

In animal models, clomiphene exerts an estrogenic effect on the pituitary and directly stimulates gonadotropin release, independently of its action on GnRH.(3) In addition clomiphene exerts a direct ovarian effect, perhaps a synergistic action with gonadotropins on ovarian enzyme systems. As estrogen does, clomiphene directly enhances FSH stimulation of LH receptors in granulosa cells.(7) In contrast, in the uterus, cervix, and vagina, clomiphene acts primarily as an antiestrogen. Thus vaginal cornification is attenuated, and the effect of estrogen on cervical mucus and endometrium is antagonized, potentially important actions affecting implantation and early embryonic development.(8) The mixed agonist-antagonist actions of clomiphene vary from species to species and from tissue to tissue.

Clomiphene has no progestational, corticotropic, androgenic, or antiandrogenic effects. Clomiphene does not interfere with adrenal or thyroid function. While the effect of the drug is brief, only 51% of the oral dose is excreted after 5 days, and radioactivity from labeled clomiphene appears in the feces up to 6 weeks after administration. Significant plasma concentrations of the active zu isomer can be detected up to 1 month after treatment with a single dose of 50 mg.(9)

This long half life of clomiphene has further theoretical concern. Clomiphene has been detected both in the serum and in follicular fluid obtained from in vitro fertilization patients on the day of ovulation.(10) The presence of clomiphene at this time and during the luteal phase could have unwanted effects. In vitro, clomiphene inhibits progesterone production by luteal granulosa cells in a fashion that suggests that clomiphene, by virtue of its anti-estrogenic action, interferes with the induction of LH receptors.(11) Because this inhibition is reversed by human chorionic gonadotropin (HCG), pregnancy and the appearance of HCG may prevent this unwelcome effect.

In rats and rabbits, a dose-dependent increase in the incidence of fetal malformations is seen when clomiphene is given during the period of organogenesis. Clomiphene has been found to cause disruptions of the organization of the uterine mesenchyme and tubal epithelium in human fetal reproductive tissue transplanted to athymic nude mice.(12) Extremely high doses inhibit fetal development. In these experiments, exposure took place at later periods of gestation that those associated with clomiphene exposure when the drug is taken for the induction of ovulation. Although clomiphene therapy should be withheld if there is any possibility of pregnancy, there is no good evidence that clomiphene is teratogenic in humans. Furthermore, infant survival and performance after delivery are normal.

Selection of Patients

Absent or infrequent ovulation is the chief indication for clomiphene therapy. It is the physician's responsibility to rule out disorders of pituitary, adrenal, and thyroid origin requiring specific treatment before initiating clomiphene therapy. A complete history and physical examination are mandatory, but only a minimum of laboratory procedures is necessary. Liver function evaluation should precede clomiphene therapy if history and physical examination findings suggest liver disease. The vast majority of patients are healthy women suffering only from infertility secondary to oligoovulation or anovulation.

If periods are infrequent, it is not absolutely necessary to document infrequent or absent ovulation by basal body temperature records and endometrial biopsy. An endometrial biopsy is a wise precaution in a patient who has been anovulatory for a long period of time because of the tendency for these patients to develop hyperplasia and even carcinoma of the endometrium. It is also wise to precede therapy with an evaluation of the semen, to avoid an unnecessary waste of time and effort in the presence of azoospermia. A dedicated effort must be made to detect galactorrhea, and the prolactin level must be measured. Galactorrhea or hyperprolactinemia dictate a different therapeutic approach: bromocriptine. The remainder of the infertility workup in a patient with no previous medical or surgical problems is deferred until after a trial of clomiphene therapy. Because approximately 75% of pregnancies occur during the first 3 treatment cycles, the infertility workup is pursued only after the patient has responded with 3 months of ovulatory cycles and has not become pregnant.(13) This is appropriate because clomiphene is simple, safe, and cost-effective.

Despite the antiestrogen action of clomiphene the incidence of poor cervical mucus on the postcoital test is only 15%.(14) Estrogen (0.625 to 2.5 mg conjugated estrogens daily) can be administered from day 10 to day 16 (for 1 week starting the day after the last day of clomiphene administration) to improve mucus production. High doses of estrogen do not interfere with the gonadotropin response, ovulation, or the pregnancy rate.(15) Another alternative is to proceed with intrauterine inseminations of washed sperm, bypassing the cervix.

Cases of ovarian failure are unresponsive to any form of ovulation induction. Therefore, the presence of ovarian tissue capable of responding to gonadotropins must be documented. This is only a problem in the patient with amenorrhea, since the presence of menstrual bleeding confirms the function (although perhaps limited) of the hypothalamic-pituitary-ovarian axis. The patient with amenorrhea who fails to produce a withdrawal bleed after a course of a progestational agent (Provera, 10 mg daily for 5 days) must be further evaluated (see Chapter 5). A case has been made by others for the usefulness of an ovarian biopsy, perhaps via the laparoscope, to establish the presence of competent ovarian tissue. It is our practice, however, to rely on the radioimmunoassay of gonadotropin levels and the response to Provera, thus avoiding unnecessary surgical and anesthetic risks, to accurately rule out hypergonadotropic hypogonadism (ovarian failure). Attempts at medical induction of ovulation in these patients would be a waste of time and money except in a few very rare cases of ovarian failure as discussed in Chapter 5.

The patients most likely to respond to clomiphene display some evidence of pituitary-ovarian activity as expressed in the biologic presence of estrogen (spontaneous or withdrawal menstrual bleeding). These are anovulatory women who have gonadotropin and estrogen production, but do not cycle, or women with inadequate luteal phases. If the mechanism of an inadequate corpus luteum is inadequate FSH stimulation during the follicular phase, it makes sense to treat this condition with clomiphene. Clomiphene does not prolong the luteal phase (as progesterone supplementation does). This is an important advantage, avoiding the anxiety and heightened monthly emotional response of infertile couples.

The patient who is deficient in gonadotropin secretion and, as a result, is hypoestrogenic, cannot be expected to respond to further lowering of the estrogen signal, and thus should not respond to clomiphene. However, this principle is not completely applicable to clinical practice. An occasional patient who is, by all criteria, hypoestrogenic, will respond. Therefore, any otherwise medically uncomplicated patient with infertility secondary to lack of ovulation is a candidate for clomiphene therapy unless galactorrhea or hyperprolactinemia is present. In addition, treatment is indicated in order to improve the timing and frequency of ovulation to enhance the possibilities of conception in the patient who ovulates only occasionally.

To our knowledge, the use of drugs for induction of ovulation does not improve the quality of the ovum, and the chance of pregnancy is not improved in women who ovulate regularly and spontaneously. Although superovulation is advocated by some prior to embarking upon in vitro fertilization, it remains to be seen whether superovulation increases the pregnancy rate in couples with unexplained infertility. There is one special instance where this restriction may not apply. Certain religious requirements, such as in orthodox Judaism, interfere with the normal reproductive process. In the devout orthodox Jewish couple, intercourse is prohibited in the presence of menstrual flow and for 7 days following its conclusion. In some women menstrual flow is prolonged or the follicular phase is shortened, so that coitus cannot take place until after ovulation. In the usual mode of treatment, medication is begun on day 5 of the cycle. Ovulation can be delayed to a more appropriate time by starting clomiphene later, usually on day 7 or 8 of the cycle. Ovulation can be expected in the interval 5-10 days after the last day of medication. This manipulation has its limitations. Administration too late in the cycle, beyond day 9, may have no effect. It is appropriate to use clomiphene to achieve an increased frequency and regularity of ovulation in patients with oligoovulation. Clomiphene is also useful to regulate the timing of ovulation in women undergoing insemination.

The question is often asked whether the indications for clomiphene therapy should be extended to include the initiation of cyclicity in the oligoamenorrheic patient who does not seek fertility. In our opinion, this is an inappropriate use of clomiphene for several reasons: 1) the effectiveness of clomiphene is restricted to the cycle in which it is used and it should not be expected to induce cyclicity following the conclusion of treatment, 2) the use of clomiphene may aggravate the clinical problems of acne and hirsutism during the treatment cycle by increasing LH stimulation of ovarian steroid production, and 3) the inability to induce cyclicity can be so discouraging to the patient that her acceptance of the drug will be impaired at some future date when it is legitimately offered as a fertility agent for the induction of ovulation.

How to Use
Clomiphene

A program of clomiphene therapy is begun on the 5th day of a cycle following either spontaneous or induced bleeding. The initial dose is 50 mg daily for 5 days. There is no advantage to beginning with a higher dose for the following two reasons: 1) In a random distribution of our patients begun with initial doses of either 50 mg or 100 mg daily, the pregnancy rate was identical; and 2) the highest incidence of side effects in our experience occurs at the 50 mg dose, and at 100 mg, patients may develop more serious reactions. About 50% of patients conceive at the 50 mg dose, and another 20% at 100 mg.(13,14) An occasional patient will be exceptionally sensitive to clomiphene and can achieve pregnancy at the reduced dose of 25 mg.

Beginning clomiphene on the 5th day is a method arrived at empirically; however, we can now offer a rational explanation based on current physiology. The clomiphene-induced increase in gonadotropins during days 5-9 occurs at a time when the dominant follicle is being selected. Beginning clomiphene earlier can be expected to stimulate multiple follicular maturation resulting in a greater incidence of multiple gestation. Indeed, clomiphene is administered earlier in in vitro fertilization programs in order to obtain more than one oocyte. Better ovulation rates have been documented starting clomiphene on days 3, 4, or 5 of the cycle, compared to days 2 and 6.(16)

If ovulation is not achieved in the very first cycle of treatment, dosage is increased to 100 mg. Thereafter, if ovulation and a normal luteal phase are not achieved in any cycle, dosage is increased in a staircase fashion by 50 mg increments to a maximum of 200-250 mg daily for 5 days. The highest dose is pursued for 3-4 months before considering the patient to be a clomiphene failure. The quantity of drug and the number of cycles go beyond those recommended by the manufacturer. However, in our experience those recommendations are inappropriately limiting. We have achieved a 15% pregnancy rate at the 150 mg and 200 mg dose levels.(13)

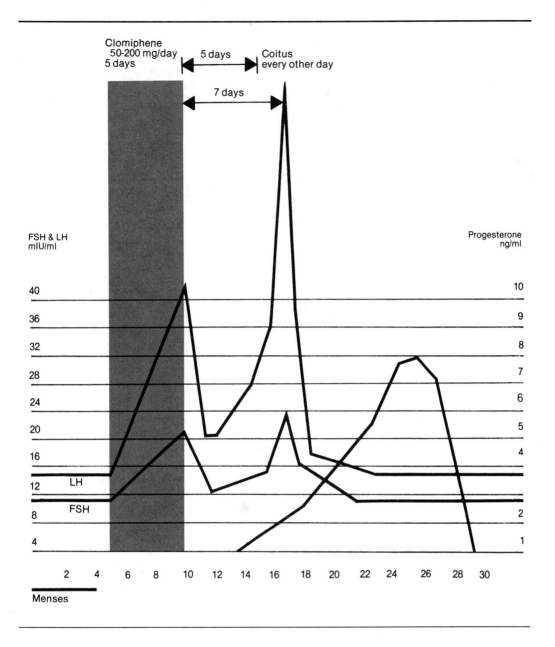

There is a significant correlation between body weight and the dose of clomiphene required for ovulation.(17,18) One must adhere to the usual regimen, however, because the weight cannot be used to predict prospectively the correct ovulatory dose. In other words, some obese women ovulate at the same low dose which achieves ovulation in thin women. Clomiphene is not stored in adipose tissue, and the increased dose often necessary in obese women is more likely due to a more intense anovulatory state with higher androgen levels producing a more resistant hypothalamic-pituitary-ovarian axis.

At the present time there is no clinical or laboratory parameter which can predict the dose of clomiphene necessary to achieve ovulation. Androgen and estrogen levels do not show any correlation with the dose of clomiphene which proves successful.(18)

Following the 5-day course of clomiphene, the ovulatory surge of gonadotropins may occur anywhere from 5 to 10 days after the last day of clomiphene administration. The patient is advised to have intercourse every other day for 1 week beginning 5 days after the last day of medication. In view of the role prostaglandins play in the physical expulsion of an oocyte, it is prudent to advise patients involved in programs of ovulation induction to avoid the use of agents which inhibit prostaglandin synthesis.

After the first treatment cycle the patient is evaluated for side effects, residual ovarian enlargement, and basal body temperature changes. In recent years, we have found it unnecessary to perform a pelvic examination every month because significant ovarian enlargement is encountered infrequently and it is usually symptomatic. It is more economical, for both patient and physician, to mail the temperature chart to the office and several days later plan by telephone for the following month. Cysts within a reasonable size range (3-6 cm) do not require a rest from treatment; they do not respond to further stimulation.

A basal body temperature record is necessary to follow the response. If an inadequate luteal phase is evident, (temperature elevation less than 11 days duration) the amount of clomiphene is increased to the next dose level. If the patient is already at the maximal level, human chorionic gonadotropin (HCG) is added as discussed below. Biphasic changes are taken as an indication of ovulation and success. Maintenance of the temperature elevation beyond the expected time of menses is the earliest practical indication of success and pregnancy.

When the temperature chart is inconclusive or when the patient is not pregnant despite a period of apparently normal ovulations, an endometrial biopsy is indicated to document the adequacy of the luteal phase. One should also consider ultrasonographic monitoring for treatment failures, looking for follicles which do not reach mature size or the luteinized unruptured follicle.

When inadequate luteal function is documented during clomiphene treatment, an increase in dosage is the logical solution. If this fails, the choice is between progesterone supplementation or treatment with Pergonal. We favor Pergonal treatment because it is possible that the luteal defect is the result of the antiestrogenic action of clomiphene on endometrial receptor levels; hence, progesterone treatment would be ineffective. Keep in mind the effect of excess androgens (which may also be exerted at the endometrial level). When androgens are elevated, suppression with dexamethasone should be tried in combination with clomiphene treatment before proceeding to Pergonal.

The additional use of HCG is limited to those cases in which there is a failure to ovulate at the maximal dose level or, when at that level, a short luteal phase is demonstrated. The rationale is to improve on the midcycle LH surge; therefore, 10,000 IU of HCG can be given as a single intramuscular dose on the 7th day after clomiphene when follicular maturation is at its peak. Because premature HCG administration may interfere with normal ovulation by down regulating LH receptors, more accurate timing of HCG administration may be desirable. This requires either measurement of the blood estradiol level or estimation of follicular size (18-20 mm diameter) by sonography. When HCG is administered, intercourse is advised for that night and for the next 2 days. In our experience, the addition of HCG has not had a significant impact on the pregnancy rate.

Care should be taken to review with the patient and her husband the pathophysiology of her condition, the principles of treatment, the prolonged course of therapy which may be necessary, and possible complications. Repeated failures accumulate frustration and despair in the couple, making each successive cycle of treatment more difficult. The anxiety and stress may hinder coital performance, and it is not uncommon for a couple to have difficulty performing scheduled intercourse.

Results

In properly selected patients, 80% can be expected to ovulate, and approximately 40% become pregnant. The percent of pregnancies per induced ovulatory cycle is about 20-25%. The multiple pregnancy rate is approximately 5%, almost entirely twins; there have been rare cases of quintuplet and sextuplet births. In our own experience in recent years, with standardization of therapy, the incidence of twins has decreased.

The abortion rate is not increased. Most importantly, the incidence of congenital malformations is not increased, and infant survival and performance after delivery are no different from normal.(19)

The discrepancy between ovulation rates and pregnancy rates is mainly due to 2 factors, the presence of other causes of infertility and a lack of persistence. In those patients with no other cause of infertility, the conception rate approaches a normal rate of 80-90%.(14,20) The pregnancy rate per ovulatory cycle equals the normal rate. The pregnancy rate in 70 of our patients who received therapy sufficient to ovulate in at least 3 cycles was 55.7%, the same pregnancy rate after 3 months of exposure in the general population.(13) With additional treatment cycles, the pregnancy rate decreases although the ovulatory rate remains high. Approximately 15% of patients treated with the higher doses of 150-250 mg will become pregnant.(13) Therefore there may be no need to attribute negative effects of clomiphene on oocyte, endometrium, the corpus luteum, and an early embryo.

If all factors are corrected, and conception has not occurred in 6 months, prognosis is poor. In one large series, only 7.8% of those who had one or more factors in addition to anovulation became pregnant.(14)

Complications

Side effects do not appear to be dose-related, occurring more frequently at the 50 mg dose. Patients requiring the high doses are probably less sensitive to the drug. The most common problems are vasomotor flushes (10%), abdominal distention, bloating, pain, or soreness (5.5%), breast discomfort (2%), nausea and vomiting (2.2%), visual symptoms (1.5%), headache (1.3%), and dryness or loss of hair (0.3%).

591

Visual symptoms include blurring vision, scotoma (visual spots or flashes), or abnormal perception. The cause of these symptoms is unknown, but in every case studied thus far, the visual symptoms have disappeared upon discontinuation of the medication, and no permanent effects have been reported. Usually these symptoms disappear within a few days, but may take 1 or 2 weeks.

Significant ovarian enlargement is associated with longer periods of treatment, and is infrequent (5%) with the usual 5-day course. Maximal enlargement of the ovary usually occurs several days after discontinuing the clomiphene (in response to the increase in gonadotropins). If the patient is symptomatic, pelvic examination, intercourse, and undue physical exercise should be avoided because the enlarged ovaries are very fragile. Ovarian enlargement dissipates rapidly and only rarely is a subsequent treatment cycle delayed.

What to Do with Clomiphene Failure

There are several options available for the 10-20% of women who fail to become pregnant with clomiphene up to the highest dose with added HCG. These include the addition of dexamethasone, extending the duration of clomiphene treatment, considering the empiric use of bromocriptine, and finally, going on to the use of human menopausal gonadotropins (Pergonal).

First, make sure galactorrhea has not been overlooked and a prolactin level has been obtained. The good results with bromocriptine make it essential that this cause of anovulation be detected.

Approximately 30% of patients who have evidence of ovulation with clomiphene but fail to achieve pregnancy do become pregnant when treated with Pergonal. After 6-9 months of clomiphene therapy, and in the absence of any other infertility factors, we proceed to one of the available options.

The Addition of Dexamethasone to Clomiphene. Patients with hirsutism and high circulating androgen concentrations are more resistant to clomiphene.(21-23) Dexamethasone, 0.5 mg at bedtime to blunt the nighttime peak of ACTH, is added to decrease the adrenal contribution to circulating androgens, and thus diminish the androgen level in the microenvironment of the ovarian follicles. Higher ovulation and conception rates are achieved with this treatment when the circulating level of dehydroepiandrosterone sulfate (DHAS) is greater than the upper limit of normal. The dexamethasone is maintained daily until pregnancy is apparent. The dose of clomiphene is returned to the starting point of 50 mg, and increased in incremental fashion as needed.

Extended Clomiphene Treatment. Two approaches have been reported for extending clomiphene treatment. We have very little experience with either. In the first, 250 mg of clomiphene are given for 8 days, followed by 10,000 IU HCG 6 days later. Three pregnancies were achieved out of 25 treatment cycles.(24) In another series, the clomiphene dose was increased every 5 days, with some patients receiving up to 25 days of consecutive treatment, the last 5 days at 250 mg daily.(25) Eight of 21 patients conceived and, in those patients who responded, measurement of gonadotropin revealed sustained elevations in FSH. This latter approach requires estrogen monitoring with discontinuation of the clomiphene when an increase in estrogen is detected. No patient ovulated after more than 21 days of treatment. A simple approach is to extend the duration of clomiphene treatment until a follicle of 18 mm diameter (on ultrasound) is obtained, then administer HCG. But extended clomiphene treatment is a lot of hassle for few results; couples might as well move on to Pergonal.

The Addition of Bromocriptine to Clomiphene. While the use of bromocriptine to induce ovulation is clearly indicated in the presence of galactorrhea or hyperprolactinemia, its use in the clomiphene failure patient with a normal prolactin and no galactorrhea is controversial. Anovulatory patients with normal levels of prolactin do respond to bromocriptine, but the effectiveness of this treatment has not been established by controlled studies. Nevertheless, the clinical response is occasionally impressive.

Bromocriptine

Elevated prolactin levels interfere with the normal function of the menstrual cycle by suppressing the pulsatile secretion of GnRH. This is manifested clinically by a spectrum, ranging from a subtle inadequate luteal phase to total suppression and hypoestrogenic amenorrhea. Regardless of the prolactin level, we interpret the presence of galactorrhea to indicate excessive prolactin stimulation. We screen all patients with galactorrhea or any ovulatory disorder with an assessment of the prolactin level. After a consideration of the problems of amenorrhea, galactorrhea, and the pituitary adenoma (as discussed in Chapter 5 and Chapter 9), bromocriptine emerges as the drug of choice for the induction of ovulation in these patients.

Ovulatory dysfunction in the presence of galactorrhea responds well to bromocriptine, even if the prolactin level is normal.(26) Either biologic activity is not being detected by the radioimmunoassay, or a random blood sample fails to reveal subtle elevations in prolactin.

Bromocriptine is examined in detail in Chapter 5, but it would be helpful to review pertinent details here. Bromocriptine is a dopamine agonist that directly inhibits pituitary secretion of prolactin. Suppression of prolactin levels restores CNS-pituitary gonadotropin function and also appears to increase ovarian responsiveness. The increase in ovarian responsiveness is seen in patients with normal prolactin levels and no galactorrhea. This is the apparent mechanism for an increase in sensitivity to clomiphene when bromocriptine is added to the therapeutic regimen. In women with persistent anovulation and polycystic ovaries, LH secretion is decreased by bromocriptine treatment, thus providing a rationale for why it might enhance the ovulatory response in these patients.(27)

The gastrointestinal and cardiovascular systems react to the dopaminergic action of bromocriptine, and, therefore, the side effects are mainly nausea, diarrhea, dizziness, headache, and fatigue. Side effects can be minimized by slowly building tolerance toward the usual dose, 2.5 mg b.i.d. We start treatment with an initial dose of 2.5 mg at bedtime. If intolerance occurs, the tablet can be cut in half and a slower program, developed by the patient, can be followed to work up to the standard dose. Usually, the second dose is added after 1 week, at breakfast or at lunch. In some patients, elevated prolactin levels can be reduced to normal levels with very small doses of bromocriptine, as little as 0.625 or 1.25 mg.(28)

The usual regimen is to administer bromocriptine daily until it is apparent the patient is pregnant, as usually determined by the basal body temperature chart. Although there has been no evidence of any harmful effects on the fetus, some patients and physicians prefer to avoid taking bromocriptine in the luteal phase, and, therefore, during early pregnancy. The drug is stopped when a temperature rise occurs, and resumed when menses begin.

Ovulatory menses and pregnancy are achieved in 80% of patients with galactorrhea and hyperprolactinemia. Response is rapid, and, therefore, if there is no indication of ovulation (a rise in the basal body temperature) within 2 months, clomiphene is added to the regimen. The starting dose of clomiphene is 50 mg daily for 5 days, given and increased in the usual fashion.

As discussed in Chapter 5, once pregnant, the majority of women with a pituitary-secreting adenoma remain asymptomatic. Women with both microadenomas and macroadenomas may undergo uneventful pregnancies. It is extremely rare for a patient to develop a problem which results in perinatal damage or serious maternal sequelae. Surveillance during pregnancy need only consist of an awareness for the development of symptoms, headaches and visual disturbances. Assessment of visual fields, prolactin assay, and sella turcica changes by limited CT scanning can await the onset of suspicious symptoms. Tumor expansion (and its symptoms) promptly regress with bromocriptine treatment. No adverse effects of bromocriptine on the pregnancy or the newborn have been reported.

Resolution of galactorrhea or hyperprolactinemia may occur spontaneously after a pregnancy. Perhaps a tumor can undergo infarction in response to the expansion and shrinkage during and after pregnancy, or the condition was associated with dysfunction of the hypothalamus, now corrected.

Bromocriptine for Euprolactinemic Women. There has been a growing clinical experience indicating successful induction of ovulation and achievement of pregnancy with bromocriptine in the absence of galactorrhea and with a normal prolactin level. Some anovulatory women with normal prolactin levels who ovulated in response to bromocriptine have been found to have elevated nocturnal peaks of prolactin.(29) The mechanism of action may be an increase in follicular responsiveness either due to suppression of prolactin or suppression of LH (a known action of dopamine). A decrease in LH may alter local follicular steroidogenesis in such a way to create a more favorable microenvironment. The method of administration is the same as above. If, after 2 months of treatment, there is no response, clomiphene is reinitiated, working up again from the starting dose of 50 mg daily. While it is our impression that this is successful in a significant number of patients, it has been shown that bromocriptine has nothing to offer for ovulatory women with unexplained infertility.(30) On the other hand, bromocriptine or bromocriptine plus clomiphene treatment of ovulatory women *with galactorrhea* (and normal prolactin levels) yielded higher pregnancy rates when compared to a control group.(31) Once again the importance of detecting galactorrhea is emphasized.

Human Menopausal Gonadotropins (Pergonal)

Pergonal (human menopausal gonadotropins) is a purified preparation of gonadotropins extracted from the urine of postmenopausal women. The generic name is menotropins. The commercial preparation contains 75 units of FSH and 75 units of LH. The potency is expressed in terms of international units based on an international reference preparation. A significant factor in the use of Pergonal is its high cost, approximately $30/ampule. Treatment may cost from $500 to $1000/cycle for the drug alone. Pergonal is inactive orally and, therefore, must be given by intramuscular injections.

Selection of Patients

Not only because of its expense, but because of its greater complication rate, patients should not receive Pergonal without a very careful evaluation. An absolute requirement is the demonstration of ovarian competence. Abnormally high serum gonadotropins with a failure to demonstrate withdrawal bleeding indicate ovarian failure and preclude induction of ovulation except in those special cases of ovarian failure as discussed in Chapter 5. Successful induction of ovulation and pregnancy have been reported in women with apparent ovarian failure, treated with a combination of estrogen (to suppress FSH to normal levels) and Pergonal. Our own experience with this approach has been disappointing, and the chance of achieving pregnancy must be very low.

A thorough infertility investigation must be performed. In addition to the demonstration of ovarian competence, tubal and uterine pathology should be ruled out, anovulation documented, and semen analysis obtained. Nongynecologic endocrine problems must be treated. Hypogonadotropic function (low serum gonadotropins), including galactorrhea syndromes, requires evaluation for an intracranial lesion, with a sella turcica x-ray and measurement of prolactin levels. It is imperative to take all steps necessary to exclude treatable pathology to which anovulation is secondary.

In our practice we first offer a course of clomiphene, not only because of the cost and complications associated with Pergonal, but also because some apparently hypogonadotropic patients will unpredictably respond to clomiphene.

Because some patients cannot tolerate bromocriptine, it is important to know that hyperprolactinemia has no adverse effect on response to Pergonal.(32)

How to Use Pergonal

Instruction and counseling of the couple are essential. A thorough understanding of the need for daily treatment and frequent observation is necessary prior to initiating therapy. As part of this instruction, the husband may be taught to administer injections. Daily recording of the basal body temperature and body weight is important for proper management. The couple should be told about the need for scheduled intercourse, the possibility that more than one course of treatment may be necessary, and the expense of the treatment. Above all, the patient must be prepared for the anguish that accompanies failure. Because this is a pressure-packed situation, unexpected impotence is occasionally encountered on the days of scheduled intercourse.

In the past there were 2 commonly used techniques of Pergonal administration, the variable and the fixed dosage methods. Pregnancy rates with the fixed dosage method are unacceptably low, and the variable dosage method should be used to achieve follicular growth and maturation. Follicle stimulation is achieved by 7-14 days of continuous Pergonal, beginning with 2 ampules daily. Response is judged by the degree of estrogen produced by the growing follicles. The patient is monitored periodically with the measurement of the 24-hour urinary excretion of total estrogens or the blood estradiol level. The patient is seen on the 7th day of treatment and a decision is made to continue or increase the dose. After the 7th day, the patient is seen anywhere from daily to every 3rd day. Patients with polycystic ovaries are handled more gingerly because they are more responsive. These patients are usually started on 1 ampule daily and monitoring begins on the 5th day of treatment.

Pergonal comes as a dry powder in a sealed glass ampule, along with a second ampule containing 2 ml of diluent. One ampule of Pergonal requires 1 ml of diluent. When 2 ampules are to be administered, solution with 1 ml is accomplished in the first vial of Pergonal, and the solution is then deposited in the second vial. Thus, when giving 2 ampules of Pergonal the contents of 2 vials are dissolved in a total of 1 ml of diluent. When 4 ampules are given, a total of 2 ml of diluent are used. Should 6 ampules of Pergonal be required, 3 ampules are dissolved in 1.5 ml of diluent and two injections are administered, each in the upper outer quadrant of each buttock. The HCG injection comes as a vial containing 10,000 units as a dry powder. One ml of the accompanying diluent is used for administration.

It cannot be emphasized too strongly that dosage administration and the judicious use of estrogen measurements depend upon the experience of the physician administering Pergonal. When estradiol and ultrasound monitoring indicate that the patient is ready to receive the ovulatory stimulus, 10,000 units of HCG are given as a single dose intramuscularly. Because of its structural and biologic similarity to LH, HCG, readily available from human pregnancy urine and placental tissue, is used to simulate the midcycle LH ovulatory surge. Neither manipulation of HCG dosage nor time of administration has been successful in changing the rates of multiple gestation and hyperstimulation.

The patient is advised to have intercourse the day of the HCG injection and for the next 2 days. In view of the fragility of hyperstimulated ovaries, further intercourse as well as strenuous physical exercise should be avoided.

Pregnancy is usually achieved with the administration of 2 ampules/day for 7-12 days. The best results are obtained when the treatment period covers 10-15 days; when less than 10 days, the spontaneous abortion rate is increased.(33) In general there is a direct relationship between dose and body weight, however, the same empiric approach is needed even in obese patients.(34) In some individuals, presumably with extremely hyposensitive ovaries, adequate follicular stimulation requires doses up to 4, 6, and more ampules/day. In this group of amenorrheic women massive doses of gonadotropins are necessary, and with proper monitoring, pregnancy can be achieved safely. The range between the dose which does not induce ovulation and the dose which results in hyperstimulation is narrow. The situation is made even more difficult because the ovaries may react differently to essentially similar doses from month to month. Close supervision and experience in the use of Pergonal are necessary to avoid difficulties.

Estrogen Monitoring. The use of estrogen measurements is necessary to choose the correct moment for administering the ovulatory dose of HCG in order to prevent hyperstimulation. The cervical mucus begins to change rapidly when estrogen levels begin to rise. After a moderate rise in estrogen, however, there are no additional significant changes in the mucus. In addition, the response of the cervical glands varies considerably among individuals. The cervical assessment can therefore alert the clinician to an estrogen change, but it cannot be relied on for precise timing to avoid excessive stimulation. On day 7 of the therapeutic cycle urine or blood is assayed for estrogen. Depending on the findings, the dosage of Pergonal is individualized for the duration of the cycle. With experience, the physician can avoid daily estrogen measurements although sometimes this is necessary.

What should the urinary estrogen level be? Below 100 μg/24 hours, a significant but not maximal pregnancy rate can be achieved. Over 200 μg/24 hours, a significant rate of hyperstimulation is encountered. Between 100 and 200 μg/24 hours, hyperstimulation or multiple ovulation may be encountered, but also the maximal pregnancy rate is achieved. To project dosage requirements, a useful fact to keep in mind is that once the phase of rapidly increasing estrogen production is reached, the urinary estrogen level will approximately double each day.

What should the blood estrogen level be? Because the blood estradiol is determined on a single sample of blood, the timing of the sampling with relationship to the previous injection of Pergonal becomes a significant variable. When Pergonal injections are given between 5 and 8 PM and blood samples are obtained first thing in the morning, an estradiol window of 1000-1500 pg/ml is optimal.(35) The risk of hyperstimulation is significant from 1500 to 2000 pg/ml, and as a general rule, over 2000 pg/ml, HCG should not be given, and the ovarian follicles should be allowed to regress. Careful correlation of estrogen levels with the ultrasonographic picture allows a more aggressive approach. Haning has calculated that an upper limit for estradiol of 3800 pg/ml for anovulatory women (with polycystic ovaries) and 2400 for women with hypothalamic amenorrhea gives a risk of severe hyperstimulation of 5% in pregnant cycles and 1% in nonconception cycles.(36)

Attempting to reproduce the normal midcycle levels of estrogen does not achieve a maximal pregnancy rate and higher levels are required. The relative safety of this approach was seen in our series, where only 2 of 24 patients with estradiol levels over 1000 pg/ml developed hyperstimulation and it was moderate in both cases.(35) When a patient nears ovulation on the weekend and estrogen monitoring is unavailable, timing of the HCG administration can be predicted fairly accurately by plotting the estradiol values on semilogarithmic paper. The rate of increase in estradiol is the same in spontaneous and induced cycles, and does not differ in cycles which result in multiple gestation.(37) The level which is reached at the time of HCG administration is more critical than the slope of increase. Once a linear rise of estradiol is established, there is no need to increase the dose.

Ultrasound Monitoring. Ultrasound assessment of the growth and development of the ovarian follicle indicates the degree of follicular maturity and capability.(38) During normal cycles, the growing cohort of follicles can be first identified by ultrasonography on days 5 to 7 as small sonolucent cysts. The dominant follicle will become apparent by day 8-10. The maximal mean diameter, indicating ovum maturity, of the preovulatory dominant follicle varies from 20 to 24 mm (range 18-28 mm), Individual women tend to produce the same maximal diameter on repeated cycles. Subordinate follicles rarely exceed 14 mm in diameter. In 5-11% of cycles, two dominant follicles develop.

During the 5 days preceding ovum expulsion, the dominant follicle exhibits a linear growth pattern of approximately 2 to 3 mm per day, followed by rapid exponential growth during the last 24 hours prior to ovulation. *Ultrasonographic surveillance of ovaries reveals that mittelschmerz is associated not with follicular rupture, but with the rapid expansion of the dominant follicle, thus the pain precedes follicular rupture.*

Ovulation is associated with complete emptying of the follicular contents in 1 to 45 minutes. Fluid can be frequently detected in the cul-de-sac. The follicle either disappears or more commonly appears as a smaller, irregular cyst which diminishes in size over the next 4-5 days.

In response to clomiphene treatment, follicles pursue a linear, but generally accelerated, rate of growth compared to spontaneous cycles.(39) The maximal diameter of clomiphene-induced preovulatory follicles is similar to that seen with spontaneous cycles, 22-23 mm, but ovulation can be successfully induced with HCG administration when the diameter reaches 18-20 mm (by the time of ovulation, the follicle will have grown another 2-3 mm).

With Pergonal, the maximal follicular diameter (15-18 mm) is smaller than that seen during spontaneous and clomiphene-induced cycles. When follicles reach this size, ovulation will occur approximately 36 hours after HCG is administered.

Ultrasound monitoring does not eliminate the risk of multiple gestation or hyperstimulation. It is claimed that a higher pregnancy rate can be achieved when ultrasound is combined with estrogen monitoring.(40) The guiding principle has been to administer HCG when mature follicles correlate with an estrogen level of 400 pg per follicle. The 400 pg principle only applies when there are several leading follicles, not when many intermediate (9-16 mm) and small (<9 mm) follicles are present. As a general rule, hyperstimulation is associated with the presence of more follicles. We believe that HCG should not be administered if there are more than 3-4 follicles 14 mm or greater in diameter (offering some protection against multiple gestation and hyperstimulation). Mild hyperstimulation has been associated with an increased number of intermediate size follicles, and severe hyperstimulation with an increase in small follicles.(41,42) A large number (11 or more) of smaller follicles also should preclude HCG administration.

Serial ultrasound observation of ovarian cycles has raised many questions. Alleged asynchronies have been identified involving the estradiol surge, the gonadotropin surge, deficient luteinization, and the growth and disappearance of follicles.(43) A new syndrome has emerged, the luteinized unruptured follicle syndrome. This condition, in which the follicle becomes luteinized without release of the ovum, cannot be diagnosed by the usual standard but indirect methods of ovulation assessment.(44) This phenomenon occurs in both fertile and infertile women, in perhaps as many as 5-10% of cycles. The actual relationship of these observations to infertility remains to be determined.

Results

The most significant aspect of this method of treatment is that it does achieve pregnancy in an otherwise untreatable situation. In general, more than 90% of patients with competent ovaries will ovulate in response to Pergonal and a pregnancy rate of approximately 50-70% can be achieved. In patients with hypothalamic amenorrhea, the pregnancy rate per cycle is 25-30% with a 1% rate of hyperstimulation. The average number of treatment cycles required is 3. As with clomiphene, there is a normal incidence of congenital malformations, and the children have a normal postnatal development.(19)

HCG disappears from the blood with an initial component having a half-life of about 6 hours and a second, slower, component with a half-life of about 24 hours. It is this relatively slow half-life which enables a single injection of 10,000 IU to maintain the corpus luteum until pregnancy takes over. The HCG concentration after the ovulation injection should be less than 100 mIU/ml by day 16 after the injection. A β-subunit assay of HCG at this time or one of the urine assays performed 2-4 weeks after the HCG injection are reliable tests for pregnancy.

Prior to the present era of more careful monitoring, the multiple pregnancy rate was reported as approximately 30% (triplets or more, 5%). Currently, the multiple pregnancy rate is about 10%.(40) The multiple pregnancies are secondary to multiple ovulations, and therefore the siblings are not identical. The rate of spontaneous occurrence of twins is only about 1% and that of triplets 0.010-0.017% of the pregnant population. Dizygotic twinning varies among different populations and is inherited through the mother. The monozygotic twinning rate is about 0.3-0.4%, fairly constant, and uninfluenced by heredity. Induction of ovulation is known to increase the frequency of monozygotic twinning by 3 fold.(45) It is not known whether the multiple pregnancy rate with Pergonal is significantly affected by a maternal history of twinning.

Fetal loss due to prematurity in the multiple pregnancies has been a serious problem. In addition, the abortion rate with Pergonal is somewhat higher (25%), probably a combination of the effect of age, multiple pregnancies, and recognition of early abortions.(46)

Therapeutic abortion in the case of triplets or more is an option, but it would be surprising if patient and physician would choose this treatment. On the other hand, selective reduction of the number of embryos in multiple pregnancy has been accomplished.(47,48) Under ultrasound guidance, transcervical aspiration of a gestational sac can be accomplished or a cardiotoxic drug can be transabdominally injected into, or adjacent to, the fetal heart. The transcervical procedure is best performed between the 8th and 9th weeks of gestation and the transabdominal procedure between the 11th and 12th weeks. The moral and ethical aspects of this decision are significant, but in view of the potential problems associated with a multiple birth, this is a reasonable alternative for some.

The likelihood of ovulation is dose related, and complications are likewise dose related. In general, 3 therapeutic cycles are required to achieve pregnancy. The rate of serious hyperstimulation has been 1%, but proper monitoring has reduced this complication to a rare happening. After at least one Pergonal-induced pregnancy the spontaneous pregnancy rate reaches 30% after 5 years. (49) Most of the pregnancies occur within 3 years of the Pergonal pregnancy.

Clomiphene-Pergonal Sequence

The combination of both clomiphene and Pergonal was explored in order to minimize the cost of Pergonal alone. As long as treatment is monitored with estrogen levels the side effects and complications should not be dissimilar to those with Pergonal alone. It has not been demonstrated that patients unresponsive to Pergonal alone would respond to the sequence method, and there is no logical reason to assume that this would be true.

The usual method of treatment is to administer clomiphene 100 mg for 5-7 days, then to immediately proceed with Pergonal beginning with 2 ampules per day. Estrogen levels are monitored as usual. This method may decrease the amount of Pergonal required by approximately 50%; however, the same risks of multiple pregnancy and hyperstimulation can be expected. This reduced requirement for Pergonal is found only in those patients who demonstrate a positive withdrawal bleeding following progestin medication or who have spontaneous menses. (50)

GnRH Agonist Combination

Recognizing that women with significant estrogen and gonadotropin levels (especially anovulatory women with polycystic ovaries) do not respond well to Pergonal, attention was turned to a method which could turn off a woman's endogenous reproductive hormone production. The availability of GnRH agonists provided such a method. As you will recall, continuous stimulation with a GnRH agonist will result in the down regulation of GnRH receptors on the anterior pituitary, followed by suppression of gonadotropin secretion. This approach is especially effective for women who either show no response to exogenous gonadotropins or who develop premature spontaneous LH and progesterone rises. Indeed, the major effect appears to be the prevention of premature luteinization which is a major reason for decreased success with Pergonal in women with polycystic ovaries.

Buserelin can be administered 100-150 ug intranasally every 4 hours or 250 ug subcutaneously on a daily basis, and combined with Pergonal or purified FSH to achieve pregnancy or to stimulate multiple follicular development for in vitro fertilization.(51,52)

We and others have used leuprolide acetate (Lupron). (53) Lupron is administered daily (0.5 mg subcutaneously) for 2 weeks. By this time, down regulation has effectively occurred. Pergonal is then begun in the usual fashion and the Lupron treatment maintained until the HCG is administered. With this combination, it is not unusual to require higher doses of Pergonal. Clinical studies may reveal that shorter periods of exposure to the agonist will be as effective.

Hyperstimulation
Syndrome

Ovarian hyperstimulation may be life threatening. In mild cases the syndrome includes ovarian enlargement, abdominal distension, and weight gain. In severe cases, a critical condition develops with ascites, pleural effusion, electrolyte imbalance, and hypovolemia with hypotension and oliguria.(54) The ovaries are tremendously enlarged with multiple follicular cysts, stromal edema, and many corpora lutea.

The basic disturbance is a shift of fluid from the intravascular space into the abdominal cavity creating a massive third space. The resulting hypovolemia leads to circulatory and excretory problems. The genesis of the ascites is unclear. The very high level of estrogen secretion by the ovaries may be the primary factor, inducing increased local capillary permeability and leakage of fluid from the peritoneal capillaries as well as the ovaries. The leakage of fluid is also critically related to the mass, volume, and surface area of the ovaries. Therefore, the larger the ovaries and the greater the steroid production, the more severe the condition. Experiments in animals have implicated a role for histamine and prostaglandins.

The loss of fluid and protein into the abdominal cavity accounts for the hypovolemia and hemoconcentration. This in turn results in low blood pressure and decreased central venous pressure. The major clinical complications are increased coagulability and decreased renal perfusion. Blood loss as the cause of the clinical picture can be easily ruled out since a hematocrit will reveal hemoconcentration. The decreased renal perfusion leads to increased salt and water reabsorption in the proximal tubule producing oliguria and low urinary sodium excretion. With less sodium being presented to the distal tubule, there is a decrease in the exchange of hydrogen and potassium for sodium, resulting in hyperkalemic acidosis. A rise in the blood urea nitrogen (BUN) is due to decreased perfusion and increased urea reabsorption. Because it is only filtered, creatinine does not increase as much as the BUN. Thus, the patient is hypovolemic, azotemic, and hyperkalemic. In response to these changes, aldosterone, plasma renin activity, and antidiuretic hormone levels are all elevated.(55)

Treatment is conservative and empiric. Although both antihistamines and indomethacin have been demonstrated to ameliorate the hyperstimulation in animal studies, their efficacy and safety in early human pregnancy are unknown. When a patient displays excessive weight gain (usually 20 or more pounds), hemoconcentration (hematocrit over 50%), oliguria, dyspnea, or postural hypotension, she should be hospitalized. Pelvic and abdominal examination are contraindicated in view of the extreme fragility of the enlarged ovaries. Ovarian rupture and hemorrhage are easily precipitated.

Upon admission, the patient is put on bed rest, with daily body weights, strict monitoring of intake and output, and frequent vital signs. Serial studies of the following are obtained: hematocrit, BUN, creatinine, electrolytes, total proteins with albumin-globulin ratio, coagulation studies, and urinary sodium and potassium. The electrocardiogram is utilized to follow and evaluate hyperkalemia. Fluid and salt are rigidly restricted because of the third spacing effect. As long as the BUN remains stable, an abnormally low urine output can be tolerated.(55) Potassium exchange resins may be necessary. Diuretics are without effect and, indeed, may be disadvantageous. The fluid in the abdominal cavity is not responsive to diuretic treatment, and diuresis may further contract the intravascular volume and produce hypovolemic shock or thrombosis. Arterial thrombosis has been reported.

In severe cases, life-threatening adult respiratory distress syndrome can occur.(56) This condition is associated with a 50% mortality rate. The use of one of the inhibitors of prostaglandin synthesis is worth trying. In addition, chlorpheniramine maleate, an H-1 receptor blocker, appears to maintain membrane stability allowing the use of fluids and mannitol to retain intravascular volume.(57)

The possibility of ovarian rupture should always be considered, and serial hematocrits may be the only clue to intraperitoneal hemorrhage. Of course, a falling hematocrit accompanied by diuresis is an indication of resolution, not hemorrhage. Laparotomy should be avoided in these precarious patients. If surgery is necessary, only hemostatic measures should be undertaken and the ovaries should be conserved if possible, since a return to normal size is inevitable.

The key point is that the hyperstimulation syndrome will undergo gradual resolution with time. In a patient who is not pregnant, the syndrome will cover a period of approximately 7 days. In a patient who is pregnant and in whom the ovaries are restimulated by the emerging endogenous HCG production, the syndrome will last 10-20 days.

The syndrome will not develop unless the ovulatory dose of HCG is given. Thus, the major emphasis in recent years has been to utilize monitoring to avoid hyperstimulation. The relationship between estrogen levels and hyperstimulation is not a perfect one. Hyperstimulation has been found with relatively low estrogen levels, and high estrogen is not necessarily followed by hyperstimulation. As a general rule, the more follicles present (on ultrasound examination) the greater the risk for hyperstimulation. But this too is not a perfect correlation. Nevertheless, monitoring is the major available deterrent to a potentially life-threatening situation.

What to do with the Pergonal Failure	If funds and emotional reserves are sufficient, a repeat course of therapy is permissible after a review of the etiologic basis for infertility. The effectiveness of treatment does not diminish with repeated cycles. Conception rates remain about the same. If a couple can handle it, they should persist if no other infertility problems are present. Guidance to adoption services and emotional support continue to be part of the physician's obligation.
Purified FSH	Purified FSH (Metrodin) is separated from LH by immunochromatography. One ampule contains 75 IU of FSH and less than 1 IU of LH. Because some LH presence is necessary for ovarian follicular steroidogenesis, growth, and development, it's not surprising that purified FSH is not useful in women with severe hypothalamic amenorrhea.
	Daily low doses of FSH can achieve pregnancy in women with polycystic ovaries; unfortunately this requires daily intramuscular injections for 30 or more days. Higher doses of FSH are associated with a risk of hyperstimulation despite only a modest rate of ovulatory response. Therefore purified FSH must be administered in a regimen similar to that of Pergonal, and the problems and results are also similar.(58) While the results in women with polycystic ovaries are good, it is not clear that this method is superior to Pergonal.
Gonadotropin Releasing Hormone (GnRH)	The advantage in the utilization of GnRH lies in the difficulty in producing hyperstimulation. An excessive amount of GnRH, as in the studies discussed in Chapter 2, results in down regulation of its own receptor. In addition, the multiple pregnancy rate with GnRH should be identical to the normal rate. Because GnRH serves largely a permissive role, the internal feedback mechanisms between the ovary and pituitary should be operative, yielding follicular growth and development similar to a normal menstrual cycle in response to the "turning on" of the system by GnRH.
	GnRH is administered constantly in a pulsatile fashion by a programmable portable minipump. Induction of ovulation with the GnRH pump is most effective in women with hypothalamic amenorrhea (absence of menstrual bleeding following a progestin challenge). However, it has been successful in some anovulatory women with polycystic ovaries. The GnRH pump is a safer, less expensive alternative for these patients than Pergonal. The GnRH pump is also effective in women with hyperprolactinemia, providing another good alternative if bromocriptine cannot be tolerated.
	GnRH is available in crystalline form which when reconstituted in the aqueous diluent is stable for at least 3 weeks at room temperature. The pump must be worn constantly around the clock, requiring some ingenuity for bathing and sleeping. GnRH can be administered by either the intravenous or subcutaneous routes. The subcutaneous route requires a higher dose. Failure with subcutaneous administration is associated with a polycystic ovary-like picture, with high LH levels, anovulation, and even symptoms of androgen excess. This is not surprising in that subcutaneous administration results in an absorption curve with a broad base without a definite peak. For intravenous administration, heparin is added to the GnRH solution in a concentration of 1000 U/ml. We favor start-

603

ing with the subcutaneous route (placing the needle in the anterior abdominal wall) because it is easier for the patient; if a good response is not immediately obtained, then switch to the intravenous route. The needles are left in place until there are signs of local reaction.

While some argue in favor of near-physiologic duplication of the pulse frequency, similar results can be obtained with empiric 90 minute cycles throughout treatment. The dose for subcutaneous administration is 20 μg per bolus, for intravenous administration, 5 μg per bolus. If the patient fails to respond, the dose should be increased by 5 μg increments.

After ovulation, the luteal phase is maintained by either continuing the pump or administering HCG (1500 IU intramuscularly at the time of the temperature rise and then every 3 days for 3 doses). In our experience most patients would rather discontinue the pump.

One of the reasons that the GnRH pump is less expensive is that it reproduces physiologic hormonal events and intensive monitoring is not necessary. The main problem is knowing with some accuracy when to have intercourse. Usually ovulation occurs by 14 days of treatment, but the range extends from 10 days to 22 days. Intercourse every other day during this period of time can be a formidable challenge. Ultrasonic monitoring of follicular development may be required, or more conveniently, the couple could use one of the urinary LH test kits to detect the LH surge and have intercourse for 2-3 days beginning the day of the color change.

Side effects with the GnRH pump are minimal, principally related to pump functioning and local reactions to the needle placement. The patient must be educated to pay close attention to proper function of the pump and maintenance of the GnRH reservoir. Hyperstimulation and multiple births have been encountered, but this is rare and associated with higher than recommended doses. The risk of dangerous hyperstimulation is essentially zero. Several cases of allergic response with the development of circulating antibodies have been reported.

The pregnancy rate in women with hypothalamic (hypogonadotropic) amenorrhea is 30-35% of treatment cycles which approximates the pregnancy rate of normal couples.(59) Persistence with repeated cycles is rewarded with high cumulative pregnancy rates.

The inconvenience and mechanical problems of the pump may be overcome in the future by the utilization of a long-acting GnRH analog which may be administered intranasally several times a day. The potential safety and simplicity of GnRH administration are powerful attractions.

Ovarian Wedge Resection	The purpose of wedge resection of the ovaries is to remove a significant amount of steroid-producing tissue. Documentation of hormonal changes following wedge resection indicates that the only important change is a sustained reduction in testosterone levels. This suggests that the barrier to ovulation is the intraovarian, atresia-promoting effects of the high testosterone production. Removal of androgen-producing tissue effectively lowers this barrier, and ovulatory cycles may ensue.

The response to ovarian wedge resection is variable. Some patients resume ovulation permanently. However, most patients return to their anovulatory state. Some patients fail to respond at all. Furthermore, the surgical procedure carries with it the potential problem of postoperative adhesion formation.

The operative risk, the variable response, and the possibility of postoperative adhesion formation are the liabilities of wedge resection. These must be weighed against the excellent results obtained with medical induction of ovulation (approximating the normal conception rate when anovulation is the only fertility problem present). It should truly be a rare patient in whom wedge resection of the ovaries is necessary. An alternative with the possibility (not yet demonstrated) of a lesser liability is cautery or aspiration of multiple cysts in polycystic ovaries by means of the laparoscope.(60) This appears to be associated with the same decrease in androgens as observed with wedge resection and can be followed by ovulation and pregnancy.

References

1. **Ernst S, Hite G, Cantrell JS, Richardson A Jr, Benson HD,** Stereochemistry of geometric isomers of clomiphene: A correction of the literature and a reexamination of structure-activity relationships, J Pharm Sci 65:148, 1976.

2. **Clark JH, Markaverich BM,** The agonistic-antagonistic properties of clomiphene: A review, Pharmacol Therap 15:467, 1982.

3. **Adashi EY,** Clomiphene citrate-initiated ovulation: A clinical update, Seminars Reprod Endocrinol 4:255, 1986.

4. **Kerin JF, Liu JH, Phillipou G, Yen SSC,** Evidence for a hypothalamic site of action of clomiphene citrate in women, J Clin Endocrinol Metab 61:265, 1985.

5. **Judd SJ, Alderman J, Bowden J, Michailov L,** Evidence against the involvement of opiate neurons in mediating the effect of clomiphene citrate on gonadotropin-releasing hormone neurons, Fertil Steril 47:574, 1987.

6. **Miyake A, Tasaka K, Sakumoto T, Kawamura Y, Nagahara Y, Aono T,** Clomiphene citrate induces luteinizing hormone release through hypothalamic luteinizing hormone-releasing hormone in vitro, Acta Endocrinol 103:289, 1983.

7. **Kessel B, Hsueh AJW,** Clomiphene citrate augments follicle-stimulating hormone-induced luteinizing hormone receptor content in cultured rat granulosa cells, Fertil Steril 46:334, 1987.

8. **Birkenfeld A, Beier HM, Schenmker JG,** The effect of clomiphene citrate on early embryonic development, endometrium and implantation, Human Reprod 1:387, 1986.

9. **Mikkelson TJ, Kroboth PD, Cameron WJ, Dittert LW, Chungi V, Manberg PJ,** Single-dose pharmacokinetics of clomiphene citrate in normal volunteers, Fertil Steril 46:392, 1986.

10. **Oelsner G, Barnea ER, Mullen MV, Mikkelson TJ, Tarlatzis BC, Naftolin F, DeCherney AH,** Simultaneous measurements of clomiphene citrate in plasma and follicular fluid in women undergoing IVF & ET, Program, American Fertility Society, Abstract 39, 1986.

11. **Lavy G, Fazio D, Polan ML,** Human chorionic gonadotropin reverses the inhibitory effect of clomiphene citrate on progesterone production by granulosa-luteal cells obtained following different ovarian stimulation protocols, Program, American Fertility Society, Abstract 40, 1986.

12. **Cunha GR, Taguchi O, Namikawa R, Nishizuka Y, Robboy SJ,** Teratogenic effects of clomiphene, tamoxifen, and diethylstilbestrol on the developing human female genital tract, Human Pathol 18:1132, 1987.

13. **Gorlitsky GA, Kase NG, Speroff L,** Ovulation and pregnancy rates with clomiphene citrate, Obstet Gynecol 51:265, 1978.

14. **Gysler M, March CM, Mishell DR Jr, Bailey EJ,** A decade's experience with an individualized clomiphene treatment regimen including its effect on the postcoital test, Fertil Steril 37:161, 1982.

15. **Taubert H-D, Dericks-Tan, JE,** High doses of estrogens do not interfere with the ovulation-inducing effect of clomiphene citrate, Fertil Steril 27:375, 1976.

16. **Ruby M, Wu CH, Dein RA,** The therapy initiation day and the outcome of clomiphene and short-course menotropin induction of ovulation, Program, American Fertility Society, Abstract 187, 1986.

17. **Shepard MK, Balmaceda JP, Leija CG,** Relationship of weight to successful induction of ovulation with clomiphene citrate, Fertil Steril 32:641, 1979.

18. **Lobo RA, Gysler M, March CM, Goebelsmann U, Mishell DR Jr,** Clinical and laboratory predictors of clomiphene response, Fertil Steril 37:168, 1982.

19. **Lunenfeld B, Blankstein J, Kotev-Emeth S, Kokia E, Geier A,** Drugs used in ovulation induction. Safety of patient and offspring, Human Reprod 1:435, 1986.

20. **Hammond MG, Halme JK, Talbert LM,** Factors affecting the pregnancy rate in clomiphene citrate induction of ovulation, Obstet Gynecol 62:196, 1983.

21. **Lobo RA, Paul W, March CM, Granger L, Kletzky OA,** Clomiphene and dexamethasone in women unresponsive to clomiphene alone, Obstet Gynecol 60:497, 1982.

22. **Daly DC, Walters CA, Soto-Albers CE, Tohan N, Riddick DH,** A randomized study of dexamethasone in ovulation induction with clomiphene citrate, Fertil Steril 41:844, 1984.

23. **Hoffman D, Lobo RA,** Serum dehydroepiandrosterone sulfate and the use of clomiphene citrate in anovulatory women, Fertil Steril 43:196, 1985.

24. **Lobo RA, Granger LR, Davajan V, Mishell DR Jr,** An extended regimen of clomiphene citrate in women unresponsive to standard therapy, Fertil Steril 37:762, 1982.

25. **O'Herlihy C, Pepperell RJ, Brown JB, Smith MA, Sandri L, McBain JC,** Incremental clomiphene therapy: A new method for treating persistent anovulation, Obstet Gynecol 58:535, 1981.

26. **Padilla SL, Person GK, McDonough PG, Reindollar RH,** The efficacy of bromocriptine in patients with ovulatory dysfunction and normoprolactinemic galactorrhea, Fertil Steril 44:695, 1985.

27. **Falaschi P, Rocco A, del Pozo E,** Inhibitory effect of bromocriptine treatment on luteinizing hormone secretion in polycystic ovary syndrome, J Clin Endocrinol Metab 62:348, 1986.

28. **Soto-Albers CE, Daly DC, Walters CA, Ying YK, Riddick DH,** Titrating the dose of bromocriptine when treating hyperprolactinemic women, Fertil Steril 43:485, 1985.

29. **Suginami H, Hamada K, Yano K, Kuroda G, Matsuura S,** Ovulation induction with bromocriptine in normoprolactinemic anovulatory women, J Clin Endocrinol Metab 62:899, 1986.

30. **Weight CS, Steele SJ, Jacobs JS,** Value of bromocriptine in unexplained primary infertility: A double-blind controlled trial, Brit Med J 1:1037, 1979.

31. **DeVane GW, Guzick DS,** Bromocriptine therapy in normoprolactinemic women with unexplained infertility and galactorrhea, Fertil Steril 46:1026, 1986.

32. **Farine D, Dor J, Lupovici N, Lunenfeld B, Mashiach S,** Conception rate after gonadotropin therapy in hyperprolactinemia and normoprolactinemia, Obstet Gynecol 65:658, 1985.

33. **Gindoff PR, Jewelewicz R,** Use of gonadotropins in ovulation induction, N Y State J Med 85:580, 1985.

34. **Chong AP, Rafael RW, Forte CC,** Influence of weight in the induction of ovulation with human menopausal gonadotropin and human chorionic gonadotropin, Fertil Steril 46:599, 1986.

35. **Haning RV Jr, Levin RM, Behrman HR, Kase NG, Speroff L,** Plasma estradiol window and urinary estriol glucuronide determination for monitoring menotropin induction of ovulation, Obstet Gynecol 54:442, 1979.

36. **Haning RV Jr, Boehnlein LM, Carlson IH, Kuzma DL, Zweibel WJ,** Diagnosis-specific serum 17β-estradiol (E_2) upper limits for treatment with menotropins using a ^{125}I direct E_2 assay, Fertil Steril 42:882, 1984.

37. **Wilson EA, Jawad MJ, Hayden TL,** Rates of exponential increase of serum estradiol concentrations in normal and human menopausal gonadotropin-induced cycles, Fertil Steril 37:46, 1982.

38. **Ritchie WGM,** Ultrasound in the evaluation of normal and induced ovulation, Fertil Steril 43:167, 1985.

39. **Leerentueld R, Van Gent I, Der Stoep M, Wladimiroff J,** Ultrasonographic assessment of Graffian follicle growth under monofollicular and multifollicular conditions in clomiphene citrate stimulated cycles, Fertil Steril 43:565, 1985.

40. **March CM,** Improved pregnancy rate with monitoring of gonadotropin therapy by three modalities, Am J Obstet Gynecol 156:1473, 1987.

41. **Tal J, Paz B, Samberg I, Lazarov N, Sharf M,** Ultrasonographic and clinical correlates of menotropin versus sequential clomiphene citrate: Menotropin therapy for induction of ovulation, Fertil Steril 44:342, 1985.

42. **Blankstein J, Shalev J, Sasdon T, Kukia EE, Rabinovici J, Pariente C, Lunenfeld B, Serr DM, Mashiach S,** Ovarian hyperstimulation syndrome: Prediction by number and size of preovulatory follicles, Fertil Steril 47:597, 1987.

43. **Elissa MK, Sawers RS, Docker MF, Lynch SeS, Newton JR,** Characteristics and incidence of dysfunctional ovulation patterns detected by ultrasound, Fertil Steril 47:603, 1987.

44. **Hamilton C, Wetzels L, Evens J, Hoogland H, Mvijtjens A, DeHaan J,** Follicle growth curves and hormonal patterns in patients with the luteinized unruptured follicle syndrome, Fertil Steril 43:541, 1985.

45. **Derom C, Derom R, Vlietink R, Van Den Berghe H, Thiery M,** Increased monozygotic twinning rate after ovulation induction, Lancet i:1236, 1987.

46. **Bohrer M, Kemmann E,** Risk factors for spontaneous abortion in menotropin-treated women, Fertil Steril 48:571, 1987.

47. **Evans MI, Fletcher JC, Zador IE, Newton BW, Quigg MH, Struyk CD,** Selective first-trimester termination in octuplet and quadruplet pregnancies: clinical and ethical issues, Obstet Gynecol 71:289, 1988.

48. **Berkowitz RL, Lynch L, Chitkara U, Wilkins IA, Mehalek KE, Alvarez E,** Selective reduction of multifetal pregnancies in the first trimester, New Eng J Med 318:1043, 1988.

49. **Ben-Rafael Z, Mashiach S, Oelsner G, Farine D, Lunenfeld B, Serr DM,** Spontaneous pregnancy and its outcome after human menopausal gonadotropin/human chorionic gonadotropin-induced pregnancy, Fertil Steril 36:560, 1981.

50. **March CM, Tredway DR, Mishell DR Jr,** Effect of clomiphene citrate upon amount and duration of human menopausal gonadotropin therapy, Am J Obstet Gynecol 125:699, 1976.

51. **Shaw RW, Ndukwe G, Imoedemhe DAG, Bernard A, Burford G, Bentick B,** Endocrine changes following pituitary desensitization with LHRH-agonist and administration of purified FSH to induce follicular maturation, Brit J Obstet Gynaecol 94:682, 1987.

52. **Weise HC, Fiedler K, Kato K,** Buserelin suppression of endogenous gonadotropin secretion in infertile women with ovarian feedback disorders given human menopausal/human chorionic gonadotropin treatment, Fertil Steril 49:399, 1988.

53. **Dodson WC, Hughes CL, Whitesides DB, Haney AF,** The effect of leuprolide acetate on ovulation induction with human menopausal gonadotropins in polycystic ovary syndrome, J Clin Endocrinol Metab 65:95, 1987.

54. **Engel T, Jewelewicz R, Dyrenfurth I, Speroff L, Vande Wiele RL,** Ovarian hyperstimulation syndrome: Report of a case with notes on pathogenesis and treatment, Am J Obstet Gynecol 112:1052, 1972.

55. **Haning RV Jr, Strawn EY, Nolten WE,** Pathophysiology of the ovarian hyperstimulation syndrome, Obstet Gynecol 66:220, 1985.

56. **Zosmer A, Katz Z, Lancet M, Konichezky S, Schwartz-Shoham Z,** Adult respiratory distress syndrome complicating ovarian hyperstimulation syndrome, Fertil Steril 47:524, 1987.

57. **Kirshon B, Doody MC, Cotton DB, Gibbons W,** Management of ovarian hyperstimulation syndrome with chlorpheniramine maleate, mannitol, and invasive hemodynamic monitoring, Obstet Gynecol 71:485, 1988.

58. **Claman P, Seibel MM,** Purified human follicle-stimulating hormone for ovulation induction: A critical review, Seminars Reprod Endocrinol 4:277, 1986.

59. **Wong PC, Asch RH,** Induction of follicular development with luteinizing hormone-releasing hormone, Seminars Reprod Endocrinol 5:399, 1987.

60. **Greenblatt E, Casper RF,** Endocrine changes after laparoscopic ovarian cautery in polycystic ovarian syndrome, Am J Obstet Gynecol 156:279, 1987.

609

21   In Vitro Fertilization

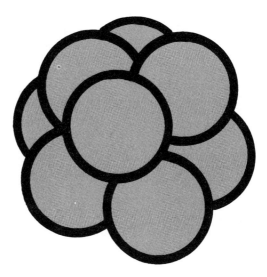

It has been over a decade since the birth of the first child conceived by in vitro fertilization (IVF). During the intervening years the number of IVF programs has increased to over 150 in the United States alone, technology has evolved, the success rate has improved, and the number of indications for IVF has increased. Furthermore, procedures that utilize some, but not all, of the methodology of IVF have become a part of clinical practice.

The momentous work of Edwards and Steptoe was developed over more than 10 years. Success was achieved by utilizing a nonstimulated cycle with timing of oocyte retrieval based on measurements of luteinizing hormone (LH) at 3-hour intervals. The very low success rate associated with that approach led to the use of clomiphene and human menopausal gonadotropins (Pergonal) to stimulate the development of multiple ovarian follicles. For convenience, injections of human chorionic gonadotropin (HCG), whose biologic activity mimics that of LH, were utilized to allow more certain timing of oocyte retrieval. This combination of controlled hyperstimulation of the ovary and substitution of exogenous HCG for the endogenous LH surge is now utilized by most IVF programs, and the rising success rate since the initial clinical experience can be attributed, in part, to multiple egg recoveries mediated by the various hyperstimulation protocols.

Numerous volumes have been published which extensively cover all aspects of IVF, and it is not our purpose to duplicate that effort. Rather, this chapter will focus on the evolving techniques and will review briefly the place of IVF in the treatment of nontubal disease.

Patient Selection	Initial experience involved women with tubal disease, but early in the 1980s, the treatment was extended to individuals with male factor infertility, unexplained infertility, endometriosis, and immunologic causes for infertility.(1) In addition, successful pregnancies have been reported following the transfer of embryos that developed from IVF, to women with premature ovarian failure.(2) Women with severe pelvic adhesive disease who were denied IVF in the past because their ovaries could not be visualized by laparoscopy now can be treated by ultrasonically-guided oocyte retrieval.
Stimulation Protocols	Basic stimulation protocols have utilized clomiphene alone, combinations of Pergonal and clomiphene, or Pergonal alone. The least successful have been those that used clomiphene alone. Clomiphene and Pergonal have been combined in endless variations and dosages, but basically the drugs are given at the same time or in sequence with clomiphene followed by Pergonal. Use of both medications for IVF has been popular in Europe and Australia, whereas the use of Pergonal only, pioneered by the Joneses' group in Norfolk, Virginia, has been more popular in the United States.(3) Concern has been voiced concerning a possible deleterious effect of clomiphene on oocyte maturation, and there is evidence that clomiphene can disrupt mesenchymal organization in human fetal female tract tissue transplanted and maintained in athymic nude mice.(4,5) This has fueled speculation that clomiphene may limit the success of IVF and that Pergonal only protocols may yield superior results. At this date, the evidence against clomiphene is not strong, but there is no denying that the trend in the United States has been toward the Pergonal only protocols.

The majority of Pergonal protocols use either 2 or 3 ampules (150-225 IU) of the drug daily for 5 days, starting on day 3 of the cycle with a further 1 to 3 days of Pergonal at variable doses. Excellent results can be achieved with either the 2 or 3 ampule dose of Pergonal although some believe that greater success can be obtained with the 2 ampule regimen.(6) Attempts to substitute pure follicle-stimulating hormone (FSH) for Pergonal for all or a portion of a cycle provide, at best, only a marginal advantage over Pergonal.

The introduction of gonadotropin releasing hormone (GnRH) agonist prior to and concomitant with Pergonal stimulation has provided one anticipated and one unexpected advantage.(7) It eliminates the possibility of premature LH surges and, in addition, it has provided some increase in the success rate of IVF. The GnRH agonist, given either by subcutaneous injection or by nasal spray, can, in prescribed doses, cause a down regulation of the pituitary instead of the normal stimulatory effect. FSH and LH secretion are decreased and ovarian follicle activity follows suit. The waves of oocytes that begin growth are inhibited. Therefore, when stimulation with Pergonal is initiated, the ovary is in a resting state. It is uncertain why this may confer an advantage during IVF. In addition to preventing premature LH surges and premature luteinization (and progesterone production), it may decrease LH stimulation of ovarian androgen production (which can interfere with follicular development).

Monitoring	Most programs use both measurements of serum estradiol and ultrasound imaging of ovarian follicles to monitor the ovarian response

to stimulation. The goal of stimulation is to achieve the growth of a lead follicle to at least 16-17 mm diameter, and at least 2 or 3 other follicles with diameters of 14 mm or greater, combined with estradiol levels of approximately 300 pg/ml per large (14 mm or greater) follicle. Once this rate of stimulation is achieved a single injection of 5,000 or 10,000 IU of HCG is given to induce final follicular maturation. The time interval between the last Pergonal injection and the HCG is considered to be critical, but unfortunately there is disagreement on how long an interval is best. The values given for follicle size and estradiol levels on the day of decision for HCG injection are only rough guidelines, because ultrasound measurements may differ among observers and machines. In addition, each program must establish, based on its own experience, its criteria for determining the adequacy of follicle size. Moreover, estradiol assays will differ from one laboratory to another, and comparisons therefore are difficult. Estradiol levels per follicle can vary widely and still be compatible with successful IVF. Some programs measure the estrogen level on the day following HCG, and if there is a marked drop in the value at that time, retrieval is canceled because that pattern is associated with a poor chance for pregnancy.

The introduction of vaginal ultrasound imaging, which eliminates the need for a full bladder, has improved greatly the visualization of ovarian follicles and allowed more accurate measurements. It also has enhanced patient comfort compared to abdominal ultrasound which requires a full bladder.

Oocyte Retrieval

Just prior to HCG injection, a serum LH can be drawn and compared to values earlier in the cycle. This will enable the physician to identify those women who have initiated a premature LH surge (LH value 2.5 times baseline). While oocytes often can be harvested in these women, the pregnancy rates are much lower than if an LH surge has not occurred. Without frequent (every 3 hour) sampling of LH, the onset of the surge cannot be identified with some precision, and this timing is critical for obtaining a reasonable level of success. LH sampling is not required in women who are treated with GnRH agonists.

Oocyte retrieval is performed approximately 35 hours after the HCG injection, which places the retrieval just prior to the time of ovulation. The HCG injection allows for confidence in this precise timing. Just as diagnostic vaginal ultrasound imaging has replaced abdominal ultrasound, so has ultrasonically-guided retrieval replaced, to a large degree, laparoscopic oocyte retrieval. Both transabdominal-transvesical ultrasound-guided retrieval and transvaginal retrieval were pioneered in Europe, and they share the advantage of not requiring the general anesthesia needed for most laparoscopic oocyte retrievals.(8,9) Because of the ease of imaging and significantly less pain, the transvaginal approach is the preferred method. Intravenous medication in the form of fentanyl and midazolam can be used. Because of the risk of respiratory depression, the slow administration of small doses and monitoring of the patient with a pulse oximeter are wise precautions. A number 16 or number 17 needle is placed down a sterile needle guide that is attached to the upper side of the vaginal ultrasound transducer. A line on the monitor screen indicates the path the needle will traverse once it enters the abdominal cavity and the ovary. The ultrasound transducer is

613

manipulated to position a follicle along this pathway. Usually only one puncture of each ovary is needed to allow sequential aspiration of all the follicles that are 12 mm or larger. Accessibility of the ovaries is a problem in only a few patients. Most women will experience only slight to moderate pain during the procedure, although an occasional woman will have a high level of pain despite analgesia. Rare complications of the procedure are intraabdominal bleeding or introduction of infection into the ovary and pelvis. Recovery from transvaginal follicle aspiration is usually rapid without the side effects associated with general anesthesia.

Oocyte Culture

Skill is required to identify the oocytes under either a dissecting or an invert microscope. Often these can be seen easily in their cumulus masses but upon occasion they are obscured by cells and by blood. Critical is the minimizing of exposure of the oocytes to ambient temperature and room air. Transfer of oocytes immediately following retrieval into a microscope-equipped isolette with controlled temperature and an atmosphere of 5% CO_2 in air may be beneficial. (10)

One of the major breakthroughs in IVF was the discovery that sperm should not be added to the eggs immediately after retrieval, and that oocytes have a higher chance for fertilization if insemination follows retrieval by 4 to 6 hours.(11) Furthermore, if the oocytes are immature, much longer (12 to 30 hours) periods of incubation prior to insemination lead to better rates of fertilization. Maturity of the oocyte is determined by the morphology of the surrounding cumulus-corona cell complex or by the presence or absence of the germinal vesicle and the first polar body.(12)

Sperm are prepared by washing, centrifugation, overlaying the sperm pellet with media and retrieval of the sperm that swim up into the media. Isolation of the most motile sperm also can be accomplished by separating the specimen on columns of liquid albumin or on Percoll gradients.

A variety of media has been used for embryo culture, with Ham's F10 the most popular in the United States. Work with mouse embryos revealed that other media were more successful than Ham's F10 in supporting development from the 2 cell to the blastocyst stage.(13) Despite this finding, similar results are obtained in human IVF with Ham's F10 and a number of other media.

The media for IVF are supplemented with a protein source, most commonly maternal serum or fetal cord serum. Less frequently, albumin is used. A higher pregnancy rate was achieved in Australia when fetal cord serum was the supplement compared to cases where maternal serum was used.(14) The fetal cord sera should be screened by testing their ability to support development of preimplantation mouse embryos as well as their freedom from HIV and hepatitis viruses. The complexity of the serum supplements, whether they are fetal or maternal, raises concern that they may contain factors that are deleterious to embryos. Protein-free media would obviate this problem, and pregnancies have been achieved with protein-free media.(15) Despite this success, most programs continue to use protein-supplemented Ham's F10.

Fertilization

Approximately 50,000-100,000 sperm are added to each dish containing an oocyte. The day after insemination, cumulus cells that remain attached to the zona pellucida are dislodged and the egg is examined for evidence of fertilization (the presence of 2 pronuclei).

Transfer

Embryos have been transferred successfully at any stage from the pronuclear to the blastocyst, although most commonly, they are transferred when development is between the 4 and 10 cell stage, approximately 48-80 hours after retrieval. Transfer of more than one embryo increases the chances for pregnancy, but in general no more than 4 or 5 embryos are transferred. Supplementary embryos can be cryopreserved and transferred in later cycles if the initial cycle is unsuccessful. The multiple pregnancy rate with transfers of more than one embryo is approximately 20%.

There does not seem to be any advantage of placing the patient in knee-chest compared to lithotomy position for transfer. Ancillary medications given around the time of transfer, such as prostaglandin inhibitors, tranquilizers, or antibiotics are of uncertain value. It is common practice to supplement the luteal phase with progesterone, although limited studies indicate that this may not be necessary.(16) Progesterone vaginal suppositories, 25 mg b.i.d., or progesterone in oil 12.5 to 25 mg IM once daily, are given for 12 days starting on the day of transfer. An alternative therapy is the use of HCG, 1500 IU every 3 or 4 days for 3 doses. The value of luteal phase supplementation may be in question, but there is no doubt that it provides some psychologic support for both patient and physician. If the woman is not receiving HCG, an initial quantitative HCG measurement can be obtained 9 days after transfer. If the test is positive, a follow-up test is obtained 3 days later. This will establish the trend of the HCG and provide some prognostic information.

Results

A certain skepticism has arisen concerning the pregnancy rates reported by IVF programs. Competition for patients is seen as the motivation for some of the exaggerations and half-truths contained in public statements and letters to referring physicians.(17) An associated problem is determining what constitutes a pregnancy.(18) A slight, unsustained rise in the HCG is properly termed a "chemical pregnancy" and it should not be counted as a success. To avoid confusion, only those pregnancies that contain identifiable products of conception or a fetus with a heart beat on ultrasound examination should be considered a pregnancy for reporting purposes. Hopefully, as the field matures, the most important statistic, which is the number of live births, will be the one used for comparison. Another problem relating to comparison of IVF statistics is the denominator, with some programs using number of cycles initiated, others number of patients who have gone to retrieval, and still others, and most commonly, number of patients who have gone to embryo transfer.

Meldrum et al, with meticulous attention to detail, have achieved pregnancy rates per transfer of more than 30%, and they have outlined the elements of a successful program.(19) Most of the better programs will have clinical pregnancy rates per transfer around 20%. Surprisingly, 5% of pregnancies achieved through IVF are ectopic. On the other hand, it is not surprising that 25% of clinical pregnancies result in spontaneous abortions because that is close to the expected rate.

A major factor influencing IVF results is the gross inefficiency of human reproduction in vivo. A number of studies have attested to the low fecundability of humans. (18) Only 25-30% of normal women who attempt pregnancy in a given cycle are successful. There is a large loss of embryos prior to or around the time of implantation in vivo, and thus, many women have pregnancy losses without realizing that they have been pregnant because the menstrual period comes at the normal time. It can be concluded that many sperm and many oocytes, even from individuals who are fertile, do not have the ability to contribute to a normal pregnancy. This affects the success of both in vivo and in vitro fertilization.

Whereas the chance for success in successive IVF cycles does not change appreciably, women who commit themselves to 3 to 6 cycles of IVF will have a good chance of achieving pregnancy. The cumulative pregnancy rates of the Norfolk Group for 1 to 6 cycles of treatment were: 13.5%, 25.3%, 38.5%, 47%, 49.3%, and 57.8%.(20) The figures exclude cases of male infertility. Most individuals will find the emotional, physical, and financial consequences of going beyond 3 to 6 cycles too difficult.

IVF for Male Factor

IVF has become an accepted treatment for male factor infertility when it does not respond to other therapies. However, fertilization is approximately one-half that obtained in patients with tubal disease. If fertilization is achieved, the chances for pregnancy following embryo transfer are equal to those obtained in women with tubal disease. A major decrease in fertilization with IVF has been observed only if the number of motile sperm dropped below 6 million/ml or there were less than 40% normal forms in the specimen. (21) Others report that counts below 10 million/ml or motilities below 30% reduce appreciably the chances for fertilization.(22) The group from Norfolk used the following criteria for accepting male infertility patients into their IVF program:(23)

1. Greater or equal to 1.5 million rapidly motile sperm in the swimup fraction.

2. Sperm penetration assay greater than 10%.

3. Sperm penetration assay greater than or equal to 50% of control.

4. Normal sperm acrosin level.

Others have not found the sperm penetration assay to be of help in choosing which males with compromised semen specimens are good candidates for IVF.(24) In addition, the usefulness of the acrosin assay is unproven.

IVF for Endometriosis

Individuals with mild to moderate endometriosis do well in IVF programs, although one report suggested that this is true only if the endometriosis has been treated.(25) The results with severe endometriosis, on the other hand, are not good. There may be a problem with decreased oocyte recovery because of adhesions. Beyond this, there also appears to be decreased numbers of follicles in women with severe endometriosis and even when comparable numbers of embryos are transferred, the pregnancy rate is decreased. Only a 2% pregnancy rate was achieved in a group with the most severe endometriosis.(26)

Other Indications

The experience using IVF for immunologic infertility is limited. If the problem lies with the male then semen is obtained by masturbation into media to dilute out the antigens carried by the seminal plasma. If sperm antibodies are in the woman's serum, it should not be used to culture the eggs and the sperm. With unexplained infertility the results may be as good as those obtained in cases of tubal disease.

Other Techniques

In addition to IVF, individuals with unexplained infertility have been offered a number of tactics to overcome hypothesized problems with gamete transport. For gamete intrafallopian transfer (GIFT), Asch and co-workers use minilaparotomy or laparoscopy to aspirate oocytes following hyperstimulation of the ovary.(27) After the oocytes are identified in the laboratory they are taken up into a transfer catheter which also contains 100,000 sperm separated by the swim-up technique. The transfer catheters are guided into the distal 1.5 to 2 cm of a fallopian tube and the contents gently discharged. Usually 2 oocytes are placed in each tube. Extra eggs obtained by aspiration can be utilized for IVF. Success with GIFT is variable but many centers report pregnancy rates around 30%. Ectopic pregnancy occurs from 3 to 8 percent of the time. In a variation of GIFT, oocytes are obtained by vaginal aspiration, fertilized in vitro, and then 1 day later placed in the fallopian tubes by the GIFT technique.

Other recent attempts to overcome problems of gamete transport include injections of washed sperm into the peritoneal cavity at the time of ovulation, and cannulation of the fallopian tube via the cervix, using ultrasound guidance, as a conduit for injecting sperm (or embryos) directly into the tube. A fertilized human ovum can be removed by uterine lavage from a donor and placed transcervically in the uterus of an infertile recipient.(28)

Not all of these newer methods have been subjected to close scrutiny and appropriate studies. They have, however, attracted wide attention and an assessment of their value may be forthcoming.

Conclusion

The new reproductive techniques and the technology associated with in vitro fertilization have been presented in a somewhat mechanistic way in this chapter. This should not obscure the fact that this is an emotionally trying experience for almost everyone undertaking therapy. Psychological stresses are acute and anxiety is accentuated with each step of the process despite the fact that couples enter treatment knowing that there is a limited chance for success. However, they invariably harbor some optimism over their chances, and thus, failures at every stage are exceptionally difficult for both patients and physicians. Support groups such as those organized by Resolve are helpful for almost every couple going through an IVF or associated program.

References

1. **Mahadevan MM, Trounson AO, Leeton JF,** The relationship of tubal blockage, infertility of unknown cause, suspected male infertility, and endometriosis to success of in vitro fertilization and embryo transfer, Fertil Steril 40:755, 1983.

2. **Chan CLK, Cameron IT, Findlay JK, Healy D, Leeton JF, Lutjen PJ, Renous PM, Rogers PA, Trounson AO, Wood EC,** Oocyte donation and in vitro fertilization for hypergonadotropic hypogonadism: Clinical state of the art, Obstet Gynecol Survey 42:350, 1987.

3. **Jones HW Jr, Jones GS, Andrews MC, Acosta A, Bundren C, Garcia J, Sandow B, Veeck L, Wilkes C, Witmyer J, Wortham JE, Wright G,** The program for in vitro fertilization at Norfolk, Fertil Steril 38:14, 1982.

4. **Laufer N, Pratt BM, DeCherney AH, Naftolin F, Merino M, Markert CL,** The in vivo and in vitro effects of clomiphene citrate on ovulation, fertilization, and development of cultured mouse oocytes, Am J Obstet Gynecol 147:636, 1983.

5. **Cunha GR, Taguchi O, Namikawa R, Nishizuka Y, Robboy SJ,** Teratogenic effects of clomiphene, tamoxifen, and diethylstilbestrol on the developing human female genital tract, Human Path 18:1132, 1987.

6. **Ben-Rafael Z, Benadiva CA, Ausmanas M, Barber B, Blasco L, Flickinger GL, Mastroianni L Jr,** Dose of human menopausal gonadotropin influences the outcome of an in vitro fertilization program, Fertil Steril 48:964, 1987.

7. **Neveu S, Hedon B, Bringer J, Chinchole JM, Arnal F, Humeau C, Cristol P, Viala JL,** Ovarian stimulation by a combination of a gonadotropin-releasing hormone agonist and gonadotropins for in vitro fertilization, Fertil Steril 47:639, 1987.

8. **Lenz S,** Ultrasonic-guided follicle puncture under local anesthesia, J In Vitro Fert Embryo Transfer 1:239, 1984.

9. **Dellenbach P, Nisand I, Moreau L, Feger B, Plumere C, Gerlinger P,** Transvaginal sonographically controlled follicle puncture for oocyte retrieval, Fertil Steril 44:656, 1985.

10. **Gerrity M, Shapiro S,** The use of a mobile laboratory cart in a successful university-based human in vitro fertilization program, Fertil Steril 43:481, 1985.

11. **Trounson AO, Mohr LR, Wood C, Leeton JF,** Effect of delayed insemination on in vitro fertilization, culture and transfer of human embryos, J Reprod Fertil 64:285, 1982.

12. **Veeck L,** Extracorporeal maturation: Norfolk, 1984, Ann NY Acad Sci 442:357, 1985.

13. **Dandekar PV, Glass RH,** Development of mouse embryos in vitro is affected by strain and culture medium, Gamete Res 17:279, 1987.

14. **Leung PCS, Gronow MJ, Kellow GN, Lopata A, Speirs AL, McBain JC, duPlessis YP, Johnston I,** Serum supplement in human in vitro fertilization and embryo development, Fertil Steril 41:36, 1984.

15. **Caro CM, Trounson A,** Successful fertilization, embryo development, and pregnancy in human in vitro fertilization (IVF) using a chemically defined culture medium containing no protein, J In Vitro Fertil Embryo Transfer 3:215, 1986.

16. **Leeton J, Trounson A, Jessup D,** Support of the luteal phase in in vitro fertilization programs: Results of a controlled trial with intramuscular Proluton, J In Vitro Fertil Embryo Transfer 2:166, 1985.

17. **Soules MR,** The in vitro fertilization pregnancy rate: Let's be honest with one another, Fertil Steril 43:511, 1985.

18. **Jones HW Jr, Acosta AA, Andrews MC, Garcia JE, Jones GS, Mantzavinos T, McDowell J, Sandow BA, Veeck L, Whibley TW, Wilkes CA, Wright GL Jr,** What is a pregnancy? A question for programs of in vitro fertilization, Fertil Steril 40:728, 1983.

19. **Meldrum DR, Chetkowski R, Steingold KA, deZiegler D, Cedars MI, Hamilton M,** Evolution of a highly successful in vitro fertilization-embryo transfer program, Fertil Steril 48:86, 1987.

20. **Guzick DS, Wilkes C, Jones HW Jr,** Cumulative pregnancy rates for in vitro fertilization, Fertil Steril 46:663, 1986.

21. **Yovich JL, Stanger JD,** The limitations of in vitro fertilization in males with severe oligospermia and abnormal sperm morphology, J In Vitro Fertil Embyro Transfer 1:172, 1984.

22. **Battin DA, Vargyas J, Sato F, Brown J, Marrs RA,** In vitro fertilization rates of male factor patients, Fertil Steril 41:42S, 1984.

23. **Acosta AA, Chillik CF, Brugo S, Ackerman S, Swanson RJ, Pleban P, Yuan J, Haque D,** In vitro fertilization and the male factor, Urology 28:1, 1986.

24. **Margalioth EJ, Navot D, Laufer N, Lewin A, Rabinowitz R, Schenker JG,** Correlation between the zona-free hamster egg sperm penetration assay and human in vitro fertilization, Fertil Steril 45:665, 1986.

25. **Wardle PG, Foster PA, Mitchell JD, McLaughlin EA, Sykes JAC, Corrigan E, Hull MGR, Ray BD, McDermott A,** Endometriosis and IVF: Effects of prior therapy, Lancet i:276, 1986.

26. **Mastson PL, Yovich JL,** The treatment of infertility associated with endometriosis by in vitro fertilization, Fertil Steril 46:432, 1986.

27. **Asch RH, Balmaceda JP, Ellsworth LR, Wong PC,** Preliminary experiences with gamete intrafallopian transfer (GIFT), Fertil Steril 45:366, 1986.

28. **Bustillo M, Buster J, Cohen S, Thorneycroft IH, Simon JA, Boyers SP, Marshall JR, Seed RW, Louw JA, Seed RG,** Nonsurgical ovum transfer as a treatment in infertile women, JAMA 251:1171, 1984.

22   Clinical Assays

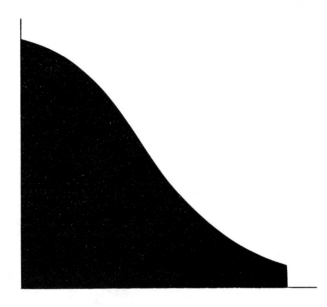

The purpose of this chapter is to review the laboratory assays which are commonly used in clinical gynecologic endocrinology. With this information, the clinician will have confidence in the selection of specific laboratory tests, and will be secure in the personal interpretation of the data.

Classically, hormones were measured in blood by bioassays, i.e. dose-response measurements based upon organ responses in animals. Some of the principles fundamental to endocrinology were established by such methods. However, bioassay methods, although adequate for qualitative statements, are relatively imprecise, nonspecific, time-consuming, expensive, and require too large an amount of the biologic sample in order to meet the quantitative requirements of modern research and clinical practice. Assays with far greater sensitivity and precision have been developed. These new methods depend upon the use of radioactive tracers and the delicate measurement of radioactivity. The most recent and popular techniques are the methods of saturation analysis.

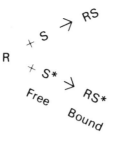

Saturation Analysis (Radioimmunoassay, Competitive Protein Binding)

Basic Principles

The methods of saturation analysis yield greater simplicity, sensitivity, and precision. Reactions in saturation analysis follow the law of mass action. A protein or antibody (R) is mixed with a substance (S) for which it has specific binding sites, forming a complex, RS. The radioactive form of the substance (S*) also forms a complex, RS*. Since the number of binding sites on the protein or antibody is limited, the labeled and unlabeled compound, S and S*, will compete for binding sites in proportion to their concentrations. Since the binding reagent, R (protein or antibody), is kept constant, increasing the unlabeled compound, S, will displace more and more labeled tracer, S*. Plotting the change in either bound or unbound (free) tracer, S*, against the amount of unlabeled compound, S, added will produce a standard curve. The amount of radioactivity bound or free in the presence of an unknown level of compound will reveal the concentration of the compound when compared to the standard curve. The requirements for saturation analysis are, therefore, either a suitable binding protein, or an antibody, and a labeled pure form of the compound to be measured.

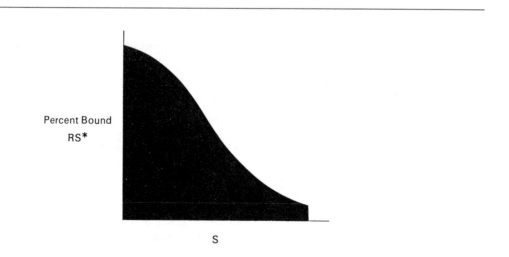

Methodology

A purified, labeled amount of the substance to be measured is added to the biologic sample (e.g. plasma) to be assayed. The radioactive tracer equilibrates with the unlabeled and unknown amount of compound in the sample. The sample is now mixed with an appropriate solvent to extract the desired compound and tracer. The extraction process usually removes several compounds which may interfere with the assay, and separation (purification) of the desired substance is frequently necessary. A chromatographic separation utilizing thin layer chromatography or column chromatography is used for most steroid assays.

The next step is to mix the extracted compound with a specific reagent. In the case of radioimmunoassay, this reagent is an antiserum, and in the case of competitive protein binding, this reagent is a protein which has affinity for the compound to be measured. The combination of the compound with this reagent (antiserum or specific protein) is called binding. Since the compound is in equilibrium with a small amount of labeled compound, the labeled compound will bind to the reagent in proportion to the amount of unlabeled compound present. This is the fundamental principle: the distribution of bound and unbound radioactivity is dependent upon the total concentration of the compound in the system. Measurement of the radioactivity, therefore, can be utilized to calculate the unknown amount of compound in the system.

Since steroid compounds are not antigenic, the production of a specific antiserum depends upon the linkage of a steroid to a large protein molecule. The protein molecule is antigenic in itself, but when combined with a steroid, the steroid-protein complex (hapten) stimulates a variety of antibodies, some of which recognize and are specific for the steroid. Thus, when the steroid-protein complex is injected into an animal the antiserum formed may be utilized as a reagent (R) for measurement of the steroid (S) in the technique of saturation analysis.

For example, a testosterone-bovine albumin conjugate can be formed by covalently linking testosterone to albumin at the 3 position via an oxime linkage to *o*-carboxymethyl hydroxylamine.

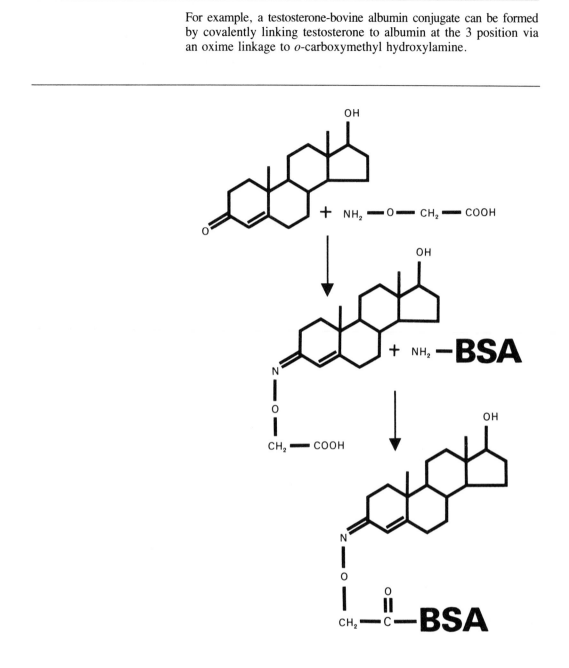

The cross-reactions to the antiserum produced with the above conjugate vary, and this antiserum may be used to measure testosterone and dihydrotestosterone, but the testosterone and dihydrotestosterone must be separate by some chromatographic means.

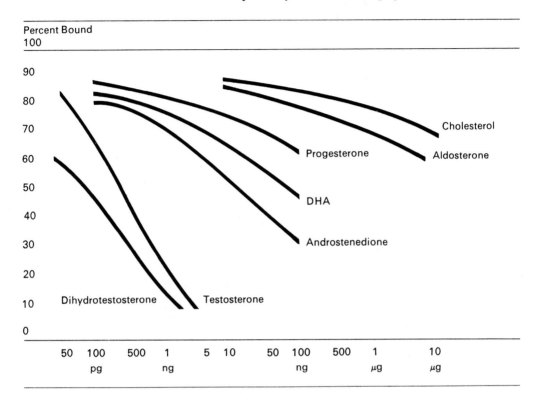

Monoclonal Antibodies. Antibodies are produced by the B lymphocytes present in the bone marrow, spleen, lymph nodes, and other lymphoid glands. Monoclonal antibodies are homogeneous, eliminating the heterogeneity and variability associated with antiserum obtained by the regular immunization process. An animal is first immunized against an antigen (anti-X in the illustration). The antibody can be derived from specific cells in the spleen or elsewhere, or from the B lymphocytes. Production of monoclonal antibodies depends upon the development of a hybridoma cell line. Usually a tumor cell is fused with the cell from the animal, for example, a combination of a myeloma and lymphocytes. The tumor cell can be maintained in culture essentially forever. The medium is manipulated so that only the fused hybridoma cells grow. For example in the illustration, the tumor B lymphocytes have a defective secondary pathway for the synthesis of nucleic acids. Therefore only those cells fused to normal lymphocytes will continue to grow in the medium which contains an inhibitor of the main biosynthetic pathway for nucleic acids. The normal lymphocytes die after only a few days in culture.

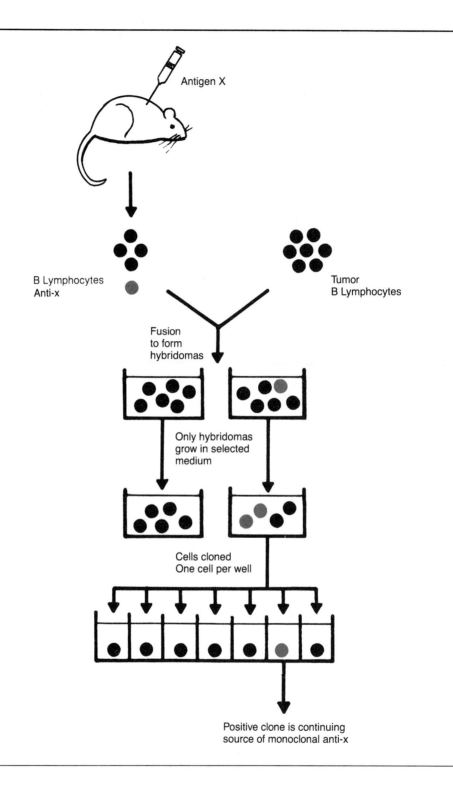

Antigen X

B Lymphocytes
Anti-x

Tumor
B Lymphocytes

Fusion
to form
hybridomas

Only hybridomas
grow in selected
medium

Cells cloned
One cell per well

Positive clone is continuing
source of monoclonal anti-x

The supernatant in each well is tested for the presence of the antibody. Ultimately a well will contain only a single cell line producing homogeneous, identical, monoclonal antibodies.

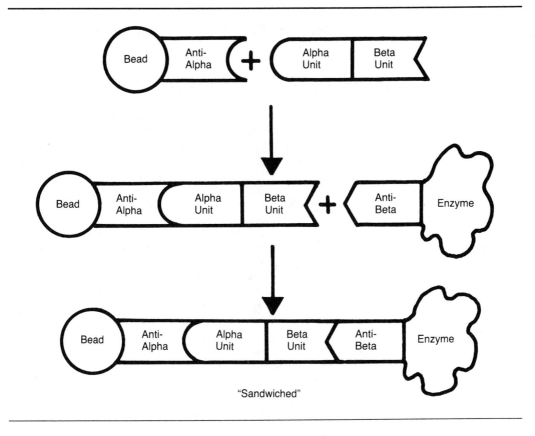

"Sandwiched"

The ELISA technique. ELISA stands for enzyme-linked immunosorbent assay, also known as the sandwich technique. This method does not require a radioactive tracer. A monoclonal antibody is coupled to an enzyme, e.g. horseradish peroxidase, which provides a color endpoint which can be measured by spectrophotometry. For the measurement of the glycopeptides (HCG, LH, TSH), this technique uses two monoclonal antibodies, one against the alpha subunit and coupled to a bead or a plastic tube, and the other antibody against the beta subunit is coupled to the enzyme. The antibody to the alpha subunit binds the intact glycoprotein molecule; the beta subunit antibody and the enzyme then sandwich the intact molecule by binding to the exposed beta subunit. The result is obtained by comparing the enzyme reading on the spectrophotometer to a standard curve. Attaching antibodies to other active substances (e.g. a chemiluminescent substance) can be expected to yield new and more economical methods.

Problems. These methods are not without problems. Utmost precision and care in technique are necessary. An unknown variation in technique may completely disrupt an assay. The periodic appearance of the well-known laboratory ''gremlin'' may be traced to a simple thing like the water supply or a change in glassware-washing routine. The accuracy of the results depends upon:

1. Specificity of the antibody or protein for the hormone to be measured.

2. Purity and specificity of the radiolabeled tracer.

627

3. Purity and availability of the standard reference hormone.

4. Sensitivity and precision of the assay.

5. Intra-assay and inter-assay experimental error.

If cross-reaction of the binding protein exists for other hormones, these cross-reacting substances must be removed. The radiolabeled tracer must have a high specific radioactivity, and purity is essential to ensure that it behaves identically as the substance being measured. Experimental error between assays as well as within an assay is an important determinant of assay reliability. A coefficient of variation of less than 15% for each is considered acceptable.

Measurement of Pituitary Gonadotropins

In the case of polypeptide hormones (gonadotropins), radioimmunoassay techniques are based upon the use of antibodies prepared by injecting the protein hormone of one species into another. The protein hormones vary in their physicochemical characteristics and amino acid composition from species to species, and, therefore, antibodies for use in radioimmunoassay are formed when protein hormones are administered cross-species. A highly specific antiserum can be produced to be utilized as the binding reagent. This specificity may make chromatographic separation that ordinarily follows extraction unnecessary.

Normal serum levels for pituitary gonadotropins during the normal menstrual cycle are illustrated:

For clinical purposes, the following ranges are useful:

Clinical State	Serum FSH	Serum LH
Normal adult female	5–20 mIU/ml, with the ovulatory midcycle peak about 2 times the base level	5–20 mIU/ml with the ovulatory midcycle peak about 3 times the base level
Hypogonadotropic state: Prepubertal, hypothalamic and pituitary dysfunction.	Less than 5 mIU/ml	Less than 5 mIU/ml
Hypergonadotropic state: Postmenopausal, castrate and ovarian failure	Greater than 40 mIU/ml	Greater than 40 mIU/ml

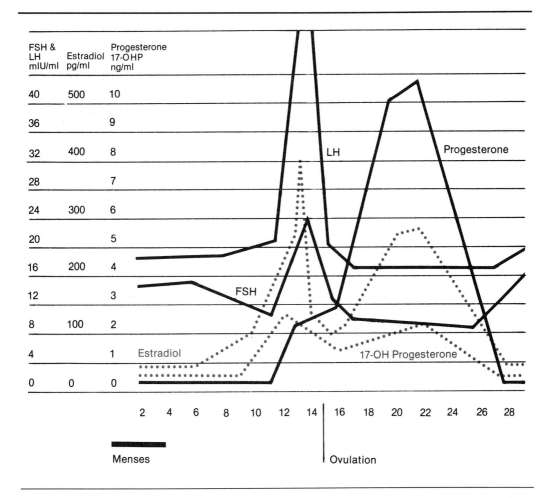

FSH & LH mIU/ml	Estradiol pg/ml	Progesterone 17-OHP ng/ml
40	500	10
36		9
32	400	8
28		7
24	300	6
20		5
16	200	4
12		3
8	100	2
4		1
0	0	0

LH

Progesterone

FSH

Estradiol

17-OH Progesterone

2 4 6 8 10 12 14 16 18 20 22 24 26 28

Menses

Ovulation

Measurement of Blood Steroids

The normal levels for total plasma estrogens or estradiol, and plasma progesterone during the normal menstrual cycle have been illustrated. Variation is seen from individual to individual, however, and the following ranges in gonadal steroids are normally reported:

	Estradiol	*Progesterone*	*Testosterone*
Follicular phase	25–75 pg/ml	Less than 1 ng/ml	20–80 ng/dl
Midcycle peak	200–600 pg/ml		20–80 ng/dl
Luteal phase	100–300 pg/ml	5–20 ng/ml	20–80 ng/dl
Pregnancy: 1st trimester	1–5 ng/ml	20–30 ng/ml	
Pregnancy: 2nd trimester	5–15 ng/ml	50–100 ng/ml	
Pregnancy: 3rd trimester	10–40 ng/ml	100–400 ng/ml	
Postmenopause	5–25 pg/ml	Less than 1 ng/ml	10–40 ng/dl

The radioimmunoassay of 17-hydroxyprogesterone has replaced measurement of the urinary pregnanetriol level for the diagnosis of adrenal enzyme deficiency. Dramatic differences exist between normal individuals and patients with adrenal hyperplasia. Levels from 5 to 2000 times greater than normal have been observed.

17-Hydroxyprogesterone	
Children	3–90 ng/dl
Adult females	
Follicular phase	15–70 ng/dl
Luteal phase	35–290 ng/dl

The radioimmunoassay of dehydroepiandrosterone sulfate (DHAS) has replaced the measurement of urinary 17-ketosteroids for the routine evaluation of adrenal androgen production. A random sample is sufficient, needing no corrections for body weight, creatinine excretion, or random variation. Variations are minimized because of its high circulating concentration and its long half-life. It is a direct measure of adrenal androgen activity correlating clinically with the urinary 17-ketosteroids. As with urinary 17-ketosteroids, aging is associated with a decrease in DHAS, accelerating after menopause and becoming almost undetectable after age 70.

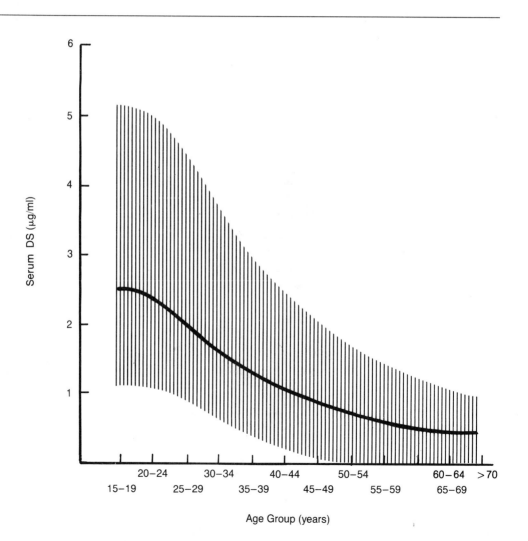

Urinary Steroid Assays	The measurement of estrogen in a 24-hour urine collection can be utilized during administration of human menopausal gonadotropins (Pergonal).	

Total Urinary Estrogen	
Prepubertal	0–5 μg/24 hr
Follicular phase	10–25 μg/24 hr
Midcycle peak	35–100 μg/24 hr
Luteal phase	25–75 μg/24 hr
Postmenopausal	5–15 μg/24 hr

Pregnanediol is the main urinary metabolite of progesterone, although it accounts for only 7-20% of total progesterone production. Measurement of pregnanediol in a 24-hour urine sample has been used in the past to document pregnancy and especially the well-being of an early pregnancy. However, with the advent of the measurement of plasma progesterone, the use of urinary pregnanediol has waned.

Urinary Pregnanediol	
Follicular phase	Less than 1 mg/24 hr
Luteal phase	2–5 mg/24 hr
Pregnancy: 20 weeks	40 mg/24 hr
Pregnancy: 30 weeks	80 mg/24 hr
Pregnancy: 40 weeks	100 mg/24 hr

Pregnanetriol is the urinary metabolite of 17-hydroxyprogesterone, and was used for the diagnosis of adrenal hyperplasia (the adrenogenital syndrome). Very little pregnanetriol is found in the urine of normal adults, but with the increased production of 17-hydroxyprogesterone due to an enzyme deficiency in the adrenal gland (adrenogenital syndrome), increased urinary excretion of pregnanetriol will occur.

Urinary Pregnanetriol	
Children	Less than 0.5 mg/24 hr
Adults	0.2 to 2–4 mg/24 hr, the upper limit varying among laboratories

631

Measurement of Human Chorionic Gonadotropin

Secretion of human chorionic gonadotropin (HCG) by the syncytio-trophoblast cells of the placenta is predominantly into the maternal circulation. The assay of HCG in maternal urine has been the basis of pregnancy tests for many years. Aschheim and Zondek originated the bioassay pregnancy test in immature mice (the A-Z test) in the late 1920's.

The biologic tests for HCG depended upon the response of ovaries or testes in immature animals. This response was due to the gonadotropic properties of HCG and was measured either in terms of increased gonadal weight or hyperemia, or the secondary response in sex organs due to the increased gonadal steroidogenesis induced by the HCG. The expulsion of ova or sperm in amphibia was widely utilized as an end point for HCG. These biologic assays have now been succeeded by immunoassays for HCG in urine and blood.

HCG is similar to LH in its structure and thus antibodies to one cross-react with the other. The sensitivity of most commercial assays in the past had to be limited in order to avoid false positive tests due to cross-reactivity with LH. Modern assays utilizing highly specific monoclonal antibodies against HCG have a greater sensitivity. The greatest sensitivity and specificity is found with the radioimmunoassay for the β subunit of HCG.

β-HCG can be detected in the blood 9-11 days after the LH peak, 7-9 days after ovulation. A concentration of 100 mIU/ml is reached about the date of expected menses. Most radioimmunoassays for the β subunit of HCG have a lower sensitivity of 2-5 mIU/ml.

Peak levels of HCG (approximately 100,000 mIU/ml) occur at 10 weeks of gestation, declining and remaining at approximately 10,000-20,000 mIU/ml by 12-14 weeks. Evaluation of a patient following a spontaneous or therapeutic abortion is occasionally a difficult problem. The urinary pregnancy test will be negative 3 weeks after abortion.

There are two clinical conditions in which blood HCG titers are very helpful, trophoblastic disease and ectopic pregnancies. Following molar pregnancies, in patients without persistent disease, the HCG titer should fall to a nondetectable level by 16 weeks. Patients with trophoblastic disease show an abnormal curve (a titer greater than 500 mIU/ml) frequently by 3 weeks and usually by 6 weeks.

Virtually 100% of patients suspected of an ectopic pregnancy, but not having the condition, will have a negative blood HCG assay. A positive test can also be utilized in diagnosis. The HCG level increases at different rates in normal and ectopic pregnancies. In a normal pregnancy the HCG should approximately double every 2 days. An HCG above 6000 mIU/ml is usually associated with an intrauterine pregnancy. When the HCG titer is below 6000 mIU/ml and abdominal ultrasound examination fails to identify an intrauterine pregnancy, a patient may be managed expectantly if the HCG titer doubles in 2 days. If the titer does not double, laparoscopy is indicated. Laparoscopy is also indicated when the titer is above 6000 mIU/ml and ultrasound shows no evidence of an intrauterine pregnancy.

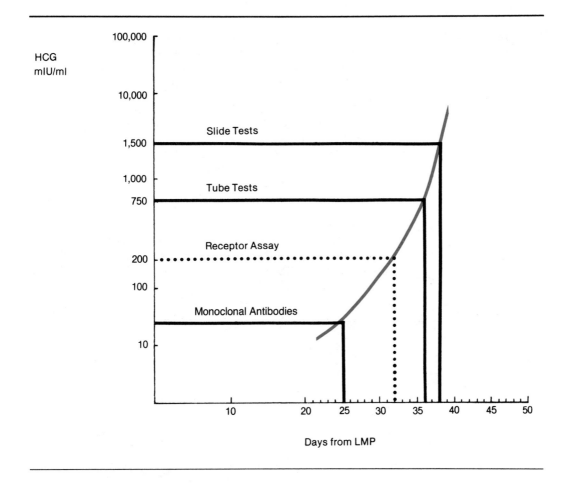

In clinical practice, these guidelines are not always so clear and definitive. The rate of HCG increase changes with advancing gestational age and increasing HCG concentrations. While the HCG level approximately doubles every 2 days below a level of 1200 mIU/ml, from 1200-6000 mIU/ml, it takes nearly 3 days to double, and above 6000 mIU/ml, about 4 days. In addition the zone at which a gestational sac is seen by ultrasound varies for different assays and different reference preparations. One should be sure that the discriminatory zone of 6000 mIU/ml applies to your local assay. Furthermore, vaginal ultrasonography is more sensitive; the discriminatory zone is considerably lower as gestational sacs can be identified with HCG concentrations below 1000 mIU/ml.

Measurement of 17-Ketosteroids 17-Ketogenic Steroids, and 17-Hydroxycorticosteroids

These assays provide essential clinical information, yet misunderstanding of their meaning and limitations is still common. A basic appreciation for the methods and what they measure is necessary for the proper interpretation of these urinary assays.

A 24-hour urine specimen is required to avoid the variations in steroid excretion which occur throughout a day. Refrigeration is essential to avoid degradation of metabolites. It is wise to obtain a urinary creatinine as a check of the validity of the 24-hour collection. Urinary creatinine excretion is a reflection of body muscle mass and remains relatively constant, approximately 1000 mg/24 hours.

The name "17-ketosteroids" is descriptive, designating compounds with a ketone group at the 17 position (C-17). The 17-KS are composed of the major urinary androgenic metabolites, but testosterone itself is not a 17-KS, and significant levels of testosterone may be associated with normal levels of 17-KS.

17-keto group

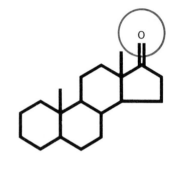

The commonly measured 17-ketosteroids are also known as the neutral 17-KS. Other compounds have a ketone group in the 17 position, but are not "neutral," for example, estrone. Estrone, due to its phenolic structure in ring A, is acidic, and therefore is removed from the urinary extract when washed with alkali in the procedure.

The 17-KS are divided into two groups: the major part being 11-deoxy-17-KS produced by the gonads and adrenal cortex, and the 11-oxy-17-KS, produced *only* by the adrenal cortex.

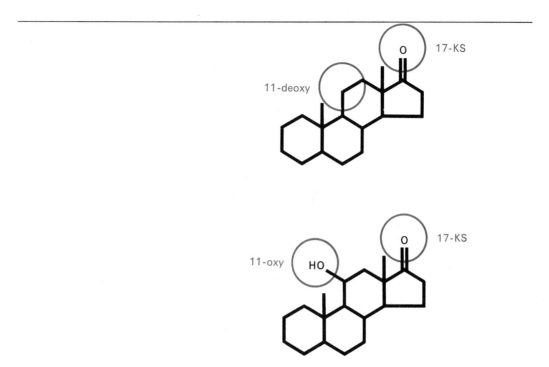

The three major urinary 11-deoxy-17-KS, and therefore, the three major urinary metabolites of androgens are: dehydroepiandrosterone (DHA), etiocholanolone, and androsterone. Note that the only difference between etiocholanolone and androsterone is the stereochemistry at the 5 position: alpha (α) in androsterone and beta (β) in etiocholanolone.

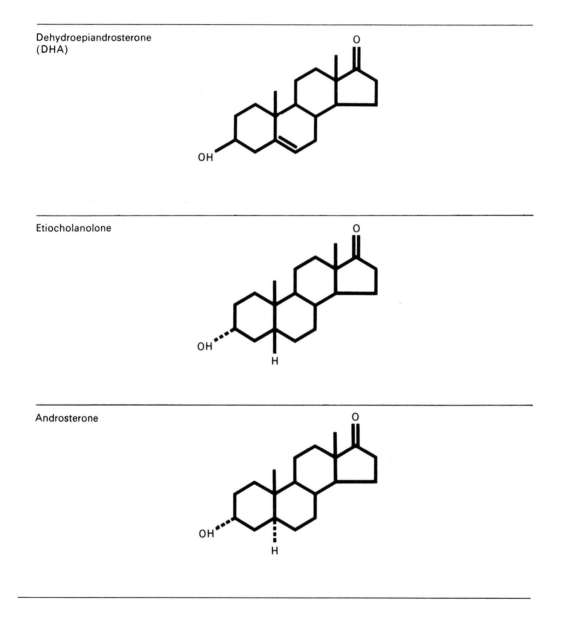

Dehydroepiandrosterone (DHA)

Etiocholanolone

Androsterone

The major 11-oxy-17KS are of adrenal origin: 11-hydroxyetiocholanolone and 11-ketoetiocholanolone (metabolites of corticosteroids), and 11β-hydroxyandrosterone (metabolite of 11β-hydroxyandrostenedione).

11β-Hydroxyandrosterone

11-Hydroxyetiocholanolone

11-Ketoetiocholanolone

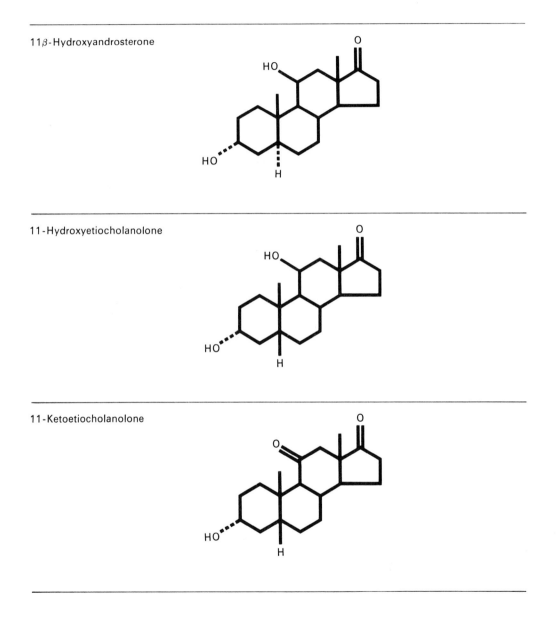

The majority of methods in clinical use for the assay of 17-KS include five major steps:

1. Hydrolysis of the 17-KS conjugates by acid to liberate the free steroids for extraction.

2. Extraction with organic solvents.

3. Removal of acidic material by washing with alkali.

4. Development of color, usually by the Zimmermann reaction (17-KS will give a purple color when treated with dinitrobenzene in the presence of alkali).

5. Measurement by colorimetric methods.

Normal 17-KS

The normal level of 17-ketosteroid excretion in a female is 10 ± 3 mg/24 hours. It should be kept in mind that excretion of 17-KS in the urine changes with age. This can be especially important in the evaluation of an elderly woman.

17-KS
mg/24 hrs

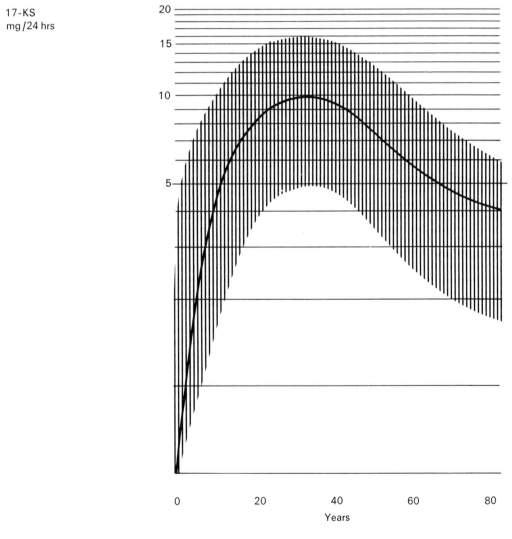

Years

As stated above, the urinary 17-KS arise from precursors secreted by the adrenal cortex and the ovaries. In addition, a certain minimum of nonspecific pigments is present in every urine sample. The composition of normal 17-KS excretion is illustrated.

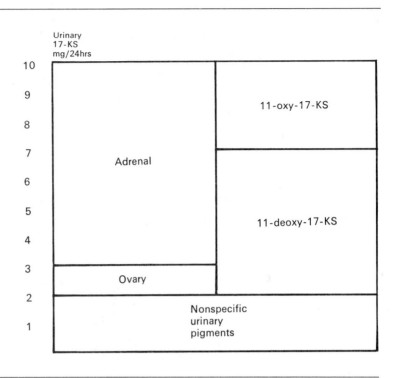

17-Ketogenic Steroids and 17-Hydroxycortico-steroids

17-Ketogenic steroid and 17-hydroxycorticosteroid (17-OHC) determinations measure urinary metabolites of glucocorticoids. There are significant differences in the two tests because more metabolites are measured by the 17-KG test.

The 17-KG and 17-OHC assays require the presence of a 17α-hydroxyl group. The mineralocorticoids (deoxycorticosterone (DOC), corticosterone (Compound B), and aldosterone) do not have a 17-hydroxyl group, and therefore are not measured in 17-KG and 17-OHC assays.

17-hydroxyl group

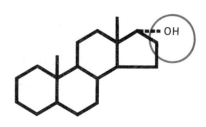

Desoxycorticosterone
(DOC)

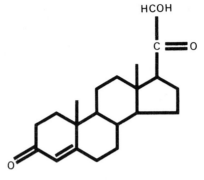

Corticosterone
(B)

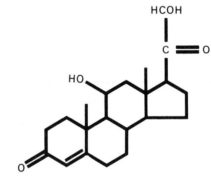

Aldosterone

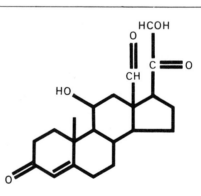

The principal glucocorticoid in the human is cortisol (hydrocortisone, Compound F). Cortisone (Compound E) is a metabolite of cortisol in the human.

Cortisol

Cortisone

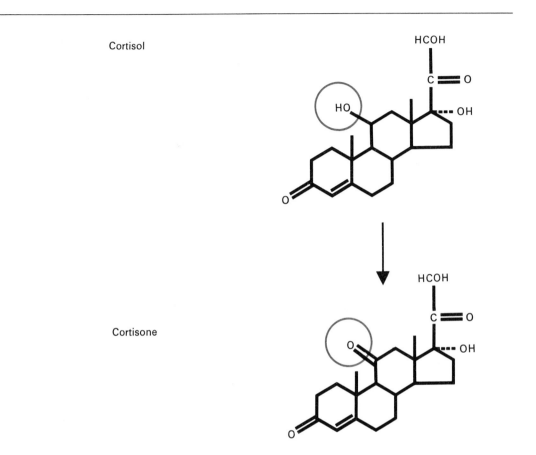

Enzymatic reductions produce the principal urinary metabolite of cortisol: tetrahydrocortisol.

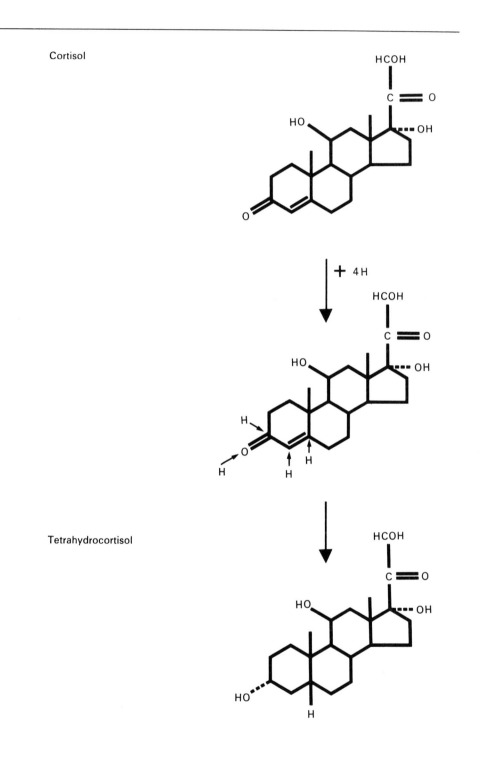

Cortisol

+ 4 H

Tetrahydrocortisol

A similar reduction sequence applies to cortisone, yielding tetrahydrocortisone. Further reduction of tetrahydrocortisol and tetrahydrocortisone involves the ketone at the carbon-20 position, yielding cortol and cortolone.

Tetrahydrocortisol

Cortol

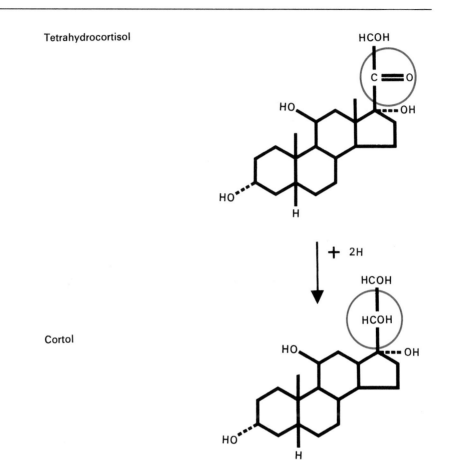

The Porter-Silber reaction produces a color with phenylhydrazine and sulfuric acid. The reaction requires an alpha ketolic group plus the 17-hydroxyl group. Therefore, a hydroxyl group must be at C-21 and C-17, and a ketone must be present at C-20. This reaction measures the 17-hydroxycorticosteroids, abbreviated as 17-OHC.

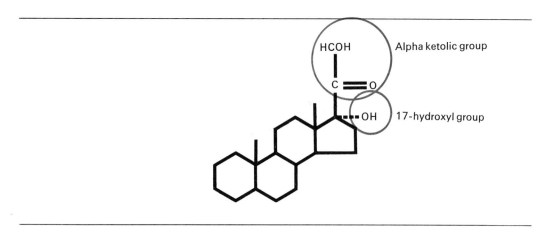

The 17-OHC assay, therefore, cannot measure cortol and cortolone, the further reduction products of tetrahydrocortisol and tetrahydrocortisone, because the C-20 group is reduced and is not a ketone. Nor can the 17-OHC assay measure pregnanetriol since the a-ketolic group is not present.

Pregnanetriol

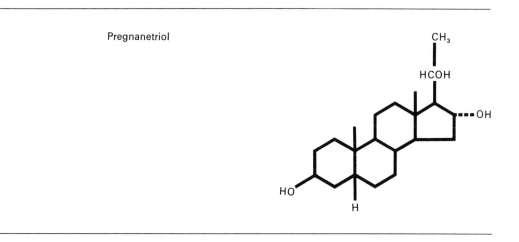

Normal 17-OHC   The normal urinary content of 17-hydroxycorticosteroids is 7 ± 3 mg/24 hours.

The 17-ketogenic (17-KG) steroids are compounds which, when oxidized with sodium bismuthate ($NaBiO_3$), give rise to 17-ketosteroids (17-KS), which can then be measured by the Zimmermann reaction. The initial measurement of 17-KS is subtracted and the difference represents the 17-KG steroids. The requirement is a 17-hydroxyl group and a second hydroxyl group on either the C-20 or the C-21 position.

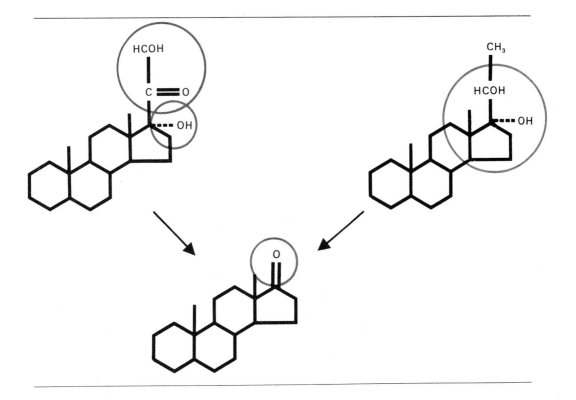

Therefore, the following compounds are measured: tetrahydrocortisol, tetrahydrocortisone, cortol, cortolone, and pregnanetriol (the latter three compounds are not measured in the 17-OHC assay). The compounds missing a 17-hydroxyl group, mainly mineralocorticoids (DOC, corticosterone, and aldosterone) will not be measured by either 17-OHC or 17-KG procedures.

Normal 17-KG

The normal urinary content of 17-KG is 10 ± 3 mg/24 hours. The measurement of additional steroids, when compared to the 17-OHC assay, may be troublesome in the adrenogenital syndrome where pregnanetriol excretion is elevated. Therefore, the 17-KG in the adrenogenital syndrome may be high, while the 17-OHC will be normal.

One should also keep in mind that values change with age.

17-OHC
mg/24hrs

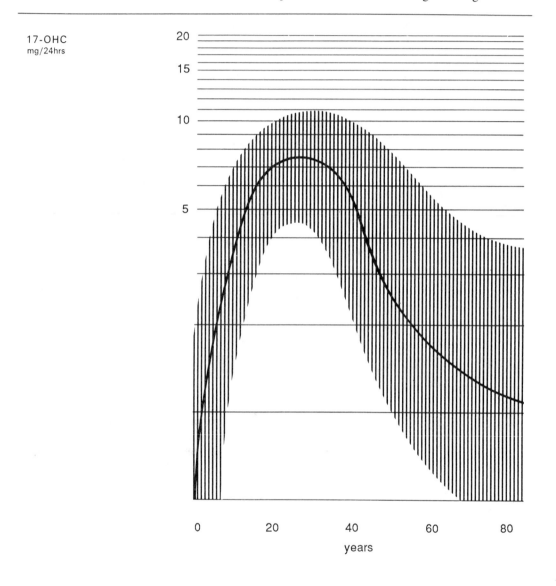

Adrenal Tests

The 24-Hour Urinary Free Cortisol. This measurement accurately reflects the daily production rate and the amount of cortisol which is free and active in the circulation. The normal value ranges from 20 to 90 μg/24 hours.

The Blood Cortisol Level. ACTH is secreted in a pulsatile fashion with the pulses being more frequent and of greater magnitude in the early morning hours, shortly before waking. A nadir in secretion is reached in the evening. Blood levels of ACTH and cortisol are highest in the early morning and lowest in the evening. When the sleep-awake cycle is altered, the diurnal rhythm shifts over about a week's time to resume the same sleep-awake pattern. A 8 AM, the normal plasma cortisol concentration ranges from 10 to 25 μg/dl. At 8 PM, the level is about half the morning concentration, and at 10 PM the level is usually less than 12 μg/dl.

The ACTH Stimulation Test. This is a test for adrenal reserve. Adrenal glands not exposed to ACTH over a long period of time will not have a normal response. Synthetic ACTH is injected in a bolus of 0.25 mg. The plasma cortisol should increase 2-3 times over baseline at 30 and 60 minutes.

The Metyrapone Test. This is a test for hypothalamic-pituitary-adrenal function (a test of ACTH reserve). Metyrapone blocks 11β-hydroxylase enzyme activity in the adrenal gland, thus interfering with cortisol production. After a baseline 24-hour urinary 17-hydroxycorticosteroid or plasma 11-deoxycortisol is obtained, metyrapone is given orally, 750 mg every 4 hours for 6 doses. The 17-OHC should at least double during the 24 hours of metyrapone administration or the next day. A plasma 11-deoxycortisol at 8 AM, 4 hours after the last dose of metyrapone, should exceed 10 μg/dl.

Thyroid Gland

Thyroid hormone synthesis depends in large part upon an adequate supply of iodine in the diet. In the small intestine iodine is absorbed as iodide, and is transported to the thyroid gland. Plasma iodide enters the thyroid under the influence of thyroid stimulating hormone (TSH), the anterior pituitary thyrotropin hormone. Within the thyroid gland, iodide is oxidized to elemental iodine which is then bound to tyrosine. Monoiodotyrosine and diiodotyrosine combine to form thyroxine (T_4) and triiodothyronine (T_3). These iodinated compounds are part of the thyroglobulin molecule, the colloid which serves as a storage depot for thyroid hormone. TSH induces a proteolytic process which results in the release of iodothyronines into the bloodstream as thyroid hormone. In the blood, thyroid hormone is tightly associated with a group of proteins chiefly thyroxine-binding globulin (TBG). Estrogen produces a rise in thyroxine-binding globulin capacity, and, therefore, thyroid function tests are affected by pregnancy and estrogen-containing medication. With the increase in TBG capacity, the maintenance of an euthyroid state depends upon the concept that free thyroxine concentration (unbound and metabolically active thyroid hormone) is within the normal range.

Although T_4 is secreted at 20 times the rate of T_3 it is T_3 which is responsible for most if not all the thyroid action in the body. T_3 is 3-4 times more potent than T_4. About one third of the T_4 secreted each day is converted in peripheral tissues, largely liver and kidney, to T_3, and about 40% is converted to the inactive, reverse T_3.

There are at least two reasons why T_3 is more active than T_4. The cellular nuclear receptor for thyroid hormone has about a 10-fold higher affinity for T_3 than T_4, and blood proteins which restrict the entry of thyroid hormone into cells bind T_4 more tightly than T_3.

One would think that measurement of T_3, therefore, would be the most accurate appraisal of thyroid function. Because of the peripheral source of T_3, however, it is not a direct reflection of thyroid secretion. In addition T_3 levels may be normal despite the presence of a goiter with elevated TSH and depressed T_4 concentrations. T_4 plays the instrumental role in TSH regulation. Thyroid hormones regulate TSH by both suppressing thyroid releasing hormone (TRH) secretion and affecting the pituitary sensitivity to TRH (by reducing the number of TRH receptors). While some tissues depend mainly on the blood T_3 for their intracellular T_3, the brain and the pituitary depend on their own intracellular conversion of T_4. The measurement of T_4 and TSH, therefore, provides the most accurate assessment of thyroid function.

The modern assessment of thyroid function is relatively easy. The confusing array of tests previously available (protein-bound iodine, T_3 uptake, free thyroxine index) has been replaced by the radioimmunoassay of free T_4, TSH, and T_3. The free T_4 level has a different range of normal values from laboratory to laboratory. The serum TSH ranges from 0.5 to 3.5 μU/ml. The radioimmunoassay of T_3 is unnecessary on a routine basis, but important for the occasional case of hyperthyroidism due to excessive production of T_3 with normal T_4 levels (T_3 toxicosis). The normal range for serum T_3 is 80-180 ng/dl.

Drugs taken orally for cholecystograms inhibit the peripheral conversion of T_4 to T_3, and can disrupt normal thyroid levels (giving elevated T_4). This effect can last 30 days after administration.

In early hypothyroidism, with undetectable symptoms or signs, a compensated state can be detected by an elevated TSH and normal T_4 (called subclinical hypothyroidism). With progressive deterioration, a progressively lower T_4 is apparent.

In subclinical hypothyroidism, the therapeutic decision is easy: replacement thyroid medication should be prescribed to return TSH levels to normal, even though T_4 levels are already normal. This avoids the appearance of a goiter and the progressive development of clinical hypothyroidism. In addition some patients in retrospect (after treatment) recognize improved and physical and mental well-being. With only very slight elevations of TSH, it is reasonable not to treat, and to check thyroid function every year to detect further deterioration.

The best preparation for hormone replacement is T_4. Mixtures of T_4 and T_3, such as desiccated thyroid, provide T_3 in excess of normal thyroid secretion. It is better to provide T_4 and allow the peripheral conversion process to provide the T_3. Likewise, for suppression of TSH after treatment of thyroid carcinoma or nodular thyroid disease, the drug of choice is T_4, thyroxine. Both TSH and T_4 should be measured when monitoring treatment because TSH alone cannot detect overdosage.

The Sensitive TSH Assay. New methods of measuring TSH incorporating monoclonal antibodies are capable of quantitating both the upper and lower limits of normal. Such assays will reveal subnormal (less than 0.5 μU/ml) levels of TSH in patients with hyperthyroidism or thyroid carcinoma.

TSH Level	Free T$_4$ level	Clinical Diagnosis
Elevated	Normal	Subclinical Hypothyroidism
Elevated	Low	Hypothyroidism
Low	Elevated	Hyperthyroidism

Index

Page numbers in *italics* denote figures; those followed by "t" denote tables

Abortion
  endometriosis and, 559
  precipitated by luteectomy, 508
  rates of, 505, 535
  recurrent
    alloimmune factors, 538
    autoimmune factors, 537–538
    hormonal treatment, 536–537
    infertility and, 516, 535–536
Acanthosis nigricans, 218
Acromegaly, 188
  hirsutism and, 240
Acrosome, *504*, 504
Activation, 26–28
Activin, 103–104
Adenylate cyclase
  composition of, 44
  desensitization of, 46
  in estradiol synthesis, 2–3
  mediating action of tropic hormones, 44–46
  regulation of, 44–46, *45–46*
Adipose tissue. *See also* Obesity
  development of fat cells, 452
  functions of, 448
  mechanism for mobilizing energy, 448
  physiology of, 448–451, *449–450*
Adoption, 539
Adrenal gland
  effect of oral contraceptives, 475–476
  fetal, 324–326
    DHAS production, 321–326
    functions, 326
    gluco- and mineralocorticoid production, 320
  hyperplasia, 244–245, 386–394, *388*
    associated metabolic disorders, 387
    diagnosis, 392t, 392–393
    enzyme deficiencies, 244–245
      20-22-desmolase, 391
      11β-hydroxylase, 390
      17α-hydroxylase, 390
      21-hydroxylase, 244–245, 387, 389
      3β-hydroxysteroid dehydrogenase, 390
    forms of, 244
    genetics, 244, 391, 391t
    genitalia in, 386
    pathophysiology, 387
    prevalence, 245
    treatment, 393–394
    virilization in, 386
  tests
    ACTH stimulation test, 647
    blood cortisol level, 647
    24-hour urinary free cortisol, 647
    metyrapone test, 647
Adrenarche, 83, 410–411
Adrenocorticotropic hormone (ACTH), 63–64
  fetal, 324–325
  in hirsutism, 241–242
  human chorionic, 335

  secretion by pituitary tumor, 188
  stimulation test, 647
    for hirsutism, 248
Agonadism, 400
Albicantia, 126
Albumin, as protein carrier, 2, 16
Aldosterone, structure, *640*
Alloimmunity, recurrent abortion and, 538
Amenorrhea, 137, 165–205
  anosmia and, 203–204
  danazol treatment and, 557
  definition, 166
  disorders associated with specific menstrual
      compartments, 180–196
    anorexia nervosa, 197–200
    Asherman's syndrome, 180–181
    effect of radiation and chemotherapy, 187–
      188, 188t
    empty sella syndrome, 178, 195–196
    gonadal agenesis, 186–187
    hypothalamic, 196
    mosaicism, 186
    Mullerian agenesis, 182–183, 185t
    Mullerian anomalies, 181
    pituitary tumors, 171, 179, 188–196
    premature ovarian failure, 187
    resistant ovary syndrome, 187
    testicular feminization, 183–184, 185t
    Turner's syndrome, 185–186
    weight loss, 197–200
    XY gonadal dysgenesis, 186
  due to testicular feminization, 395
  estrogen-progestestin test, 172
  evaluation of, 167–173
    step 1, 167–171, *169–170*
    step 2, 172
    step 3, 172–173
  exercise and, 200–203
    anorectic reaction, 203
    critical weight hypothesis, 200–201, *201*
    runner's "high", 202
    stress and energy expenditure, 201–202
  galactorrhea and, 167, 291, 292, 294, *295*
  gonadotropin levels, 172t, *173*
    high, 172–175
  hormone replacement therapy, 204–205
  hypothalamic, 179
  in polycystic ovary syndrome, 226
  postpill, 204, 480–481
  primary and secondary, 166
  while on low-dose oral contraceptives, 485–486
American Fertility Society classification of endo-
     metriosis, 550, *551*
Amniocentesis
  for diagnosis of hypothyroidism, 342
  indicated by high maternal serum AFP, 336
Amniotic fluid
  arachidonic acid levels, 362
  cortisol levels, *360*, 361

estrogen levels, 328
iodothyronine levels, 342
progesterone levels, 319
prolactin levels, 337-338
Androgen insensitivity syndromes, 184, 394-398, *396*
complete: testicular feminization, 395-396
incomplete, 396-397
5α-reductase deficiency, 397-398
responses to androgen in target cells, 394-395, *395*
Androgens. *See also* specific androgens and their metabolites
abnormal synthesis, 398-399
adrenarche, 83, 410-411
decidualized endometrium due to high levels of, 171
effect on hair, 236
effect on SHBG production in liver, 237
effect on testosterone binding capacity, 21
excess. *See* Adrenal gland,hyperplasia
mechanism of action, 29
metabolism, 20-23, *22*
in patients with persistent anovulation, 220, 223
preovulatory production of, 106
protein binding of, 233, 237
role in CNS development, 385
role in early follicular development, 94, *94*
role in genital development, 383
sources of circulating, 16
stimulation of libido, 106-107
structure, *4*
Androstane, steroid nucleus, 4, *4*
3α-Androstanediol glucuronide, 238-239
Androstenedione
conversion to estrogen correlated with body weight, 129
as major androgen product of ovary, 20
menstrual midcycle increase in, 14
in patients with persistent anovulation, 220
postmenopausal levels, 128
production of, 18
structure, *12*
Androsterone, 636
structure, *636*
Angiogenic growth factor, 100
Angiotensin II, role in pregnancy, 369, *370*
Anorchia, 400-401
Anorectics, 456
Anorexia nervosa, 197-200
associated dysfunctions, 199
diagnosis, 197
gonadotropin levels, 199
symptoms and signs, 198
treatment, 199-200
vs. anorectic reaction, 203
Anosmia, amenorrhea and, 203-204
Anovulation, 213-228
decidualized endometrium and, 171
establishing by progestational challenge, 170
evaluation for pituitary tumor, 171
with galactorrhea, 171
hirsutism and, 238
infertility and, 519
link to endometrial and breast cancer, 170
obesity and, possible mechanisms, 216, 217
pathogenesis, 213-218
abnormal feedback signals, 215-217
loss of FSH stimulation, 215-216, *216*
loss of LH stimulation, 216-217

central defects, 214-215, *215*
local ovarian conditions, 217-218
polycystic ovary and, 220-227. *See also* Ovary-,polycystic
in postmenarchal cycles, 416-417
precise etiology, 219
progestational therapy, 171
lack of withdrawal bleeding, 171-172, *172*
quantity of withdrawal bleeding, 171
Antibiotics, effect on oral contraceptive efficacy, 485
Antibodies, monoclonal, 625-627, *626*
Antral follicle, *93*, 95-105
Apoproteins, 9
Arachidonic acid
amniotic fluid levels, 362
role in prostaglandin synthesis, 352-354, 362, 364
Arginine vasopressin, 70, *71*
Arginine vasotocin, 81
Aromatization, *12*, 13, 15, 29-30, 92, 94-95, 125
Asherman's syndrome, 180-181
Aspirin, effect on platelets, 356-357, *357*
Atherosclerosis
obesity and, 446, 455
role of cholesterol, 9-11, 143-144
Atrial natriuretic peptide, in pregnancy, 338
Atrophic changes, menopausal, 136, 145, 151
Autocrine communication, 2
Autoimmune disease
ovarian failure and, 175, 176
recurrent abortion and, 537-538

Basal body temperature, 527-528, *529*
as guide for timing of therapeutic insemination, 578-579
Bayley-Pinneau tables, 431, 438t-443t
Betamethasone, effect on maternal estriol level, 326
Birth control pills. *See* Contraceptives,steroid
Bleeding
breakthrough
estrogen, 272
with medroxyprogesterone acetate, 488
progesterone, 272, 278, 280
while on low-dose oral contraceptives, 486-487
dysfunctional uterine. *See* Dysfunctional uterine bleeding
why anovulatory bleeding is excessive, 275
withdrawal
estrogen, 272
progesterone, 171-172, 272
Body mass index nomogram, 446, *447*
Breast, 283-310
abnormal sizes and shapes, 285, *285*
accessory nipples, 285
best time to examine, 284
fibrocystic changes, 299
galactorrhea. *See* Galactorrhea
growth and development, 283-284
lactation. *See* Lactation
mammary gland
early differentiation, *285*
ejection of milk, 288
maternal drugs in breast milk, 288
mastalgia, 296
microcalcifications, 308
Breast cancer, 297-307
anovulation and, 170, 227

average size when detected, 308
doubling time, 308
effects of estrogen, 29, 149
estrogen window etiologic hypothesis, 303–304
Halsted surgical procedure, 298
histology of axillary lymph nodes, 297–298
mammographic detection. *See* Mammography
mortality data, 297, *297*
needle aspiration of lumps, 306–307
oral contraceptives and, 475
prevalence, 149, 297
progestational protection against, 305
receptors and clinical prognosis
  estrogen receptors, 305–306
  progesterone receptors, 305–306
  receptor assay to determine management, 306
relation to woman's age, 297
risk factors, 149, 298–303, 310
  alcohol in diet, 300
  benign breast disease, 299
  classification of breast biopsy tissue, 299
  endocrine factors, 300–303
    adrenal steroids, 300
    birth control pills, 302–303
    DES exposure, 303
    endogenous estrogen, 300–301
    exogenous estrogen, 301
    thyroid, prolactin, various nonestrogen drugs, 302
  familial tendency, 300
  fat in diet, 300
  ovarian activity, 299
  reproductive history, 298
screening recommendations, 310
stepwise progression vs. systemic disease concepts, 298
survival rates, 297–298
treatment, 306–307, *307*
Bromocriptine
dosage, 593
for euprolactinemic women, 594–595
failure to suppress amniotic fluid prolactin, 286–287
for galactorrhea, 179, 192, 214, 295–296, 593–594
for inadequate luteal phase, 530–531
for mastalgia, 296
for ovulation induction, 593–595
  addition to clomiphene, 593
  ovulation and pregnancy rates with, 594
pharmacology, 191
for pituitary adenomas, 177, 179, 191–193, 214
  dosage, 192
  for patients seeking pregnancy, 192
  treatment results, 192
  tumor regression, 192–193
for premenstrual syndrome, 131
side effects, 191–192, 593
Bulimia, 198
Buserelin, combined with human menopausal gonadotropins for ovulation induction, 600–601

CA-125 assay, for endometriosis, 549
Calcitonin, for osteoporosis, 141
Calcium
as intracellular mediator, *34*, 34–35
osteoporosis and, 138–139, *140*
for patients not on estrogen replacement therapy, 154, 205

for patients on estrogen replacement therapy, 139, *140*, 153
role in parturition, 365–366
supplementation unmasking hyperparathyroidism, 154
Call-Exner bodies, 124, 125
Calmodulin, 34–35, *35*
Cancer
breast. *See* Breast cancer
cervical, 475
endometrial
  development in anovulatory patient, 170
  estrogen replacement therapy and, 148–149
  intraepithelial, 274
  oral contraceptives and, 474
lung, gonadotropin production and, 173
ovarian
  androgen-producing tumors, 241, 242, 251–252
  estrogen excess and, 146
  oral contraceptives and, 474–475
  precocious puberty and, 420–421
  premature ovarian failure and, 175
testicular, 183–184
Carbamazepine, effect on oral contraceptive efficacy, 485
Carbohydrates
components of tropic hormones, 36–38
effect of oral contraceptives on metabolism of, 477–478
Cardiovascular disease
related to estrogen loss, 136, 142t, 142–145, 143t
  reduced risk related to estrogen replacement therapy, 142–143
steroid contraceptives and, 469–470
  risk of death, 471–473
Catecholestrogens, 67, *68*
Central nervous system differentiation, 385
Cervix
cancer, oral contraceptives and, 475
infection, 521
  oral contraceptives and, 479
Cesarean section, correlation with respiratory distress syndrome, 343
Chemotherapy, effect on ovary, 188
Chlamydia, 521, 523, 570
Chloasma, oral contraceptives and, 479
Chlorpromazine, to stimulate lactation in adoptive mothers, 288
Cholecystokinin, 62
Cholesterol
conversion to pregnenolone, 13
dietary modifications for high levels, 154
relationship with cardiovascular disease, 9–11
role in steroidogenesis, 7–11, 42
structure, *4, 12*
Chylomicrons, 7
Cimetidine, for hirsutism, 257
Circadian cycle, of major sex hormones in female, 21
Clathrins, *39, 40*
Climacteric. *See also* Menopause
estrogen withdrawal, 135–137
problems of estrogen deprivation, 137–146
Clomid. *See* Clomiphene citrate
Clomiphene citrate, 527
addition of bromocriptine, 593
addition of dexamethasone, 592
addition of HCG, 590–591
dosage, 588

correlation with body weight, 589
to elevate sperm count, 571
extended treatment, 592–593
failure, 591–593
fetal malformations and, 586
half-life, 585
how to use, 588–591, *589*
to increase FSH in polycystic ovary syndrome, 226
to initiate cyclicity when pregnancy is not desired, 588
mechanism of action, 585
ovulation and pregnancy rates with, 591
patient monitoring, 590
patient selection, 586–588
sequential treatment with human menopausal gonadotropins, 600
side effects, 591–592
structure, 584, *584*
to treat inadequate luteal phase, 530
treatment complications, 591–592
treatment results, 591
use in in vitro fertilization, 612
use of basal body temperature chart, 590
Clonidine, for hot flushes, 154
Coagulation, disseminated intravascular, 371
Colles fracture, 138
Colostrum, 286
Contraceptives, steroid, 461–492
  for anovulatory, amenorrheic patient, 171
  beginning postpartum, 484
  benefits of, 485
  capsules implanted under skin, 490
  choice of pill, 483–484
  contraindications, 488
    absolute, 481
    relative, 482
  Depo-Provera as alternative to, 488–490, *489*
  for dysfunctional uterine bleeding, 276–278, *277*
  effect of antibiotics, 485
  failure, 484
  for hirsutism, 252–253, *253*
  injectable, 490
  metabolic effects, 469–481
    adrenal gland, 476–477
    breast discomfort, 479
    carbohydrate metabolism, 477–478
    cardiovascular disease, 469–470
      risk of death, 471–473
    cervicitis, 479
    chloasma, 479
    decreased libido, 480
    depression, 480
    diabetes, 477–478
    eye disorders, 480
    galactorrhea, 291
    gallbladder disease, 479
    gastrointestinal disorders, 479
    hematologic effects, 479
    hypertension, 473–474
    liver, 478
      adenomas, 478–479
    oncogenic potential, 474–476
    relief of dysmenorrhea, 480
    thyroid, 477
    urinary tract infection, 479
    vascular headache, 470
    viral diseases, 479
    vitamin metabolism, 479–480
    weight gain, 479

minipill, 483, 490
multiphasic preparations, 466, 483
  effectiveness, 468, 468t
  mechanism of action, 466–468
  ovarian cysts and, 483
  to treat endometriosis, 554, 557
for older woman, 487–488
oncogenic potential
  breast, 302–303, 475–476
  cervix, 475
  endometrium, 474
  ovary, 474–475
patient monitoring, 482–483
  laboratory surveillance, 483
pelvic inflammatory disease and, 480
pharmacology, 461–468
  estrogen component, 461–462, *462*
  progestin component, 462–466, *463*, *465*
for postcoital contraception, 490
postpill amenorrhea, 204, 480–481
for premenstrual syndrome, 131, 480
problems with low-dose pills, 485–487
  amenorrhea, 485–486
  breakthrough bleeding, 486–487
progestin-impregnated vaginal rings, 490
relation to smoking in women over 35, 470, 487–488
safety, 485
safety of, 461
for teenagers, 484
Cooperativity, 28
Coronary heart disease
  risk factors for, 10
  role of cholesterol, 9–11
Corpus luteum, 126
  aging of, 126
  degeneration of, 214
    mechanism of, 113
    timing of, 113
  dependence of pregnancy on, 318, 320, 508
  dependence on LH, 112
  HCG stimulation of, 320
  luteolytic action of prostaglandins, 357–358
  steroidogenesis in, 45, 114
Corticoids, structure, *4*
Corticosteroid binding globulin, role in blood transport of steroids, 16
Corticosteroids, effect on maternal estriol level, 326
Corticosterone, structure, *640*
Corticotropin-like intermediate lobe peptide, 63–64
Corticotropin releasing hormone (CRH), 66
Cortisol
  deficiency in adrenogenital syndrome, 387, 393
  growth suppression of, 431
  levels associated with labor, *360*, 361
  measurement of
    blood levels, 647
    24-hour urinary free levels, 647
  production and clearance in obesity, 453
  structure, *641–642*
Cortisone, structure, *641*
Cortol, structure, *643*
Coumadin, effect on oral contraceptive efficacy, 485
Cushing's syndrome, 188
  causes, 241
  CT scanning for adrenal tumors, 242
  dexamethasone suppression test, 241–242

diagnosis, 241–242
hirsutism and, 240, 241–242
Cyclic adenosine 3'5'-monophosphate
  activation by tropic hormones, 31–35, *32–34*
  in estradiol synthesis, 3
Cyclic guanosine 3'5'-monophosphate, 34
Cyproterone acetate
  for hirsutism, 257
  structure, *256*
Cystitis, 136, 145

Danazol
  actions of, 554–555
  contraindications, 555–556
  for endometriosis, 554–558
    dosage, 556–557
    prior to surgery, 553
    treatment of mild disease, 556
  hirsutism and, 240
  for mastalgia, 296
  metabolism, 555
  side effects, 555
  structure, *555*
Dehydroepiandrosterone (DHA), 636
  blood level rise in initiation of puberty, 82
  in hirsutism, 238, *238*
  in patients with persistent anovulation, 220
  postmenopausal levels, 129
  source of, 236, *237*
  structure, *12, 636*
Dehydroepiandrosterone sulfate (DHAS)
  levels of
    after menopause, 129
    blood rise in initiation of puberty, 82
    in hirsutism, 238, *238*, 242–244, *243*
    in patients with persistent anovulation, 220,
      226
    in polycystic ovary syndrome, 244
    relation to aging, 630, *630*
  measurement by radioimmunoassay, 630, *630*
  production by fetal adrenal gland, 321–326
  source of, 236, *237*
  suppression by progestational therapy, 254–255
Deoxycorticosterone (DOC)
  in pregnancy, 320
  structure, *640*
Depo-Provera. *See* Medroxyprogesterone acetate
Depression
  medroxyprogesterone acetate and, 488, 558
  oral contraceptives and, 480
20-22-Desmolase deficiency, 391
Dexamethasone
  addition to clomiphene for ovulation induction,
    592
  effect on maternal estriol level, 326
  for hirsutism, 257
Dexamethasone suppression test, 241–242
DHA. *See* Dehydroepiandrosterone
DHAS. *See* Dehydroepiandrosterone sulfate
  (DHAS)
DHT. *See* Dihydrotestosterone
Diabetes mellitus
  effect of oral contraceptives, 477–478
  infertility and, 570
  obesity and, 453
Diethylstilbestrol (DES)
  female exposure in utero
    breast cancer risk, 303
    hysterosalpingography technique for, 525
  male exposure in utero, 569

structure, *584*
to treat endometriosis, 554
Dihydrotestosterone (DHT)
  blood levels of, 23
  derivation of, 21
  in hirsutism, 238–239
  mechanism of action, 29–30
Dilantin, hirsutism and, 240
Dilatation and curettage
  for Asherman's syndrome, 181
  for dysfunctional uterine bleeding, 276, 281
  as part of infertility investigation, 539
Dilators, to create functional vagina, 182
Dopamine
  effect on GnRH, 56, 58–60, *59*
  as prolactin inhibiting hormone, 53, 59, 288–289
Down's syndrome, maternal serum AFP level and,
  336
Dynorphins, 62
Dysfunctional uterine bleeding, 265–281
  in adolescents, 280
  categories, 265
  definition, 265
  endometrium. *See also* Endometrium
    histologic changes during ovulatory cycle,
      266–270, 266–271
    hyperplasia vs. neoplasia, 274
    responses to steroid hormones, 272–274, *273*
    teleologic theory of menstrual events, 271
  evaluation of, 147
  follow-up assessment, 281
  perimenopausal, 146–147
  treatment, 147, 150, 276–279
    antiprostaglandins, 279
    combined birth control pills, 276–278, *277*
    dilatation and curettage, 276, 281
    estrogens, 278, 280
    key points in, 279, 279t
    objective of, 276
    progestins, 276
  vs. normal estrogen-progesterone withdrawal
    bleeding, 272–273, 280
  why anovulatory bleeding is excessive, 275
    alternate hypothesis, 275
Dysmenorrhea, 133–134
  associated symptoms, 133
  endometriosis and, 549
  primary vs. secondary, 133
  relieved by oral contraceptives, 480
Dyspareunia, in climacteric, 145

Eating disorders
  anorexia nervosa, 197–200
  bulimia, 198
Electrolysis, for hirsutism, 253, 258
ELISA. *See* Enzyme-linked immunosorbent assay
Embryo
  implantation of, 506–509
  loss associated with in vitro fertilization, 506
  transfer, 615
Empty sella syndrome, 178, 195–196
Endocytosis, 39, 44, 319
Endometriosis, 547–559
  American Fertility Society classification, 550,
    551
  diagnosis, 549–550
    CA-125 assay, 549
    examination, 549–550
    symptoms and signs, 549
  etiology, 547–548

hormonal treatment, 553–558
  combination birth control pills, 554, 557
  danazol, 554–558
    for mild disease, 556
    prior to surgery, 553
  DES, 554
  GnRH agonist, 558
  long-term, 559
  methyltestosterone, 554
  Provera, 558
hormone replacement after surgery, 559
infertility and, 550, 552
  prevention of, 559
male, 548
ovulation and, 559
prevalence, 548
recurrence, 558
sites of, 548
spontaneous abortion and, 559
surgical treatment, 552–553
in vitro fertilization and, 559, 617
Endometrium
  Asherman's syndrome, 180–181
  biopsy, 528, 586
  cancer
    development of in anovulatory patients, 170
    estrogen replacement therapy and, 148–149
    hyperplasia vs. neoplasia, 274
    intraepithelial neoplasia, 274
    oral contraceptives and, 474
  decidualized, 171
  histologic changes during ovulatory cycle, 266–270, 266–271
    implantation phase, 268–269
    menstrual endometrium, 266
    phase of endometrial breakdown, 269–271
    proliferative phase, 267
    secretory phase, 268
  myoma, 281
  polyps, 281
  responses to steroid hormones, 272–274, 273
    estrogen breakthrough bleeding, 272
    estrogen withdrawal bleeding, 272
    progesterone breakthrough bleeding, 272
    progesterone withdrawal bleeding, 272
  teleologic theory of menstrual events, 271
  when to perform biopsy, 155, 227
Endorphins, 62–65
  in menstrual cycle, 65, 102
  in pregnancy, 338
Enkephalins, 62–65
  in pregnancy, 338
Enzyme-linked immunosorbent assay technique, 627, 627–628
Epidermal growth factor, 100
17-Epitestosterone, structure, 5
Estes procedure, 502
Estetrol, 328
Estradiol. See also Estrogen
  assay in premature ovarian failure, 176
  blood levels of, 629t
  bound vs. free, 3
  clearance from circulation, 3
  effect on follicular development, 125, 217
  effect on FSH, 14
  metabolism, 2, 16
  micronized, 153
  postmenopausal levels, 129
  postovulatory levels, 109
  in pregnancy, 323–324

production in normal, nonpregnant female, 18
role in ovulation, 213–214, 217
secretion in bloodstream, 3
sources of, 2
structure, 12
Estrane, steroid nucleus, 4, 4
Estratest. See Methyltestosterone
Estriol
  breast cancer and, 300
  metabolism, 16
  in pregnancy, 323–324
    assays to measure fetal well-being, 326–328, 327
    relation to birth weight, 326
Estrogen
  abnormal clearance and metabolism of, 215
  blood level rise in initiation of puberty, 82
  breast cancer and, 29, 300–301
    estrogen window etiologic hypothesis, 303–304
  breast development at puberty and, 284
  conjugated, 151, 153
    for Asherman's syndrome, 181
    to treat poor cervical mucus, 521
  content in birth control pills, 461–462, 462
  declining levels leading to menopause, 128
  deprivation, problems of, 137–146
    altered menstrual function, 137
    atrophic changes, 145–146
    cardiovascular effects, 142–145
    menopausal syndrome, 146
    osteoporosis, 138–142
    vasomotor symptoms, 137–138
  for dysfunctional uterine bleeding, 278
  effect on hair, 236
  excess, problems of, 146–147
    mechanisms of increase, 146
  extraglandular production of, 129–130, 216, 216
  mechanism of action, 27–29
  metabolism, 16–18, 17–18
  monitoring levels for timing of ovulation induction, 597–598
  persistent secretion of, 215
  for postcoital contraception, 358, 491
  postmenopausal levels, 129–130, 134
  in pregnancy, 321–323, 321–324
    amniotic fluid measurements, 328
    assays to measure fetal well-being, 326–328, 327
    late pregnancy increase in, 360, 360–364, 363
    measurement of, 326–328, 327
  production from androstenedione correlated with body weight, 129
  for progestin breakthrough bleeding, 278, 280
  progressive withdrawal, 135–137
  in relation to follicle
    attrition, 135–136
    growth, 125–126
    maturation and availability, 127, 127–128
    selection for ovulation, 126
  relative potencies, 151
  replacement therapy, 134–135
    addition of progestin, 140
    for amenorrhea, 204–205
    choice of drugs, 151t, 151–152
    classic sequential treatment method, 152–153
    continuous/combined treatment method, 153
    contraindications, 147, 154

effect on lipid profile, 143–144, 152, 153–154, 154t
osteoporosis and, 139–141
for premature ovarian failure, 176
problems with, 147–149
recommendations for use, 150–151, 155
risk of heart disease and, 142–143
route of administration, 152
requirements for bone growth, 415
role in luteolysis, 358
structure, *4*
uninterrupted, in patients with persistent anovulation, 220, 227
urinary levels of, 631t
Estrone
levels of, after menopause, 129
metabolism, 16
in patients with persistent anovulation, 220
in pregnancy, 323–324
structure, *6, 12*
Ethinyl estradiol, 151
content in birth control pills, 461–462
structure, *462*
Ethiodol, 525–526
Ethisterone, 462
structure, *463*
Ethynodiol diacetate, structure, *465*
Etiocholanolone, 636
breast cancer and, 300
structure, *636*
Exercise, for osteoporosis, 141–142

Fallopian tube
damage leading to infertility, 519, 524–525
egg transport in, 501–503
Feminization, testicular, 183–184, 185t
androgen intracellular mechanism in, 30–31
clinical manifestations, 183
incomplete, 184
testes in, 183–184
Ferguson reflex, 72
Fertilization
in vitro, 611–618
alternate techniques, 617
embryo loss and, 506
embryo transfer, 615
for endometriosis, 617
endometriosis and, 559
fertilization, 615
history, 611
for male factor infertility, 576–577, 616
monitoring ovarian response to stimulation, 613
oocyte culture, 614
oocyte retrieval, 613–614
other indications for, 617
patient selection, 612
results, 615–616
stimulation protocols, 612
in vivo, 503–505
acrosome reaction, 504
cortical reaction, 504
failures associated with, 505
zona reaction, 503
α-Fetoprotein, 336
indicating fetal abnormalities, 336
Fetus
adrenal gland, 324–326
DHAS production, 321–326
functions, 326

gluco- and mineralocorticoid production, 320
AFP levels indicating abnormalities, 336
cortisol levels, 343–344
effect of postcoital estrogen, 491
effect of prostaglandins on circulation, 358–359
lung maturation, 342–344
sexual differentiation. *See* Sexual differentiation
thyroid gland, *339–341,* 339–342
Fibroblast growth factor, 100
Flufenamic acid, for dysmenorrhea, 133
Fluoride, for osteoporosis, 139
9-Fluorohydrocortisone, for adrenogenital syndrome, 393
Follicle
antral, *93,* 95–105
atresia, 92, 106
in adult life, 124, 125
in fetal life, 124
attrition leading to menopause, 128, 135
dominant
feedback system, 100–102
growth factors, 100
selection of, 98–99
formation stages
adult, 125–126
fetal, 122–124, *123*
luteinized unruptured, 534, 599
microenvironment of, 96t
preantral, 92–95, *93*
preovulatory, *93,* 105–107
primordial, 92, *93*
steroidogenesis, 11–15, *12*
two-cell mechanism of, 14–15, *15,* 96, *96,* 223, 226
Follicle stimulating hormone binding inhibitor, 104
Follicle stimulating hormone (FSH)
activation of aromatization, 92
in amenorrheic patients
high levels, 173–176
low levels, 177
normal levels, 177
anovulation due to loss of stimulation, 215–216
levels of
after menopause, 128
after orchiectomy, 566
normal serum, 628t, *629*
in perimenopausal period, 128, 174
with pituitary adenoma, 173
in polycystic ovary syndrome, *222,* 222–223
midcycle surge
functions of, *109,* 109–110
mechanism of, *77–78,* 78–79
purified, for ovulation induction, 603
role in follicular growth, 125–126
role in steroidogenesis, 2, 14–15, *15*
secretion at puberty, 82–84
stimulation of spermatogenesis, 566
Follicular fluid, 95–96, *97,* 102–104
Folliculostatin, role in menstrual cycle, 103
Fractures, osteoporosis and, 138–139
FSH. *See* Follicle-stimulating hormone

G protein, 44
Galactorrhea, 291–296
amenorrhea and, 167, 291, 292, 294, *295*
bromocriptine therapy, 179, 192, 214, 295–296, 593–594
caused by drug inhibition of PIF, 291–292

definition, 291
differential diagnosis, 291–292, *293*
endometriosis and, 549
evaluation of, 167–173
hemodialysis and, 292
hypothyroidism and, 292
nonpituitary tumors and, 292
pituitary tumors and, 189–190, 292
spontaneous resolution after pregnancy, 594
stress and, 292
Galactosemia, high gonadotropins in, 175
Gallbladder
effect of estrogen replacement therapy, 147
effect of oral contraceptives, 479
Gamete intrafallopian tube transfer (GIFT), 576, 617
Gap junctions, 92–93, 365
Genitalia
ambiguous. *See also* Hermaphrodite; Pseudo-hermaphrodite
assignment of sex of rearing, 405–406
diagnosis, 403–405, *404*
differentiation, 382–383, *383–384*
Glucagon, in obesity, 453
Glucocorticoids
association with induction of labor, 359–360
to enhance fetal lung maturation, 344
production of, 20
Glucose
effect of oral contraceptives, 477
functions of, 448
release of free fatty acids, 449–450, *449–450*
Glucosiduronate, structure, *23*
GnRh. *See* Gonadotropin releasing hormone
Gonadocrinins, 104
"Gonadostat"
in infancy and childhood, 409–410
in puberty, 411–412
Gonadotropin releasing hormone-associated peptide (GAP), 53, 59
Gonadotropin releasing hormone (GnRH), 35–36
agonists
combined with human menopausal gonado-tropins for ovulation induction, 600–601
contraceptive effects, 492
for endometriosis, 558
for precocious puberty, 423–424
use in in vitro fertilization, 612
antagonists, contraceptive effects, 492
effect on pituitary gonadotropins, 53, 74–76, *75*
effects of dopamine and norepinephrine, 56, 58–61, *59–61*
half-life of, 56
luteolytic action of, 46
ovulation and, 73–79, *74–75, 77–78*
for ovulation induction, 603–604
placental, 336
role in initiating puberty, 412–413
secretion of, 56–57, *56–57*
control of pulses, 58–61, 68, *69*
modified by feedback effects, 56
opioid peptides affecting, 66
at puberty, 83
pulsatile discharge, 56–57
timing of pulses, 58
stimulating prolactin secretion, 60
structure, 53, *53*
tuberoinfundibular tract, 54, *55, 56, 59*
Gonadotropin releasing hormone-like peptides, 104

Gonadotropins. *See also* Follicle stimulating hormone; Luteinizing hormone
in amenorrheic patient, 172t, 172–178, *173*
high levels, 173–177
low levels, 177–178
normal levels, 177
assay in premature ovarian failure, 176
big, 37
in galactosemia, 175
hypogonadotropic hypogonadism, 179
levels of
in anorexia nervosa, 199
effect of danazol, 554
in infancy and childhood, 409–412
normal serum, 628t, *629*
in polycystic ovary syndrome, *222,* 222–223
measurement by radioimmunoassay, 628
production associated with lung cancer, 173
pulsatile release of, 57
in resistant ovary syndrome, 174
role in steroidogenesis, 2–3
secretion through fetal life, childhood, puberty, 81–84, *83*
stimulation leading to precocious puberty, 419–420
Gonads
abnormal development, 386, 399–401, 400t
agenesis, 186–187
agonadism, 400
differentiation of, 380–382
dysgenesis, 401–403
amenorrhea and, 185
Noonan's syndrome, 402–403
pure, 402
XY, 186
effect of radiation and chemotherapy, 187–188, 188t
streak, 382, 401–402
Granulosa cells
effect of FSH, 14–15
FSH receptors on, 92–93, 97
LH receptor development, 98–99
in luteal phase, 111
in polycystic ovary, 226
postovulatory changes, 126
proliferation in follicular phase, 93, 95
steroidogenesis, 14–15
Growth factors, 100
Growth hormone, 35
effect of opioid peptides, 67
in obesity, 453
secretion by pituitary tumor, 188
Growth problems, adolescent, 430–433
short stature, 431–432
tall stature, 432–433
use of Bayley-Pinneau tables, 431, 438t-443t
Guaifenesin, to treat poor cervical mucus, 521
Guanosine 5'-triphosphate (GTP), activation and uptake of, 44

Hair. *See also* Hirsutism
biology of growth, 234–236
determinants of length, 235
differences in follicle concentration between racial and ethnic groups, 234
effect of castration on growth, 236
effects of endocrine problems, 236
factors influencing growth, 235–236
growth phases, 235
hormonal effects on, 236

hypertrichosis, 236
lanugo, 234
nonhormonal influences on growth, 236
periods of shedding, 235
sexual, 235–236
terminal, 236
vellus, 236
HCG. *See* Human chorionic gonadotropin
HDL—cholesterol. *See* Lipoproteins
Headache
in climacteric, 136
vascular, and oral contraceptives, 470
Hermaphrodite, true, 385. *See also* Pseudohermaphrodite
Hernia uterine inguinale, 399
Hip fracture, 138
Hirsutism, 233–258, 244–245. *See also* Hair
ACTH stimulation test, 248
androgen-producing tumors and, 251–252
anovulation and, 238, 240
adrenal involvement, 249
congenital adrenal hyperplasia and, 244–245
diagnostic workup, 241
due to methyltestosterone therapy, 155
evaluation of, 239–240
limitations/pitfalls, 258
17-hydroxyprogesterone level, 246, *247–248*
idiopathic, 257–258
oral contraceptives and, 480
other manifestations of increased androgens,
239–240
in polycystic ovary syndrome, 226
postmenopausal, 130
rare causes of, 240
screen for Cushing's syndrome, 241–242
testosterone levels in, 21, 233, *250*, 251
treatment, 252–257
cimetidine, 257
combination type oral contraceptives, 252–
253, *253*
cyproterone acetate, *256*, 257
dexamethasone, 257
duration of, 254, *255*
electrolysis, 253–254, 258
medroxyprogesterone acetate, 253
spironolactone, 256, *256*
surgical, 255
Histamine, role in embryo implantation, 508
Hormones. *See also* specific hormones and
classes
biosynthesis, metabolism, mechanism of
action, 1–46
definition of, 1–2
levels after menopause, 128–130
steroid
blood levels, 629t
measurement by radioimmunoassay, 629–
630
blood transport of, 16
bound vs. free, 16
conversion in peripheral tissues, 16–18, *18–19*
endometrial responses to, 272–274, *273*
excretion of, 23
mechanism of action, 24–31
classic receptor model, 24–26, *25*
new concept, 26–31, *27–28, 30*
nomenclature, 4–6
nucleus, 4, *4*
sampling blood levels of, 21
structure, 4–6, *4–6*

synthesis, 2, 11–15, 20–21
urinary levels, measurement of, 631, 631t
tropic
heterogeneity of, 36–38
mechanism of action, 31–35
regulation of, 36–46
Hot flushes, 136, 137–138, 150
clonidine for, 154
medroxyprogesterone acetate for, 154
HPL. *See* Human placental lactogen
Human chorionic adrenocorticotropin hormone,
335
Human chorionic gonadotropin (HCG), 329–332
added to clomiphene for ovulation induction,
590–591
dependence of corpus luteum on, 330
distinction from LH, 330
in ectopic pregnancy, 632
half-life, 329
injection in in vitro fertilization, 613
levels of, 330
measurement of, 632–633
production by conceptus at time of implantation, 508
role in maintaining luteal function, 113–114
role in steroidogenesis, 330
in steroidogenesis, 14
to simulate midcycle LH surge, 596
stimulation of corpus luteum, 320
subunits of, 36, *37*, 38, 329–330
to treat poor cervical mucus, 521
in trophoblastic disease, 330–331, 632
use of blood titers, 330–331
Human chorionic thyrotropin, 335
Human lymphocyte antigens, recurrent abortion
and, 538
Human menopausal gonadotropins
for ovulation induction, 595–603
abortion rate, 599
administration techniques, 596
combined with clomiphene, 600
combined with GnRH agonist, 600–601
dosage, 596–597
relation to body weight, 596
estrogen monitoring, 597–598
failure, 603
how to use, 595–599
multiple gestations, 598–599, 599–600
ovulation and pregnancy rates with, 599
patient selection, 595
results, 599–600
ultrasound monitoring of follicles, 598–599
to treat inadequate luteal phase, 530
to treat poor cervical mucus, 521
use in in vitro fertilization, 612
Human placental lactogen (HPL), 35, *332–334,*
332–335
clinical uses of assay, 335
half-life, 332
lactogenic effect of, 286
maternal levels in multiple gestations, 332
physiologic function, 333–335
production of, 286
Hydrocortisone, for adrenogenital syndrome, 393
11β-Hydroxyandrosterone, 637
structure, *637*
17-Hydroxycorticosteroids
measurement of, 639–644
normal urinary content, 644
11-Hydroxyetiocholanolone, 637

structure, *637*
Hydroxyindole-*o*-methyltransferase, 80–81
11β-Hydroxylase deficiency, 245, 249, 390
17-Hydroxylase deficiency, 175, 390
21-Hydroxylase deficiency, 244–245, 387, 389
  classification, 389
  clinical forms, 387
  incidence, 391
  inheritance pattern, 389
  prenatal diagnosis, 391
17-Hydroxypregnenolone, structure, *12*
17-Hydroxyprogesterone (17-OHP)
  in evaluation of hirsutism, 241
  level in hirsutism, 246, *247–248*
  measurement by radioimmunoassay, 630, 630t
  ovulatory levels of, 110
  in patients with persistent anovulation, 220
  to screen for congenital adrenal hyperplasia, 391–392
  structure, *12*
3β-Hydroxysteroid dehydrogenase deficiency, 245, 249, 390
Hypercalcemia, 139
Hypercortisolism, 141
Hyperparathyroidism, 141
  unmasked by calcium supplementation, 154
Hypertension
  estrogen replacement therapy and, 144–145
  obesity and, 446
  oral contraceptives and, 473–474
  pregnancy-induced, 368–373
Hyperthecosis, 255
  polycystic ovary and, 224
Hyperthyroidism, 649t
  estrogen excess and, 146
  trophoblastic disease and, 335
Hypoglycemia, in pregnancy, 333–334
Hypogonadism
  eugonadotropic
    frequency, 429
    lab assessment, 430
  hypergonadotropic
    frequency, 428
    lab assessment, 429
  hypogonadotropic, 179
    anovulation and, 219
    frequency, 429
    lab assessment, 430
  impaired GnRH secretion and, 53
Hypospadias, 379, 385
  infertility and, 570
Hypothalamus
  dysfunction leading to anovulation, 214
  GnRH secretion, 54–57
  hypophyseal portal circulation, 52, *52*
  neurohormones of, 52–53
Hypothyroidism, 649t
  amenorrhea and, 169
  breast cancer and, 302
  galactorrhea and, 169, 292
  newborn screening for, 342
  obesity and, 453
  precocious puberty and, 420
  short stature and, 431
  subclinical, 648
Hysterosalpingography, 524–526
  necessary films, 524–525
  oil- vs. water-soluble dyes, 526
  risk of infection, 524
  techniques for dye injection, 525

  as therapy for infertility, 525–526
  timing of, 524
Hysteroscopy, 526
  for treatment of Asherman's syndrome, 181

Ibuprofen, for dysmenorrhea, 133
Ichthyosis, due to placental sulfatase deficiency, 328–329
Immunotherapy, for recurrent abortion, 538
Implantation of embryo, 506–509
Indomethacin
  for dysmenorrhea, 133
  effect on fetal breathing, 362
  for persistent ductus patency, 359
  as prostaglandin inhibitor, 356
  to stop premature labor, 362
Infertility
  causes, 518
    deferring pregnancy, 514
    endometriosis, 550, 552
    inadequate luteal phase, 528–531
    luteinized unruptured follicle, 534
    male factors, 518–519
    mycoplasma, 531, 570
    ovulatory disorders, 519, 527
    poor cervical mucus, 521
    sexually transmitted disease, 516, 570
    sperm allergy, 532–533
    tubal damage, 519, 524–525
    woman's age, 514–516
  counseling of couple, 518
  epidemiology, 513–514
  investigation of female, 518–540
    basal body temperature, 527–528, *529*
    endometrial biopsy, 528
    endoscopy, 534–535
    hysterosalpingography, 524–526
    hysteroscopy, 526
    postcoital test, 519–524
    progesterone levels, 528
  investigation of male, 565–573
    semen analysis, 567–568
    sperm penetration assay, 572–573
    urologic evaluation, 570–572
      anatomic abnormalities, 570
      endocrine disorders, 570–571
      varicocele, 571–572
  myths regarding, 539–540
  physician's role in, 517–518
  reasons for concern with, 516–517
  recurrent abortion and, 516, 535–538
  time required for conception, 519t
  treatment
    bromocriptine, 530–531
    clomiphene citrate, 527, 530
    human menopausal gonadotropin, 530
    hysterosalpingography, 525–526
    progesterone, 530
  U.S. decline in fertility, 513–514
  when to advise adoption, 539
Inhibin, role in menstrual cycle, 103
Insemination
  intrauterine, 574–576
    because of poor cervical mucus, 521
    effect of woman's age, 576
    indications for, 574
    pregnancy rates after, 575
    pretreatment of semen, 576
    superovulation and, 576
    swim-up technique, 574–576

timing methods for, 575
therapeutic, 573–574
    with donor sperm, 577–579
        choice of donor, 577–578
        technique, 579
        timing of, 578–579
    effect of maternal age on conception rate, 515
Insomnia, in climacteric, 136
Insulin, 35
    effect of oral contraceptives, 477
    effects of obesity, 218, 453
    maternal, effect of HPL, 333–334
    resistance, hyperthecosis and, 224
    role in breast development, 284
Insulin-like growth factor I (somatomedin-C), 100, 218
    in pregnancy, 335
    role in pubertal growth spurt, 414–415
Intrauterine device, 491–492
    infections and amenorrhea, 181
In vitro fertilization. See Fertilization in vitro
Iodine, thyroid hormone synthesis and, 647
Isositol trisphosphate, 34

Kallman's syndrome, 66, 203–204
Kartagener's syndrome, 501
Karyotype, investigation in treatment of recurrent abortion, 535–536
11-Ketoetiocholanolone, 637
    structure, 637
17-Ketogenic steroids
    measurement of, 639, 645
    normal urinary content, 646, 646
Ketoprofen, for dysmenorrhea, 133
17-Ketosteroids
    in adrenogenital syndrome, 392, 392t
    in hirsutism, 241–244
    measurement of, 634–639
    neutral, 634
    normal excretion, 638, 638
        composition of, 639, 639
    structure, 634
Klinefelter's syndrome, infertility and, 570

Labor
    cortisol levels, 360, 361
    oxytocin levels, 73, 365
    premature, treatment by prostaglandin inhibition, 359, 366
    role of prostaglandins in induction of, 359
Lactation, 286–290
    cessation of, 289
    contraceptive effect of, 289–290
    effect of prolactin releasing factor, 289
    effect of steroid contraceptives, 484
    hormonal requirements for, 286–288
    inappropriate. See Galactorrhea
    initiating in adoptive mothers, 288
    "letdown" response, 288
    maintenance of milk production, 287
    maternal drugs in breast milk, 288
    mechanism of milk ejection, 288
    oxytocin effect, 73, 288
    protective effect against breast cancer, 298
    suppression of prolactin inhibiting factor, 288–289
LDL—cholesterol. See Lipoproteins
Leuprolide acetate, for ovulation induction, 600–601
Levonorgestrel, effect on lipid profile, 144

Leydig cells, 381–383, 565–566
LH. See Luteinizing hormone
Libidinal changes
    in climacteric, 136
    hormonal therapy for, 155
    oral contraceptives and, 480
Lipase, 449–450
Lipoproteins
    in androgenized women with polycystic ovaries, 227–228
    as carrier for cholesterol, 7–9, 8–9
    categories of, 7
    constituents of, 9
    definition, 7
    effect of Depo-Provera, 488–489
    effect of estrogen, 143–144, 152, 153–154, 154t
    effect of steroid contraceptives, 472–473
    fetal LDL levels, 324–325
    LDL and its receptor, 42, 42–44
    protective nature of HDL, 10
    removal of LDL from blood, 9–10
    role in atherosclerosis, 9–11, 143–144
β-Lipotropin, 63
Liver
    disease and estrogen excess, 146
    effects of oral contraceptives, 478–479
        adenomas, 478–479
Lub's syndrome, 396
Lungs
    cancer, gonadotropin production and, 173
    fetal maturation, 342–344
        correlation with lecithin/sphingomyelin ratio, 343
        pregnancy abnormalities affecting, 343
        pulmonary surfactant, 342–343
Lupron. See Leuprolide acetate
"Lupus" anticoagulant, 371–372
Luteal phase, 111–112, 111–114
    inadequate, 528–531
        recurrent abortion and, 536–537
Luteinization inhibitor, 104
Luteinization stimulator, 104
Luteinized unruptured follicle syndrome, 534, 599
Luteinizing hormone (LH)
    in amenorrheic patients
        high levels, 173–176
        low levels, 177
        normal levels, 177
    anovulation and, 215, 216–217
    characteristics of pulses, 58
    hot flushes and, 137
    levels of
        after menopause, 128
        normal serum, 628t, 629
        in perimenopausal period, 128
        in polycystic ovary syndrome, 222, 222–223
    midcycle surge
        abrupt stop of, 110
        events stimulated by, 107
        mechanism of, 76–77, 77–78
        time to menses, 113
        timing of, 107
    role in follicular maturation, 125
    role in steroidogenesis, 2, 14, 14–15, 15, 45
    secretion in puberty, 82–84
    subunits of, 36, 37, 38
Luteinizing hormone receptor binding inhibitor, 104

Magnetic resonance imaging, to evaluate Mullerian anomalies, 181
Mammography, 308–310, *309*
    for DES-exposed women, 303
    effectiveness, 309
    false negative rate, 308
    patient age for, 309
    radiation from, 308
    vs. other diagnostic modalities, 308
Marijuana use, fertility and, 61, 569
Mastalgia, 296
Mayer-Rokitansky-Kuster-Hauser syndrome, 182–183
McCune-Albright syndrome, precocious puberty and, 421
Medroxyprogesterone acetate, 153. *See also* Progestins
    as alternative to oral contraceptives, 488–490, *489*
    amenorrhea after discontinuing, 204
    for anovulation, 227
    for Asherman's syndrome, 181
    for dysfunctional uterine bleeding, 147
    effect on lipid profile, 144
    for endometriosis, 558
    for hirsutism, 253
    for precocious puberty, 423
    for premenstrual syndrome, 132
    for progestational challenge, 170–171
    protective endometrial effect of, 148–149
    for vasomotor symptoms, 154
Mefenamic acid, for dysmenorrhea, 133
Megestrol acetate, effect on lipid profile, 144
Melanocyte stimulating hormone, 63–64, 324
Melatonin, 80–81
Menarche, 83
    age of, 414, *416*, 416
    critical weight hypothesis, 414
    estrogen production for, 128
    relation to percent body fat, 414
    relationship with growth spurt, 416
Menopausal syndrome, 146
Menopause, 128
    age of, 134
    estrogen-progestin replacement therapy, 134–135
    lack of follicles, 128
    life expectancy after, 134, *135*
    premature, 175
Menotropins. *See* Human menopausal gonadotropins
Menstrual cycle
    follicular phase, 91–107. *See also* Follicle
    GnRH release and, 58, 68, *69*
    histologic changes in endometrium during, 266–271. *See also* Endometrium
    hyperprolactinemia and disturbances of, 294
    key events in, 114
    length of, 272
    luteal phase, *111–112*, 111–114
    normal serum gonadotropin levels, 628t, *629*
    opioid peptides and, 65–67, *66*
    ovulation, 107–110
    pattern of gonadotropin secretion, 100–102
        FSH pulsatile pattern, 102
        LH pulsatile pattern, 101
        midcycle surge, 76–79, *77–78*
    during perimenopausal period, 128
    regulation of, 91–114

symptoms related to estrogen deprivation, 136, 137
Menstruation. *See also* Amenorrhea; Menstrual cycle; Ovulation
    amount of blood loss, 272
    basic principles of, 166–167
    compartmental system of, 167, *168*
    teleologic theory of, 271
Mestranol
    content in birth control pills, 461–462
    structure, *462*
Metabolic clearance rate, definition of, 17
Methylprednisolone, for sperm allergy, 533
Methyltestosterone
    for decreased libido, 155
    for endometriosis, 554
    hirsutism and, 240
Methylxanthines, mastalgia and, 296
Metrodin. *See* Follicle stimulating hormone, purified
Metyrapone test, 647
Microangiopathy, 371
Mineralocorticoids, production of, 20
Monoamine oxidase inhibitors, for premenstrual syndrome, 131
Mosaicism, 186
Mucus, cervical
    cyclical changes in, 519
    evaluation in postcoital testing, 519–521
    fern pattern of, *520*
    pH, 523
    poor, treatment of, 521
    stretchability of, 520
Mullerian duct structures
    agenesis, 182–183, 185t
    anomalies, 181
    differentiation, 382
Mullerian inhibiting factor
    abnormal, 399
    antitumor effects, 399
Multiple myeloma, 141
Myalgia, in climacteric, 136
Mycoplasma
    as cause of infertility, 531, 570
    doxycycline treatment, 531
Myocardial infarction, steroid contraceptives and, 469

Naloxone, 64–67
Naproxen, for dysmenorrhea, 133
Neuroendocrinology, 51–84
    brain and ovulation, 73–79, *74–75*, *77–78*
    brain peptides, 62–67
    catecholestrogens, 67, *68*
    GnRH secretion, 56–61
        control on pulses, 58–61
        effects of dopamine and norepinephrine, 56, 58–61, *59–61*
        hypothalamus and, 54–55
        pulsatile nature of, 57
        timing of pulses, 58
    gonadotropin secretion through fetal life, childhood, puberty, 81–84, *83*
    hypothalamic-hypophyseal portal circulation, 52, *52*
    neurohormone concept, 52–53
    pineal gland, 79–81
    posterior pituitary pathway, 70–73, *71*
    tanycytes, 70, *70*
Neurophysins I and II, 70–72

Neurosecretion, 54
Neurotensin, 62
Noonan's syndrome, 402–403
Norepinephrine, effect on GnRH, 56, 60–61, *60–61*
Norethindrone, 153
  content in birth control pills, 462–466
  effect on lipid profile, 144
  structure, *463, 465*
Norethindrone acetate, structure, *465*
Norethynodrel, structure, *465*
Norgestrel, structure, *465*
19-Nortestosterones, 462, 466

Obesity, 445–458
  anatomic, 454–455
    android, 454
    gynoid, 454
    waist:hip ratio, 454–455
  anovulation and, 216, 217, 226
  associated endocrine changes, 453–454
  atherosclerosis and, 446
  body mass index, 446, *447*
  brain center and, 451
  breast cancer and, 299
  conversion of androstenedione to estrogen correlated with, 129
  definition, 446
  endometrial cancer and, 129
  estrogen excess and, 146
  experimental, 455
  genetic influences, 452–453
  ideal weight, 446
  insulin resistance and, 218
  management of, 455–458
    anorectics, 456
    diet, 455–456
    exercise, 457t, 457–458
  measurement of body fat, 446
  physiology of adipose tissue, 448–451, *449–450*
  psychologic factors and, 451–453, *452*
  relationship to mortality, 445
Oocyte
  culture, 614
  retrieval for in vitro fertilization, 613–614
Oocyte maturation inhibitor, 104
Opiates, endogenous
  body functions affected by, 65
  classes of, 64
  effect on oxytocin, 73
  effect on prolactin, 67
  effect on TSH, 67
  exercise-induced increase in, 66–67
  menstrual cycle and, 65–67, *66*
  in pregnancy, 338
  receptors, 64–65
  regulation of production, 62
  sources of, 62
Oral contraceptives. *See* Contraceptives, steroid
Osteoporosis, 136, 138–142, 204
  disabilities of, 138
  estrogen loss and, 138
  estrogen replacement therapy for, 139–140, 152
  etiology, 138
Ovary, 121–155
  adult, 124–126
  anovulation, 217–218. *See also* Anovulation
  corpus luteum, 126. *See also* Corpus luteum
  cysts
    multiphasic oral contraceptives and, 483
    precocious puberty and, 421

distinction from adrenal gland, 11
effect of radiation and chemotherapy, 187–188, 188t
embryology and differentiation, 122–124, 381–382
  differentiation and cortical supremacy stage, 122
  indifferent gonadal stage, 122
  stage of follicle formation, *123,* 123–124
  stage of oogonal multiplication and maturation, 122–123
enlargement with clomiphene therapy, 592
failure
  anovulation and, 219
  premature
    adrenal failure and, 176
    amenorrhea and, 187
    biopsy vs. empirical treatment, 176
    conditions associated with, 175
    estrogen replacement therapy for, 176
    exogenous gonadotropin stimulation, 176–177
    need for chromosome evaluation, 175
    recommended blood tests, 176
    resumption of normal function, 176
follicle growth, 125–126
follicle maturation/availability and estrogen production, *127,* 127–128
hormone production after follicle exhaustion, 128–130
hyperstimulation syndrome, 601–602
neonatal, 124
oophorectomy and breast cancer risk, 299
oophorectomy and heart disease risk, 143
ovulation, 126. *See also* Ovulation
polycystic, 220–227, *225*
  cause, 220
  clinical manifestations, 226–227
  decidualized endometrium and, 171
  decreased SHBG in, 221, *222,* 223
  gonadotropin levels, 222, *222*
  histology, 224
  hyperthecosis and, 224
  inherited, 226
  insulin resistance and, 218
  morphology, 224
  in relation to two-cell theory of steroidogenesis, 223, 226
  therapy, 227
  treatment with GnRH agonist, 221, *221*
resistant (insensitive), 187
  amenorrhea and elevated gonadotropins with, 174
tumors
  androgen-producing, 241, 242, 251–252
  estrogen excess and, 146
  oral contraceptives and, 474–475
  precocious puberty and, 420–421
wedge resection, 605
Ovulation, 107–110, 126
  brain and, 73–79, *74–75, 77–78*
  declining frequency of, 127, 134
  endometriosis and, 559
  induction of, 583–605
    bromocriptine, 593–595
    clomiphene citrate, 584–593
    GnRH, 603–604
    human menopausal gonadotropins, 595–603
    hyperstimulation syndrome, 601–602
    ovarian wedge resection, 605

purified FSH, 603
return after weaning, 290
superovulation, 576
timing of, 107
Ovum
effect of drugs for ovulation induction, 587
fertilizable life span, 503
function of zona pellucida, 503
transport of, 501–503
Oxytocin, 35, 67, 104
effect of opioid peptides, 73
"letdown" response due to release of, 288
levels during pregnancy, 73
release due to suckling, 287
role in parturition, 365
role of, 71–73
structure, 70, *71*

Paracrine communication, 2
Pelvic inflammatory disease
infertility and, 524
oral contraceptives and, 480
Peptides. *See also* specific peptides
brain, 62–67
endogenous opioid, 62–67. *See also* Opiates
Pergolide, for prolactin-secreting adenomas, 193
Pergonal. *See* Human menopausal gonadotropins
Phenobarbital, effect on oral contraceptive efficacy, 485
Phenytoin, effect on oral contraceptive efficacy, 485
Phospholipase C, 34
PIF. *See* Prolactin inhibiting factor
Pineal gland, 79–81
relationship with light, 80
role in humans, 79, 81
Pituitary gland. *See also* Sella turcica
effects of transplantation to ectopic sites, 52
hypopituitarism and short stature, 431
non-neoplastic masses, 188–189
posterior pathway, 70–73, *71*
in primary hypothyroidism, 169
tumors
evaluation of amenorrheic patient, 171, 179, 188–196
prolactin-secreting adenomas, 189–195
bromocriptine therapy, 191–193, 295–296
cause of amenorrhea, 190
galactorrhea and, 189, 294–295
gonadotropin levels, 173
incidence, 189
long-term follow-up, 194
oral contraceptives and, 480
pergolide therapy, 193
pregnancy and, 194–195
results of surgery, 190–191
summary, 193–194
transsphenoidal surgery, 190, 295
x-ray evaluation of sella turcica, 177–179, *178*
Placenta
progesterone synthesis, *318*, 318–319
protein hormones
human chorionic adrenocorticotropin hormone, 335
human chorionic gonadotropin, 329–332
human chorionic thyrotropin, 335
human placental lactogen, 332–335
other peptides, 336
Placental protein 12, 104
Placental sulfatase deficiency, 328–329

Platelet-derived growth factor, 100
Platelets
adhesion and aggregation of, 355
effect of aspirin, 356–357, *357*
function of, 355
Polycystic ovary syndrome. *See* Ovary,polycystic
Polyglandular syndrome, 175
Polyhydramnios
prolactin levels in, 338
treatment with prostaglandin inhibition, 366
Polyostotic fibrous dysplasia, precocious puberty and, 421
Porter-Silber reaction, 644
Postcoital test, 519–524
evaluation of cervical mucus, 519–521
normal numbers of sperm in, 521–522
prognostic value of, 522
timing of, 519
Preantral follicle, 92–95, *93*
Prednisone, for sperm allergy, 533
Pregnancy, 317–344
achievement after bromocriptine therapy for pituitary adenoma, 194–195
achievement following Asherman's syndrome, 181
"chemical," in in vitro fertilization, 615
dependence on corpus luteum, 318, 320, 508
ectopic
blood HCG assay, 331
IUD use and, 491
effect on hair growth, 236
effects of danazol, 555
endogenous opiates and, 338
estrogens in, *321–323*, 321–324
amniotic fluid measurements, 328
estetrol measurement, 328
measurement of, 326–328, *327*
fetal-placental unit
DHAS production, 324–326, *325*
estrogen synthesis, *321–322*, 321–323
progesterone synthesis, *318*, 318–320
α-fetoprotein, 336
hirsutism and, 240
hypoglycemia in, 333–334
with IUD in place, 491
lactation. *See* Lactation
luteoma during, 240
molar, 331, 335
oxytocin levels, 73
perinatal thyroid physiology, *339–341*, 339–342
placental sulfatase deficiency, 328–329
progesterone in, *318–319*, 318–320
prolactin secretion in, 337–338
protein hormones of placenta, 329–336
human chorionic adrenocorticotropin hormone, 335
human chorionic gonadotropin, 329–332
human chorionic thyrotropin, 335
human placental lactogen, 332–335
other peptides, 336
role of relaxin, 337
toxemia of, 368–373. *See also* Toxemia of pregnancy
virilization during, 240
Pregnancy-associated plasma protein A, 104
5α-Pregnane-3,20-dione, in pregnancy, 320
Pregnane, steroid nucleus, 4, *4*
Pregnanediol
in progesterone metabolism, 19, *20*
urinary excretion levels, 19, 631t

Pregnanetriol
in progesterone metabolism, 20
structure, *644*
urinary levels of, 631t
Pregnenolone
conversion to dehydroepiandrosterone, 13
conversion to progesterone, *12*, 13
Premenstrual syndrome, 130–132
definition, 130
etiology, 131–132
prevalence, 131
symptoms, 130–131
treatment, 131
Primidone, effect on oral contraceptive efficacy, 485
Primordial follicle, 92, *93*
Pro-oxyphysin, 70
Pro-pressophysin, 70
Production rate, definition of, 17
Prodynorphin, 62
Proenkaphalin A, 62, 64
Proenkaphalin B, 62
Progestational challenge
in amenorrhea, 167, 170–171
in hirsute patient, 241
Progesterone
for anovulation, 171
antagonism, for contraception, 492
decidualized endometrium due to high levels of, 171
functions in pregnancy, 320
levels of
in amniotic fluid, 319
assessment in infertility evaluation, 528
blood, 629t
in luteal phase, 112–113
myometrial, 319
at ovulation, 107–108
in pregnancy, *318–319*, 318–320
metabolism, 19–20, *20*
micronized, effect on lipid profile, 144
parenteral, in oil, for progestational challenge, 170
for premenstrual syndrome, 131
preovulatory production of, 105–106
production rate of, 19
protective effects
in breast, 170–171, 305
in endometrium, 170–171
role in parturition, 360–362
structure, *5–6, 12*
suppression of lactation, 287
synthesis, 463–464
as therapy for recurrent abortion, 536–537
to treat inadequate luteal phase, 530
Progestins
added to estrogen replacement therapy, 140
classic sequential treatment method, 152–153
continuous/combined treatment method, 153
effect on blood pressure, 144–145
effect on bone, 140
protective breast effects, 149
protective endometrial effects, 148–149
for women under 40, 150
content in birth control pills, 462–466, *463, 465*
for dysfunctional uterine bleeding, 147, 150, 276
in early postmenopause, 150
effect on hair, 236
for endometrial intraepithelial neoplasia, 274

structure, *4*
Prolactin, 35, 99. *See also* Pituitary gland
breast cancer and, 302
decidual synthesis of, 287
effect of opioid peptides, 67
effect on breast development, 284
effects of suckling, 287
levels of
in amniotic fluid, 286–287
greater than 100, 178–179
high
leading to anovulation, 214
leading to galactorrhea, 291–296. *See also* Galactorrhea
during pregnancy, 286–287
in primary hypothyroidism, 169
at weaning, 290
measurement in amenorrhea, 167
role in milk biosynthesis, 287
secretion, 52
in pregnancy, 337–338
effect of bromocriptine, 337
stimulation by GnRH, 60
suppression by dopamine, 53, 59
Prolactin inhibiting factor (PIF), 53, 59
drug suppression of, 291–292
effect of stress on, 292
suppression by suckling, 288–289
Prolactin releasing factor, 289
Proopiomelanocortin, 62–67, *63*, 104
Propylthiouricil, maternal, effect on fetal thyroid hormones, 340
Prorenin, 104
in pregnancy, 338
Prostacyclin (PGI$_2$)
aggregation balance, *355*
defensive role of, 355–356
role in parturition, 364
sources of, 354–355
toxemia of pregnancy and, 370–373
Prostaglandin synthetase inhibitors, 356–357, *357*
for Asherman's syndrome, 181
aspirin, 356–357
benefits, 134
contraindications, 133
for dysfunctional uterine bleeding, 279
for dysmenorrhea, 132, 133t, 133–134
to inhibit premature labor, 359, 366
for polyhydramnios, 366
side effects, 133
Prostaglandins, 351–373
biosynthesis, 352–354, *353–354*
cyclooxygenase pathway, 354, *354*
lipoxygenase pathway, 353, *353*
role of arachidonic acid, 352–354
for cervical ripening, 366–367
E, inhibition of uterine contractions, 133
effect on fetal circulation, 358–359
F$_{2\alpha}$
dysmenorrhea due to, 133
luteolytic action of, 46, 357–358
history, 351–352
I$_2$, 354–356. *See also* Prostacyclin
induction of follicle wall rupture, 108–109, 126
for induction of labor, 366–367
inhibition, 356–357
levels of
in endometriosis, 550
in labor, 364
metabolism, 356

for postpartum hemorrhage, 367
role in cyclic AMP mechanism, 33–34
role in embryo implantation, 508
role in luteal regression, 357–358
role in parturition, 359–366, *360, 363*
role in regulating blood flow in pregnancy, 367–368
side effects, 367
for therapeutic abortion, 367
those relevant to reproduction, 354
thromboxanes, 354–356
toxemia of pregnancy and, 368–373
Proteolytic enzymes, activation at ovulation, 108
Pseudocyesis, 61
Pseudohermaphrodite
female, 386–394, *388*
associated metabolic disorders, 387
caused by danazol, 555
definition, 385
20-22 desmolase deficiency, 391
diagnosis, 392t, 392–393
genetic aspects, 391, 391t
genitalia in, 386
11β-hydroxylase deficiency, 390
17α-hydroxylase deficiency, 390
21-hydroxylase deficiency, 387–389
3β-hydroxysteroid dehydrogenase deficiency, 390
pathophysiology, 387
treatment, 393–394
virilization in, 386
male, 394–399
abnormal androgen synthesis, 398–399
abnormal Mullerian inhibiting factor, 399
androgen insensitivity syndromes, 394–398
incomplete insensitivity, 396–397
5α-reductase deficiency, 397–398
testicular feminization, 395–396
definition, 385
etiology, 394
gonadotropin resistant testes, 399
Pseudohypoparathyroidism, 44
Pseudomenopause, 554
Pseudopregnancy, 554
Puberty
adrenarche, 83, 410–411
age of, 414
age of onset, 83
breast development, 83
effect of estrogen, 284
premature, 410
decreasing depression of "gonadostat", 411–412
delayed, 428–430
causes, 428
diagnosis, 428
lab assessment, 429–430
relative frequency of abnormalities, 428–429
treatment, 430
developmental stages, 414
gonadarche, 410–411
gonadotropin secretion in, 82–84
growth acceleration and, 414–415, *415*
growth of pubic hair, 83
hypothalamic pituitary gonadal changes, 82–84
menarche, 83, 414, *416*, 416
period of infancy and childhood, 409–410
precocious, *418*, 418–427
causes, 419
classification, 419t

diagnosis, 422–423
due to availability of sex steroids, 420–421
due to cerebral problems, 420
due to stimulation of gonadotropin secretion, 419–420
lab findings in, 421t
prognosis, 424–425
pseudo-, 420–421
special cases of, 422
treatment, 423–424
prepubertal period, 410–413
pubic hair growth, 414
role of GnRH, 412–413
summary of events, 417
Tanner staging, 425t, *426–427*
timing of, 413

Quingestanol acetate, structure, *465*

Radiation
effect on ovary, 187–188, 188t
for prolactin-secreting adenomas, 191
as risk factor for breast cancer, 304
Receptors, cellular. *See also* specific compounds
class I, 41
class II, 41
coupling, 44–45, *45*
estrogen and progesterone, breast cancer and, 305–306
hormone complex, 1-3, 24–26, 44–45
internalization of, 38–41, *41*
lateral migration, 39, *39*
LDL, *42*, 42–44
mediated endocytosis, 39, 44
monoclonal antibodies to, 26
opioid, 64–65
processing, 29
recycling, 26
steroid, 14, 26–29
up and down regulation, 38–44
5α-Reductase
deficiency, 397–398
increased activity in hirsutism, 238–239
Reifenstein syndrome, 396
Relaxin, 337
Replenishment, 26, 28
Reserpine, breast cancer and, 302
Respiratory distress syndrome, 342–343
correlation with lecithin/sphingomyelin ratio, 343
Rheumatoid arthritis, estrogen replacement therapy and, 145
Rifampin, effect on oral contraceptive efficacy, 485
RU 486, 492
Rubin's test, 524
Runner's "high", 202

Saturation analysis, *622–627*, 622–628
basic principles, 622
methodology, 623–628
Scarification, 126
Schistosomiasis, uterine, amenorrhea and, 181
Secretion rate, definition of, 17
Sella turcica
abnormal, evaluation of, 179
empty sella syndrome, 178, 195–196
evaluation in galactorrhea, 167, 171
evaluation with elevated prolactin, 171
in premature ovarian failure, 169

in primary hypothyroidism, 169
x-ray evaluation, 177–179
Semen. *See also* Sperm
abnormalities, 568
analysis, 523, 567–568
normal values, 568
liquification, 567
Serophene. *See* Clomiphene citrate
Serotonin, effect on GnRH, 60
Sertoli cells, 566
Sex hormone binding globulin (SHBG)
binding capacity in men and women, 237
binding of testosterone, 233
breast cancer and, 301
decreased in polycystic ovary syndrome, 221, 222, 223
estrogen excess and, 146
factors affecting level of, 16
levels in obese women, 217
as protein carrier, 2, 16
Sexual differentiation, 379–406
abnormal, 385–406. *See also* Pseudohermaphrodite
adrenogenital syndrome, 386–394
assignment of sex of rearing, 405–406
diagnosis of ambiguous genitalia, 403–405, *404*
female masculinization due to excess maternal androgens, 394
gonadal dysgenesis, 401–402
gonadogenesis, 394–401
male pseudohermaphrodite, 394–399
true hermaphrodite, 401
normal, *380*, 380–385
CNS differentiation, 385
duct system differentiation, 382
establishment of genetic sex, 380
external genitalia differentiation, 382–383, *383–384*
gonadal differentiation, 380–382
SHBG. *See* Sex hormone binding globulin
Sheehan's syndrome, 180, 189
postpartum failure to lactate in, 287
Sialic acid, 102
increased, in gonadotropin molecules, 177
Sickle cell disease, effect of medroxyprogesterone acetate, 489
Skin atrophy, 136, 145
Smoking
early menopause and, 134
effect on fecundity, 519
osteoporosis and, 139, 141
steroid contraceptives and, 470
Somatomedin-C. *See* Insulin-like growth factor I
Somatostatin, 62
Sperm
allergy, 532–533
treatment, 533
antibody testing, 523, 532–533
attrition in number of, 500
capacitation, 500–501
decrease in count, 567–568
determination of motility, 568
donor, 577–579
effect of coital timing on number, 569
effect of heat, 569
effect of marijuana use, 569
effect of radiation or environmental toxins, 569
effect of zona pellucida on, 503
evaluation of morphology, 568

immobilization test, 532
intrauterine insemination of, 521, 574–576
penetration assay, 533, 572–573
in postcoital testing, 519–524
normal number, 521–522
preparation of, in in vitro fertilization, 614
transport of, 499–500
washing, 533
Spermatogenesis, 566
Spermicides, 523
Spinal compression fracture, 138
Spironolactone
for fluid retention, 132
for hirsutism, 256
structure, *256*
Steroidogenesis, 11–15, *12*
of corpus luteum, 45, 114
fetal-placental, 317
reactions during, 13
stimulation of, 2
two-cell system, 14–15, *15*, 96, *96*, 223, 226
two-pathway theory, 13
Stress, estrogen excess and, 146
Stroke, steroid contraceptives and, 470
Surfactant, pulmonary, 342–343
Swyer syndrome, 400
Syndrome of inappropriate antidiuretic hormone secretion, 72

Tamoxifen, for mastalgia, 296
Tanner staging, 425t, *426–427*
Tanycytes, 70, *70*
Testes
abnormalities and infertility, 570
bilateral dysgenesis, 400
components of, 565
differentiation, 381
gonadotropin resistant, 399
regulation of, 565–567
in testicular feminization, 183
Testes-determining factor, 381
Testosterone
bound vs. free, 233
effect of androgens on binding capacity, 21
effect on hair, 236
levels of
blood, 629t
fetal, 82
in hirsutism, 21, 233, *250*, 251
postmenopausal, 128
for mastalgia, 296
menstrual midcycle increase in, 14
in patients with persistent anovulation, 220
production rate of, 21, 236
sources of, 236, *237*
in hirsutism, 238, *238*
structure, 5, *6*, *12*
Tetrahydrocortisol, structure, *642–643*
Theca cells, steroidogenesis, 14–15
Thelarche, 83
Thromboembolic disease, steroid contraceptives and, 469
Thromboxanes, 354–356
effect of aspirin, 356–357
sources of, 354–355
Thyroid hormones, 647–649
effect of drugs taken for cholecystograms, 648
effect of oral contraceptives, 477
fetal, *339–341*, 339–342
effect of maternal propylthiouricil, 340

fetal/newborn changes in, 341–342
measurement by radioimmunoassay, 648–649
placental transfer of, 339
postnatal surge of, 340–341, *341*
structure, *339*
Thyroid stimulating hormone (TSH)
  assay of, 649, 649t
  effect of opioid peptides, 67
  fetal, 339–341
  measurement in amenorrhea, 167, 169–170
  postnatal surge of, 340–341, *341*
  release due to suckling, 287–288
Thyrotoxicosis, 141
Thyrotropin releasing hormone (TRH), 53, 62
  stimulation of prolactin response, 179
Tolfenamic acid, for dysmenorrhea, 133
Toxemia of pregnancy, 368–373
  causes of, 368
  impaired blood flow and, 368
  prostaglandins and, 368–373
Transcortin, role in blood transport of steroids, 16
Transformation, 24
Transforming growth factor, 100
Translocation, 24
TRH. *See* Thyrotropin releasing hormone
Trophoblast, 507
Trophoblastic disease, blood HCG assay, 330–331, 632
Tuberculosis, amenorrhea and, 181
Turner's syndrome, 166, 185–186, 401–402
  gonadotropin secretion in, 83

Ureaplasma urealyticum, as cause of infertility, 531
Urethra, problems in climacteric, 136, 145
Urinary tract
  infection and oral contraceptives, 479

problems in climacteric, 136, 145
Uterine hernia syndrome, 399
Uterus. *See* Dysfunctional uterine bleeding; Endometriosis; Endometrium

VACTERL malformations, 485–486
Vagina
  agenesis of, 182–183
  atrophy in climacteric, 136, 145
Varicocele, infertility and, 571–572
Vas deferens, abnormalities and infertility, 570
Vasoactive intestinal peptide (VIP), 62
Vasomotor symptoms, 136, 137–138, 150
Vasopressin, 67
  arginine, 70
    structure, 70, *71*
  role of, 71–72
Vertebral compression fracture, 138
Virilism, 175, 233
Vitamin B6, for premenstrual syndrome, 131
Vitamin E, for mastalgia, 296
Vitelline membrane, 505
Vulva, atrophy in climacteric, 136

Weight. *See also* Obesity
  gain
    with medroxyprogesterone acetate, 488
    oral contraceptives and, 479
  ideal, 446
  loss
    amenorrhea and, 197–200
    improving ovulatory function in obese women, 217
Wolffian duct structures
  development of, 23
  differentiation, 382

Zona pellucida, functions of, 503